ADULT AUDIOLOGIC REHABILITATION

ADULT AUDIOLOGIC REHABILITATION

Joseph J. Montano, Ed.D.
Jaclyn B. Spitzer, Ph.D.

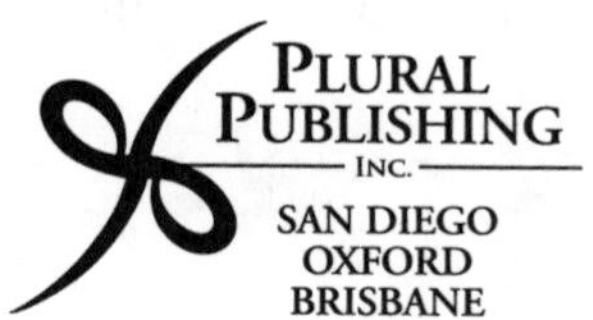

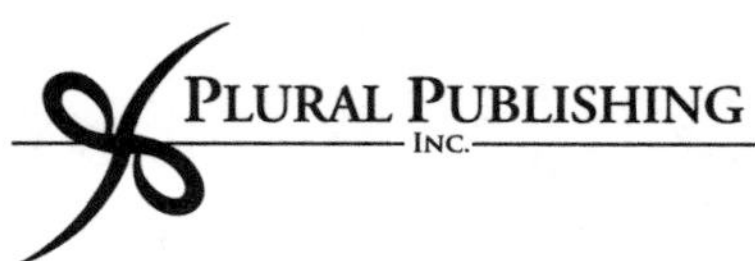

5521 Ruffin Road
San Diego, CA 92123

e-mail: info@pluralpublishing.com
Web site: http://www.pluralpublishing.com

49 Bath Street
Abingdon, Oxfordshire OX14 1EA
United Kingdom

Typeset in 10½/13 Palatino by Flanagan's Publishing Services, Inc.
Printed in the United States of America by Bang Printing

Library of Congress Cataloging-in-Publication Data

Adult audiologic rehabilitation / [edited by] Joseph J. Montano & Jaclyn B. Spitzer.
p. ; cm.
Includes bibliographical references and index.
ISBN-13: 978-1-59756-250-8 (alk. paper)
ISBN-10: 1-59756-250-5 (alk. paper)
1. Audiology. 2. Hearing disorders—Patients—Rehabilitation. I. Montano, Joseph J. II. Spitzer, Jaclyn Barbara.
[DNLM: 1. Rehabilitation of Hearing Impaired. 2. Adult. 3. Hearing Aids. 4. Hearing Impaired Persons—psychology. WV 270 A244 2009]
RF290.A38 2009
617.8—dc22

2008052902

CONTENTS

FOREWORD

I had my first experience with the concept and practice of Audiologic Rehabilitation (AR) when I was admitted as a patient to the AR program at Walter Reed Army Hospital in January 1952. Essentially, this was the type of program from which the profession of Audiology would later emerge (see Alpiner & McCarthy, Chapter 1, this volume). For the two months I was there, I was exposed to the best clinical practices that existed at the time. Classes were conducted by former teachers of the deaf, speech correctionists, and lipreading teachers (the term "speechreading" had not yet been coined). For the most part, the lessons consisted of various speechreading and visual training exercises, supplemented by some "auditory training" sessions (following a classic "Carhart" approach). These two activities basically defined AR at the time. Also included in the program were occasional didactic lectures on various topics (e.g., the audiogram, anatomy and physiology of the auditory system, etc.). Appointments for hearing aid fittings and follow-ups were spaced throughout the two-month period. The hearing aids provided us were monaural body-worn vacuum tube aids, and we were told that we were lucky to have them. Patients just a few years earlier were issued a duo-pack hearing aid, which required separate packs for the battery and the amplifier, with a rather large wire connecting the two.

In retrospect, although we couldn't really appreciate it at the time, those of us who were able to participate in that program indeed were very lucky to be where we were, receiving the kind of care we did. I don't think the full reality of what a hearing loss would mean in our lives was fully understood by any of us. It was very easy to underestimate the full and eventual impact of a hearing loss. At any rate, in that setting and at that time, the issues facing someone with an "invisible" hearing loss paled in comparison to what we saw of the men with combat injuries at the main hospital. Complaints and self-pity were simply not acceptable reactions. Although we didn't choose to attend the program, being there turned out to be a turning point, at least in my life.

In the company of others, I learned to accept myself and the reality of my hearing loss, perhaps the most significant goal in any AR program. Although this was not an explicit objective of the program, it arose naturally as a consequence of being somewhat sequestered for two months with a group of young men with similar problems. Later, as a professional audiologist, I thought of that program as a kind of AR Camelot—the ultimate model to which we could aspire but never really attain. Still the question does arise: Were there any lessons we could take from our early romance in "Camelot" and apply them in this day and age? I think there are.

The first is that the hearing aid selection procedures (primitive as they were) were viewed as an ongoing process (as I recall, one appointment a week was scheduled over an 8-week period) and completely integrated with the rest of the AR program. Questions about hearing aids, difficult listening situations, speechreading issues, and so forth, could arise—formally or informally—throughout the day. From a conceptual point of view, hearing aids were not separated from the rest of the AR activities that took place. This is somewhat at variance with how AR is now generally practiced. Currently, hearing aids are selected and several follow-up appointments are scheduled. But the need for, and provision of, any other type of AR service is completely happenstance—sometime yes, sometimes no, sometimes this, and sometimes that. Not so in Camelot; all was integrated into a single curriculum.

The second important lesson I think we can apply is that the group experience was perhaps the most valuable benefit of the program. I doubt that this was an explicit goal of the program. It was, rather, a fallout benefit which proved to be profoundly effective despite being inadvertent. Just the fact of being part of a group, of sharing our experiences and concerns with other young men in the same situation, helped us to accept the reality of our condition. We would joke with one another about "being on the air," to the point where the daily use of a hearing aid was common—and expected. As a profession, we are now keenly aware of the advantages of group management; the fact that I can still feel its impact some 57 years later is a testament to the power, and effectiveness, of a group program.

A third observation regarding the Walter Reed program is that it wasn't voluntary. We were simply transferred there, with no option to refuse. But I think it worked. Many men who in other settings would have to be dragged kicking and screaming into a therapy room, or more realistically simply would not go, were enrolled and then benefited from the inclusion in spite of themselves. Clearly, this is not exactly a formula that can be applied in any other kind of situation! We don't draft people into an AR program. It does suggest, however, that even people who are reluctant to engage in a therapy program can be helped, as long as they can somehow be convinced or cajoled to participate.

I do believe that this can be somewhat achieved if a short-term group AR program were considered to be a routine component of the hearing-aid selection process. In other words, just as a client's hearing status is expected to be evaluated by an audiologist prior to the hearing aid fitting, so too should such a program be instituted subsequent to a hearing aid selection. People would be free to ignore the recommendation, of course—we are not a totalitarian society—but, for example, how many people ignore their orthopedist's suggestion for a course of physical therapy after a surgical procedure? I think we can agree, not very many. Clearly, the perception of need is completely different in these two situations, which I believe is due to a society that trivializes the possible consequences of a hearing loss and underestimates what can be achieved with an AR program. Even a short-term posthearing aid selection AR program can pay big dividends for many people with hearing loss.

What was provided in the Walter Reed AR program has not been, and could not be, replicated in its entirety anywhere else. At the time it was developed, during WW II, nothing and no expense was too much for "the boys." In retrospect, however, it now does seem like overkill; it is likely that the same results could have been achieved with a somewhat truncated program, or one constituted a bit differently. But we have no way of knowing now. We have no objective evidence of the program's efficacy (though I would gladly provide my personal testimonial regarding its effectiveness). We didn't have the scholarly insights and information on AR that exist currently. During that era, AR meant being fit monaurally with a body-worn, vacuum tube hearing aid and attending speechreading and occasional auditory training classes—period. Now, on the other hand, we have a comprehensive body of information applicable and relevant to the entire AR process. And, it seems, that just about all of it is included in this book.

When Dr. Montano and Dr. Spitzer forwarded the detailed outline to me, my initial response was, "Wow!" I jumped at the opportunity to write the Foreword. I have spent my entire professional life dealing one way or another with AR, but until I saw the outline of topics contained in this book, I never really appreciated how much we have changed and developed since the early days. The authors selected to write the chapters are a compilation of the "best and the brightest" that the profession has to offer. The book is divided into four logical sections, each one of which deals comprehensively with a different aspect of AR.

The first section of the book lays the groundwork. In this introductory portion, AR itself is precisely defined (we will see that it involves more than is at first apparent) and placed in a historical framework. Perhaps because of my own history, I find this a very appealing topic; we really don't know where we are or where we're going unless we can appreciate where we've been. This section does that for us. It provides a frame of reference we can use when we examine any efforts in this area, our own as well as those of others. In addition, the importance of the contributions of the World Health Organization and the impact of hearing-loss on self-perception are highlighted and provide a critical foundation for the provision of AR services.

The broad area of assessment is covered in the second section. One convincing indicator of how far the profession has progressed is that three of the topics in this section—self-assessment, quality of life, and implantable technologies—did not even exist 50 years ago. The fact that people with hearing impairment could, and should, personally rate the communicative and social effects of their own hearing loss seems obvious to us now, but not so years ago. Now, on the other hand, self-assessment scales are a component in every "best practice" recommendation.

Insofar as quality of life is concerned, of course, people years ago were aware that a hearing loss could affect it, but the idea that quality of life considerations could and should be formally assessed never seemed to arise. Now, as the profession finds it necessary to justify the expense of hearing aids and therapeutic procedures to third party payers, the positive impact of our management efforts do have to be quantitatively demonstrated. The administrators who manage the purse strings will not be satisfied with only our personal assurance that some procedure or device is helpful. They want to see the evidence before any financial outlay is approved.

Also included in this second section is a chapter on hearing aids, an area that is clearly a central component of any AR effort. We've come a long way since the original Carhart procedure for the comparative evaluation of hearing aids, abetted by the ubiquitous question "How does that sound?" As this chapter indicates, the vast improvements in technology that have occurred have been accompanied by concurrent developments in assessment techniques. In other words, it's not enough to point to some new and impressive technology as an indicator of progress; it is also necessary to corroborate its merits in behavioral terms. Not every technical advance is accompanied by listening improvements.

The third section constitutes the bulk of the book. In it, we see not only the traditional concepts of speechreading and auditory training upgraded and cloaked in modern dress, but also full coverage of the relevant psychosocial issues (counseling, the group process, consumer advocacy) and specific therapeutic techniques (music therapy, repair strategies). The inclusion of these areas is another reminder of how our approach to AR has changed since the early days. The chapter on Assistive Listening Technology reminds us how much communication can be enhanced by the direct transmission of a talker's voice to a hard-of-hearing listener. I know that whenever I use an assistive listening device, I am reminded anew of the great help that these systems can provide someone with a hearing loss—and how much they are underemployed by people with hearing loss.

A review of special issues in AR is provided for us in the last section. New information and insights have given rise to additional areas of professional responsibility. One of these is the manifestation, evaluation, and management of people with central auditory processing (CAP) problems. The case is made that this is a rehabilitation issue that the profession of Audiology must address. The evidence presented in this section will help lay the necessary evidential and conceptual groundwork for the involvement of audiologists in this area. Finally, lest we forget that human beings are our core concern, the rehabilitation of older adults is discussed in this section. We are an increasingly aging society, and older people present issues that may, and probably will, differ in some respect from those observed in younger people with hearing loss.

In brief, this book presents an impressive display of the concepts and content areas that now constitute AR. The authors selected to write the various chapters are well known in their own countries and internationally. What they have presented is the current state of the art—a compilation of information, insights, practices, and concepts that were unheard of when I was a patient, and even later when I myself started practicing as an Audiologist. As a body of knowledge, Audiologic Rehabilitation has been a growing reality. Still, in spite of all that has changed, we should remind ourselves what has not changed, and that is the impact of a hearing loss upon the life and well-being of the afflicted person. We are still going to see the same reactions from people that we saw years ago, from denial to isolation. And it is still going to take conscientious, caring, and competent clinicians to provide the services, so well documented in these pages, that these people need.

The challenge that now confronts the profession is to employ this vast body of knowledge for the benefit of adults with hearing loss. Knowing more does not mean that we are doing more. Certainly knowledge is a prerequisite to action, which this book amply provides us, but somehow this knowledge has to find its way to people. There is still an inadequate public appreciation of the consequences of this "invisible" handicap. Impaired hearing is still more often a subject for so-called "humor" than for empathy and assistance. A public understanding of the potential consequences of a hearing loss—realizing that it is not a joke—is *the* prerequisite for hearing loss to receive the same kind of public support that other disabilities now receive via third-party payments. The kind of public support I envision goes beyond support for various kinds of devices and would include individual, group, and self-administered (possibly home-based) AR therapies. Support groups, too, like the Hearing Loss Association of America (HLAA), can play a significant role in the broader goal of helping people live with a hearing loss.

Ironically, it seems that the latest major development in hearing rehabilitation—cochlear implants—seems to be stimulating a modern resurgence of the traditional AR therapies. There is a recognition that new implant users require more than the device itself. Although most of this recent interest seems focused on helping these people to adjust to the new and strange auditory sensations produced by a cochlear implant (i.e., auditory training), there also appears to be an increased appreciation of AR as a concept that potentially applies to all people with hearing loss. In my judgment, the fact that the medical profession is now involved with implants, to an extent they never were with hearing aids, has provided additional impetus for follow-up AR therapy. A surgeon "prescribing" a course of therapy (probably conducted by the audiologist or speech-language pathologist) imbues the process with an authority that currently is lacking when a nonphysician makes the same recommendation. Like it or not, it is the reality.

There is one final comment I'd like to make about AR: It can be fun. Plus, it is an area for which audiologists and speech-language pathologists bear the uncontested, primary professional responsibility. It affords these professionals an opportunity to interact with their clients on a more personal, human level. Now they can switch their focus from the hearing loss to the hearing problem, away from the audiogram and to the human being with the hearing loss. It can be a very rewarding, and sometimes surprisingly enjoyable experience. I do believe that professionals so involved will find that they now enjoy their work even more than they did before. So jump in, the water's fine.

Mark Ross, Ph.D.

PREFACE: GOALS AND TOPICS

The seeds for this book were planted in 2003 when it was learned that Jerry Alpiner and Patti McCarthy were not intending to prepare a revised edition of their classic Audiologic Rehabilitation (AR) textbook, *Rehabilitative Audiology: Children and Adults*. The Alpiner, then subsequent Alpiner/McCarthy, textbook had been a staple of AR graduate education in Audiology and Speech-Language Pathology since the 1970s. Its absence would indeed create a void in the education of audiologists.

During the same period of time, the profession of Audiology was undergoing a metamorphosis. Based on our self-directed initiative, we had become a doctoral entry-level profession and programs had begun developing a doctoral-level curriculum. Therefore, a growing need for intermediate and advanced textbooks was developing and additional textbooks would have to be created.

The third observation that influenced our decision to pursue the creation of this book was the limited availability of AR literature in American professional journals, although international publications appeared to be more inclusive of this area of practice and research. This impression became reinforced by a series of AR workshops developed through the Hearing Rehabilitation Foundation (HRF). The HRF sponsored four biennial International conferences (2003, 2005, 2007, and 2009) on Adult AR. The conferences brought together researchers and practitioners from four continents to provide global insight into the manifestations of hearing loss. The contributions of our colleagues across the world have been prominent and influential to the state of practice in AR.

With these three issues in mind, we decided to tackle the creation of an advanced AR textbook with an international perspective. Although Alpiner and McCarthy addressed both children and adults in their book, we felt that, given the changing milieu with technologic developments and demographic shifts in society, it was appropriate to focus the scope of this book to adults.

Our concept of a fully functional doctoral-level audiologist required a sophisticated, in-depth background of information not sufficiently addressed in any existing textbook. What information does a doctoral-level audiologist need to develop the perspective to care for an individual with hearing loss? What knowledge will subserve the necessary skills development for advanced practice of AR? Although there might not be universal agreement to the answers to these questions, we believe that the audiology doctoral student must be cognizant of a wide range of information to provide an advanced level of rehabilitative management to their clients/patients. It is in this endeavor that we distinguish ourselves from other specialties that also work with persons with hearing loss, and where we combine the unique skills that make us essential in the long-term planning for living with this sensory deficit.

Therefore, we chose to include topic areas that are not only clinical but delve into the underlying issues surrounding hearing loss in adults. To develop the doctoral-level audiologist, we need a long-term perspective to define the subject matter and have insight into its history. We gathered together expert opinions and research-based formulations in chapters on such significant aspects of living with hearing loss as stigma, the viewpoint of the consumer, classification of function, self-perception, and impact on quality of life. Crucial elements of service provision in AR are covered in chapters dedicated to counseling, visual speech perception, auditory training, special needs of older adults, and central auditory processing. We chose to include information on dimensions of service that are not as widespread in their distribution in the field, such as utilization of music, tinnitus management, conversation repair strategies, and group processes. The influence of technology is seen in chapters relating to amplification and hearing aid verification, hearing assistive technology systems, and assessment for implantable devices. We believe that our field is in critical need of research and literature support of AR practices and efficacy, and thus we have included expert guidance on evidence-based practice and future research needs.

An underlying concept of this text is that AR is an expanding aspect of our discipline. Changes are taking place, not only in our credentials and in our knowledge base, but in our scope of practice as we define it. The scope of rehabilitative services is inclusive rather than exclusive. The role of technology in the current practice of AR is apparent, but, as seen in our text, it should be only the means, rather than the end, to the larger picture of rehabilitative planning for individual patients. Learning about and applying technology is intriguing and seductive, and we must always be aware of the potential for mistaking recommendations for devices as an endpoint in formulating plans. As we remain sensitive to this sometime temptation, the reader will note the powerful emphasis throughout this text on the information necessary to develop excellence in counseling.

As you read through this book, you will be struck by the frequent references to the World Health Organization International Classification of Function. This is an example of a change in professional mindset from the medically based categorization of hearing loss as disease to a more eclectic classification that embodies functional consequences of impairment on the individual within the context of lifestyle and environment. This classification system is quickly becoming accepted and applied as can be seen through the numerous literature references within this text.

We have also made some "nontraditional" choices for inclusion in this textbook. Including a substantial chapter on tinnitus management reflects our certainty that audiologists will be progressively more and more involved in providing care to tinnitus sufferers. In the past, there has been little emphasis in coursework on tinnitus treatment options, as well as little guidance for the practitioner in the counseling process. By including a chapter on this topic, we hope that the nature of the discussion of AR will be extended to include tinnitus treatment as a standard part of AR courses.

In the chapter on music therapy with cochlear implantees, Geoff Plant makes the point that musical enjoyment is crucial to the quality of life. The inclusion of this "nontraditional" chapter is intended to stimulate students and clinicians to view music as an integral aspect of therapeutic planning. Furthermore, we suggest that music as a stimulus for assessment and rehabilitation should not be restricted to use with persons with implanted sensory devices; rather, it should be considered as an element in AR for many persons as a positive force from which they can derive auditorially based learning and pleasure.

Another "nontraditional" chapter is the section on AR and central auditory processing. When combined with the chapter on rehabilitative needs of the elderly, we are preparing the reader for the upcoming explosion of aging Baby Boomers and the extended longevity being seen in many westernized nations. The fully functional audiologist will need to recognize the influences of normal aging and differentiate those from central auditory processing deficits, and be prepared to modify therapeutic approaches to accommodate such differences.

The topics we chose to include in this text are ones we believed would represent the current state of AR, and, perhaps, shape its future. Limits in a book's length, time constraints, and author availability precluded the inclusion of some topics that we nonetheless recognize as important. In particular, balance and vestibular rehabilitation was not addressed, and we believe it is a topic of importance for the future. In addition, this is one of those areas where our scope of practice currently is not clear, with other professionals involved in the day-to-day management of the dizzy patient. We also chose not to include material on specific devices, such as hearing aids and cochlear implants, as we believed that entire texts have been devoted to these topics, and that the concepts and methodologies we explore are the true focus of AR.

We also highlight strongly the importance of research on evidence-based practice in this text.

Several authors comment that they await further validation of techniques or think that such demonstrations are forthcoming in their selected content focus. It is incumbent on a doctoral profession to produce evidence of the efficacy of their techniques and to further the scope of knowledge of their field. Thus, we hope that by stimulating the present generation of audiology students, we will also be contributing to the impetus for them to carry out this type of research, so necessary for the future growth of the field.

Joseph J. Montano and Jaclyn B. Spitzer

ACKNOWLEDGMENTS

This project would never have seen the light of day were it not for Mickey Stewart and Sam Selesnick, my colleagues at Cornell, who persuaded me to join their faculty in 2006 and have shown limitless support and encouragement; the members of the Department of Hearing and Speech; and my dear friend Jaci Spitzer who said to me, when I casually mentioned this idea for a textbook on AR, "Let's do it." Without her, there would be no book. Thanks.

Joseph J. Montano

This project was supported by the faculty at Columbia University, most especially Lanny Garth Close, and the members of the Department of Speech and Hearing of New York Presbyterian Hospital, ever watching my back. Thank you for every day.

Jaclyn B. Spitzer

CONTRIBUTORS

Harvey B. Abrams, Ph.D.
Associate Chief of Staff for Research and Development
Research and Development Service
Bay Pines VA Healthcare System
Bay Pines, Florida
Chapter 6

Zvia Admon, L.L.M.
Legal Consultant for the Israeli Ministry of Justice
Commission for Equal Rights of People with Disabilities
Tel Aviv, Israel
Chapter 15

Jerome G. Alpiner, Ph.D.
Professor Emeritus
University of Colorado
Centennial, Colorado
Chapter 1

Scott J. Bally, Ph.D.
Gallaudet University
Department of Hearing, Speech and Language
Washington, D.C.
Chapter 13

Ruth Bentler, Ph.D.
Professor
Department of Speech Pathology and Audiology
University of Iowa
Iowa City, Iowa
Chapter 8

Orna Eran, Ph.D.
Consultant and Audiological Scientist for the Israeli Government Ministries Ministry of Defense
Bureau for Disabled Persons Rehabilitation;
Ministry of Justice Commission for Equal Rights of People with Disabilities;
The National Insurance Institute of Israel
Tel Aviv, Israel
Chapter 15

Sue Ann Erdman, M.A.
Audiologic Rehabilitation Counseling and Consulting Services
Jenson Beach, Florida
Chapter 9

Jean Pierre Gagné, Ph.D.
Professor titulaire
École d'orthophonie et d'audiologie
Centre de recherche de l'Institut universitaire de gériatrie de Montréal
Université de Montréal
Montréal, Québec, Canada
Chapters 3 and 4

Louise Hickson, Ph.D.
Acting Head of School
School of Hearing and Rehabilitation Sciences
University of Queensland
Brisbone, Queensland, Australia
Chapter 18

Theresa Hnath Chisolm, Ph.D.
Professor and Chair
Department of Communication Sciences and Disorders
Tampa, Florida
Chapter 6

Mary Beth Jennings, Ph.D.
Assistant Professor
National Centre for Audiology
Faculty of Health Sciences
University of Western Ontario
London, Ontario, Canada
Chapters 3 and 4

Jack Katz, Ph.D.
Auditory Processing Service
Prairie Village, Kansas
Chapter 21

Patricia B. Kricos, Ph.D.
Professor
Department of Communication Sciences and Disorders
Gainesville, Florida
Chapter 19

Charissa R. Lansing, Ph.D.
Associate Professor
Department of Speech and Hearing Science
Associate Professor, Beckman Institute
University of Illinois at Urbana-Champaign
Champaign, Illinois
Chapter 11

Christopher Lind, Ph.D.
Senior Lecturer in Audiology
Course Coordinator-Master of Audiology
Department of Speech Pathology and Audiology
Flinders University
Adelaide, South Australia, Australia
Chapter 10

Dean M. Mancuso, Au.D.
Manager, Aural Rehabilitation
Columbia University Medical Center of New York Presbyterian Hospital
New York, New York
Chapter 7

Patricia A. McCarthy, Ph.D.
Professor
Program Director-Audiology
Department of Communication Disorders & Sciences
Rush University Medical Center
Chicago, Illinois
Chapter 1

Joseph J. Montano, Ed.D.
Associate Professor of Audiology in Clinical Otolaryngology
Weill Cornell Medical College
Cornell University
Director, Audiology and Speech Pathology Division
New York, New York
Preface and Chapter 2

Craig W. Newman, Ph.D.
Section Head, Audiology
Head and Neck Institute
Cleveland Clinic
Professor, Cleveland Clinic Lerner College of Medicine of Case Western Reserve University
Cleveland, Ohio
Chapter 20

William Noble, Ph.D.
Professor
Discipline of Psychology
University of New England
Armidale, New South Wales, Australia
Chapter 5

Geoff Plant, O.A.M.
Rehabilitation Specialist
Clinical Research Department
MED-EL Worldwide Headquarters
Arlington, Massachusetts
Chapter 17

Anne T. Pope
President
Hearing Loss Association of America
New York, New York
Chapter 16

Mark Ross, Ph.D.
Professor Emeritus
University of Connecticut
Storrs, Connecticut
Foreword

Jennifer Henderson Sabes, M.A.
Research Audiologist
University of California, San Francisco
San Francisco, California
Chapter 12

Sharon A. Sandridge, Ph.D.
Director, Audiologic Clinical Services
Co-Director, Tinnitus Management Clinic
Co-Director, Audiology Research Lab
Head and Neck Institute
Cleveland Clinic
Professor, Cleveland Clinic Lerner College of Medicine of Case Western Reserve University
Cleveland, Ohio
Chapter 20

Kenneth Southall, M.Sc.
Centre de recherche
Institut universitaire de gériatrie de Montréal
Affilié à l'Université de Montréal
Montréal, Québec, Canada
Chapters 3 and 4

Jaclyn B. Spitzer, Ph.D.
Professor
Clinical Audiology and Speech Pathology
in Otolaryngology/Head and Neck Surgery
Columbia University College of Physicians and Surgeons
Director, Audiology and Speech Pathology Division
Columbia University Medical Center
New York, New York
Professor
Department of Communication Sciences and Disorders
Montclair State University
Montclair, New Jersey
Preface and Chapter 7

Carren J. Stika, Ph.D.
Adjunct Faculty
San Diego State University
School of Speech, Language and Hearing Sciences
San Diego, California
Chapter 16

Robert W. Sweetow, Ph.D.
Director of Audiology
Professor of Otolaryngology
University of California, San Francisco
San Francisco, California
Chapter 12

Linda M. Thibodeau, Ph.D.
Head, Au.D. Program
University of Texas at Dallas
Callier Center for Communication Disorders
Advanced Hearing Research Center
Dallas, Texas
Chapter 14

Barbara E. Weinstein, Ph.D.
Executive Officer
Clinical Doctoral Programs
Graduate Center
City University of New York
New York, New York
Chapter 22

Yu-Hsiang Wu, M.D., Ph.D.
Postdoctoral Research Scientist
Department of Communication Sciences and Disorders
University of Iowa
Iowa City, Iowa
Chapter 8

This book is dedicated to my wife Patricia and our children: Katie, Daniel, Lauren, Laura, and AJ who somehow put up with my antics and continue to love me, and, to my former students at Long Island University/C.W. Post who were the true inspiration for this book.

Joe Montano

I dedicate this book to Elaine Rubinson, whose frustration and tears burned me, and whose strength taught me. Further, to Harriet and Victor Rubinson, who also lived the stories and sometimes pain and joy of Elaine, and to Raquel, who knew her grandmother all too little, I am glad you endured all with me.

Jaclyn B. Spitzer

Part I

Developing a Knowledge Base: Introduction and Background

1

History of Adult Audiologic Rehabilitation: The Past as Prologue

Jerome G. Alpiner
Patricia A. McCarthy

The more things change, the more they remain the same. This French proverb comes to mind when looking at audiologic rehabilitation (AR) from a historical perspective. Indeed, although technology and techniques have evolved over time, the raison d'etre for adult audiologic rehabilitation has remained the same, that is, improvement of human communication. In 1973, Toubbeh validated this goal of audiologic rehabilitation by stating, "Human communication is action, it is culture, it is the *history* of man, it is the fabric of all societies, its absence negates man's existence." This impressive quote, made over 36 years ago, reminds us that improvement of human communication in those with hearing loss is a vital pursuit for the individual as well as society. So although individuals, society, and technology have changed dramatically over the past century, the purpose and goals of audiologic rehabilitation have remained steadfast.

What can be learned by examining the history of adult audiologic rehabilitation? It is a well-accepted maxim among historians that understanding the past is fundamental to understanding the present. Furthermore, our future practice can be shaped by reflecting on our roots. Understanding our history perhaps can provide us a baseline on which to grow as audiologic rehabilitation evolves into a sophisticated 21st century evidence-based treatment process. Certainly, the knowledge and skills used in the contemporary practice of adult audiologic rehabilitation are not the result of magical events but the rather product of building a profession by complementing each generation's progress. In this chapter, we explore the contributions of these previous generations and consider their impact on the present and future practice of adult audiologic rehabilitation. As shown in Figure 1–1, centuries of progress have provided underpinnings for the current practice of audiologic rehabilitation.

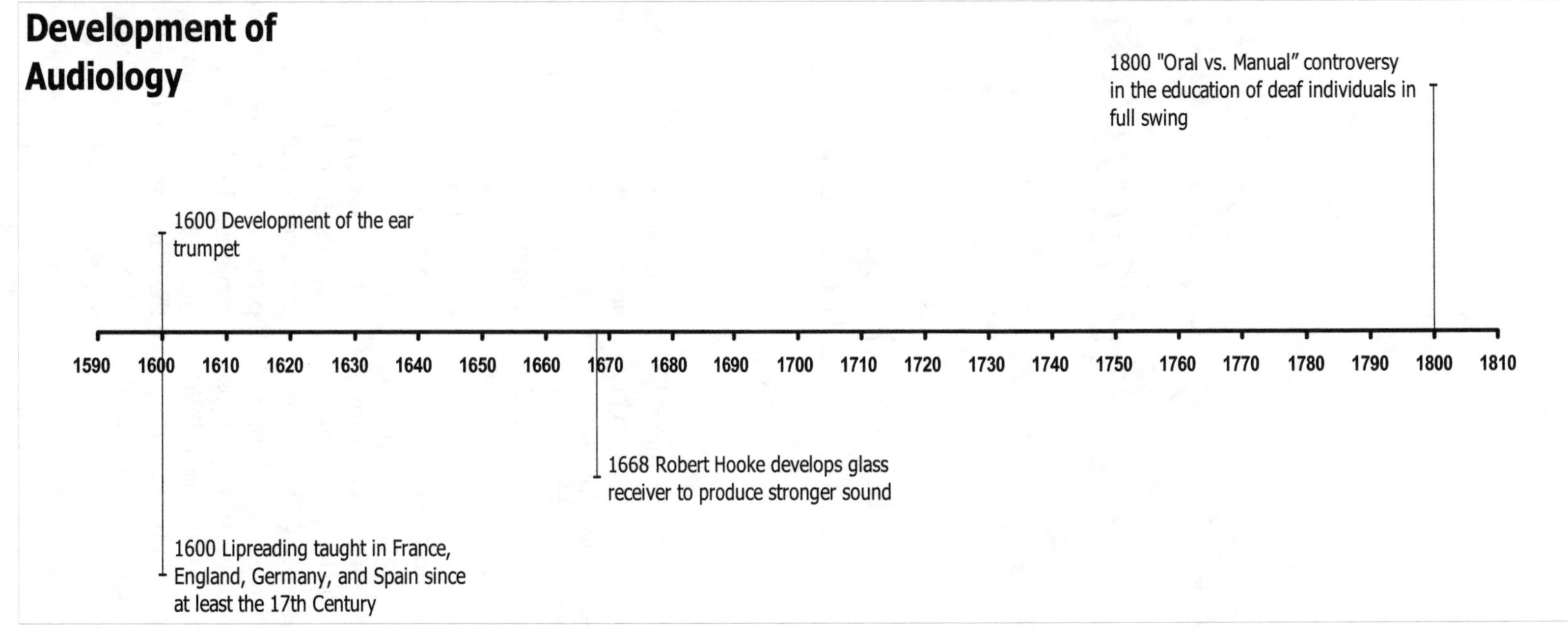

Figure 1–1. Time line 1.

What Do We Call It Anyway?

Over the years, the terminology used to describe the rehabilitation process has assumed many names, thus leading to confusion among the public, the profession, and third party payers. Through the years there have been various squabbles, so to speak, about what the identifying term should be. Some terminology examples include aural rehabilitation, rehabilitative audiology, auditory rehabilitation, audiologic rehabilitation, lipreading, speechreading, auditory training, and hearing therapy. Titles of textbooks, journal articles, and professional presentations verify this lack of agreement.

Much of the disagreement about terminology centers around use of the term "aural rehabilitation," which implies a process focused on hearing per se. The argument posits that the process of improving the communication of adults with hearing loss is a holistic approach that extends well beyond simply improving hearing. For example, strictly speaking, even lipreading would not be part of "aural" rehabilitation because it is primarily a visual process. Therefore, the quest to use a more representative term than aural rehabilitation has ensued.

It was not until World War II when a military aural rehabilitation program was started that the term "audiology" came into existence. At that point in history, audiology was defined by the Veterans Administration (VA; Newby, 1964). The VA defined an audiologist as "one who is concerned with the assessment of hearing, and the habilitation and rehabilitation of children and adults with hearing impairment." Even at that time, there was concern about the lack of audiologists to provide service in aural rehabilitation. At the same time, there appeared to be a division between educational services and the provision of audiology services for individuals with hearing impairment. There also was concern about emphasis on audiology diagnostic services rather than on aural rehabilitation. Despite this, the term aural rehabilitation continued to be used widely to describe a process distinct from diagnostic audiology.

The American Speech-Language-Hearing Association (ASHA, 1984) offered its definition of aural rehabilitation as referring to "services and procedures for facilitating receptive and expressive communication in individuals with hearing impairment. These services and procedures are intended for those persons who demonstrate a loss of hearing sensitivity" (p. 1). This definition is not so much what aural rehabilitation is but refers more to the procedures performed. ASHA then describes specific procedures, which can be found in the guidelines. The main categories are (1) Identification and evaluation of sensory capabilities, (2) Interpretation of results, counseling, and referral, (3) Intervention for communication difficulties, (4) Re-evaluation of the client's status, and (5) Evaluation and modification of the intervention program.

One major reason for describing procedures as well as training requirements for aural rehabilitation is the interdisciplinary nature of the field whereby speech-language pathologists can perform these activities without a Certificate of Clinical Certification in Audiology (CCC-A) or an audiology license. In fact, there are some Medicare and third-party payers guidelines that will only reimburse speech-language pathologists, not audiologists, for services typically considered under the rubric of aural rehabilitation (e.g., speechreading). In some ways, audiologists see this as a turf battle in which another profession has co-opted part of their scope of practice without the requisite training. It could be argued that if the process were called "audiologic rehabilitation," it might be more clearly seen as requiring the expertise of an audiologist. (For more information on reimbursement issues related to AR, the reader is referred to Chapter 2.)

Further confusion has arisen with the various titles used by professionals engaged in rehabilitation with adults with hearing loss. For example, many professionals desire to be called audiologists as an umbrella title that encompasses the entire scope of practice including aural rehabilitation. Others have preferred to use an adjective that specifies his or her primary expertise in the profession such as "rehabilitation audiologist" or "diagnostic audiologist." These terms typically have no basis in credentialing. Furthermore, insurance companies are more apt to reimburse when procedures are listed and the professional has certain credentials.

Terminology also can be confusing to the public and raises some interesting questions. Does aural rehabilitation include deaf individuals who might use sign language as their primary mode of communication? Do some persons hear the word oral (for aural) and think of a dentist? Does the consumer with hearing loss even know what the term "aural rehabilitation" encompasses? One speech and hearing clinic ran an advertisement in a newspaper indicating that it provided speechreading therapy. A respondent to the ad called to request an appointment for a class in speed-reading. To a certain degree, terminology has caused somewhat of an identity crisis!

Although there is no right answer as to what the process should be correctly called, audiologists in the 21st century are increasingly using the term "audiologic rehabilitation." This term gives ownership to the profession of audiology and encompasses the vast scope of the rehabilitation process. Audiologists have an extensive armamentarium of knowledge, skills, and tools that prepare them to engage successfully in the rehabilitation process. As discussed throughout this textbook, the rehabilitation process does not begin and end with surgery (cochlear implants, implantable hearing aids, etc.) or the dispensing of amplification (hearing aids, hearing assistive technology, etc.). As such, we strongly suggest use of the term audiologic rehabilitation in current practice.

From the Ear Trumpet to Lipreading (Early Origins)

In our techno-sophisticated world, the idea of using ear trumpets as amplification is archaic (Figure 1–2). Yet ear trumpets were creative developments to increase speech intensity initially used by sailors and others who needed to communicate at distances. Ear trumpets were later used to help persons with hearing impairment communicate better. One of the earliest descriptions of ear trumpets was by Jean Leurechon in his 1624 book, *Recreation Mathematique*.

Ear trumpets were generally custom-made and their use as hearing aids began around 1800

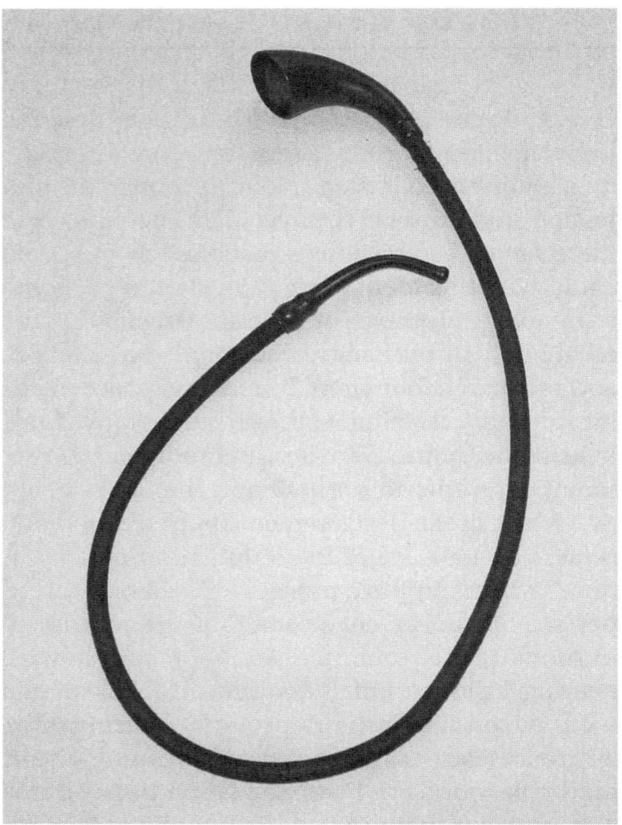

Figure 1–2. Ear horn/trumpet.

(Berger, 1984.) Hearing aid trumpet styles and prices varied as did the rate of success by the user. (It is interesting that the same could be said of hearing aids in the 21st century!) Technology in the 17th century was even of concern in the development of the ear trumpet. Robert Hooke in 1668 worked toward improving hearing by developing a glass receiver which produced stronger sound (Berger, 1984). He also produced two receivers, one which was latten, and conical in nature; the other of glass and round, both sharp at one end. The former produced a stronger sound. It appears that amplification, starting with ear trumpets, became a significant factor in helping individuals with hearing impairment.

Even before the emergence of ear trumpet amplification, lipreading played an important role in the rehabilitation and education of individuals with hearing loss. Lipreading was taught in various countries, such as France, England, Germany, and Spain since at least the 17th century. Children and adults received instruction; both analytic and synthetic methods were utilized. The analytic approach emphasized the learning of individual sounds on the lips; the synthetic approach had a more broadbased communication orientation. Some of the prominent names in the development of these approaches include, Bruhn (1955), Bunger (1961), Nitchie (1950), and the Kinzie sisters (1920). Electronic amplification technology did not exist in those days. Therefore, lipreading served as one of the only viable methods for teaching the "deaf and dumb" (Peet, 1851). For a comprehensive and fascinating review of lipreading the reader is referred to *The Story of Lipreading* by DeLand (1931).

By the 19th century, the "oral versus manual controversy" in the education of deaf individuals was in full swing. Advocates of oralism relied on lipreading as a major communication mode so that "deaf" individuals could learn to function in a hearing society. Advocates of manualism decried the poor verbal and written language skills of deaf individuals who relied purely on oralism. They argued that use of American Sign Language would allow deaf individuals to develop language and communication skills. By the mid-20th century, however, much of the passion for this controversy dissipated with the development of powerful, miniaturized hearing aids brought about by the development of the transistor in 1949 (www.pbs.org, 1999). Adults with moderate-to-severe hearing losses who had previously functioned as deaf individuals could now benefit from both powerful gain hearing aids and lipreading.

Although lipreading schools and teachers have become a thing of the past, the role of visual cues in communication cannot be underemphasized in adult audiologic rehabilitation in the 21st century. Best practice hearing aid fitting protocols stress the synergistic benefits of bisensory stimulation that result from amplification and the use of visual cues in communication. (Note: In keeping with the authors' discussion of consumer confusing terminology, the term lipreading is often used interchangeably with the term speechreading. Although speechreading is meant to be more inclusive, both identifiers refer to visual communication. The reader is referred to Chapter 11 in this text for a review of the contemporary research related to lipreading and visual communication.)

World War II Era: Birth of Audiology (Figure 1–3)

If they were still alive, those responsible for the creation of audiology as a profession might be chagrined that some 60 years later, audiologists have strayed so far from our rehabilitative roots. Indeed, the profession was created in response to the needs of the World War II "aural casualties requiring rehabilitative measures" (Truex, 1944). In response to these needs, both the Army and Navy developed "Aural Rehabilitation Centers"; three by the Army (Deshon, Borden, and Hoff General Hospitals) and one by the Navy (Philadelphia Naval Hospital) (Spencer, 1946; Truex, 1944). Raymond Carhart, the acknowledged "father of audiology," served in the Army Medical Corps (1944–1946) as the Director of the Acoustics Clinics in the Veterans Rehabilitation Center of Deshon General Hospital before beginning the first academic program in audiology at Northwestern University in 1947 (Olsen, Rose, & Hedgecock, 2003).

The "listening clinics" were created to "place these people back into effective communication with their fellows and their environment" (Spencer, 1946). The rehabilitative process began with a hearing examination and fitting of the "most satisfactory" hearing instrument. But this was truly just the beginning of the eight-week process. An intense "course of instruction" was designed for each patient to reorient him to sounds transmitted by the hearing instrument. Use of the term "reorient" suggests an understanding that fitting the hearing aid was the only first step in the process. Special instruction was needed because of the "cerebral reorientation to the auditory stimuli of auditory noises" that accompanies hearing aid use (Truex, 1944). The curriculum included daily individual and group lip-reading instruction, counseling regarding personal, economic, or domestic problems, maintenance of contacts with the patient's family, and bridging the gap between the

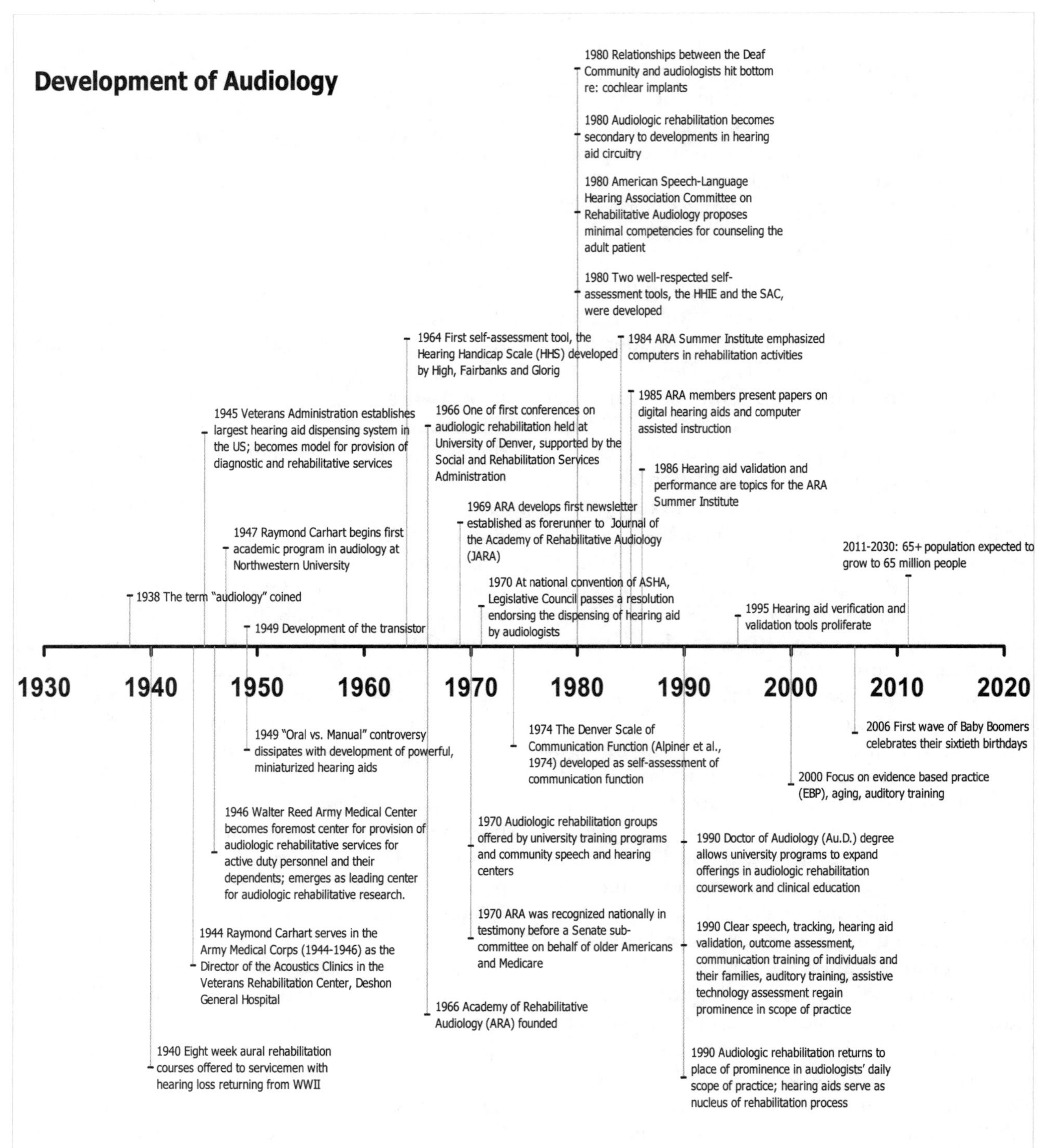

Development of Audiology
1980 Relationships between the Deaf Community and audiologists hit bottom re: cochlear implants
1980 Audiologic rehabilitation becomes secondary to developments in hearing aid circuitry
1980 American Speech-Language Hearing Association Committee on Rehabilitative Audiology proposes minimal competencies for counseling the adult patient
1980 Two well-respected self-assessment tools, the HHIE and the SAC, were developed
1964 First self-assessment tool, the Hearing Handicap Scale (HHS) developed by High, Fairbanks and Glorig
1984 ARA Summer Institute emphasized computers in rehabilitation activities
1985 ARA members present papers on digital hearing aids and computer assisted instruction
1945 Veterans Administration establishes largest hearing aid dispensing system in the US; becomes model for provision of diagnostic and rehabilitative services
1966 One of first conferences on audiologic rehabilitation held at University of Denver, supported by the Social and Rehabilitation Services Administration
1986 Hearing aid validation and performance are topics for the ARA Summer Institute
1969 ARA develops first newsletter established as forerunner to Journal of the Academy of Rehabilitative Audiology (JARA)
1947 Raymond Carhart begins first academic program in audiology at Northwestern University
2011-2030: 65+ population expected to grow to 65 million people
1970 At national convention of ASHA, Legislative Council passes a resolution endorsing the dispensing of hearing aid by audiologists
1938 The term "audiology" coined
1995 Hearing aid verification and validation tools proliferate
1949 Development of the transistor
1930
1940
1950
1960
1970
1980
1990
2000
2010
2020
1949 "Oral vs. Manual" controversy dissipates with development of powerful, miniaturized hearing aids
1974 The Denver Scale of Communication Function (Alpiner et al., 1974) developed as self-assessment of communication function
2006 First wave of Baby Boomers celebrates their sixtieth birthdays
2000 Focus on evidence based practice (EBP), aging, auditory training
1946 Walter Reed Army Medical Center becomes foremost center for provision of audiologic rehabilitative services for active duty personnel and their dependents; emerges as leading center for audiologic rehabilitative research.
1970 Audiologic rehabilitation groups offered by university training programs and community speech and hearing centers
1990 Doctor of Audiology (Au.D.) degree allows university programs to expand offerings in audiologic rehabilitation coursework and clinical education
1970 ARA was recognized nationally in testimony before a Senate sub-committee on behalf of older Americans and Medicare
1944 Raymond Carhart serves in the Army Medical Corps (1944-1946) as the Director of the Acoustics Clinics in the Veterans Rehabilitation Center, Deshon General Hospital
1990 Clear speech, tracking, hearing aid validation, outcome assessment, communication training of individuals and their families, auditory training, assistive technology assessment regain prominence in scope of practice
1966 Academy of Rehabilitative Audiology (ARA) founded
1940 Eight week aural rehabilitation courses offered to servicemen with hearing loss returning from WWII
1990 Audiologic rehabilitation returns to place of prominence in audiologists' daily scope of practice; hearing aids serve as nucleus of rehabilitation process

Figure 1–3. Time line 2.

Veteran's Facility and the "civilian agencies that will continue any additional rehabilitative measure that might be needed" (Truex, 1944). The fact that a hearing-impaired veteran might need "additional rehabilitative measures" beyond the eight week course is evidence that rehabilitative measures were respected and essential in the 1940s. Six decades later, even a few hours of post-hearing-aid-fitting rehabilitation is rare.

Hearing aid satisfaction and outcome measurement were critical parts of the rehabilitation process. The Army and Navy programs administered satisfaction questionnaires and reported that "94% of the boys" were still using their hearing aids three months to two years postfitting (Spencer, 1946). Captain Grant Fairbanks reported that more than 350 hearing aid prescriptions were possible with various combinations of microphones, receivers, amplifiers, and batteries. Yet there still were complaints like "I can hear everything in the room except the guy I'm trying to listen to" (Spencer, 1946), thus supporting the adage that the more things change, the more they stay the same.

Even in the 1940s, unrealistic hearing aid expectations were prevalent as some patients wanted "miracles from their hearing aids" (Spencer, 1946). Auditory training ("expertly supervised listening") was designed to help patients adjust to electronic amplification and to improve sound perception and discrimination. Groups of 6 to 10 participated in Army and Navy listening clinics that provided a variety of sound experiences including phoneme discrimination tasks, music, radio programs, and speeches. A primary goal of these groups was to help "a man outgrow the negativism of deafness" (Spencer, 1946). Attention was also given to vocational/occupational issues presented by hearing loss. (Note: For more information on the stigma associated with hearing loss, the reader is referred to Chapter 4.)

Motivation for engaging in the rehabilitation process was an issue for these early military programs. In order to combat the pessimism and fatigue of soldiers and sailors with hearing impairment returning from World War II, some interesting motivational methods were employed. For example, an "orientation girl" was used to brief the new patient and because he could not "hear the bugle," a "pretty WAC" would wake him in the morning. Furthermore, lipreading teachers were mostly women who were "easier to look at" and "vocally better groomed" (Spencer, 1946). Certainly recognizing the role of motivation was laudable despite the rather sexist methods employed!

So, compared to the rehabilitative processes offered in the 1940s, what new concepts or strategies have emerged in the past six decades? The Aural Rehabilitation Centers designed by the Army and Navy addressed amplification, adjustment, and "cerebral reorientation" to hearing aids, motivation, expectations, self-assessment, auditory training, lipreading, counseling, family support, psychosocial and vocational issues, group sessions, and the need for follow-up rehabilitation. The new hearing aid user in the early 21st century who is receiving all of those services is indeed rare.

Post-WWII: Walter Reed Army Medical Center and Veterans Administration

The provision of audiologic rehabilitation services during and post-World War II established it as a priority for service personnel and veterans with hearing loss. Since that time, hearing loss has continued as a major health concern during both peace and war times. As such, many of the major trends in audiologic rehabilitation have emerged as the result of the efforts of the Veterans Administration (VA) and the Walter Reed Army Medical Center (WRAMC). The VA established the largest hearing aid dispensing system in the United States and became the model for provision of diagnostic and rehabilitative services to eligible veterans with hearing loss. The WRAMC became the foremost center in the provision of audiologic rehabilitative services for active duty personnel and their dependents and emerged as the leading center for audiologic rehabilitative research. In the 21st century, these agencies continue to lead the way in research and development of rehabilitative technology, methods, amplification, service delivery, and outcome measurement.

What's Happening in the 1960s

American adult audiologic rehabilitation was enhanced in 1966 with the emergence of the Academy of Rehabilitative Audiology (ARA). Prior to this time there had been no major effort to establish a formal organization to emphasize the rehabilitation aspect of audiology. The name itself helped to institutionalize the concept of "audiologic" in lieu of "aural" rehabilitation.

The impetus for development of ARA came from a group of audiologists, led by John O'Neill and Herbert Oyer, who were concerned about the lack of interest in aural rehabilitation programs including in the training of university students. As a result of this concern, the Academy of Rehabilitative Audiology (ARA) was inaugurated in 1966 with assistance from the Federal Office of Vocational Rehabilitation in Washington, D.C. The purpose of the academy was to generate interest in AR and offer a mechanism for interest and participation in this area of the profession.

Interestingly, various issues that have faced AR since its inception mirror the activities of the ARA. There seemed to be turf concerns regarding the ownership of audiologic rehabilitation between rehabilitation and clinical audiologists. In order to track the development of aural rehabilitation, the ARA approved a position for an archivist. In her role as archivist, Skalbeck (1984) provided a rationale for the transition of AR through the years. She stated, "If you subscribe to Santayana's warning that those who do not know history are destined to repeat it, there should be merit for old and new members, and perhaps other audiologists to review where we have been and where we think we are going."

Audiology continued to grow at a logarithmic pace during the years from 1966, particularly in the development of diagnostic techniques. Unfortunately, there appeared to be a continuing decline in interest related to the remediation aspects of audiology. Some colleagues even took a position that it was more important to test than to engage in audiologic rehabilitation. There seemed to be a widespread attitude that, if rehabilitation was ignored, the use of diagnostic equipment and techniques would become more professional and valued. Surveys of audiology journals illustrated the trend of publishing many more diagnostic articles than rehabilitative.

Institute on Aural Rehabilitation

One of the early conferences on audiologic rehabilitation was held at University of Denver in 1966 supported by the Social and Rehabilitation Services Administration with Jerome Alpiner serving as project director (Alpiner, 1966). Representatives from throughout the United States attended. The institute focused on significant areas of AR for audiologists and helped define and encourage their role in the rehabilitation process.

This was a landmark and exciting conference for advocates of audiologic rehabilitation. It is worth noting that this event was held several years *before* ASHA approved the dispensing of hearing aids by audiologists. This was a time in which we were excited about developing ways to help those adults with hearing loss—after they purchased aids from dispensers (hearing aid dealers at this time). Some of the relevant topics included lipreading, auditory training, social/psychological factors, vocational programs, closed circuit and commercial television training, and research in aural rehabilitation. An interesting exercise would be to survey today's audiologists to determine if the above procedures are provided in their practices. Additionally, it would be enlightening to know how many patients either receive any of these services as part of hearing aid fitting or after fitting follow-up.

An ARA newsletter was established prior to development of the *Journal of the Academy of Rehabilitative Audiology (JARA)*. Three articles appeared in the April 1969 issue. Brainard (1969) reported on an investigation of the relationship between performance on a filmed lipreading test and analysis of the visual environment. Lovering (1969) reported on visual acuity and lipreading performance and reported that lipreading scores will degenerate as a function of visual distraction. Kitchen (1969) studied the relationship of visual synthesis to lipreading performance. Oyer (1969) reported the establishment of a laboratory at Michigan State University that was solely for the purpose of scientific studies in aural rehabilitation. And so it was! AR was on its way as an identified, valued aspect of the profession.

The 1970s: Things Are a Changin'

Probably the one of the most significant decision ever to be made by ASHA was to allow audiologists to sell hearing aids. This senior author was on the ASHA Executive Board at the time and recalls that the exchanges were emotional, to the extent that one member indicated a resignation would be forthcoming if the resolution passed. It passed; he did not resign.

Prior to ASHA's decision to permit the dispensing of hearing aids, there was a Fourth of July approach in which both sides were quite adamant, emphatically holding a position that audiologists should not be able to dispense hearing aids. Siegenthaler (1972) took the position that audiologists should not dispense hearing aids. Several of his major points at the time included:

1. The clinical audiologist, who is free from maintaining his income by the sale of hearing aids is in a proper position to offer services (AR) whereas another group (hearing aid dealers), should dispense hearing aids on the basis of the audiologist's recommendations.
2. If audiologists dispensed hearing aids, some predicted the demise of hearing aid dealers as well as audiologists. Audiologists would lose the subsidies from universities and government agencies over a period of time. Meanwhile, hearing aid dealers would lose their business because audiologists will go into private practice and dispense aids from their officers.
3. Audiology technicians will be trained to do basic audiometrics submitting results, for example, to otolaryngologists. Perhaps the technicians even would be franchised to dispense hearing aids. It was pointed out that some otolaryngologists would train their nurses to do the basic testing. Siegenthaler also indicated that the Rehabilitation Services Administration (RSA) had awarded a grant to the National Association of Speech and Hearing Agencies to train armed services medical corpsmen to be audiometric technicians.
4. The issues were complex and somewhat confusing regarding who would perform the various audiology procedures.

Harford (1972) took the position in favor of dispensing of hearing aids by audiologists. At the national convention of ASHA in 1971, the Legislative Council passed a resolution endorsing the dispensing of hearing aid by audiologists. The resolution was then submitted to the Executive Board. A statement of rationale was presented to answer the basic question: "Why should ASHA change its Code of Ethics to allow the dispensing of hearing aids by its members who are audiologists if they wish to do so?" A brief review of these responses follows:

1. There was an increased concern in the 1960s and 1970s that audiologists were not able to fulfill their obligations to the hearing impaired. There was a feeling that the hearing delivery system should be expanded to dispensing hearing aids in order to provide comprehensive audiologic rehabilitation services.
2. There needed to be a more efficient system for hearing aid delivery beyond recommending the aids to be fit by hearing aid dealers.
3. A number of audiologists had given up their ASHA certification in order to become directly involved in the hearing aid fitting process. This was an extremely significant move by some audiologists
4. A number of audiologists felt that they would be better able to research the effectiveness of hearing aids and other wearable amplification devices as part of the AR process.

Changes in the ASHA Code of Ethics significantly influenced the training of audiologists, the breadth of the job market, the financial implications of the profession, and service delivery to hearing-impaired adults in the United States. Ask yourself what you would be doing today if audiologists were not able to dispense hearing aids!

The 1970s were, in many ways, a decade when audiologic rehabilitation practice patterns were established and audiologic rehabilitation was respected as integral part of audiology practice. In 1973, Garwood, Bergman, Dixon, and Haspiel reported on the roles assumed by audiologists and concluded that there was one common thread that should hold audiologists together, "their practice and engagement in the aural rehabilitation process." Regardless of roles assumed by audiologists as administrators, clinicians, academicians, private practitioners, or government employees, rehabilitation of individuals with hearing loss was the uniting goal of the profession.

The emphasis on rehabilitation was particularly evident in university training programs. In the 1970s most audiologic rehabilitation groups were offered by university training programs and community speech and hearing centers. The usual format was for six week programs (once a week) with groups of about six or seven individuals. Most university programs were either free or required a nominal charge, which probably did not cover the overhead of the clinic. Group sessions were supervised by university instructors with clinical practicum students actively involved in this clinical learning model. The typical format for these group sessions generally included lipreading, auditory training, and some hearing aid orientation. Counseling was included to allow participants to engage in dialogue regarding their communication situations. Community programs generally charged, although nominally, and the services provided were similar to the university programs.

Interest in outcome measurement was prevalent in the 1970s although that terminology was not yet in the audiologist's lexicon. Pre and post-lipreading tests were typically given to document improvement accrued as a result of group AR. The limitations of lipreading testing often made this an exercise in frustration given ceiling effects and the inherent difficulty of creating a reliable, valid assessment of visual communication ability. However, a 1977 study by Binnie suggested that there were positive outcomes associated with these group rehabilitation sessions. Individuals enrolled in a university AR group at Purdue University were given a lipreading pretest during the first group session. At the end of the program, these same participants were given a lipreading post-test. Not surprisingly, there was little measured improvement in lipreading skills. In addition, participants also were given a questionnaire probing whether they felt their communication had improved as a result of these group sessions. Interestingly, the participants overwhelmingly responded that their communication and their confidence in communicating had improved dramatically. So despite no measurable changes in lipreading ability, participants in group AR self-reported marked improvement in communication abilities. These intriguing results suggested that something positive other than improvement in lipreading skills was occurring as the result of the rehabilitation process.

Even in the 1970s, audiologists were frustrated by adults with hearing loss who could improve their communication efforts via rehabilitation but chose not to do so. Based on their observations that adults with hearing loss frequently did not follow through with AR recommendations, Oyer et al. (1976) sought to determine some of the reasons for this lack of follow-up. A questionnaire was sent to 45 adults who had been evaluated and advised to participate in rehabilitation programs yet chose not to participate. A review of their results and insights into audiologic service delivery suggests their conclusions were not only relevant in the 1970s but also in the early 21st century. Some examples include:

1. Audiologists are unable to demonstrate the worth of AR and the changes that it can bring about.
2. The flexibility in scheduling AR programs for working people should be studied.
3. Audiologists do not differentiate and place in proper perspective the relative values of ampli-

fication derived from a hearing aid and the further refinements to be achieved through auditory training and lipreading.

4. Perhaps audiologists need to enlist the support of family members, friends, or other significant persons to aid in encouraging the hearing impaired to participate in AR. It is possible that insufficient attention is given to familiarizing these people with the communication problem, the limitations of hearings aids, and the difficulty in hearing aid adjustment.

Thirty years later, the challenge of engaging adults with hearing loss in the AR process has become more complex. As in the 1970s, audiologists often short-sell the value and impact of the rehabilitation process. For example, few audiologists involved in hearing aid fittings offer group rehabilitation sessions despite the evidence that suggests this model reduces hearing handicap (Preminger, 2003) and is cost effective (Northern & Beyer, 1999). Furthermore, those audiologists who do offer group sessions are challenged to find ways to encourage individuals to attend. In many ways, adult group rehabilitation as a treatment model is less accepted in the 21st century than it was in the 1970s. Furthermore, while giving lip service to the value of rehabilitation, audiologists three decades later often fail to convince individuals of the value of rehabilitation, continue to report that they do not have the time to offer rehabilitation, and appear to be unconvinced of its value in the hearing aid fitting process despite compelling evidence to the contrary (Chisholm et al., 2007).

During the 1970s, the Academy of Rehabilitative Audiology continued to emphasize AR as a flexible product that could be infused into any type of audiologic practice. For the first time, the ARA was recognized nationally to provide testimony before a Senate subcommittee on behalf of older Americans and Medicare. Furthermore, Hardick (1976) reported on expert testimony provided to the ENT Committee of the Food and Drug Administration (FDA) on standards for auditory training. A significant recommendation was licensing providers of auditory training the same as hearing aid dispensers. During this time, initial discussions began regarding the need for audiologists to be licensed to make them more "recognized" and accountable.

A New Approach in 1970s and 1980s: Self-Assessment

One day in the 1970s, the senior author of this chapter (then a university professor) posed a question to his doctoral students, "When audiologists make recommendations to patients, do they really objectively know that individual's communication function, aside from the numerical evaluation scores?" The lively, ensuing discussion encompassed such issues as how the patient got along at home, at work, in social contacts, in all everyday living situations. The discussion, as well as others that were occurring among those interested in AR, focused on the growing belief that audiology test scores were not the only index to determine the rehabilitative needs of adults with hearing loss. Certainly, obtaining numerical audiologic data was one critical part of the rehabilitation process but the next step was to think of the ways to assess what impact the hearing loss had on the individual's life. As such, an emerging focus of the 1970s was how to assess communication function beyond the audiogram.

There were initial attempts to address this issue as early as the 1940s. The Social Adequacy Index was designed by Davis (1948) to examine the relationship between speech reception thresholds and discrimination scores. It was felt that more information about the connection between hearing loss and understanding speech was needed. In 1964, The Hearing Handicap Scale (HHS) was developed by High, Fairbanks, and Glorig to assess the effects of hearing loss on everyday living activities. Although a ground-breaking effort, the HHS was criticized for it lack of validity and failure to address vocational and psychological effects of hearing loss However, these early pioneers provided impetus for the numerous assessment procedures that followed in the 1970s.

As researchers began to develop self-assessment tools to identify the effects of hearing loss on the individual, it became clear that audiologists approached self-assessment in many different ways. Some were interested in using the procedures for research purposes. Others focused on assessment results as outcome measures by comparing a patient with himself pre- and postaudiologic rehabilitation. Tools were developed for specific populations including the elderly. Noble and Atherley (1970) devised the Hearing Measurement Scale (HMS) to assess handicap resulting from industrial noise exposure. Interestingly, the seven subcategories in the HMS laid the groundwork for future self-assessment tools developed over the next three decades. They include:

1. Speech-hearing
2. Acuity for nonspeech sound
3. Localization
4. Reaction to handicap
5. Speech distortion
6. Tinnitus
7. Personal opinion of hearing loss

The Denver Scale of Communication Function (Alpiner et al., 1974) approached self-assessment from a communication function standpoint. It was designed to help the audiologist make a subjective assessment of communication attitudes of adults with acquired hearing loss for more effective rehabilitative planning. It is based on the assumption that lipreading tests failed to measure improvement in communication function. Responses were made using a seven-point scale from agree to disagree. Some examples of items in the DSCF include:

The members of my family are annoyed with my hearing loss.

People sometimes avoid me because of my hearing loss.

Since I have trouble hearing, I hesitate to meet new people.

Hutton (1980) developed the Hearing Problem Inventory (Atlanta) to help the audiologist design an individualized rehabilitative program for patients. The instructions to clients stated "We want you to know about you and your problems. In this way we can do a better job of solving your specific problems." Interestingly, Hutton was one of the first to determine that a critical domain in assessing hearing aid satisfaction is hearing aid wear time. Hours of hearing aid use has since been included in such self-assessment tools as the International Outcomes Inventory (Cox & Alexander, 2002) and the Glasgow Hearing Aid Benefit Profile (Gatehouse, 1999).

Another variation of self-assessment was devised by Sanders (1975). Three profile questionnaires probe Communicative Performance in Home Environments, Occupational Environments, and Social Environments, with a four-point response scale format (little or no difficulty to great difficulty). A useful feature of these scales is that they assess how often each particular situation occurs for the individual thus allowing relevant responses to each item. Interestingly, over 20 years later, Gatehouse (1999) incorporated this concept into the Glasgow Hearing Aid Benefit Profile by asking "Does this situation happen in your life?" for each item.

A different twist on self-assessment, incorporating a family member's responses, was developed in the late 1970s by this chapter's authors. The McCarthy-Alpiner Scale of Hearing Handicap (1980) (M-A Scale) was designed to assess the psychological, social, and vocational effects of hearing loss from the perspective of the individual with hearing loss compared to a family member, allowing the audiologist to examine responses for counseling purposes (McCarthy & Alpiner, 1983). Use of this scale provides a platform for determining the attitudes of family members that can contribute to a counseling-based rehabilitation plan.

Two well-respected self-assessment tools, the HHIE and the SAC, were developed in the early 1980s. The Hearing Handicap Inventory for the Elderly (HHIE) and the screening version (HHIE-S) (Ventry & Weinstein, 1982, 1983) include items that assess the social and emotional handicapping effects of hearing loss. Even today, they are used widely in research and clinical practice. The 10-item HHIE-S, in particular, has been used not only as a screening instrument and rehabilitative assessment tool for the elderly, but also to document handicap reduction with hearing aid use and as a valid outcome measurement tool. The Self-Assessment of Communication (SAC), another screening tool, was designed to measure the communication ability of hearing-impaired adults also has a companion scale, the Significant Other Assessment of Communication (SOAC) (Schow & Nerbonne, 1982). Many modifications of both of these tools have been published over the last few decades including the Hearing Handicap Inventory for Adults (HHIA) (Newman, Weinstein, Jacobson, & Hug, 1991) and the adaptation of the SAC/SOAC for use with adolescents (Elkayam & English, 2003).

Another important development in the realm of self-assessment was the Communication Profile for the Hearing Impaired (CPHI) developed by Demorest and Erdman (1987). This profile provides an in-depth analysis of adjustment to hearing loss in four main areas: communication performance, communication environment, communication strategies, and personal adjustment. The CPHI was originally standardized on over 900 active and retired military personnel and was later standardized further with a variety of clinical population (Erdman & Demorest, 1998).

As the concept of the patient self-assessing his or her difficulties caught on as an adjunct to the audiometric evaluation, self-assessment tools have continued to proliferate. Many of the originally developed assessment tools are still used whereas new tools have been developed to reflect the trends of the day (hearing aid benefit and satisfaction, quality of life, etc). Since 1990, Robyn Cox has consistently contributed some of the best designed and pertinent self-assessment tools used in audiology. These include the Abbreviated Profile of Hearing Aid Benefit-APHAB (Cox & Alexander, 1995), the Expected Consequences of Hearing Aid Ownership-ECHO (Cox & Alexander, 2000), and the Satisfaction with Amplification in Daily Living-SADL (Cox & Alexander, 2001). The previously mentioned Glasgow Hearing Aid Benefit Profile-GHABP (Gatehouse, 1999), The Client Oriented Scale of Improvement-COSI (Dillon et al., 1999), and the International Outcome Inventory for Hearing Aids—IOI-HA (Cox, Stephens, & Kramer, 2002) represent the next generation of self-assessment tools since the initial efforts of the 1970s.

The past and present roles of self-assessment methodology were summarized in a meaningful way by Ross (1987):

> In the past 17 years, we have seen an ever burgeoning array of self-assessment scales. Their purpose is to evaluate a client's rehabilitative needs by assessing communication handicap, performance, environment, and strategies. On reviewing such scales, I find myself impressed with their scope and sensitivity. We are not only at the threshold of really defining the communication problems experienced by specific clients and developing realistic therapeutic strategies, but we also have a tool by means of which we can begin to assess the validity of our results. (p. 17)

The 1980s: The Traditional Approach Gives Way to Counseling

By the 1970s and 1980s, the traditional approach to audiologic rehabilitation had changed little since the early days (McCarthy & Culpepper, 1987). As a result, it is fair to say that not all audiologists or hearing aid vendors were using the traditional approach as an integral part of their hearing aid fittings. The role of rehabilitation was becoming secondary to the amazing developments in hearing aid circuitry that were emerging. This attitude was widespread and exemplified in this anecdote. A local hearing vendor was invited to speak to an audiology class about the hearing aid fitting process. (Recall the model of the audiologist doing the HAE and the hearing aid vendor "selling" the device.) The vendor agreed to discuss hearing aids but was negative on the role of the rehabilitation process. His rationale was that, if one discussed anything other than the hearing aid itself, the patient would think the hearing aids were "not perfect." Unfortunately, this attitude still exists to some degree in the 21st century. Many hearing impaired consumers' expectations for hearing aids are too high as a result of marketing and advertising; they often expect a "miracle." Meanwhile, emphasis on the need for rehabilitation to improve communication is ignored or given little attention.

The decline of the traditional approach also was influenced by audiologists' frustration with lack of reimbursement for these services. The traditional approach included a comprehensive audiologic evaluation, an assessment of lipreading function, planning for group and/or individual therapy sessions, implementation of therapy, post-therapy evaluation, prognosis, and recommendations. Although audiologists could be reimbursed for hearing aids (typically as a self-pay prosthetic device), they could not be reimbursed by a third party payer for hearing aids or such rehabilitative services as lipreading or auditory training. Furthermore, only "speechreading" was identified as a reimbursable service by Medicare; and even then, only speech-language pathologists were specified as providers (Madell & Montano, 2000). Although the codes have been rewritten recently, reimbursement for audiologic services, with the exception of rehabilitation following cochlear implantation, remains elusive today.

Another factor contributing to the decline of the traditional approach to AR was the lack of candidacy or discharge criteria needed for decision-making in the treatment process. Obviously not all patients are candidates for AR and for those who are candidates, how much rehabilitation is enough? In 1981, Tulko and Santore suggested a method for determining candidacy based on an assessment of the patient's communication ability at the time of the evaluation. Interestingly, their method did not catch on nor was it validated. Yet, several decades later, determining candidacy for audiologic rehabilitation remains a dilemma for audiologists. Furthermore, development of discharge criteria is a critical need in the 21st century if audiologic rehabilitation is to become a reimbursable service in the future.

With the decline in the traditional approach, audiologists began to embrace a counseling approach to rehabilitation in the 1980s. Vernon and Oettinger (1989) argued that the term "hearing loss" had true significance because the longer an individual experiences a hearing impairment, the more it is perceived as a true "loss." Audiologists began to realize that they often were the initial "listeners" to patients experiencing a loss of hearing. Consequently, audiologists began to address the psychological, emotional, social, and vocational implications of hearing loss and to realize that they had the responsibility to determine the extent of these issues for the individual and his and her family.

Sanders (1975) helped to define the audiologist's role in counseling by suggesting that it can be divided into two areas: informational and personal-adjustment counseling. He described informational counseling as "when the audiologist provides the client with an understanding of the hearing impairment, its consequences and the role of amplification." Personal adjustment counseling was described as "when the audiologist assists the client in finding a solution to her/his problem and achieving independence."

During the 1980s, there was a proliferation of books, articles, and conferences proffered to upgrade audiologists' skills and knowledge of the theory, content, and action of the counseling process (Wylde, 1987). Counseling assumed such importance within the profession that the American Speech-Language-Hearing Association Committee on Rehabilitative Audiology (1980) proposed minimal competencies and described four objectives for counseling the adult patient: (1) Enhancement of the individual's welfare; (2) Assistance in the resolution of pertinent problems; (3) Stimulation and motivation to achieve; and (4) Improvement of self-concept and social relationships.

Despite the upsurge in interest in counseling in the 1980s as part of the rehabilitation process, not all audiologists embraced it as a requisite part of the scope of practice. There was a pervasive feeling among many audiologists that engaging in diagnostic evaluations with sophisticated equipment was higher level than engaging in the counseling process. Furthermore, there also were those audiologists who wished to provide counseling but did not because it was not reimbursable. Consequently, the "time as money" factor ruled out counseling for many patients.

The 1980s and 1990s: The Deaf Community and Audiology

It is perhaps ironic that audiologists, as hearing health professionals, traditionally have known so little about deafness as a culture. A quotation from the 1980s describes one Deaf individual's perceptions of audiologists:

> I hope that the next time I have to take a hearing test with an audiologist, I hope he or she will have the patience with us because we deaf people have patience to take hearing tests over and over again for the rest of our lives. If people want to become audiologists, they need to understand our sensitivity and our behavior toward them because there are times when we hate to take those hearing tests. To some of us, a hearing test is not important especially to me. Audiologists are wonderful people to work with if they have the time and patience for us . . . " (Rohland & Meath-Lang, 1984, pp. 148–149)

Prevalent attitudes of the Deaf Community towards audiologists in the 1980s can be seen in the work of Rohland and Meath-Lang (1984) who analyzed essays written by 193 Deaf individuals. They found a positive attitude toward audiologists when they were able to use sign language. However, many essays expressed negative feelings towards audiologists in the form of anger, mistrust, and misperceptions about the reasons for being tested. Audiologists generally were viewed in a negative way.

Relationships between the Deaf community and audiologists have had a history of mistrust and frustration for many years but hit bottom during the 1980s and 1990s when cochlear implants were first approved by the FDA. Many Deaf individuals, as well as their family members, took the position of desiring to live in a Deaf culture (note capitalization of Deaf) and viewed cochlear implants as a threat to that culture. American Sign Language (ASL) was touted as the "natural" language of the Deaf and a symbol of the culture. Initial responses to the new technology caused suspicion that audiologists and physicians were trying to "medicalize" deafness and wipe out the Deaf culture. Audiologists denied these claims and showed little patience with parents who refused cochlear implants for their children.

During the 1980s and 1990s, the Deaf community and audiologists were moving on diverse paths. As audiologists became experts in cochlear implant evaluations, programming, and rehabilitation, the Deaf community embarked on somewhat of a civil rights movement. The Deaf demanded that they no longer be treated like second class citizens in every aspect of their lives. For example, they demanded that for the first time in history, the president of Gallaudet University must be a member of the Deaf Community. Given these developments, it is not surprising that relationships between the Deaf and audiologists were strained during this period. With the new millennium, however, the anger and suspicion on both sides dissipated and were replaced by cooperation and increased trust. (These issues are illustrated beautifully in a poignant, true-life film titled *Sound and Fury*, a 2001 Academy Award nominee for Best Documentary. *Sound and Fury: Six Years Later* (2006) further documents the family's struggles with the decision to implant their children and ultimately themselves.)

The 1980s to 1990s: ARA Contributions

During the last two decades of the 20th century, The Academy of Rehabilitative Audiology (ARA) continued it efforts to strengthen audiologic rehabilitation as a professional entity with credibility. A review of some of ARA activities of this period suggests the Academy was leading the way with innovations in audiologic rehabilitation. For example, in the early 1980s an ARA sponsored ASHA Convention presentation focused on the training necessary to provide AR services whereas the 1984 ARA Summer Institute emphasized computers in rehabilitation activities. By 1985, ARA members were preparing papers on digital hearing aids and computer-assisted instruction. Amplification, validation and performance were topics for the ARA Summer Institute in 1986. In 1988, a major ARA presentation dealt with digital signal processing of video signals. These presentations certainly demonstrate that AR had progressed beyond just lipreading and auditory training.

By the end of the 20th century, the ARA annual meeting was no longer planned as a Summer Institute but held in the fall to attract a larger audience. The ARA leadership has been successful in putting together meeting programs with speakers from diverse backgrounds who bring fresh and alternative perspectives to the AR process. The ARA has become an inclusive, eclectic forum for the exchange of ideas that has broadened the definition of AR and strengthened it as a clinical process.

End of the 20th Century: Focus on the Aging Population

Three large-scale demographic population trends in the late 20th century required audiologists rethink the role of AR with the aging population. First, the increased longevity of the World War II generation meant that many individuals were living well into their eighties and nineties. For example, in 1980 the 85+-year-old population in the United States was 2.2 million; by 2000, that population was 4.3 million and expected to increase over the next several decades (U.S. Dept of Health and Human Services, 2004). Second, the number of aging Baby Boomers who would evolve into "Senior Boomers" in the early 21st century was staggering. In fact, by 2006 the first wave of Baby Boomers had celebrated their sixtieth birthdays. Between 2011 and 2030, the 65+-population was expected to grow to 65 million people, representing a 75% increase (Hodge, 2006). Third, the aging American population was becoming more racially and ethnically diverse than ever before (McCarthy, 2006). For example, the older Hispanic population was estimated to increase from about 2 million in 2003 to 8 million in 2030 (He, Sengupta, Velkoff, & DeBarros, 2004). Consequently, by the end of the 20th century, audiologists were faced with dramatically changing caseloads that would require innovative approaches to meet the needs of this expanding population.

As the American population "grayed," audiologists began to recognize that the normal aging process could undermine the effectiveness of AR (McCarthy & Culpepper, 1987). Audiologists understood that anatomic, physiologic, social, and psychological changes of aging were negatively impacting methodologies that were successful with the "younger" population. Furthermore, hearing aid success with some aging patients could be limited by visual problems, psychosocial and cognitive issues, and touch sensitivity. Audiologists began to learn that money, mobility, and family relationships were part of the AR process. Consequently, it became clear that assessment tools were needed that would provide a holistic profile of aging patients that would encompass these variables.

One of the first tools that focused on the needs of aging individuals was developed by the senior author of this chapter. The Denver Scale of Communication Function for Senior Citizens Living in Retirement Centers was designed to make each item in the scale relevant to the individual by posing a primary question followed by a probe effect and an exploration effect (Zarnoch & Alpiner, 1977). Alpiner (1982) was concerned with the effects of the environment on the communication of aging individuals living in extended care facilities. A novel aspect of this scale was the checklist for identification of environmental noise in a nursing home setting including noise levels and architectural obstructions, both internal and external, for each area of the nursing home. The goal was to create a favorable listening environment for residents by eliminating or reducing noise. A second checklist evaluated the physical environment for excessive ambient noise, personal safety, and furniture arrangement.

The Hearing Handicap Inventory for the Elderly (HHIE), discussed earlier in this chapter, assessed both social and emotional effects of hearing impairment in the noninstitutionalized older person (Ventry & Weinstein, 1982). Alpiner and Baker (1981) developed the Communication Assessment Procedure for Seniors (CAPS) to evaluate attitudes and communication status in specific situations. This interview type scale also probed the aging individual's interest in rehabilitation.

Another innovative approach to audiologic rehabilitation for the aging population was the establishment of an Elderhostel focusing on hearing loss. Elderhostels had been in existence since 1975 and typically provided learning opportunities for seniors in a residential setting. In the 1980s, an Elderhostel at Gallaudet University was developed specifically for older adults with hearing impairment (Bally & Kaplan, 1988). The Gallaudet program provided information about hearing loss for hearing-impaired seniors and significant others, adjustment and coping strategies, consumerism and self-help, and an individualized AR program. This unique program allowed in-depth AR as well as peer and family support.

For decades, audiologists had used the term "phonemic regression" (Gaeth, 1948) to describe the inordinately poor speech recognition abilities of presbycusic patients. By the 1990s, a debate ensued regarding the factors that contributed to this poor speech perception. Three hypotheses were used to explain the speech understanding problems of the elderly (Humes, 1996). The peripheral hypothesis suggested that the speech recognition problems of elderly could be explained by aging changes in the auditory periphery. The central auditory hypothesis focused on the structural and functional changes in the auditory pathways of the brainstem. The cognitive deficit suggested that cognitive deficits contributed to the poor speech understanding of the elderly population. A number of studies were published that provided evidence for each of these hypotheses.

Audiologists had a vested interest in this research because of the implications for rehabilitation of the aging presbycusic population. For example, the efficacy of putting hearing aids on elderly patients with central auditory processing problems was debated in the 1990s. Some studies suggested that older individuals with central auditory processing disorder would not benefit from amplification (Chmiel & Jerger, 1996). Furthermore, estimates of the prevalence of CAPD in the elderly population were as high as 70% for individuals over 60 years (Stach, Spretnjak, & Jerger, 1990). Others, however, argued that diagnosing CAPD in the aging population was difficult because of these intervening variables and lack of a reliable sensitive test battery. By the early 21st century, it was well accepted that each of these complex factors could variably influence the speech perception abilities of aging individuals. As such, rehabilitative methods that focus on auditory and cognitive skills, such as the LACE (Sweetow, 2005), are being developed to meet the unique needs of the aging population.

1990s: "Rehab" Returns

By the 1990s, audiologic rehabilitation had returned to a place of prominence in many audiologists' daily scope of practice. Mueller (1998) summarized this evolution, " . . . slowly we're starting to recognize that rehabilitative audiology is indeed more . . . that hearing aid fitting is indeed rehabilitative audiology . . . the "hearing aid fitters" are joining hands with the people formerly described as into rehab . . . " (p. 10).

This return to our "roots" was precipitated by several developments in the profession. First, despite amazing developments in amplification technology, audiologists recognized that hearing aids were not a magic cure-all for communication problems caused by hearing impairment. As Mark Ross emphasized, "The overwhelming majority of people being fitted with hearing aids for the first time need help. They can all benefit from services that transcend what the hearing aid alone can provide . . . " (Carmen & Ross, 2000, p. 59). Second, with the advent of high-end digital amplification, meeting patients' expectations became more important than meeting "targets" during hearing aid fittings. Assessing patients' expectations before engaging in the hearing aid fitting process was seen as preemptive. Third, the importance of rehabilitation with cochlear implants suggested commensurate rehabilitation might be warranted for new hearing aid users. Gagné and Tye-Murray

(1994) summarized this by stating, "Adult audiologic rehabilitation has evolved considerably in recent years. Changes in the services provided to clients have been influenced by technological advances, clinical experience, and a growing body of research literature in our field as well as in related disciplines."

Graduate coursework in the 1990s reflected the increasing knowledge and skills necessary to provide AR. By the 1990s, a typical course syllabus for an adult rehabilitative audiology course included these course objectives: The student will demonstrate (1) A functional understanding of the full scope of audiologic rehabilitation in adults; (2) Knowledge of self-assessment tools and interpretation; (3) Knowledge of the psychosocial effects of hearing loss; and (4) Knowledge of amplification and assistive listening device assessment, evaluation and technology. Furthermore, the newly developed Doctor of Audiology (Au.D.) allowed university programs to expand their offerings in audiologic rehabilitation coursework and clinical education.

With the hearing aid as the nucleus of the audiologic rehabilitation process, audiologists in the 1990s expanded their repertoire of rehabilitative services. These included clear speech, tracking, hearing aid validation, outcome assessment, communication training of individuals and their families, auditory training, assistive technology assessment, fitting and evaluation, vestibular rehabilitation, tinnitus management, rehabilitation following implantation, and counseling.

In 1994, the late Carl Binnie, made three predictions to provide a forecast for the evolution of AR. He projected that the population of the United States would grow to 280 million persons, with about 24 to 28 million with hearing loss. The second prediction was that by the year 2000, 75% of all hearing instruments would be digitally programmable, allowing the audiologists to adjust signal processing. By the year 2000, computer-based instruction would assume a significant role in audiologic rehabilitation. Clearly, his prescient predictions have been realized.

Can we predict the future of AR with the same accuracy? Perhaps not. But the historical review provided in this chapter suggests that the past is our prologue. Returning to a patient-centered rehabilitative profession, rather than a device-centered profession, and focusing on improved communication will ensure that audiology will meet the hearing health care needs and expectations of our patients in the 21st century.

References

Alpiner, J. G. (1966). *Proceedings of the Institute on Aural Rehabilitation*. Denver, CO.

Alpiner, J. G. (1982). Rehabilitation of the geriatric client. In J. G. Alpiner (Ed.), *Handbook of adult rehabilitative audiology* (pp. 160–205). Baltimore: Williams & Wilkins.

Alpiner, J. G. (1992). Archives report. *Journal of the Academy of Rehabilitative Audiology*, *24*, 16.

Alpiner, J. G., & Baker, B. (1981). Communication assessment procedures in aural rehabilitation process. *Seminars in Speech and Language*, *1*(2), 189–204.

Alpiner, J. G., Chevrette, W., Glascoe, G., Metze, M., & Olsen, B. (1974). *The Denver Scale of Communication Function*. University of Denver, CO.

American Speech-Language-Hearing Association. (1984). *Definition of and competencies for aural rehabilitation* [Relevant paper]. Available from www.asha.org/policy.

American Speech-Language-Hearing Association, Committee on Rehabilitative Audiology. (1980). Proposed minimal competencies necessary to provide aural rehabilitation. *ASHA*, *22*, 461.

Bally, S. J., & Kaplan, H. J. (1988). The Gallaudet University aural rehabilitation Elderhostels. *Journal of the Academy of Rehabilitative Audiology*, *21*, 99–112.

Berger, K. W. (1984). *The hearing aid, operation and development* (3rd ed.). Livonia, MI: National Hearing Aid Society.

Binnie, C. A. (1977). Attitude changes following speechreading training. *Scandinavian Audiology*, *6*, 13–19.

Binnie, C. A. (1994). The future of audiologic rehabilitation: Overview and forecast. *Journal of the Academy of Rehabilitative Audiology*, *27*, 12–24.

Brainard, S. (1969). An investigation of the relations between performance on a filmed lipreading test and analysis of the visual environment. *Journal of the Academy of Rehabilitative Audiology*, *11*(2), 8–9.

Bruhn, M. E. (1955). *The Mueller-Walle method of lipreading for the hard of hearing* (7th ed.). Washington DC: Volta Bureau.

Bunger, A. M. (1961). *Speech-reading—Jena method.* Danville, IL: The Interstate Press.

Carmen, R., & Ross, M. (2000). Profiles in AR: First in a series Richard Carmen interview Mark Ross. *Hearing Journal, 53*(3), 54–62.

Chisholm, T., Johnson, C., Danhauer, J., Portz, L., Abrams, H., Lesner, S., et al. (2007). Systematic review of health related quality of life and hearing aids: Final report of the American Academy of Audiology Task Force on the health-related quality of life benefits of amplification in adults. *Journal of the American Academy of Audiology, 18*, 151–183.

Chmiel, R., & Jerger, J. (1996). Hearing aid use, central auditory disorder and hearing handicap in elderly persons. *Journal of the American Academy of Audiology, 7*(3), 190–202.

Cox, R., & Alexander, C. (2002). The international outcome inventory for hearing aids (IOI-HA): Psychometric properties of the English version. *International Journal of Audiology, 41*, 30–35.

Cox, R. M., & Alexander, G. C. (1995). The abbreviated profile of hearing aid benefit (APHAB). *Ear and Hearing, 16*, 176–186.

Cox, R. M., & Alexander, G. C. (2000). Expectations about hearing aids and their relationship to fitting outcome. *Journal of the American Academy of Audiology, 11*, 368–382.

Cox, R. M., & Alexander, G. C. (2001). Validation of the SADL questionnaire. *Ear and Hearing, 22*, 151–160.

Cox, R. M., Stephens, D., & Kramer, S. E. (2002). Translations of the international outcome inventory for hearing aids (IOI-HA). *International Journal of Audiology, 41*(1), 3–26.

Davis, H. (1948). The articulation area and the social adequacy index for hearing. *Laryngoscope, 58*, 761–778.

DeLand, F. (1931). *The story of lipreading: Its genesis and development*. Washington DC: Volta Bureau.

Demorest, M. E., & Erdman, S. A. (1987). Development of the communication profile for the hearing impaired. *Journal of Speech and Hearing Disorders, 52*(2), 129–143.

Dillon, H., Birtles, G., & Lovegrove, R. (1999). Measuring the outcomes of a national rehabilitation program: Normative data for the client oriented scale of improvement (COSI) and the hearing aid users questionnaire (HAUQ). *American Academy of Audiology, 10*, 67–79.

Elkayam, J., & English, K. (2003). Counseling adolescents with hearing loss with the use of self-assessment/significant other questionnaires. *Journal of the American Academy of Audiology, 9*, 485–499.

Erdman, S. A., & Demorest, M. E. (1998). Adjustment to hearing impairment I: description of a heterogeneous clinical population. *Journal of Speech Language and Hearing Research, 41*(1), 107–122.

Gaeth, J. H. (1948). *A study of phonemic regression in relation to hearing loss*. Unpublished work, Evanson, IL: Northwestern University.

Gagne, J.-P., & Tye-Murray, N. (1994). Research in audiological rehabilitation. *Journal of the Academy of Rehabilitative Audiology, Monograph, Supplement 27.*

Garwood, V., Bergman, M., Dixon, J., & Haspiel, G. (1973). Roles played by audiologists. *Journal of the Academy of Rehabilitative Audiology, 6*(1), 20–21.

Gatehouse, S. (1999). Glasgow hearing aid benefit profile: Derivation and validation of a client-centered outcome measure for hearing-aid services. *Journal of the American Academy of Audiology, 10*, 80–103.

Hardick, E. (1976). Testimony to the Food and Drug Administration on standards for auditory training. *Journal of the Academy of Rehabilitative Audiology, 11*(1 & 2), 63.

Harford, E. (1972). Why audiologists should dispense hearing aids. *Journal of the Academy of Rehabilitative Audiology, 5*(1 & 2), 10–14.

He, W., Sengupta, M., Velkoff, V., & DeBarros, K. (2005). *65+ in the United States: 2005* (U.S. Census Bureau, Current Population Reports No. P23-209). Washington, DC: U.S. Government Printing Office.

High, W. S., Fairbanks, G., & Glorig, A. (1964). A scale for self-assessment of hearing handicap. *Journal of Speech and Hearing Disorders, 29*, 215–230.

Hodge, P. (2006). Living younger longer: Baby boomer challenges. *White House Conference on Aging.* Washington, DC.

Humes, L. (1996). Speech understanding in the elderly. *Journal of the American Academy of Audiology, 7*(3), 161–167.

Hutton, C. L. (1980). Responses to a hearing problem inventory. *Journal of the Academy of Rehabilitative Audiology, 13*, 133–154.

Kinzie, C. E. (1920). The Kinzie method of speech reading. *Volta Review*, *22*, 600–619.

Kitchen, D. W. (1969). The relationship of visual synthesis to lipreading performances. *Academy of Rehabilitative Audiology Newsletter*, *2*(2), 7–8.

Leurechon, J. (1624). *Recreation mathematique*. Pont-à-Mousson, France: Jean Appier Hanzelet.

Lovering, L. (1969). Visual acuity and lipreading performances. *Academy of Rehabilitative Audiology Newsletter*, *2*(2), 9–10.

Madell, J., & Montano, J. (2000). Different employment settings. In J. G. Alpiner, & P. A. McCarthy (Eds.), *Rehabilitative audiology: Children and adults* (3rd ed., pp. 60–79). Baltimore: Williams & Wilkins.

McCarthy, P. A. (2006). *The seniors of today and tomorrow. Hearing care for adults 2006*. Chicago: Phonak AG, pp. 33–38.

McCarthy, P. A., & Alpiner, J. G. (1980). *The McCarthy-Alpiner Scale of Hearing Handicap*. Unpublished manuscript.

McCarthy, P. A., & Alpiner, J. G. (1983). An assessment scale of hearing handicap for use in family counseling. *Journal of the Academy of Rehabilitative Audiology*, *16*, 256–270.

McCarthy, P. A., & Culpepper, N. B. (1987). The adult remediation process. In J. G. Alpiner & P. A. McCarthy (Eds.), *Rehabilitative audiology: Children and adults* (pp. 305–342). Baltimore: Williams & Wilkins.

Mueller, H. G. (1998). Self assessment revisited [Editorial]. *Hearing Journal*, *51*(3), 10.

Newby, H. A. (1964). *Audiology* (2nd ed.). New York: Appleton-Century-Crofts.

Newman, C., Weinstein, B., Jacobson, G., & Hug, G. (1991). Test-retest reliability of the hearing handicap inventory for adults. *Ear and Hearing*, *12*, 355–357.

Nitchie, E. H. (1950). *New lessons in lip-reading*. Philadelphia and New York: Lippincott.

Noble, W. G., & Atherly, G. R. C. (1970). The hearing measurement scale: A questionnaire for the assessment of auditory disability. *Journal of Auditory Research*, *10*, 229–250.

Northern, J., & Beyer, C. (1999). Hearing aid returns analyzed in search for patients and fitting patterns. *Hearing Journal*, *52*(7), 46–52.

Olsen, W., Rose, D., & Hedgecock, L. (2003). A brief history of audiology at Mayo Clinic. *Journal of the American Academy of Audiology*, *14*(4), 173–180.

Oyer, H. L., Freeman, D., Hardick, E., Dixon, J., Donnelly, K., Goldstein, D., et al. (1976). Unheeded recommendations for aural rehabilitation: Analysis of a survey. *Journal of the Academy of Rehabilitative Audiology*, *9*(1), 20–30.

Oyer, J. J. (1969). Professional noters. *Academy of Rehabilitative Audiology Newsletter*, *2*(2), 11.

Peet, H. P. (1851). Memoirs in the origin and the early history of the art of instructing the deaf and dumb. *American Annals of the Deaf and Dumb*, *3*, 129–161.

Preminger, J. (2003). Should significant others be encouraged to join adult group audiologic rehabilitation classes? *Journal of the American Academy of Audiology*, *14*(10), 545–555.

Rohland, P. S., & Meath-Lang, B. (1984). Perceptions of deaf adults regarding audiologists and audiological services. *Journal of the Academy of Rehabilitative Audiology*, *17*, 130–150.

Ross, M. (1987). Aural rehabilitation revisited. *Journal of the Academy of Rehabilitative Audiology*, *20*, 13–23.

Sanders, D. A. (1975). Hearing aid orientation and counseling. In M. C. Pollack (Ed.), *Amplification for the hearing impaired* (pp. 323–370). New York: Grune & Stratton.

Schow, R., & Nerbonne, M. (1982). Communication screening profile. *Ear and Hearing*, *3*, 135–147.

Siegenthaler, B. (1972). Audiologists should not dispose hearing aids. *Journal of the Academy of Rehabilitative Audiology*, *5*(1 & 2), 5–9.

Skalbeck, G. (1984). The academy of rehabilitative audiology: 1966–1976. *Journal of the Academy of Rehabilitative Audiology*, *17*, 16.

Spencer, S. (1946, August 31, 1946). New ears for the deaf. *The Saturday Evening Post*, *219*(9), 22–44.

Stach, B. A., Spretnjak, M. L., & Jerger, J. (1990). The prevalence of central presbycusis in a clinical population. *Journal of the American Academy of Audiology*, *1*(2), 109–115.

Sweetow, R. (2005). Training the adult brain to listen. *Hearing Journal*, *58*(6), 10.

Toubbeh, J. I. (1973). Prison without bars: Human communication disorders. *Rehabilitation Record*, *14*(3), 1–4.

Truex, E. (1944). The rehabilitation service for the hard of hearing at Deshon General Hospital, Butler, Pennsylvania. *Journal of the Acoustical Society of America*, *16*(1), 71–74.

Tulko, C., & Santore, F. (1981). Speechreading and auditory perception training for the adult with an acquired hearing loss. *Journal of the Academy of Rehabilitative Audiology*, *14*, 177–197.

U.S. Department of Health and Human Services (2004). *Administration on aging. Statistics: Aging into the 21st Century. Demography: Growth of the elderly population.* Available from: http://www.aoa.gov/prof/statistics/future_growth/aging21/demography.asp 2004.

Ventry, I., & Weinstein, B. (1982). The hearing handicap inventory for the elderly: A new tool. *Ear and Hearing*, *3*, 128–134.

Ventry, I., & Weinstein, B. (1983). Identification of elderly people with hearing problems. *Asha*, *25*, 37–42.

Vernon, M., & Ottinger, P. J. (1989). Psychosocial aspects of hearing impairment. In R. Schow & M. Nerbonne (Eds.), *Introduction to aural rehabilitation* (2nd ed., pp. 240–270). Austin, TX: Pro-Ed.

Wylde, M. A. (1987). Psychological and counseling aspects of the adult remediation process. In J. G. Alpiner, & P. A. McCarthy (Eds.), *Rehabilitative audiology: Children and adults* (1st ed., pp. 343–369). Baltimore: Williams & Wilkins.

Zarnoch, J. M., & Alpiner, J. G. (1977). *The Denver Scale of Communication Function for senior citizens living in retirement center.* Unpublished manuscript.

2

Defining Audiologic Rehabilitation

Joseph J. Montano

Should one query audiologists about the definition of audiologic rehabilitation (AR) it would soon become apparent that perceptions vary greatly. Some may deny they provide AR services because their clinical function is purely diagnostic, whereas others may believe that everything they do as an audiologist is rehabilitative including the assessment of hearing. AR seems to have an ambiguous nature and, although most published definitions imply it is an inclusive process, most practitioners view it as exclusive, a specialty area not within the realm of the diagnostic audiologist. It is not uncommon to hear audiologists say they do not provide AR services, even when they dispense amplification and hearing assistive technology systems. As a result, AR often is thought of as restricted to the clinical provision of services such as auditory training and speechreading. Although these procedures are certainly components of the AR process, they do not define its existence.

The origin of the field of Audiology is largely believed to be a direct outcome of the services provided to military personnel suffering from noise-induced hearing loss during World War II (Bergman, 2002; Ross, 1997). The programs that developed were rich in AR services that included hearing aids, counseling, auditory training, and speechreading. For a number of reasons, as the profession developed, emphasis shifted from rehabilitation to diagnostics. AR seemed to have gotten lost in the excitement of new technological developments such as auditory brainstem response (ABR) and otoacoustic emissions (OAEs). Even in academic programs, AR classes were limited to usually one or perhaps two, and seemed to focus primarily on speechreading and auditory training (Ross, 1997). Although AR diminished in popularity, knowledge of its value is not misunderstood. The provision of AR services, in fact, is one of the most relevant characteristics that distinguish the practice of audiologists from hearing aid specialists in the amplification arena. Ross goes on to state, "When it becomes necessary for us to justify our existence as a unique profession to various health, education and governmental agencies, we never fail to claim this activity (AR) as our own" (p. 14).

Many practitioners consider AR the foundation of our field and pursue research and practice in this area. Alpiner and McCarthy (2009) discuss the evolution of AR in the field of audiology. As we study the history of AR from its origins through the establishment of professional organizations such as the Academy of Rehabilitative Audiology and the ASHA Special Interest Division 7 (Aural Rehabilitation and Its Instrumentation), we are able to understand better the development of the definitions that provide important clinical direction.

In an attempt to define the AR process, we can consider the basic questions of its implementation: who, what, where, when, and how. Perhaps, by reviewing the existing definitions of AR and providing some basic answers to these simple questions, some light can be shed upon the AR process and an attempt can be made to unify the perceptions of audiologists. With this in mind, this chapter reviews existing definitions of AR and identifies barriers to the provision of AR services.

Who Provides Service in AR?

Many consider AR to be the true marriage of audiology and speech-language pathology, particularly in the provision of services for children with hearing loss. Membership in both ARA and ASHA Division 7 consists of both audiologists and speech-language pathologists (SLPs) with many holding degrees and certification in both professions. In view of the nature of AR, the roles of SLPs and audiologists can be complementary and cooperative (ASHA, 2001). This overlap, however, may have contributed to confusion and misunderstanding among many audiologists. AR falls within the Scope of Practice of both professions (ASHA, 2004a, 2007), and although knowledge and skills may have been delineated (ASHA, 2001), third-party reimbursement for service provision in AR is distinctly different; in fact, it is often quoted as the reason audiologists do not provide these services. Within the realm of third-party reimbursement, many AR services are covered only when performed by SLPs.

Strides have been made to improve the reimbursement of AR services for audiologists, and as a result, four new Current Procedural Terminology (CPT) codes were established in 2006. Kander and White (2006) described the following codes: 92626: Evaluation of auditory rehabilitation status; first hour; 92627: Each additional 15 minutes, on same day as 92626; 92630: Auditory rehabilitation of children and 92633: Auditory rehabilitation of adults. The codes developed for adults are more specifically aimed at adult cochlear implant recipients.

Reimbursement for AR services provided under Medicare is limited to diagnostic services only, with limited coverage for treatment. Procedures for auditory training and speechreading are still not considered covered services under Medicare for audiologists, whereas the SLP can apply codes for these services using 92507. Under Medicare, audiologists are viewed primarily as diagnostic practitioners, rather than providers of rehabilitation (White, 2006).

It is not only who provides AR service that adds to our confusion, but what the process should be called. Alpiner and McCarthy (2009) discuss the terminology paradox that is currently present in our field. The terms aural rehabilitation, audiologic rehabilitation, and most recently auditory rehabilitation often are used interchangeably. Speech-language pathologists prefer to use the term aural rehabilitation whereas audiologists have more consistently referred to these services as audiologic rehabilitation. One need only refer to the ASHA Preferred Practice Patterns (PPP) for the Profession of Speech-Language Pathology (ASHA, 2004b) and Audiology (ASHA, 2006) to illustrate the difference. PPPs for speech refer to services provided to individuals with hearing loss as aural rehabilitation whereas the Audiology PPPs use the term audiologic rehabilitation. It is for this reason that the acronym AR was employed in the ASHA (2001) knowledge and skills publication for aural/audiologic rehabilitation.

What Is AR?

This question leads to a discussion of defining AR. It was not the attempt of this author to provide a new definition of AR, but rather to clarify perhaps the underlying intention of many of our already available references. A review of the literature reveals an abundance of definitions, which seem to vary significantly when viewed in terms of history. Gagné and Jennings (2009) report that, although some definitions stress the activities associated with the rehabilitation of hearing loss, others focus on the reduction of associated disabilities and handicaps. The emphasis of AR has shifted from procedure-specific to a more patient-centered concept. Schow et al. (1993) reported on a trend of decreasing traditional treatments in AR (auditory training and speechreading) but an increasing perception by audiologists that their clinical duties include both diagnostic and rehabilitative services. Prendergast and Kelley (2002) postulate that this change is primarily due to a shift from traditional procedural AR approaches toward services designed to address emotional and social aspects of hearing loss. This belief can be substantiated when we compare the definitions used to describe AR throughout the years.

In 1971, Sanders published the first edition of his historic book, *Aural Rehabilitation*. This text, along with subsequent editions, introduced a generation of audiologists to AR. The common thread throughout the chapters of this book was the importance of an individual's overall communication ability. He reported that approaching assessment from a theoretical framework that encouraged rehabilitation was just as critical for individuals with mild-to-moderate hearing loss as it was for those with severe-to-profound loss. Assessing individual areas of strengths and weaknesses would help identify abilities that were in need of training making it possible to "circumvent the weaknesses through the development of the use of compensatory channels (p. 5)." Included in this text were chapters dedicated to topic areas such as: auditory and visual perception, amplification and hearing aids, auditory training, visual communication training, and the integration of vision and audition. The author stressed the importance of not limiting our services to just the assessment of hearing.

ASHA (1984) published a position statement that discussed the definition of and competencies for aural rehabilitation. Developed by the Committee on Rehabilitative Audiology, the paper revisited the ASHA (1974) Legislative Council resolution that reported audiologists as the primary providers of AR services and their role in the supervision of such services. However, it was felt that, in practice, the speech-language pathologist was providing a significant proportion of AR services for individuals with hearing loss. As a result, the Committee created a new definition of AR and included the components to service provision. "Aural rehabilitation refers to services and procedures for facilitating adequate receptive and expressive communication in individuals with hearing impairment" (ASHA, 1984, p. 23). The authors went on to describe the elements necessary to accomplish the goals of AR. These included evaluation of sensory capabilities, fitting of auditory and sensory aids, counseling, and referral. The importance of counseling both the individual and family regarding the impact of hearing loss began to become a prominent message in the definition of AR.

Although this position statement acknowledged the interdisciplinary nature of AR, it did nothing to help delineate the difference between the audiologists and speech-language pathologists in service delivery. In fact, it appears that one of its purposes was to negate the audiologists' primary role in AR that had been established earlier in 1974. Assumingly unintentional, the use of the terms expressive and receptive communication within the core context of the definition, although certainly accurate, may have created the appearance that AR is more directly associated with speech-language pathology. The terminology, although not exclusive to speech and language, often is associated with child language development or adult neurologic language processes. The paper appeared at a time when audiologists were seeking a more independent professional identity and was probably indirectly responsible for the increased popularity of the label audiologic rehabilitation.

Not long after the publication of this position paper, the creation of Special Interest Divisions of ASHA became a reality. These divisions were established to meet member needs for specialized areas of professional practice. Division 7 (Aural Rehabilitation and Its Instrumentation) was among the inaugural groups developed.

The Steering Committee of Special Interest Division 7 (1992) contributed an article to the ASHA magazine that focused attention on some of the beliefs of their Division and stated simply that "Audiologic rehabilitation was Audiology" (p. 18). The implication, of course, was that the entire field of Audiology was designed to be rehabilitative in nature. Their definition includes the importance of the impact of hearing loss on function within the context of the family and environment. These concepts would soon become primary objectives for AR.

Erdman (1993, 2000) stated that the "ultimate goal of rehabilitative audiology is to facilitate adjustment to the auditory and nonauditory consequences of hearing impairment" (p. 374). This brief description of AR begins to show the shifting emphasis in rehabilitation models from procedure-specific definitions to more functionally driven descriptors. Here, the author places equal value on the auditory (hearing loss degree and nature, speech perception, etc.) and nonauditory (emotional, psychosocial, vocational, etc.) implications associated with the loss of hearing ability and goes on to discuss the importance of counseling in the rehabilitation process. In fact, Erdman (2000) remarks that counseling is the "essence of successful rehabilitation" (p. 435) of AR. (For more information on counseling in AR, the reader is referred to Chapter 9 of this text.)

It became important that our profession begin to expand their definition of AR beyond the evaluation and management of hearing loss to the impact of psychosocial functioning (Ross, 1997). The increase in popularity of self-assessment measurement tools, such as the Hearing Handicap Inventory for the Elderly (HHIE) (Ventry & Weinstein, 1982), The Hearing Performance Inventory (Giolas et al., 1979) and the Communication Profile for the Hearing Impaired (CPHI) (Demorest & Erdman, 1987), provided the audiologist with an arsenal that could be used to quantify the impact of adult hearing loss. The measures could yield a basic classification function; for example, the HHIE could be used to determine a level of hearing handicap, or can be more global, such as the CPHI and provide a profile that can be used as an effective counseling tool. Regardless of measurement focus, the direction of assessment for AR was tending to shift more toward the implications of a loss of hearing on numerous domains of function.

Ross (1997) reported that the process of AR includes "any device, procedure, information, interaction, or therapy which lessens the communicative and psychosocial consequences of a hearing loss" (p. 19). He, like Erdman (1993), seems to place equal emphasis on issues related to the auditory and psychosocial aspects of functioning. Without specifying, he relegates any procedure appropriate to lessen the impact of hearing loss on communication function to AR. Certainly, one could include traditional activities such as speechreading and auditory training as treatment components but just as easily consider counseling, vocational assessment, and family intervention.

Gagné (1998) continued to emphasize function over procedure when he defined AR as the process designed to "eliminate or reduce the situations of handicap experienced by individuals who have a hearing impairment and by persons with normal hearing who interact with those individuals" (p. 70). The author was quite specific about the inclusion of others in the communication environment of the individual with hearing impairment and can be directly related to a landmark publication in development at the time by the World Health Organization.

The World Health Organization and Its Impact on the Definition of AR

In 1980, the World Health Organization published its first classification of disability with the International Classification of Impairment, Disability and Handicap (ICIDH). It attempted to unify related terminology in the realm of handicap and disability. This original paper identified "impairment" as having an impact on the organ level and "disability" as related to activities and handicap referring to one's role in society. During the late 1990s, WHO began to revisit this classification system and subsequently published the International Classification of Functioning, Disability and Health, commonly referred to as the ICF in 2001. The impact of the

WHO classifications is covered in depth in Chapter 3 of this text.

The ICF described both health and health-related domains in relationship to the body, the individual and to society at large. The primary areas of concern within the ICF are body functions and structures and what is referred to as activities and participations. The ICF describes "What a person with a disease or disorder does do or can do." Whereas the ICIDH seemed to highlight the negative consequences of impairment, the ICF emphasizes the positive (Boothroyd, 2007).

The influence of the WHO ICF can be directly observed in a publication prepared by the ASHA Working Group on Audiologic Rehabilitation (ASHA, 2001). This group was charged to update the ASHA (1984) position statement (discussed earlier) on the definition of and competencies for AR. The interdisciplinary nature of AR was evident in the group membership, which consisted of both audiologists and speech-language pathologists. Unlike the 1984 document, this group decided to address directly the issues related to the provision of services by two distinct professions and essentially created two documents within one.

The format of the 2001 publication consisted of an introduction that defined AR and provided background and history. The specific areas of basic knowledge and specific knowledge and skills are divided into two sections: (1) Knowledge and Skills for Audiologists Providing AR Services and (2) AR Knowledge and Skills for Speech-Language Pathologists. The paper specifically delineates the roles of the two professions; although collaborative, these roles are different.

The authors emphasize that AR no longer refers to simply procedural-specific treatments such as auditory training, speechreading, or even hearing aid dispensing, but rather it is a process that is broad with tentacles reaching into all aspects of a person's functioning. With this in mind, the working group offered this definition of AR:

> Audiologic/aural rehabilitation (AR) is an ecological, interactive process that facilitates one's ability to minimize or prevent the limitations and restrictions that auditory dysfunctions can impose on well-being and communication, including inter-personal, psycho-social, educational, and vocational functioning. (p. 2)

The WHO ICF (2001) terminology includes descriptors such as activity and activity limitations; participation and participation restrictions. In addition, this publication stresses the importance of contextual factors, such as environmental and personal influences, on an individual's ability to function with an impairment. The inclusion of terms such as ecological, interactive, minimize or prevent limitations (activity), and restrictions (participation) reinforce the impact of the ICF on this ASHA (2001) document.

The knowledge and skills for audiologists providing AR services addressed by ASHA (2001) include areas of general knowledge such as: psychology; human growth and development; cultural and linguistic diversity, and quantitative research methodologies to name a few. Within the area of basic communication processes, knowledge in anatomy; physiology; speech and hearing sciences; linguistics; psycholinguistics, and dynamics of interpersonal skills are recognized.

Table 2–1 includes the special areas of knowledge and skills identified in ASHA (2001). The skills described are meant to educate the audiologist on the specific areas needed to practice AR.

Table 2–1. Special Areas of Knowledge and Skills for Audiologists Providing Audiologic Rehabilitation (AR) Services

Knowledge	Skills
Auditory System Function and Disorders	Identify and describe disorders of auditory function

continues

Table 2–1. *continued*

Knowledge	Skills
Developmental Status, Cognition, and Sensory Perception	Assessment in client's preferred mode of communication; verify visual acuity; identify need for assessment of cognitive skills, sensory perception, developmental delays, academic achievement and literacy; determine need for referral
Audiologic Assessment Procedures	Case history; otoscopic exam; conduct/interpret behavioral, physiologic or electrophysiologic evaluations; administer self-report measures; conduct and assess for APD[1]; identify need for referral
Speech-Language Assessment Procedures	Identify need for and perform screenings; describe effects of hearing loss on speech and language development; provide appropriate measures of speech, language, and voice production; administer and interpret measurements of communication skills in auditory, visual, auditory-visual, and tactile modalities.
Evaluation and Management of Devices and Technologies	Electroacoustic characteristic of devices and technologies; describe, perform and interpret behavioral/psychophysical aided measures; conduct appropriate fittings; monitor fittings; perform routine visual, troubleshoot common causes of device malfunctioning; describe effects of devices on communication and psychosocial functioning; plan and implement program of orientation; conduct routine assessment of adjustment to and effective use of amplification; monitor outcomes
Effects of Hearing Impairment on Functional Communication	Identify and evaluate situational expressive and receptive communication needs; identify environmental factors that affect communication performance; identify interpersonal relations on communication function
Effects of Hearing Impairment on Psychosocial, Educational and Occupational Functioning	Describe/evaluate impact of hearing loss on psychosocial development and functioning; describe systems and methods of educational programming; describe/evaluate impact of loss on vocational status; identify effects of hearing problems on the marital dyad, family dynamics; identify need and provide for counseling in relation to hearing impairment and communication difficulties; provide assessment of family members' perception of and reactions to communication difficulties.
AR Case Management	Use effective interpersonal communication in interviewing and interacting with clients and family; describe client-centered, behavioral, cognitive, and integrative theories and methods of counseling and their relevance in AR; provide appropriate individual and group adjustment counseling; provide auditory, visual, and auditory-visual communication training; provide training in communication strategies; provide appropriate expressive communication training; provide appropriate technologic intervention; provide appropriate intervention for management of vestibular disorders; develop and implement an intervention plan; develop and implement a system for measuring and monitoring outcomes.
Interdisciplinary Collaboration and Public Advocacy	Collaborate effectively as part of multidisciplinary teams; plan and implement in-service and public information programs; plan and implement parent-education programs; advocate implementation of public law in educational, occupational, and public settings; make appropriate referrals to consumer-based organizations
Hearing Conservation/ Acoustic Environments	Plan and implement programs for prevention of hearing impairment; identify need for and provide appropriate hearing protection devices; monitor the effect of environmental conditions; measure and evaluate environmental acoustic conditions.

[1]APD = Auditory Processing Disorder.
Source: Adapted from ASHA, 2001.

As is evident through a review of this table, the list is quite inclusive and does not distinguish between services for children and adults. A similar presentation of information was developed for speech-language pathologists but is not covered in the context of this chapter.

Boothroyd (2007) advocated a holistic approach to AR. He defined this as "the reduction of hearing loss-induced deficits of function, activity, participation and quality of life through a combination of sensory management, instruction and perceptual training and counseling" (p. 63). The WHO ICF is acknowledged as a major influence on the goal of his paper. As was evident in the ASHA (2001) definition, specific terminology such as: function, activity, and participation directly align Boothroyd's philosophy with the trend in the profession to expand our views of AR. That is, a shift from primarily procedural activities to the therapeutic process aimed at reducing the impact of hearing loss on function (ASHA, 2001; Erdman, 1993, Gagné, 1998; Ross, 1997).

The Where and When of AR

AR programs have traditionally been found in settings such as university programs and Department of Veterans Affairs medical centers that not only provided clinical services but have been responsible for much of the published research in this area. Even though AR has been shown to be cost-effective (Abrams et al., 2002) and is identified as a desired service to consumers (Pope & Stika, 2009), its availability is limited in most practice settings.

AR, however, can be implemented effectively in a variety of audiology employment sectors with the use of some creative programming and clinical intuition. Madell and Montano (2000) discussed the inclusion of AR services in a variety of work settings and provided suggestions for program development. In particular, these authors encourage the provision of AR in locations such as private practice and small clinical settings, hospitals, and long-term care facilities.

Warner-Czyz (2000) provides suggestions for program designs for group AR that can be successfully implemented in hospitals, small facilities, and private practice offices. She postulates that the lack of AR services in these settings is due primarily to constraints such as time and financial concerns, lack of interest among consumers, and lack of information and confidence on the provision of services by audiologists.

Jennings and Head (1994) discussed an ecological approach to service provision for long-term care. In their model, the audiologist serves a multipurpose role and programming includes the individual along with the family, staff, and the environment. Montano (2001) encouraged the use of creative in-service programming as a means to educate staff who work closely with nursing home residents with hearing loss. In such an environment, it is unusual for staffing to include a full-time audiologist and frequently they are only available on either a part-time or consultation basis, if at all. Therefore, when present, it is necessary to recruit the existing staff who work with these clients on a day-to-day basis. This can be done by training sessions that take place not in the classroom, but rather in small hands-on groups working directly with the client. Management of hearing aids, troubleshooting techniques, and application of communication strategies are all important topics for staff training. In addition, Montano (2001) encouraged the discussion of the psychosocial impact that hearing loss may have on the residents in a nursing home. The use of hearing loss simulating software such as HELPS (Sensimetrics, 2006) can provide a means for the caregiving staff of understanding the potential issues one can face with hearing loss.

Specialized hearing and speech centers, such as the League for the Hard of Hearing, have long provided AR services for their communities. When it is not feasible to offer these services directly in one's practice, it is the responsibility of the audiologist to make the necessary and appropriate referrals for the service when available. Programs like the Gallaudet Peer Mentoring program (Bally & Bakke, 2007) have been created to train consumers as audiologist-extenders in pertinent areas related to the management of hearing loss. With this knowledge, these individuals are capable of becoming an important resource for the audiologist and can be of assistance to those as they search for self-adjustment to hearing loss. Many of the individuals who have begun to partake of this program are members of the Hearing Loss Association of America (HLAA). As a result, the trained persons can serve an additional purpose by educating individuals on the existence of self-help groups and can be a source of a wealth of information on coping with hearing loss. Barlow et al. (2007) reported that individuals with late onset of deafness reported mixed reactions to the services provided by health care providers but were enthusiastic about and greatly valued the peer support and resources they gained from programs offered by other deafened individuals. It is interesting to note, however, that the fact that such a peer-mentoring program has been established suggests that it is necessary and meeting an unmet need for consumers with hearing loss. This may be an example of the audiologist being remiss and the consumer needing to take up the slack.

Hospital settings often prove to be a challenging environment for the establishment of AR programs (Tye-Murray et al., 1994). With the major focus on medical diagnostic audiology, therapeutic intervention for hearing loss often is not available. However, given the interdisciplinary nature of the hospital environment, it could be an ideal setting for AR. Hospitals strive to provide state-of-the-art care for their patients, and the availability of technologically advanced amplification and hearing assistive technology systems (HATS) can fit nicely into a modern outpatient facility. In addition, the use of HATS for in-patients with hearing loss provides an essential AR element to the care that these individuals may receive. One resource that is particularly helpful in establishing a hospital-based program is the availability of referral personnel such as psychologists, social workers, and vocational rehabilitation specialists.

Regardless of the work environment, AR should be and, in fact can be, a part of your practice. The extent of services offered, of course, will depend largely on your work environment and the resources available to you.

At any rate, when one attempts to identify a common thread that runs through the AR definitions previously discussed, counseling appears on the forefront. The counseling process is all-inclusive and begins the moment the audiologist first greets his or her patient in the waiting room. If one keeps in mind the need to help patients adjust to hearing loss and reduce the limitations and restrictions associated with it, then counseling should take a prominent position in one's practice.

How Can We Provide AR Services?

The ability to provide services in AR may be directly associated with the delivery model used in practice. Erdman et al. (1994) characterized the service delivery models used in audiology as either medical or rehabilitation models. The medical model is considered a top-down approach where the clinician provides the assessment and determines the audiologic diagnosis and treatment options. In this model, the clinician is believed to do something "to" the patient and makes the decisions necessary for proper rehabilitation. The client's role is more passive and is directed by the clinician. It assumes that the clinician knows what is best for the client and is based on the premises that hearing loss is disease/pathologically oriented and is most often appropriate for acute conditions.

The rehabilitation model of service delivery takes a more horizontal approach and is felt to be more interactive and facilitative. Here, the clinician helps identify problems and works "with" the client toward resolution. This model is most often considered when dealing with chronic conditions and assumes the client's needs and perceptions will influence treatment strategies. In this model, the client takes a more active role in his/her own rehabilitation and its focus shifts toward functional performance including activities and participations.

Providing AR services in clinical practice frequently is more than the identification of the problem and perhaps even the provision of amplification systems to improve auditory performance. Often, hearing loss contains many layers in need of treatment. Providing a hearing aid may simply address one area without satisfactorily dealing with the embedded problems associated with adjustment to this loss. In order to provide the necessary remediation, multiple aspects of program provision may be necessary. Hearing aid delivery may fall short without the provision of hearing aid orientation. Communication strategies, speechreading, and auditory training may enhance communication performance. Perhaps, even access to peer support groups may add an important dimension to an AR program.

The effectiveness of many programs in AR has been evaluated in the research and we are now beginning to develop an arsenal of evidenced-based practice studies to justify our services. Reviews of practice areas such as counseling-based groups (Hawkins, 2005), amplification (Cox, 2005), individual auditory training (Sweetow & Palmer, 2005), and, most recently, a summary of a variety adult AR services (Hickson, 2009) are continuing to provide this important foundation. Evidence supporting the effectiveness of our services will help support the quest to find acknowledgment of the importance of AR by third-party payers.

Implementation can be difficult in many of our work environments; but even in busy hospital clinics or private practice, creative solutions can be developed to provide AR for patients. Tye-Murray et al. (1994) provided a number of suggestions for AR program provision including: home training, client libraries containing relevant reading materials and DVDs, and established assistive device centers where technology can be displayed and demonstrated.

Sweetow and Sabes (2007) identified AR as an area with an increasing degree of interest among audiologists. There is a growing interest in computer-based programs that can assist the audiologist in the provision of individualized auditory/auditory-visual training. Popularity of such programs, such as Computer-Assisted Speech Perception Testing and Training at the Sentence Level (CASPERSent) (Boothroyd, 1987), Computer-assisted Speech Training (Pichora–Fuller, & Benguerel, 1991), Listening and Communication Enhancement (Sweetow & Sabes, 2006), and Seeing and Hearing Speech (Sensimetrics, 2008), is becoming evident.

Spitzer (2000) identified emerging trends that she believed would have an impact on the provision of AR services. Technologic developments, not only in amplification options and cochlear implants but also in assessment procedures, in particular the focus on auditory processing, will influence the direction of the services we provide. The importance of processing and impaired auditory function is at the heart of an editorial presented by Pichora-Fuller (2007) where she highlights the relationship of audition and cognition and its importance to future developments of treatment and technology.

The impact of the environment on communication function is a growing concern in AR programs, and models have been established that take an ecological approach to treatment (Jennings & Head, 1994; Nobel & Hetu, 1994). Madell and Montano (2000) described a process that should include identifying the individual with hearing loss and understanding the implications; furthermore, the barriers to communication must be analyzed within the context of their environments and interactions with communication partners. Kramer et al. (2005) encouraged the use of significant others in a home education program as a component of the rehabilitation process for older adults with hearing loss. The emphasis of all these programs is the impact of the hearing loss on communication function within the environment, a concept closely aligned with the WHO's ICF.

As we look to the research, it is apparent that AR has evolved over the years and is no longer viewed as only individual therapeutic services provided to a person with hearing loss. There are many opportunities for clinicians to provide AR whether it is within their own work setting, in community-based programs or even at home through computer-generated educational software. Acknowledgment and understanding of issues surrounding successful adjustment to hearing loss will help guide the audiologist in the development of appropriate objectives for treatment.

Conclusions

As we begin to develop new AR programs or perhaps refine the ones already in existence, we tend to look toward accepted definitions to guide us.

We search for meaning, guidance, and clarity as we establish program goals and objectives. It was not the intent of this chapter to provide a new definition of AR, but rather to explore the wisdom of the many authors who have chosen to help us better understand our professional responsibilities in this arena.

The definition of AR has progressed and developed along with the culture of science and health. The breadth of services has expanded and the impact of hearing loss has been better understood. Definitions are dynamic and will continue to shift and change. In our role as audiologists, we will be directly responsible for the future of AR and, along with our consumers with hearing impairment, will provide the essence for the next generation of descriptions used to define our profession. We look to these definitions for guidance and many of our decisions are based on their existence. Therefore, embrace what we know about AR and look forward to where it will be tomorrow.

References

Abrams, H, Hnath-Chisolm, T., & McArdle, R. (2002). A cost-utility analysis of adult group audiologic rehabilitation: Are the benefits worth the cost? *Journal of Rehabilitation Research and Development*, *39*(5), 549–558.

Alpiner, J. G., & McCarthy, P. A. (2009). History of adult audiologic rehabilitation: The past as prologue. In J. J. Montano & J. B. Spitzer (Eds.), *Adult audiologic rehabilitation* (pp. 3–24). San Diego, CA: Plural.

ASHA. (1974). The audiologist: Responsibilities in the habilitation of the auditory handicapped. *Asha*, *21*, 931.

ASHA. (1984, May). Definition of and competencies for aural rehabilitation. *Asha*, pp. 37–41.

ASHA. (2001). Knowledge and skills required for the practice of audiologic/aural rehabilitation. *ASHA desk reference* (Vol. 4). Rockville, MD: Author.

ASHA. (2004a). *Scope of practice in audiology*. Available from: http://www.asha.org/policy

ASHA. (2004b). *Preferred practice patterns for the profession of speech-language pathology*. Available from: http://www.asha.org/policy

ASHA. (2006). *Preferred practice patterns for the profession of audiology*. Available from: http://www.asha.org/policy

ASHA. (2007). *Scope of practice in speech-language pathology*. Available from: http://www.asha.org/policy

Bally, S. J., & Bakke, M. H. (2007). A peer mentor training program for aural rehabilitation. *Trends in Amplification*, *11*(2), 125–131.

Barlow, J. H., Turner, A., P., Hammond, C. L., & Gailey, L. (2007). Living with late deafness: Insight from between worlds. *International Journal of Audiology*, *4*(5), 442–448.

Bergman, M. (2002). American wartime military audiology. *Audiology Today Monograph 1*, pp. 2–24.

Boothroyd, A. (1987). CASPER: A computer system for speech-perception testing and training. *Proceedings of the 10th Annual Conference of the Rehabilitative Society of North America* (pp. 428–430). Washington, DC, Association for the Advancement of Rehabilitation Technology.

Boothroyd, A. (2007). Adult aural rehabilitation: What is it and does it work? *Trends in Amplification*, *11*(2), 63–71.

Cox, R. M. (2005). Evidenced-based practice in provision of amplification. *Journal of the American Academy of Rehabilitative Audiology*, *16*, 419–438.

Demorest, M. E., & Erdman, S. A. (1987) Development of the Communication Profile for the Hearing Impaired. *Journal of Speech and Hearing Research*, *52*, 129–143.

Erdman, S. A. (1993). Counseling hearing-impaired adults. In J. Alpiner & P. McCarthy (Eds.), *Rehabilitative audiology: Children and adults* (2nd ed., pp. 374–413). Baltimore: Williams & Wilkins.

Erdman, S. A. (2000). Counseling adults with hearing impairment. In J. Alpiner & P. McCarthy (Eds.), *Rehabilitative audiology: Children and adults* (3rd ed., pp. 435–472). Baltimore: Lippincott Williams & Wilkins.

Erdman, S. A., Wark, D., & Montano, J. J. (1994). Implications of service delivery models in audiology. *Journal of the Academy of Rehabilitative Audiology*, *27*, 45–60.

Gagné, J. P. (1998) reflections on evaluation research in audiologic rehabilitation. *Scandinavian Audiology*, *49*(Suppl.), 69–79.

Gagné, J. P., & Jennings, M. B. (2009). Audiologic rehabilitation intervention services for adults with acquired hearing impairment. In. M. Valente, H. Hosford-Dunn, & R. Roeser (Eds.), *Audiology treatment* (pp. 371–400). New York: Thieme.

Giolas, T. G., Owens, E., Lamb, S. H., & Schubert, E. D .(1979). Hearing Performance Inventory. *Journal of Speech and Hearing Research, 44*, 169–195.

Hawkins, D. B. (2005). Effectiveness of counseling-based adult group aural rehabilitation programs: A systematic review of the evidence. *Journal of the American Academy of Audiology, 16*, 485–493.

Hickson, L. (2009). Evidence-based research in audiologic rehabilitation. In J. J. Montano & J. B. Spitzer (Eds.), *Adult audiologic rehabilitation* (pp. 367–380). San Diego, CA: Plural.

Jennings, M. B., & Head, B. G. (1994). Development of an ecological audiologic rehabilitation program in a home-for-the-aged. *Journal of the Academy of Rehabilitative Audiology, 27*, 73–88.

Kander, M., & White, S. (2006, March 21). Coding auditory and aural rehabilitation procedures. *ASHA Leader, 11*(4), 3, 16–17.

Kramer, S., Allessie, G. H., Dondrop, A., Zekveld, A., & Kapteyn, T. (2005). A home education program for older adults with hearing impairment and their significant others: A randomized trial evaluating short- and long-term effects. *International Journal of Audiology, 4*(5), 255–264.

Madell, J. R., & Montano, J. J. (2000). Audiologic rehabilitation in different employment settings. In J. G. Alpiner & P. A. McCarthy (Eds.), *Rehabilitative audiology: Children and adults* (3rd ed., pp. 60–82). Baltimore: Lippincott Williams & Wilkins.

Montano, J. J. (2001, November). *Knowledge and needs of nursing personnel working with older adults with hearing loss in long term care*. Poster presentation. ASHA Convention, New Orleans, LA.

Noble, W., & Hétu, R. (1994). An ecological approach to disability and handicap in relation to impaired hearing. *Audiology, 33*, 117–126.

Prendergast, S., & Kelley, L (2002). Aural rehab services and survey reports who offers which ones and how often. *Hearing Journal, 55*(9), 30–35.

Pichora-Fuller, M. K. (2007). Rehabilitative audiology: Using the brain to reconnect listeners with impaired ears to their acoustic ecologies. *Journal of the American Academy of Audiology, 18*(7), 536–538.

Pichora-Fuller, M. K., & Benguerel, A-P. (1991). The design of CAST (computer-aided speechreading training). *Journal of Speech and Hearing Research, 34*, 202–212.

Pope, A., & Stika, C. (2009). Peer support groups: Promoting treatment effectiveness in partnership with consumers. In J. J. Montano & J. B. Spitzer (Eds.), Adult audiologic rehabilitation (pp. 339–350). San Diego, CA: Plural.

Ross, M. (1997). A retrospective look at the future of aural rehabilitation. *Journal of the Academy of Rehabilitative Audiology, 30*, 11–28.

Sanders, D. (1971). *Aural rehabilitation*. Englewood Cliffs, NJ: Prentice-Hall.

Schow, R. L., Balsara, N. R., Smedley, T. C., & Whitcomb, C. J. (1993, November). Aural rehabilitation by ASHA audiologists: 1980–1990. *American Journal of Audiology*, pp. 28–37.

Sensimetrics Corporation. (2006). *HeLPS: Hearing loss and prosthesis simulator.* Somerville, MA: Author.

Sensimetrics Corporation. (2008). *Seeing and hearing speech: Lessons in lipreading and listening*. Somerville, MA: Author.

Spitzer, J. B. (2000). Toward contemporary models of adult audiologic rehabilitation. *Seminars in Hearing, 21*(3), 205–212

Steering Committee ASHA Special Interest Division 7. (1992). Spotlight on Special Interest Division 7: Audiologic rehabilitation. *Asha, 34*, 18.

Sweetow, R., & Palmer, C. V. (2005). Efficacy of individual auditory training in adults: A systematic review of the evidence. *Journal of the American Academy of Audiology, 16*, 494–504.

Sweetow, R. W., & Sabes, J. H. (2006). The need for and development of an adaptive listening and communication enhancement (LACE™) program. *Journal of the American Academy of Audiology, 17*(8), 538–558.

Sweetow, R. W., & Sabes, J. H. (2007). Technologic advances in aural rehabilitation: Applications and innovative methods of service delivery. *Trends in Amplification, 11*(2), 101–111.

Tye-Murray, N., Witt, S., Schum, L., Kelsay, D., & Schum, D. J. (1994, November). Feasible aural rehabilitation services for busy clinical settings. *American Journal of Audiology*, pp. 33–44.

Ventry, I., & Weinstein, B. (1982). The Hearing Handicap Inventory for the Elderly: A new tool. *Ear and Hearing, 3*, 128–134.

Warner-Czyz, A. D. (2000). Clinical application of adult audiologic rehabilitation programs. *Seminars in Hearing*, *21*(3), 235–244.

White, S. (2006). Third-party coverage and reimbursement for aural rehabilitation. *Perspectives on Aural Rehabilitation and Instrumentation Division*, *13*(1), 2–3.

World Health Organization. (1980). *International classification of impairment disability and handicap.* Geneva, Switzerland: Author.

World Health Organization. (2001). *International classification of functioning, disability and health.* Geneva, Switzerland: Author.

3

The International Classification of Functioning: Implications and Applications to Audiologic Rehabilitation

Jean-Pierre Gagné
Mary Beth Jennings
Kenneth Southall

Audiology originated as a health profession during World War II. Many military personnel required services for the hearing problems they incurred during the war. In the United States of America, rehabilitation services provided by the Veterans Administration were comprehensive, and included: hearing aid fitting; personal adjustment and orientation to hearing aids; auditory and speechreading training programs; training in the use communication strategies; speech correction therapy; personal psychological counseling services; and educational and vocational training (Ross, 1997). Since the early 1940s, there have been many changes in the types of rehabilitation services typically provided to individuals with hearing loss. To a large extent, the services provided have been driven by developments in technology. Generally, as technologic advances occurred, there were significant improvements in the type of amplification systems made available to people with hearing loss (Carver, 1972; Harris, 1976; Hodgson, 1986). As a result, audiologists became more involved in the prescription, fitting, dispensing, and evaluation of hearing aids. Much effort was devoted to adapt the electroacoustic performance of hearing aids to the distinct characteristics of the individuals with hearing loss. Also, several approaches were developed to optimize the amplified acoustic signals that were delivered in the ear canals of people with hearing loss, while taking into consideration many idiosyncratic physical, acoustic, and psychoacoustic properties of the hearing mechanism, as well as the perceptual system of hearing aid users.

As the availability and performance of hearing aids improved, a gradual decline in the provision of other forms of rehabilitation services (speech-perception training, communication management training, conversational fluency training, counseling, etc.) was observed. Several factors may account for this general decline in non-technologically-driven rehabilitation services. One supposition is that many audiologists are neither comfortable with nor trained to address the emotional needs and psychosocial predicaments of many people with hearing loss (Luterman, 2002). Another factor may be the significant time commitment typically associated with providing training programs. Still another factor may be the fact that, until recently, few investigators have successfully demonstrated the efficacy (and long-term benefits) of noninstrumental rehabilitation services (Gagné, 1994; Hawkins, 2005). Given the cost of health-related services, there is an increasing demand by those who pay for these services (individuals, third party payers, governmental agencies) to demonstrate the effectiveness and efficiency of treatment programs before they are incorporated into the services offered to clients (Gagné, 2000).

One reason why few investigators were able to demonstrate the benefits of rehabilitation programs may be because, at least in some cases, an inappropriate conceptual framework was applied to the development and provision of rehabilitation programs and for the type of evaluative research conducted. This observation is based on two different sources of information. First, there exist rehabilitation programs that are efficacious and effective. Expert clinicians have reported anecdotal evidence indicating that the rehabilitation services they provided to clients were beneficial. Perhaps more importantly, clients have reported satisfaction with the services they received, and claimed that many of the problems they experienced due to their hearing loss were resolved (Abrahamson, 2000; Binzer, 2003). Second, some researchers who conducted evaluative research to quantify the benefits provided by specific audiologic rehabilitation (AR) programs reported that the results of statistical analyses did not unequivocally demonstrate the benefits of those programs. However, in some cases, the large variability in the data may account for the results obtained. Specifically, some participants displayed large benefits, whereas others failed to display any improvement (or they showed decrements in performance) during the post-treatment evaluation (Gagné, 1994). Although the statistical analyses failed to reveal a significant improvement, individual participants reported that the rehabilitation program in which they took part was helpful in resolving some of the difficulties they experienced in their everyday living activities (e.g., Binnie, 1977; Gagné, 1994). It is possible that the statistically nonsignificant results reported were due, at least in part, to the fact that the dependent variables used as outcome measures were not sufficiently sensitive or specific to capture the positive effects of the training program. It is also possible that the inability to demonstrate the efficacy of the rehabilitation services is due, at least in part, to limitations in the way the rehabilitation services and research projects were conceptualized and evaluated.

The main goal of the present chapter is to describe conceptual frameworks of health that can be used to conceive, describe, apply/conduct, and analyze AR services. First, we make the case that adopting and applying a conceptual framework is a natural and essential component of AR (as it is for every other service provided by health professionals). Second, we discuss some shortcomings of applying a medical (curative) model of health as a conceptual framework for rehabilitation. Third, we describe two conceptual frameworks that have been successfully applied to the rehabilitation sciences. In both cases the models are based on classification systems adopted by the World Health Organization (WHO). They are: the International Classification of Impairment, Disabilities and Handicaps (ICIDH; WHO, 1980) and the International Classification of Functioning, Disability and Health (commonly referred to as the ICF; WHO, 2001). Fourth, we illustrate how the ICF (WHO, 2001) can be used to guide clinical intervention services and evaluative research in audiologic rehabilitation.

What Are Conceptual Frameworks? Why Are They Useful?

The way we perceive a given phenomenon is influenced by how "we view the world." The knowledge of an individual usually is organized and explained according to the relevant practices of a given society. Stated in another way, the relevant practices of a given society are used to describe and explain phenomena that exist or are thought to exist. Depending on their robustness and accuracy, those practices are considered to constitute theories, models, or in some cases they may be referred to as a conceptual framework.

In academia, most disciplines are driven by concepts, theories, or models. For example, for many physicists the big bang theory is used to explain how our universe was created, and how it is evolving as a function of time. Acousticians choose to describe and analyze sounds based on three different parameters, namely, duration, intensity, and frequency. There exist models of communication that describe and explain the rules that people intuitively use when they interact with one another.

Theories, models, and frameworks constitute the underlying bases on which science is organized and upon which science will progress. They are used to organize, describe, and investigate elements of knowledge and the constituents of a concept of interest. For example, in Chapter 4, this volume, Gagné, Southall, and Jennings (2009) described a theoretical model (Major & O'Brien, 2005) that can be used to describe and explain how the phenomenon of stigma may operate in people who have a hearing loss. Conceptual models provide precise and comprehensive definitions of concepts. Hyde and Riko (1994, p. 347) argued that "terminology is more than labels; it reflects and affects its underlying constructs and it provides a vehicle for debate and research." Moreover, conceptual models provide the basis on which various people can have common understanding and perspective. Conceptual models provide the basis on which a phenomenon is conceived, described, analyzed, understood, and explained. They constitute the basis from which research questions are identified and hypotheses are tested. In rehabilitative audiology (as in all other health disciplines), conceptual models guide the way clinical services are organized, designed, and dispensed. Furthermore, these frameworks influence the type of research that takes place within a discipline as well as how that research is organized and conducted.

Related to AR, the conceptual framework to be adopted will determine how that domain of health is conceived and perceived. Clinically, the conceptual model adopted will influence how we define AR. Furthermore, it will predicate the basis from which the type of rehabilitation services are selected and provided. Moreover, it will influence how we evaluate the effects and benefits of the services provided. From a research perspective, the conceptual framework chosen will determine the research issues to be addressed. In turn, the research question addressed, or the hypothesis tested, will influence the experimental paradigm used and the type of data analyses to be performed to test the hypotheses formulated. Moreover, it will influence the conclusions that are drawn from research investigations.

Imagine two audiologists who adhere to different conceptual frameworks of AR. The conceptual framework adopted by one audiologist may lead that person to design a program that aims to eliminate hearing loss. Based on a different conceptual framework, the goal of the other professional may be to reduce or eliminate the deleterious effects of hearing loss on the client's everyday life activities. Under such circumstances, it is likely that, for the same client, the treatment program selected by one audiologist will be different from the program selected by the other professional. Furthermore, it is very likely that the research methodology used as well as the method and criteria employed to evaluate the success of their intervention program will differ across the two professionals. As unlikely as it may seem, in AR (as in other rehabilitation sciences), dramatically different conceptual frameworks have been used to guide the types of rehabilitation services provided to people with hearing loss and to describe (quantitatively and qualitatively) the outcomes of those services. Needless to say, for a discipline to progress and improve, the conceptual frameworks underlying that discipline must be appropriate, realistic, and valid. Over the years, there has been an evolution in the types of conceptual frameworks used to characterize AR.

A Medical Model of Health

Given its long history, its importance, and the overwhelming presence of medicine in western societies, the medical model has been the predominant conceptual framework of health used in all health-related disciplines. The medical model is grounded in causal logic. Health care professionals aim to identify and thereby explain a patient's symptoms by what causes them. Stated simplistically, in a medical model of health, patients have symptoms that are caused by diseases or impairments. Based on the symptoms, a remedy or treatment is selected and applied (e.g., the prescription of some medication, surgery, a program of exercises, dietary regime, etc.). A treatment is considered successful if, after its administration, the symptoms, the disease, or the impairment disappears; the patient is cured and the person re-establishes the condition of health held before consulting the health care professional (Duchan, 2004). This conceptualization of health is very "body oriented." This model is effective when the treatment program is at the level of the cell, organ, or body structure. For example, health problems often require the elimination of a virus (e.g., an organism that causes a cold, the flu or a childhood disease), or the removal of a body part (e.g., tonsils, gallstones, tumors), or the repair of a body structure (e.g., fractured leg or arm) to restore "normal function." In a medical model of health, the goal of a treatment program is to "cure" the patient (i.e., to restore normal biological functioning or to minimize the impact of the patient's symptoms: Duchan, 2004). This way of conceiving health promotes a view of pathology as an identity in isolation from the affected individual. Such a view of health has limited relevance for chronic, progressive, and irreversible diseases, such as sensorineural hearing loss (Hyde & Riko, 1994).

The health issues addressed by professionals who provide rehabilitation services are very different from the acute health care issues that can be conceptualized within a medical model. In the domain of rehabilitation, the health problems of the people seeking help are usually chronic. That is, often the health problem is irreversible and cannot be rectified in a short period of time. Consequently, people with chronic health problems have to "learn" to live with their problems, to modify aspects of their lifestyles, and to adapt to the effects that their health condition has on their daily living activities. Often, the chronic nature of the health condition will have deleterious effects on non-body-related dimensions of the individual's personal life (e.g., at the psychological, social, economic levels and the level of leisure activities) and the social integration of that person in society.

It may not be appropriate to use a medical model to conceptualize the health (and treatment needs) of people who have chronic disorders (such as a permanent sensorineural hearing loss). At the present time, beyond the services that might initially be provided to the person with a permanent hearing loss (e.g., injection of cortisone), there is not much that can be done medically to restore the person's hearing abilities. Although a number of helpful rehabilitation services may be provided, none of those treatments are likely to "cure" the hearing loss. Thus, viewed from the perspective of the medical model of health, it is difficult to imagine rehabilitative treatment programs that would be shown to be effective. That is, at the present time, the availability of treatment programs designed to eliminate sensorineural hearing loss are limited (albeit some progress is being made; for example, perhaps in the future treatments that will regenerate hair cells at the level of the cochlea). The person has a hearing loss before the rehabilitation services are provided and will continue to have a hearing loss after having completed the rehabilitation program. Hence, if the criterion used to evaluate the benefits provided by a rehabilitation program consists of evaluating aspects of hearing impairment, it is unlikely that the program will be shown to be successful (Gagné, 1998, 2000; Gagné, McDuff, & Getty, 1999).

Although it is never explicitly stated, it can be argued that, in the past, rehabilitation services and evaluation research in AR were designed and evaluated exclusively according to a medical model of health. For example, several decades ago, the unstated goal of fitting hearing aids was to restore normal-hearing acuity. The appropriateness of a hearing aid fitting was evaluated according to the results of the aided audiogram or measures of functional aided hearing. An intervention program (i.e., fitting hearing aids) was deemed to be successful if the aided auditory detection thresholds were within the audiometric limits of normal hearing (e.g., Olsen, Hawkins, & Van Tasell, 1987; Skinner, 1988). The (unstated) premise here was that the hearing aids would "cure" the hearing loss (i.e., produce auditory detection thresholds at the level of normal hearing). Similarly, the efficacy of a speechreading training program was evaluated by comparing the speechreading proficiency of a participant before and after the speechreading program was administered (e.g., Binnie, 1977). The underlying assumption was that the "speech-perception problems" associated with hearing loss would be "cured" (or improved) if the participant displayed improvements in speechreading proficiency (or audiovisual speech perception proficiency) based on post-treatment speech-perception tests administered in a laboratory setting. The results of these investigations provided little information on how different (hopefully better) the person's speech-perception proficiency (or the conversational fluency) was while accomplishing his or her everyday living activities.

Based on the conceptual models of health that were available and used at the time, it is not surprising that the results of evaluative research investigations generally were not successful in demonstrating the benefits of audiologic rehabilitation. First, the premise underlying the conception of the health problems (i.e., the medical model) and the type of outcome measures typically used to evaluate benefit (both clinically and in research projects) were not adapted to the goals of rehabilitation. It was not until the 1980s that other conceptual models of health were developed and applied to rehabilitation sciences.

The International Classification of Impairment, Disability, and Handicap

According to the WHO (1948), health is a "state of complete physical, mental and social wellbeing and not merely the absence of disease or infirmity." This view extends the conception of health beyond the level of body parts and body functions. In 1980, the WHO proposed an international classification of health that attempted to encapsulate its conception of health and well-being. A main objective of the *International Classification of Impairment, Disabilities, and Handicap* (ICIDH) (WHO, 1980) was to propose a generic model of health and rehabilitation that would be accepted internationally and that would apply to all forms of rehabilitation services, regardless of the discipline. The ICIDH (WHO, 1980) considers the effects that diseases and disorders may have at the organic level (impairments), at the level of the individual in a real-life setting (disabilities), as well as at the sociocultural level (handicaps). The WHO (1980) definitions of impairment, disability, and handicap are provided in Table 3–1. A visual representation of the conceptual framework of health provided by the ICIDH (WHO, 1980) is shown in Figure 3–1.

According to this framework, impairments are dysfunctions in body structures or body functions that are measurable in the laboratory or clinic. For example, an individual's audiogram may reveal the presence of elevated bone conduction detection thresholds. Or, the result of laboratory experiments may demonstrate that an individual has broader than normal auditory psychophysical tuning curves. The results of both tests are indicative of a hearing impairment attributable to some pathology in the hearing system. Examples of hearing disabilities include having poor auditory localization skills and poor speech perception performances in quiet, or in noise. That is, people with hearing impairment who perform less well than matched peers with normal hearing on tasks of auditory sound localization or on speech-perception tests would be deemed to display specific hearing disabilities. A handicap is a disadvantage caused by an impairment or a disability that prevents or limits a person from fulfilling the role that would otherwise be considered normal for that individual, given the sociocultural environment in which the person lives. From an audiologic perspective, handicaps are nonauditory problems that result from hearing impairment or disability. For example, a specific job may require that workers be in regular verbal communication with each other, even though the level of noise in the work setting is very high. A person with a hearing loss may experience problems in that work setting if that individual has more difficulties than the other workers understanding speech in noise (i.e., a speech perception in noise disability). In this example, the person with hearing loss would be deemed to have an occupational handicap.

Table 3–1. Definition of Impairment, Disability, and Handicap According to the International Classification of Impairments, Disorders, and Handicaps (ICIDH: WHO, 1980)

Impairment:	any loss or an abnormality of a psychological, or anatomical structure or function.
Disability:	any restriction or inability (resulting from an impairment) to perform an activity in the manner or within the range considered normal for a human being.
Handicap:	any disadvantage for a given individual, resulting from an impairment or a disability, that limits or prevents the fulfillment of a role that is normal (depending on age, sex, and social and cultural factors) for that individual.

The following example illustrates how the domains of impairment, disability and handicap apply to audiologic rehabilitation. Meningitis, a *disease*, may damage the inner and outer hair cells at the level of the cochlea causing an auditory *impairment* (a severe bilateral sensorineural hearing loss). The *impairment* may cause the person to experience some hearing *disabilities* including the fact that the individual may perform less well on speech-perception tasks than peers who have normal hearing. Moreover, the hearing *impairment* and the hearing-related *disabilities* may cause *handicaps* that limit or prevent that person from fulfilling social roles that would be considered normal for that individual. For example, that person may have work-related handicaps due to: the inability to converse on the telephone; difficulties communicating with one other individual in a noisy work environment; difficulty in taking part in meetings in which several persons are involved. The same person may have leisure-related handicaps due to: the inability to communicate by telephone with friends; difficulty communicating with others in noisy environments such as restaurants; the inability to watch the evening news on the television (because it is not possible to understand the audio signal unless the volume is set to very loud or unless the audio signal is somehow amplified); and an inability to take part in bird-watching activities (because the person cannot hear the bird songs or localize where they are coming from).

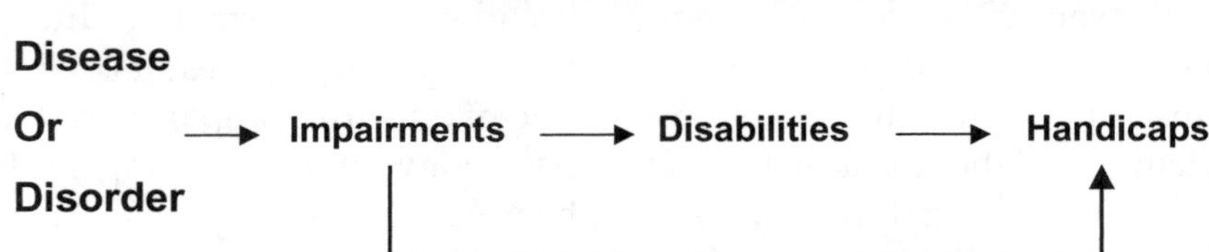

Figure 3–1. The relationship between the different components of ICIDH (WHO, 1980).

It is important to recognize that there is not a direct relationship between the domains of impairment, disability, and handicap. An impairment may not always result in a disability, and a disability does not necessarily result in a handicap (Hyde & Riko, 1994). Furthermore, two persons who have the same type and degree of hearing loss may not experience the same type (or degree) of handicaps. For example, Tom and Jerry may have a similar hearing loss. Their hearing loss may make it difficult for each of them to take part in conversations that involve two or more participants. This disability (e.g., difficulty conversing in noise) may constitute a work-related handicap for Tom because his job requires that he meet regularly with coworkers to establish their weekly sales objectives. However, Jerry may be a postman. Having difficulty conversing in noise may not be an occupational handicap for Jerry because his job does not require him to take part in meetings in which several people are involved. Two persons with different hearing loss may have the same handicap. For example, although Charlie's hearing loss may be less severe than Tom's and Jerry's, he may have the same hearing disability (difficulty conversing in noise). Moreover, that hearing disability may constitute an occupational handicap because Charlie is a waiter in a dark and noisy sports bar where he must interact with his customers.

It is important to note that, according to this conceptual framework, people with hearing loss do not have *a hearing handicap*; however, they may have a handicap due to their hearing loss. Similarly, a person with a hearing loss is not *hearing handicapped*; however, in some situations, the person may experience a handicap because of the hearing loss (Stephens & Hétu, 1991). Although not stated explicitly, according to the ICIDH (WHO, 1980) framework, a handicap is the result of an interaction between, on the one hand, impairments and disabilities and, on the other hand, the particular sociocultural and physical environment in which an activity or an event takes place (Stephens & Hétu, 1991). For example, Natasha, (a schoolguard at a crosswalk) with a mild to moderate hearing loss may have difficulty localizing sound in space. This disability constitutes a work-related handicap when she directs traffic at a busy street intersection. However, the same disability may not constitute a handicap when she converses with children while standing on the sidewalk. A useful reference, Stephens and Hétu (1991) described how the concepts of impairment, disability, and handicap apply to rehabilitative audiology.

At the time that it was proposed, the ICIDH (WHO, 1980) constituted a major breakthrough for all disciplines of rehabilitation. By extending the concept of health beyond the domains of disorders and impairments, the ICIDH framework provided rehabilitation sciences with an opportunity to develop a different conceptualization of itself and to redefine its goals. Consistent with the ICIDH model (WHO, 1980), the goal of audiologic rehabilitation can be defined as the alleviation or reduction of hearing disabilities and handicaps encountered by individuals with hearing loss (Gagné & Jennings, 2008). Within this perspective, audiologic rehabilitation services could be helpful for people with a chronic hearing loss. Whereas, AR offers little or no possibilities to cure permanent hearing impairment, some programs can be designed to reduce or eliminate hearing disabilities and handicaps. For example, within a medical (curative) model of health, the stated (or implicit) goal of providing a client with hearing aids is to restore the client's impaired hearing abilities (e.g., restoring auditory detection thresholds to normal levels). However, within the perspective of the ICIDH (WHO, 1980), the goal of providing the client with hearing aids may be to eliminate or reduce hearing disabilities (e.g., improving the detection of acoustic alerting signals, improving speech understanding in quiet and/or in noise; making it possible to localize voices or warning signals in space) or to reduce situations of handicap attributable to the hearing loss (e.g., maintaining one's occupation even though it requires conversing on the telephone; continued appreciation of one's leisurely activities such as playing scrabble with friends or watching sports programs on television). Speechreading training may not constitute an efficacious treatment if the goal of the program is to reduce the degree of hearing loss (an impairment) or to improve visual speech perception per se. However, it may constitute an efficacious program if the goal of the treatment program is to improve the client's ability to understand speech in a noisy environment (a hearing disability) such as a family dinner or at a noisy street corner. By defining the goals of rehabilitation according to disabilities and handicaps, the ICIDH makes it possible to evaluate the efficacy and the effectiveness of specific types of services or programs provided to people with specific impairments and specific needs (defined in terms of disabilities and handicap). For example, how successful is the treatment (e.g., a visual alerting device) in making the client aware that someone is ringing the doorbell? Or, how helpful is the treatment (e.g., earphones connected to a personal infrared amplification system) in enabling the client to understand the television? Conceiving audiologic rehabilitation from an ICIDH (WHO, 1980) perspective makes it possible to demonstrate some beneficial effects of rehabilitation programs. Also, it provides insights into identifying the types of programs that are most efficacious to solve specific disabilities and handicaps. For example, using a single hearing aid may constitute an efficacious treatment program if the goal of the intervention program is to improve speech comprehension in quiet. The same treatment program may not be as efficacious if the goal of the program is to improve sound localization in a noisy work environment. More importantly, the ICIDH (WHO, 1980) made it possible to demonstrate that, by reducing disabilities and handicaps, the quality of life of people with hearing loss could be improved without altering the person's disorder or impairment (Mulrow, Aguilar, Endicott, Velez, & Tuley, 1990; Mulrow, Tuley, & Aguilar, 1992).

Notwithstanding its contribution to rehabilitation sciences, there remained some confusion among researchers and professionals concerning the concepts addressed in the ICIDH model. For example, some people had difficulty establishing the line of demarcation between elements that were in the domain of impairments and those that were in the domain of disabilities (Stephens & Hétu, 1991). For example, the inability to detect a 1000-Hz pure tone presented at 40 dB HL via loudspeakers in an audiometric test booth may be taken as a measure of hearing impairment. Does the inability to detect complex tonal signals such as an FM signal centered at 1000 Hz (e.g., a signal that resembles an ambulance warning signal) in the same test setting constitute a measure of impairment or disability? Some professionals considered performance on a speech perception test administered in noise as a measure of impairment (a diagnostic sign of a cochlear hearing loss) whereas others considered the performance on the same task a measure of hearing disability (Stephens & Hétu, 1991). Similarly, there was some confusion between what was considered a disability and what was considered a handicap. For example, does having difficulty understanding speech on the telephone constitute a hearing disability or does it constitute a handicap?

Over the years, some shortcomings of the ICIDH model were identified. For example, according to Figure 3–1, which represents a schematized representation of the ICIDH, the model is unidirectional (Frattali, 1998; Threats, 2006). Specifically, disorders may lead to impairments, which may lead to disabilities. Furthermore, according to the model, impairments and disabilities may lead to handicaps. However, the model does not account for situations whereby disabilities may lead to impairments or where handicaps may lead to disabilities or impairments. In some circumstances, those possibilities may occur. For example, someone may have a hearing impairment (elevated hearing detection thresholds), which may lead to hearing disabilities (e.g., understanding speech in quiet and in noise). The hearing disability may lead to a social integration handicap (because of the difficulties associated with understanding speech, the person avoids social interactions with others). Over a period of time, the social integration handicap (staying at home alone, isolating oneself from others) may bring the person to suffer from psychological depression. How does the ICIDH model account for this situation? In this instance, some people may claim that the depression constitutes a secondary handicap (Stephens & Hétu, 1991). Others would report that the handicap (social isolation) led to the development of a new disorder, namely, depression.

Another criticism of the ICIDH model was that some elements known to influence disabilities and handicap could not be accounted for in the ICIDH framework. For example, it has been demonstrated that the physical and social environment are involved in the handicap creation process (Fougeyrollas, Bergeron, Cloutier, Côté, & St. Michel, 1998; Fougeyrollas & Majeau, 1991; Noble & Hétu, 1994). For example, it is well known that the physical environment (e.g., noise, reverberation, and poor illumination) will influence the magnitude of disability and handicap experienced by people with a sensorineural hearing loss. The social environment may also alter the degree of handicap experienced by an individual. For example, to minimize a leisure-related handicap, it would be acceptable for someone with a hearing loss to ask conversational partners to take turns and speak one at a time when playing bridge (to optimize the ability to understand speech). However, socially, it is less acceptable to make the same request (asking the people who are sitting closeby to speak one at a time) at a large sporting event, such as a football game. Recognizing the intricate interaction between the person with hearing loss and the environment (physical and social) in which a specific activity or event takes place, Noble and Hétu (1994) proposed that the concepts of hearing disability and handicap always be considered within an ecologic approach. Specifically, they described how a handicap should be defined according to the interaction that exists between the person and the environment. As illustrated in an above-mentioned example, the disabilities and handicaps experienced by Natasha, the school-guard at the crosswalk, are situation-specific (contextually determined). Investigators in other disciplines of rehabilitation also recognized the importance of the environment in describing disability and handicap (see also Fougeyrollas et al., 1998; Fougeyrollas, & Majeau, 1991; WHO, 1997, 1999, 2001).

There is evidence that personal attributes of the individual with an impairment may also have an influence on the degree of disability and handicap that is experienced. For example, a person who has a very outgoing personality may request communication partners to apply specific communication strategies in order to facilitate speech understanding (e.g., requesting conversational partners to use of clear speech). However, a shy person may refrain from making the same request. Hence, under similar communicative settings, the latter person is likely to display a greater amount of disability or handicap. In certain cultures, it is not acceptable for women to make eye contact when they interact with men. Hence, for those women, the use of visual speech cues (speechreading) to improve their speech understanding proficiency is not possible. In this instance, a person's cultural background may influence the degree of disability and handicap experienced in a given communication setting. Given these shortcomings associated with the ICIDH classification system, the WHO undertook a major revision of its conceptual framework of health.

The International Classification of Functioning, Disability, and Health

After exploring different variations of conceptual frameworks (WHO, 1997, 1991, 2001), the WHO formally proposed a revised classification system: the *International Classification of Functioning, Disability and Health* (most commonly referred to as the *International Classification of Functioning* (ICF) (WHO, 2001). Not unlike its predecessor, this classification system can be applied to all rehabilitation sciences. Furthermore, it is accepted and recognized internationally (e.g., Peterson, 2005; Peterson & Rosenthal, 2005; Smiley, Threats, Mowry, & Peterson, 2005; Threats & Worral, 2004). Thus, an important advantage of the ICF (WHO, 2001) is that it can be used to compare the results of rehabilitation research as well as aspects of clinical services across disciplines and across countries. Also like its predecessor, adopting the ICF (WHO, 2001) changes how intervention services are conceived, organized, and dispensed. Given the importance of this classification system, a description of the model follows.

The overall aim of the ICF (WHO, 2001) is to provide a common framework for describing consequences of health conditions and specifically for understanding the dimensions of health and functioning. The main elements of the ICF (WHO, 2001) are displayed in Figure 3–2 and they are defined in Table 3–2. The ICF has two domains,

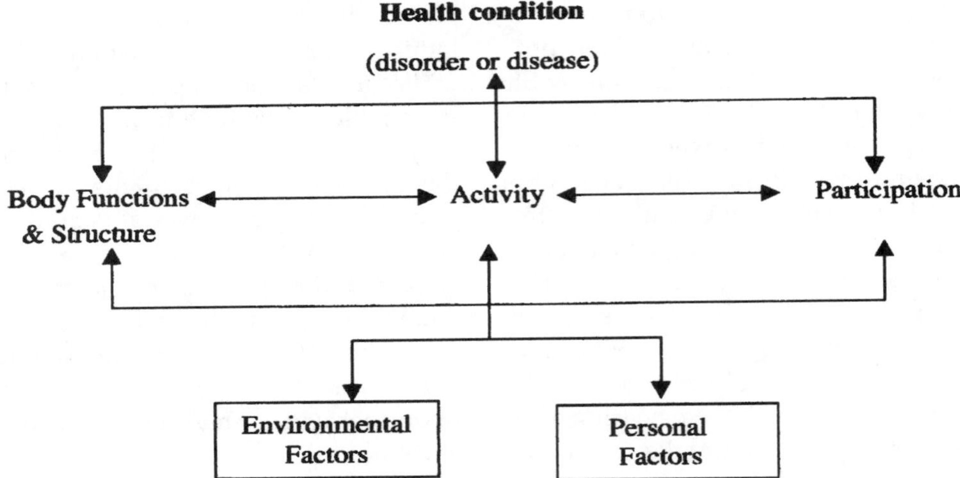

Figure 3–2. Illustration of the interactions of the concepts incorporated into the International Classification of Functioning, Disability and Health (WHO, 2001).

Table 3–2. Definitions of Terms Used in the International Classification of Functioning, Disability, and Health (ICF: WHO, 2001)

Body Functions are physiological functions of body systems (including psychological functions).

Body Structures are anatomical parts of the body such as organs, limbs, and their components.

Impairments are problems in body function or structure such as a significant deviation or loss.

Activity is the execution of a task or action by an individual.

Participation is involvement in a life situation.

Activity Limitations are difficulties an individual may have in executing activities.

Participation Restrictions are problems an individual may experience in involvement in life situations.

Environmental Factors make up the physical, social, and attitudinal environment in which people live and conduct their lives.

each with two components. One domain incorporates aspects of functioning and disability. This part includes body functions and body structures as well as activities and participation. The second part includes contextual factors, specifically environmental factors and personal factors. According to the ICF (WHO, 2001), an individual's state of health is determined by the dimensions of functioning and disability and is moderated by how these dimensions interact with each other. The schematic representation of the model indicates that the dimensions of health (body functions and body structures; activities and participations) may be influenced by one another. The model also indicates that contextual factors (environmental and personal factors) may be influenced by the dimensions of health. The WHO (2001) has designed a coding scheme to classify categories of body functions, body structures, activities, and environment (WHO, 2003). However, at the present time there no codes exist to classify personal factors. Thus, in this model, one's health condition is defined as a result of a complex relationship between functioning and disability interacting with two categories of contextual factors. For example, according to the ICF checklist (WHO, 2003) because of a severe sensorineural hearing loss (i.e., an impaired body structure, coded as s260 and a disabled body function, coded as b230) a person may not be able to use a regular telephone to communicate with others (an activity limitation coded as d3600). Consequently, that individual may not be able to perform tasks that are inherent to the job such as contacting clients and participating in conference calls with colleagues (participation restrictions). It should be noted that within the ICF framework, activity is defined as "the execution of a task or action by an individual." An activity limitation occurs when the person has difficulty executing an activity (e.g., using the telephone to communicate). Participation, on the other hand, refers to the involvement of an individual in a real life situation. A participation restriction is experienced when the person has difficulty participating in a real life situation (e.g., contacting clients by telephone or participating in work-related telephone conference calls). In the present version of the ICF (WHO 2001, 2003), activity limitations and participation restrictions are merged into a single list and both concepts share the same coding system (e.g., d1, Learning and Applying Knowledge; d2, General Tasks and Demands; d3, Communication; d7, Interpersonal Interactions and Relationships; d8, Major Life Areas; see, WHO, 2003). That is, especially for rehabilitation purposes, there are no real advantages in attempting to separate the concept of "activity" from the concept of "participation." Referring to the example above, it would be more appropriate to state that the person experienced limitations when he or she participated in certain activities such as using the telephone to call clients or to take part in telephone conference calls.

The conceptual framework underlying the ICF (WHO, 2001) differs from the original WHO classification system in some fundamental ways. One difference between the conceptual frameworks of the ICIDH (WHO, 1980) and the ICF (WHO, 2001) is that the latter allows for activity limitations and participation restrictions to cause impairments at the level of body structures and body functions. There are experimental data to support this claim. For example, experimentally investigators have shown that performance on certain listening activities such as sound discrimination tasks and speech recognition tasks (see: Gatehouse, 1989; Hurley, 1993; Palmer, Nelson, & Lindley, 1998; Robinson & Gatehouse, 1995; 1996; Silman, Gelfand, & Silverman, 1984; Willott, 1996) are poorer when the stimuli are presented in the ear in which a person (with a bilateral hearing loss) does not wear a hearing aid (hence, few or no listening activities are processed through that ear) than in the ear in which a person uses amplification (i.e., the ear that is typically used for listening). In these examples, the data can be interpreted as illustrations of activity limitations (not listening to sound in the unaided ear) that led to an impoverished body function (poorer sound processing in that ear) and maybe even a disorder in body parts (perhaps some neural degeneration along the central auditory system).

Another significant difference between the ICIDH (WHO, 1980) and the ICF (WHO, 2001) classification schemes is the importance given to the contextual factors, (i.e., personal factors and environmental factors). Clinically, it is possible to illustrate the importance that personality factors may have on creating activity limitations and participation restrictions. For example, two persons with similar hearing loss (impaired body structures and functions) may belong to different bowling teams. One person (Nancy) may be very outgoing and assertive. Whenever, a team member says something she didn't understand, Nancy politely asks the person to repeat the statement while speaking clearly and facing her ("because I have difficulty hearing"). Jack, on the other hand, is very shy and he has a passive personality. Whenever a member of his bowling team says something he doesn't understand, Jack usually just smiles and pretends he understood. In this example, differences in personality traits may account for the fact that Nancy experiences fewer activity limitations/participation restrictions than Jack during their respective bowling outings.

Similarly, environmental factors (both physical and social) may contribute to determining whether a disability is experienced. For example, due to his hearing loss, Tony may experience a participation restriction when he plays bocce ball with his friends in the afternoon, but not in the evening. The explanation is as follows. Within the neighborhood park, the bocce ball court is located just beside the waterslide playground for toddlers. During the day, because it is crowded with children, the waterslide playground is very noisy.

The noise is so loud that Tony does not understand what his playing partners say to him. However, the waterslide playground closes at 5:00 PM everyday. Tony does not experience any participation restriction when he plays bocce ball at night (after 5:00 PM) because the playing area is quiet and he has no difficulty communicating with his playing companions.

An example of how social environmental factors may influence whether a person with a hearing loss experiences a restriction while participating in a given activity may be as follows. Because of his hearing loss, Jay, who refuses to use hearing aids, often doesn't understand when people say things to him, even in relatively quiet environments. Typically, when he fails to hear someone, Jay relies on his spouse to repeat (louder and using clear speech) what the interlocutor said (Jay's spouse is his "hearing aid"). This strategy works fairly well when the couple is alone and watching a movie on the television in the living room. However, the couple cannot use the same strategy when they go to see a play or when they go to the movie theater. In those settings, it is socially unacceptable for Jay's spouse to repeat what was said to her partner.

Another benefit of the ICF (WHO, 2001) as a conceptual framework for rehabilitation is that it can be used to explain how, in certain situations, people with normal hearing may experience an activity limitation/participation restriction because another person participating in the activity has a hearing impairment. For example, Hétu (1996) reported that spouses of working men with hearing loss experienced activity limitations/participation restrictions. Specifically, it was reported that, because of their hearing loss, husbands did not enjoy participating in many social gatherings, such as visiting friends, having dinner at the restaurant, or going to plays/movies. Thus, because of the unwillingness of the husbands to participate in those activities (due to their hearing loss), the spouses also experienced a participation restriction. Hickson and Scarinci (2007) described this situation as a "third-party" disability. Their graphic representation of third party disability is displayed in Figure 3–3. As can be seen from this diagram, in a given environment, the presence of a person with an impairment (e.g., a hearing loss) may influence the health condition of a person without any impairments.

Criticism of the ICF (WHO, 2001)

The ICF (WHO, 2001) has been widely accepted by professionals in rehabilitation sciences, including audiologic rehabilitation. Nowadays, the classification system serves as the conceptual framework in most professional training programs as well as in many centers that provide rehabilitation services. However, some investigators have pointed out limitations of this classification system as a conceptual framework for audiologic rehabilitation (e.g., Noble, Tyler, Dunn, & Bhullar, 2008; Noble, 2009; Stephens & Danermark, 2005; Wade & Halligan, 2003). For example, according to Wade and Halligan (2003), a number of issues related to a person's health are not appropriately accounted for in the classification system (Table 3–3).

Noble et al. (2008) have claimed that the domain of "handicap" that was present in the ICIDH (WHO, 1980) is not clearly incorporated into the ICF (WHO, 2001) classification system. According to these authors, concepts included in the domains of activity limitations and participation restrictions do not incorporate all the dimensions that were included in domains of disability and handicap. For Noble et al. (2008), the term handicap (re: ICIDH, 1980) refers to the nonauditory manifestations (including the psychosocial consequences) of having an impairment or disabilities. According to the same authors, the term participation restriction captures only the "restriction" component of what was incorporated into the domain of handicap. Specifically, the domain of participation restriction does not incorporate the deleterious effects that a specific participation restriction may have on the individual. For example, the ICF (WHO, 2001) can account for the communication difficulties that an individual may experience when attending a social gathering (a participation restriction). However, the same domain of the classification system cannot account for the personal stress that may be present when

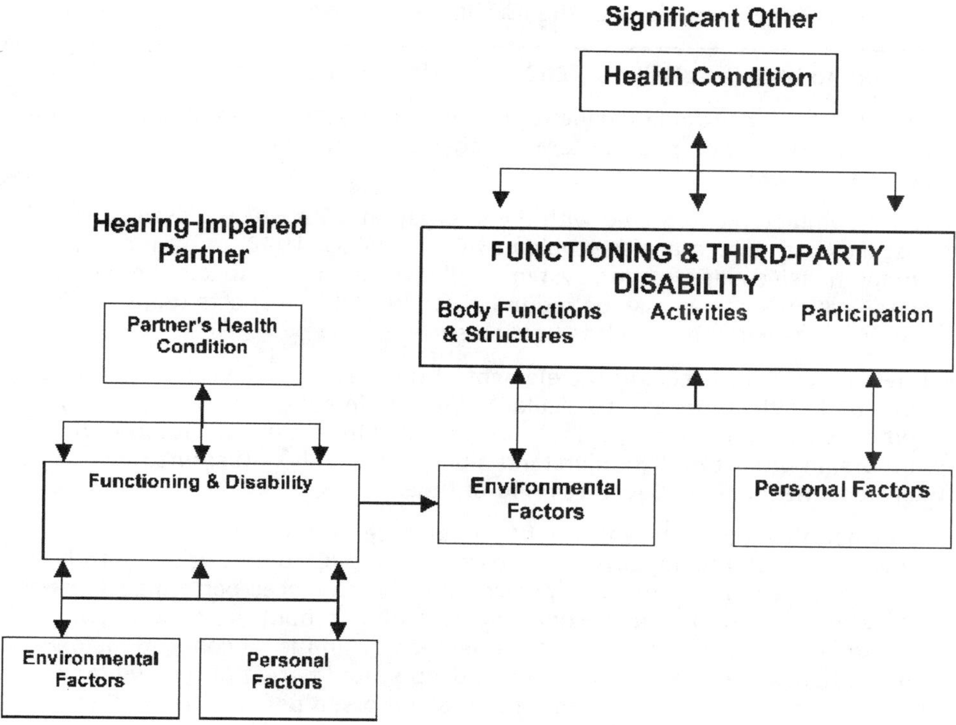

Figure 3–3. Model of the ICF (WHO, 2001) that incorporates third-party disability. (Printed with permission from Hickson and Scarinci, 2007.)

the individual takes part in such activities. Similarly, the domain of participation restriction does not account for the emotional distress that an individual may experience due to hearing loss. Without disputing the legitimacy of the issues raised by Noble et al. (2008), we would claim that the ICF (WHO, 2001) does account for these factors, albeit not within the domain of participation restriction. According to the ICF (WHO, 2001), it is possible for an activity limitation/participation restriction to create/cause a "new" impairment. Thus, according to the ICF classification, one possible consequence of an activity limitation or participation restriction (e.g., psychological or emotional distress) may be the development of a "new" impairment (e.g., pathologic anxiety, depression, etc.). In turn the "new" impairment may lead to activity limitations and/or participation restrictions (social isolation, the person decides to eliminate or reduce opportunities to participate in activities with others). Similarly, an activity limitation/participation restriction could modify aspects of an individual's personality (i.e., in the domain of personal factors). For example, an individual may become frustrated because of the difficulties encountered when conversing in a noisy environment. This frustration may lead the person to become more intolerant (a personal factor) of some communication partners.

Clinical Applications of the ICF

Using the ICF (WHO, 2001) as a conceptual framework for rehabilitation sciences, audiologic rehabilitation has been defined as intervention procedures designed: "to restore or optimize participation in activities considered limitative by persons who have a hearing impairment or by other

Table 3–3. Some Limitations of the ICF Outlined by Wade and Halligan (2003)

According to Wade and Halligan (2003), the classification system:

- Does not have neutral language (terminology) to describe body functions and body structures (i.e., positive terminology to counter the terms impairment and disabilities).
- Is not completely integrated with the International Statistical Classification of Diseases and related health problems (ICD-10, WHO, 1992) to form a comprehensive classification system of illness. In some respects the two classification systems may be redundant and in other respects there are links missing between the two classification systems.
- Does not take into account the element of time. That is, the ICF describes a person's health status at a particular point and time (i.e., the here and now) and does not capture the person's previous health status. According to these authors, in order to fully understand a person's health status, one must be consider the individual over a period of time.
- Does not attribute sufficient weight (importance) to the person ('the individual') with the impairment. In particular, the ICF does not sufficiently consider how much a "person's choice" directly influences performance in activities. Specifically, the ICF does not take into account the notion of an individual's free will. That is, in most democratic and legal conceptions of human nature there is a pervasive and deep-seated notion of free-will and individual responsibility. According to the authors, a person's free-will will have an influence on whether or not an activity limitation /participation restriction occurs as well as the magnitude of the limitations/restrictions.
- Does not implicitly take into account the role of other persons who may be involved in activity limitations and participation restrictions.
- Does not consider the phenomenon of quality of life. This is important because quality of life is a major determinant of an individual's well being.

individuals who partake in activities that include persons with a hearing impairment" (Gagné & Jennings, 2008, p. 390). Accepting the ICF as a conceptual framework for rehabilitation and agreeing with the aforementioned definition of audiologic rehabilitation has many ramifications for the way rehabilitation services are conceived, designed, organized and dispensed.

Several authors have discussed how the ICF (WHO, 2001) can be applied clinically (e.g., Gagné, 2000; Gagné & Jennings, 2008; Hickson & Scarinci, 2007; Hickson & Worral, 1997; Smiley et al., 2005; Worral & Hickson, 2003). For example, Gagné and Jennings (2008) described one approach to rehabilitation that is consistent with the ICF (WHO, 2001): a solution-centered problem-solving approach to rehabilitation. Similarly, Smiley et al. (2005) described how the ICF could be incorporated into rehabilitation programs designed for people with hearing loss. These authors used case presentations to illustrate one application of the ICF to audiologic rehabilitation. Hickson and her colleagues (Hickson & Scarinci, 2007; Worral & Hickson, 2003) outlined how the ICF can be used by those who provide rehabilitation services to older adults with hearing loss.

Perhaps one of the most positive aspects of using the ICF (WHO, 2001) as a conceptual framework for audiologic rehabilitation is that it provides a functional description of the difficulties experienced by individuals with hearing loss (or someone with normal hearing who interacts with a person who has a hearing impairment: see Gagné & Jennings, 2008). Literally, all difficulties that a person might experience due to hearing loss can be described as an activity limitation/participation restriction. Consequently, clients who seek rehabilitation services can be asked to (or shown how to) describe the effects that their hearing loss has on everyday activities. For example, Mrs. Kirk may report that the most important difficulties that she experiences due to her hearing loss are communicating with her friends at the bridge club and interacting with communication partners during social gatherings (see Appendix 3-A). Similarly, Mr. Hall might report having difficulty conversing when meeting clients (one-on-one as well as in small groups), especially in his office or at restaurants (see Case Presentation in Appendix 3-B). Involving clients in the process of identifying and describing the specific difficulties they experience in their everyday life ensures that the activity limitations/participation restrictions targeted by the rehabilitation program will be very concrete and they will consist of difficulties that the clients deem important to resolve.

Another advantage of describing difficulties in terms of activity limitations or participation restrictions is that it shifts the source of the problem (and the focus of the rehabilitation efforts) away from the person who has a hearing loss towards the problematic activity. That is, the focus of the rehabilitation program will not be the hearing loss per se (or the person with the hearing loss). Rather, the focus of the rehabilitation program is the problematic activity (i.e., making it possible for all the people involved to participate fully in the targeted activity). For example, the goal of the rehabilitation program may be to make it possible for Mrs. Kirk to participate actively in conversations at social gatherings (see Appendix 3-A). Or, the goal of the rehabilitation program may be to make it possible for Mr. Hall to minimize communication breakdowns when he negotiates with clients, either in his office or at restaurants (see Appendix 3-B). The solutions to those problems may involve the active participation of people other than Mrs. Kirk and Mr. Hall. Identifying the goals of rehabilitation in terms of activity limitations/participation restrictions may eliminate/reduce the guilt, shame (including the negative psychological impact), and responsibility that some people with hearing loss experience because they view themselves as solely responsible for communication breakdowns. Perhaps other factors, such as the environment or other persons who take part in the activity, are also partially responsible for the difficulties experienced.

Another important advantage of describing the difficulties in terms of activity limitations/participation restrictions is that it allows the people who seek rehabilitation services to identify the difficulties (limitations/restrictions) that have a direct impact on their lives. For example, Ted who has a hearing loss may not be able to have conversations with his friends when they are standing at a noisy street corner (a limitation/restriction that is very common among people with hearing loss). However, the inability to participate in that activity may not be important to him. Hence, when asked to report the most important limitations/restrictions experienced due to his hearing loss Ted would not likely report this activity as being particularly relevant. On the other hand, Alice who has a hearing loss may place a lot of importance on an activity that is problematic even though it does not occur frequently. For example, she may report that an important problem that she would like to resolve is the difficulty she has conversing with her 6-year-old grandson when they play cards. For Alice, this participation restriction may be considered a high priority for rehabilitation even though the activity itself may occur only infrequently (e.g., once every 2 or 3 weeks).

Two important points about using the ICF to identify the goals of rehabilitation program are: (1) they necessarily involve the persons consulting in the process of identifying the goals of rehabilitation as this person is best qualified to identify the most important activity limitations/participation restrictions they experience; and (2) the rehabilitation program (and more specifically the goals of the rehabilitation program) will be formulated in functional terms (everyday activities specific to the client: see, Gagné & Jennings, 2008).

Clearly defining the goal of the rehabilitation program is probably the most important component of any intervention program. If the goal of the program is unambiguously identified and described, it will be easier to select the intervention strategy that is most likely to overcome the targeted activity limitation/participation restriction. Moreover, once the program is completed, it will make it possible to evaluate the outcome of the intervention program. Essentially, the outcome of an intervention program will be assessed according to the answer given from the following question: *"Is the specific activity limitation/participation restriction targeted by the intervention program (the specific "goal") still present, or has the problem been fully (or partly) solved?"*

Using the ICF (WHO, 2001) as the conceptual framework for rehabilitation programs allows one to clearly distinguish the goals of an intervention program from the tools and the strategies selected to attain the intended goal. It is not rare for the goal of a rehabilitation program to be overshadowed by the application of the proposed treatment. For example, the rehabilitation audiologist may ascertain that wearing hearing aids would enable a client to understand the television better. In this instance, the goal of the rehabilitation program is not to fit the client with hearing aids. Rather, the goal is to make it possible for the client to understand the television. Using hearing aids constitutes the strategy (the 'intervention tool') to attain the specific goal. The outcome of the rehabilitation program will be favorable only if the client's ability to understand the television is improved; and not necessarily whether or not the client uses hearing aids. The desired outcome (understanding the television) may not be attained even though the client regularly uses hearing aids for this activity (e.g., because of background noise in the room where the client watches the television). Similarly, improving visual or audiovisual speech perception skills using hearing assistive technologies (HATs) does not constitute goals of rehabilitation programs. The goal of a rehabilitation program should not be that "the client will use hearing aids for an average of 8-hours per day" or "that the client will purchase and install a luminous alerting system to the telephone." The goal of an intervention program should be stated in terms of the client's participation in specifically identified activities (see Appendixes 3-A and 3-B).

Another positive aspect of using the ICF (WHO, 2001) is that this conceptual framework for rehabilitation makes available many different options to overcome activity limitations/participation restrictions. Recall that according to the ICF, an activity limitation/participation restriction occurs as a result of a complex interaction among several factors including: the person's impairment; the activity itself; the personal factors associated to the person with the impairment and those of other people who are involved in the activity; and the environmental factors including: the physical and the social environment, which incorporates the other people who take part in the activity (Hickson & Scarinci, 2007). If all of those factors can contribute to creating an activity limitation/participation restriction, then they might also be considered when identifying possible solutions to overcome the limitations/restrictions. That is, the possible solutions to overcoming an activity limitation/participation restriction might be one, or a combination of many of those factors. Examples of the factors that should be considered when identifying solutions to activity limitations/participation restrictions are provided in the case studies presented in the appendixes.

As discussed above, with some minor modifications, the ICF (WHO, 2001) also can be used to account for some activity limitations/participation restrictions that a person without impairment might experience. For example, Pat, who has normal hearing, might experience a limitation/restriction when he plays bridge because Charlotte, his playing partner, who has a severe hearing loss, has difficulty understanding the bids made by the other three players. Or, Louise may explain that she no longer goes to the theater (a participation restriction) because her husband, who has a severe hearing loss, will not accompany her. Or, Lou might have to forego his social dance class because his partner's hearing loss is such that she can no longer follow the beat of the music. In our view, it is legitimate (and sometimes advantageous) for an audiologist to provide rehabilitation services to someone with normal hearing who participates in activities that involve people with hearing loss. Sometimes the person referred to the audiologist will deny having problems due to hearing loss. The audiologist may ask the spouse (e.g., the wife) if she experiences any activity limitations or participation restrictions in her everyday activities; if so, the husband may be solicited as part of the solution to overcome the difficulties experienced when the couple participates in the targeted activities.

In summary, relative to a medical model of health, adopting the ICF (WHO, 2001) as a conceptual framework for audiologic rehabilitation services will have marked ramifications on how rehabilitation programs are conceived, described, provided, and evaluated. Most importantly, it likely will have a significant impact on the clients who seek rehabilitation programs. The rehabilitation programs will not focus on reducing the client's impairment (e.g., improving auditory or audiovisual speech perception performances; using effective communication strategies; refining conversational skills). Rather, the rehabilitation programs will focus on reducing or eliminating the limitations/restrictions that clients experience when they participate in certain activities that they have identified as being important to them.

Implications of Applying the ICF to Research in Rehabilitation

In the introductory section of this chapter, it was suggested that one reason that few studies have been able to demonstrate the effectiveness of AR services was that (in some cases) the conceptual framework underlying the research investigations was inappropriate. Gagné (2003) outlined four fundamental principles that should guide evaluative research in AR. A detailed discussion of these fundamental principles is beyond the scope of the present chapter. However, one principle relevant to this discussion was "*treatment programs should be selected so that they meet the goals of audiological rehabilitation and be consistent with the conceptual framework from which these goals are defined*" (Gagné, 2003, p. S105). Given that there is a wide consensus that the ICF (WHO, 2001) constitutes the most suitable conceptual framework for clinical services in rehabilitative sciences (including AR), it is logical that the same framework be used to guide evaluative research in AR.

Gagné (2000) discussed some of the implications of applying the ICF (WHO, 2001) to treatment evaluation research. He explained that the most important ramification of the ICF is that the goal of the *research* should be consistent with the (based on the same) conceptual framework that guide clinical services. From an ICF perspective, the goal of an evaluative research project must be to determine whether the treatment program under investigation eliminates (or reduces) activity limitations and/or participation restrictions rather than disorders, impairments, disabilities, or handicaps. This is not a trivial issue. This approach requires a major shift in how evaluative research should be conducted, because the way the research question is defined will influence almost all aspects of the research project, including the choice of research paradigm, the data collected, the types of analyses conducted, and the interpretation given to the data obtained. For example, conceptually there is an important difference between an investigation that aims to determine "whether a digital hearing aid (with a specific algorithm) improves speech perception in noise" and an investigation that aims to determine "whether a digital hearing aid (with a specific algorithm) will improve Mrs. Busybee's ability to converse with her friends at the bridge club." The first question is a generic question of hearing disabilities (speech perception in noise). The second question addresses the specific issue of Mrs. Busybee's participation restriction in a specific activity. It is likely that the most suitable research paradigm for a given research project will vary according to the questions posed. For example, a classical group research design conducted in the laboratory (e.g., presenting speech stimuli in noise under different experimental conditions, including one that involves the digital hearing aid under investigation) would constitute an appropriate paradigm to address the first question. Whereas, that paradigm would not be appropriate to address the second question. For the second question, a single-subject experimental design based on data obtained from questionnaires administered to (or interviews conducted with) Mrs. Busybee would constitute an appropriate experimental paradigm. Both the classical group research design and the single subject experimental design have positive aspects and negative aspects. They simply address different questions. The results obtained from the first study would make it possible to make some generalized statement concerning speech perception in noise with the hearing aid. However, it would not provide data that would help ascertain whether or not the hearing aid would resolve the specific limitations/restrictions that Mrs. Busybee experiences at her bridge club (because of the differences in noise, settings, tasks between the experimental conditions and the actual activity limitation). On the other hand, the second experimental design would make it possible to address the specific objective set for Mrs. Busybee (does it help communication at the bridge club). However, the data obtained from that investigation would not make it possible to generalize the findings (whether or not the hearing aid is useful) to other situations nor to other individuals.

A discussion of the application of experimental designs that lend themselves to treatment evaluative research that is consistent with treatment services based on the ICF (WHO, 2001) is beyond the scope of this chapter. However, there is a literature that addresses this issue (e.g., Barlow, & Hersen, 1984; Cardillo, & Smith, 1994a, 1994b; Gagné, 2003; Gagné et al., 1999; King, Leolane, & Verba, 1994; Kiresuk, Smith, & Cardillo, 1994; Kiresuk & Sherman, 1968; McReynolds & Thompson, 1986; Olswang, Thompson, Warren, & Minghetti, 1990; Smith & Cardillo, 1994). As this point relates to the present chapter, it should be noted that, in order to be useful and valid, treatment evaluative research must be consistent with the underlying conceptual framework used to provide clinical services. If it is not, the results of those investigations may not have practical clinical applications; or, even worse, the research will lead to findings and conclusions that are incorrect and invalid.

Summary

A major goal of the chapter was to point out that (whether it is officially acknowledged or not), there is always a conceptual framework underlying the rehabilitation services that audiologists provide. Another important goal was to describe some conceptual frameworks, namely, the ICIDH (WHO, 1980) and particularly the ICF (WHO, 2001), that provide a valid and useful model for AR. Adopting the ICF (WHO, 2001) requires a major paradigm shift in the way audiologists conceive rehabilitation and in the way rehabilitation services are organized and provided. However, there is little doubt that adopting the ICF (WHO, 2001) will result in the provision of better services to those who require them.

References

Abrahamson, J. (2000). Group audiologic rehabilitation. *Seminars in Hearing*, *21*(3), 227–233.

Bandura, A. (1977. Self-efficacy: Toward a unifying theory of behavioural change. *Psychological Review*, *84*(2), 191–215.

Barlow, D. H., & Hersen, M. (1984). *Single case experimental designs: Strategies for studying behavior change* (2nd ed.). New York: Pergammon Press.

Binnie, C. A. (1977). Attitude changes following speechreading training. *Scandinavian Audiology*, *6*, 13–19.

Binzer, S.M. (2003). The future of the past in aural rehabilitation. *Seminars in Hearing*, *23*(1), 3–12.

Cardillo, J. E., & Smith, A. (1994a). Psychometric issues. In T. J. Kiresuk, A. Smith, & J. E. Cardillo (Eds.), *Goal attainment scaling: Applications, theory, and measurement* (pp. 173–212). Hillsdale, NJ: Lawrence Erlbaum Associates.

Cardillo J. E., & Smith, A. (1994b). Reliability of goal attainment scores. In: T. J. Kiresuk, A. Smith, & J. E. Cardillo (Eds.), *Goal attainment scaling: Applications, theory, and measurement* (pp. 213–241). Hillsdale, NJ: Lawrence Erlbaum Associates.

Carver, W. F. (1972). Hearing aids: A historical perspective and technical review. In: J. Katz (Ed.),

Handbook of clinical audiology (pp. 567–577). Baltimore: Williams & Wilkins.

Duchan, J. (2004). Maybe the audiologists are too attached to the medical model. *Seminars in Hearing, 25*, 347–354.

Fougeyrollas, P., Bergeron, H., Cloutier, R., Côté, J., & St. Michel, G. (1998). *The Quebec Classification: Disability creation process*. Lac St-Charles, Quebec, Canada: Réseau international du processus de production de handicap.

Fougeyrollas, P., & Majeau, P. (1991). The handicap creation process: How to use the conceptual model-examples. *ICIDH International Network, 4*, 3–61.

Frattali, C. M. (1998). Outcomes measurement: Definitions, dimensions and perspectives. In C. M. Frattali (Ed.), *Measuring outcomes in speech-language pathology* (pp. 1–27). New York: Thieme Press.

Gagné J.-P. (1994). Visual and audio-visual speech-perception training. In J.-P. Gagné & N. Tye-Murray (Eds.), Research in audiological rehabilitation: Current trends and future directions [Monograph]. *Journal of the Academy of Rehabilitative Audiology, 27*, 133–159.

Gagné, J.-P. (1998). Reflections on evaluative research in audiological rehabilitation. *Scandinavian Audiology, 27*(Suppl. 49), 69–79.

Gagné, J.-P. (2000). What is treatment evaluation research? What is its relationship to the goals of audiological rehabilitation? Who are the stakeholders of this type of research? *Ear and Hearing, 21*(4), 60S–73S.

Gagné, J.-P. (2003). Treatment effectiveness research in audiological rehabilitation: Fundamental issues related to dependent variables. *International Journal of Audiology, 42*, S104–S111.

Gagné, J.-P., & Jennings M. B. (2008). Audiological rehabilitation intervention services for adults with an acquired hearing impairment. In M. Valente, H. Hosford-Dunn, & R. J. Roeser (Eds.), *Audiology Treatment* (Chapter 16, pp. 547–579) New York: Thieme Medical.

Gagné J.-P., McDuff, S., & Getty, L. (1999). Some limitations of evaluative investigations based solely on normed outcome measures. *Journal of the American Academy of Audiology, 10*, 46–62.

Gagné, J.-P., Southall, K., & Jennings, M. B. (2009). The psychological effects of social stigma, In J. J. Montano & J. B. Spitzer (Eds.), *Adult audiologic rehabilitation* (pp. 63–92). San Diego, CA: Plural.

Gatehouse, S. (1989). Apparent auditory deprivation effects of late onset: The role of presentation level. *Journal of the Acoustical Society of America, 86*, 2103–2106.

Harris, J. D. (1976). Introduction. In M. Ruban (Ed.), *Hearing aids: Current developments and concepts* (pp. 1–7). Baltimore: University Park Press.

Hawkins, D. B. (2005). Effectiveness of counselling-based adult group aural rehabilitation programs: A systematic look at the evidence. *Journal of the American Academy of Audiology, 16*, 485–493.

Hétu, R. (1996). The stigma attached to hearing impairment. *Scandinavian Audiology Supplement, 43*, 12–24.

Hickson, L., & Scarinci, N. (2007). Older Adults with acquired hearing impairment: Applying the ICF in rehabilitation. *Seminars in Speech and Language, 28*, 283–290.

Hickson, L., & Worral, L. (1997). Hearing impairment, disability and handicap in older people. *Physical and Rehabilitation Medicine, 9*(3&4), 219–243.

Hodgson, W. R. (1986). Hearing aid development and the role of audiology. In W. R. Hodgson (Ed.), *Hearing aid assessment and use in audiologic habilitation* (3rd ed., pp. 1–12). Baltimore: Williams & Wilkins.

Hurley, R. (1993). Monoraural hearing aid effect: Case presentation. *Journal of the American Academy of Audiology, 4*, 285–294.

Hyde, M. L., & Riko, K. (1994). A decision-analytic approach to audiological rehabilitation. In J.-P. Gagné & N. Tye-Murray (Eds.), Research in audiological rehabilitation: Current trends and future directions [Monograph]. *Journal of the Academy of Rehabilitative Audiology, 27*, 337–374.

King, G., Keolane, R. O., & Verba, S. (1994). *Designing social inquiry: Scientific inference in qualitative research*. Princeton, NJ: Pinceton University Press.

Kiresuk, T. J., & Sherman, R. E. (1968). Goal attainment scaling: A general method for evaluating community mental health programs. *Community and Mental Health Journal, 4*, 443–453.

Kiresuk, T. J., Smith A., & Cardillo J. E. (1994). *Goal attainment scaling: Applications, theory, and measurement*. Hillsdale, NJ: Lawrence Erlbaum Associates.

Luterman, D. M. (2002). *Counseling persons with communication disorders and their families* (4th ed.). Austin, TX: Pro-Ed.

Major, B., & O'Brien, L. T. (2005). The social psychology of stigma. *Annual Review of Psychology, 56*, 393–421.

McReynolds L., & Thompson, C. K. (1986). Flexibility of single-subject experimental designs. Part I: Review of the basics of single-subject designs. *Journal of Speech and Hearing Disorders, 51*, 194–203.

Mulrow, C. D., Aguilar, C., Endicott, J. E., Velez, R., & Tuley, M. R. (1990). Association between hearing impairment and the quality of life of elderly individuals. *Journal of the American Geriatric Society, 38*, 45–50.

Mulrow, C. D., Tuley, M. R., & Aguilar, C. (1992). Sustained benefits of hearing aids. *Journal of Speech, Language, and Hearing Research, 35*, 1402–1405.

Noble, W. (2009). Self-assessment in adult audiologic rehabilitation. In J. J. Montano & J. B. Spitzer (Eds.), *Adult audiologic rehabilitation* (pp. 95–110). San Diego, CA: Plural.

Noble, W., & Hétu, R. (1994). An ecological approach to disability and handicap in relation to impaired hearing. *Audiology, 33*, 117–126.

Noble, W., Tyler, R., Dunn, C., & Bhullar, N. (2008). Hearing handicap ratings among different profiles of adult cochlear implant users. *Ear and Hearing, 29*, 112–120.

Olsen, W. O., Hawkins, D. B., & Van Tasell, D. (1987). Representations of the long-term spectra of speech. *Ear and Hearing, 8*(5), 100S–108S.

Olswang, L. B., Thompson, C. K., Warren, S. F., & Minghetti, N. J. (1990). *Treatment efficacy research in communicative disorders*. Rockville, MD: American Speech-Language-Hearing Foundation.

Palmer, C. V., Nelson, C. T., & Lindley, G. A. (1998). The functionally and physiologically plastic adult auditory system. *Journal of the Acoustical Society of America, 103*, 1705–1721.

Peterson, D. B. (2005). International Classification of Functioning, Disability and Health (ICF): An introduction for rehabilitation psychologists. *Rehabilitation Psychology, 50*, 105–112.

Peterson, D. B., & Rosenthal, D. L. (2005). The International Classification of Functioning, Disability and Health: A primer for rehabilitation educators. *Rehabilitation Education, 19*, 81–94.

Robinson, K., & Gatehouse, S. (1995). Changes in intensity discrimination following monaural long-term use of a hearing aid. *Journal of the Acoustical Society of America, 97*, 1183–1190.

Robinson, K., & Gatehouse, S. (1996). The time course of effects on intensity discrimination following monaural fitting of hearing aids. *Journal of the Acoustical Society of America, 99*, 1–4.

Ross, M. (1997). A retrospective look at the future of aural rehabilitation. *Journal of the Academy of Rehabilitative Audiology, 30*, 11–28.

Skinner, M. W. (1988). *Hearing aid evaluation*. Englewood Cliffs, NJ: Prentice-Hall.

Silman, S., Gelfand, S. A., & Silverman, C. A. (1984). Late-onset auditory deprivation: Effects of monaural vs. binaural hearing aids. *Journal of the Acoustical Society of America, 76*, 1357–1362.

Smiley, D., Threats, T., Mowry, R., & Peterson, D. (2005). The International Classification of Functioning, Disability and Health (ICF): Implications for deafness rehabilitation education. *Rehabilitation Education, 19*(2–3), 139–158.

Smith, A., & Cardillo, J. E. (1994). Perspective on validity. In T. J. Kiresuk, A. Smith, & J. E. Cardillo (Eds.), *Goal attainment scaling: Applications, theory, and measurement* (pp. 243–272). Hillsdale, NJ: Lawrence Erlbaum Associates.

Stephens, D., & Danermark, B. (2005). The International Classification of Functioning, disability and health as a conceptual framework for the impact of genetic hearing impairment. In D. Stephens & L. Jones (Eds.), *The impact of genetic hearing impairment* (pp. 54–67). London: Whurr.

Stephens, D., & Hétu, R. (1991). Impairment, disability and handicap in audiology: Towards a consensus. *Audiology, 30*, 185–200.

Threats, T. (2006). Towards an international framework for communication disorders: Use of the ICF. *Journal of Communication Disorders, 39*, 251–265.

Threats, T., & Worrall, L. (2004). Classifying communication disability using the ICF. *Advances in Speech-Language Pathology, 6*(1), 53–62.

Wade, D. T., & Halligan, P. (2003). New wine in old bottles: The WHO ICF as an explanatory model of human behaviour. *Clinical Rehabilitation, 17*, 349–354.

Willott, J. F. (1996). Physiological plasticity in the auditory system and its possible relevance to hearing aid use, deprivation effects, and acclimatization. *Ear and Hearing, 17*(Suppl.), 66S–77S.

World Health Organization. (1948). World Health Organization constitution. Geneva, Switzerland.

Accessed on April 5, 2008 from http://www.who.int/governance/eb/who_constitution_en.pdf

World Health Organization. (1980). *International Classification of Impairments, Disabilities and Handicaps. A manual of classification relating to the consequences of diseases.* Geneva, Switzerland: Author.

World Health Organization. (1992). International statistical classification of diseases and related health problems (10th Rev. ed., ICD-10). Geneva, Switzerland: Author.

World Health Organization. (1997). *International Classification of Impairments, Disabilities and Handicaps–2 (ICIDH-2) Beta–1 draft.* Geneva, Switzerland: Author.

World Health Organization. (1999). *International Classification of Impairments, Disabilities and Handicaps–2 (ICIDH-2) Beta–2 draft.* Geneva, Switzerland: Author.

World Health Organization. (2001). *International Classification of Functioning, Disability and Health.* Geneva, Switzerland: Author.

World Health Organization. (2003). ICF CHECKLIST, *Version 2.1a, Clinician Form for International Classification of Functioning, Disability and Health.* Accessed on April 5, 2008 from http://www.who.int/classifications/icf/site/checklist/icf-checklist.pdf

Worrall, L., & Hickson, L. (2003). *Communication disability in aging: From prevention to intervention.* Clifton Park, NY: Delmar Learning.

Appendix 3-A
Case Presentation of Mrs. Kirk

Background Information

Mrs. Helen Kirk is a 75-year-old widow who moved from her house into a two-bedroom apartment 6 months ago. Mrs. Kirk reports that her family first suspected that she had a hearing loss approximately 5 years ago. She waited one year before having her hearing tested. At that time, she was advised that she had a mild-to-moderate high frequency sloping sensorineural hearing loss and would benefit from the use of amplification. She was prescribed and fitted with in-the-ear bilateral hearing aids at that time.

Description of Activity Limitations and Participation Restrictions

Mrs. Kirk uses her hearing aids, but reports having difficulty hearing conversations in groups and in background noise. She noticed that she is having more and more difficulty following conversations during her weekly bridge-club meetings. Often, she does hear her friends, and responds inappropriately. She finds that very annoying. She also reports that recently she has turned down invitations to social gatherings organized by her church because these events are noisy, and because she has difficulty understanding her friends in those settings.

Mrs. Kirk was asked to identify the possible causes for the difficulties she experienced. Specifically, she was asked to consider (1) factors related to herself, (2) factors related to people she communicates with, and (3) factors related to the setting for the bridge club and for the social gatherings she attends. After some probing from the audiologist, Mrs. Kirk was able to identify several possible causes for the difficulties experienced in each setting (Table 3A–1 below). When asked what could be done to improve communication in those settings, Mrs. Kirk reported that she had some ideas about how to deal with each situation. However, she knows that she is a relatively shy person and she does not think that she has the self confidence to follow through with any of her ideas. The pertinent information related to Mrs. Kirk's rehabilitation needs and services are summarized in the table below:

Table 3A–1. Summary of Information Related to Mrs. Kirk's Rehabilitation Program

Background Information	▪ 75-year-old woman; widow ▪ Family first suspected that she had a hearing loss approximately 5 years ago. She waited one year before having her hearing tested. ▪ Advised that she had a mild-to-moderate high-frequency sloping sensorineural hearing loss ▪ Advised she would benefit from amplification ▪ Prescribed and fitted with in-the-ear bilateral hearing aids
Activity Limitations/ Participation Restrictions	▪ Reports difficulty hearing conversations in noisy backgrounds. Two settings identified were: ▫ weekly bridge club ▫ social gatherings related to church activities
Potential Factors that Contribute to the Problems **Factors related to herself:**	▪ She is a shy person and, ▪ She does not think that she has the self-confidence required to follow through with her ideas

Table 3A–1. *continued*

Related to others:	▪ People get involved in conversations. Consequently, they do not speak one at a time and do not face her when they are talking. This makes it impossible to follow topic changes
Related to the environment at bridge club	▪ More than one person talking at once ▪ People do not necessarily look at her when they speak
Related to the environment at the social gatherings	▪ Background noise due to multiple talkers makes it impossible to follow conversation ▪ Background noise and often inadequate lighting make it impossible to follow conversation, even if only focusing on the person who is closest to her
Objectives and Structure of the Intervention Program	
Related to the bridge club	▪ Will be more assertive and request clarifications when she does not understand ▪ Will be more assertive and request that only one person speak at once ▪ Will be more assertive and request that people look at her when they speak ▪ Will identify places within the room where there is less noise and where the lighting is good for speechreading
Related to the social gatherings at the church	▪ Will be more assertive and request that communication partners move to area of room that is optimal for communication ▪ Will be more assertive and request that people speak clearly ▪ Intervention program to focus on: identifying optimal environments for communication; characteristics of assertive behaviors; building Perceived Self-Efficacy (Bandura, 1977), that is, a belief in her ability to organize and carryout out strategies to deal with the communication difficulties she experiences
Intervention Program	▪ Attend an eight-session AR group that is based on the principles of a problem-solving approach (see Gagné & Jennings, 2008) to dealing with communication difficulties and incorporating sources of efficacy beliefs ▫ Enactive mastery experiences, such as role-play ▫ Vicarious experiences, such as watching others similar to herself involved in role-play ▫ Verbal persuasion experiences, for example, • discussions with group members about how they have dealt with similar difficulties • encouragement from group members • learning relaxation techniques to focus on changing her judgment of anxiety and stress levels that occur during communication difficulties
Outcome, Impact, and Consequences of Intervention	▪ New strategies learned to deal with her communication difficulties and self-confidence gained for implementing these strategies ▪ Information received on being assertive in formulating requests from communication partners were very helpful in reducing stress associated with use of communication strategies ▪ Now accepts invitations to attend social gatherings with friends and is much more satisfied when she attends bridge club

Appendix 3-B
Case Presentation of Mr. R. Hall

Background Information

Mr. Robert Hall is a 58-year-old man who lives with his wife. Mr. Hall is employed as a corporate account manager with a major chartered bank. His work involves meeting with clients one-on-one and in groups, both in his office, in clients' offices. He also meets informally at restaurants for both lunch and dinner. Mr. Hall reports that he started to notice difficulty hearing during business meetings and in restaurants approximately 3 years ago. He had his hearing tested and the results showed that he had hearing detection thresholds within normal limits up to 2000 Hz. At higher test-frequencies, the audiogram showed a sloping moderate sensorineural hearing loss. At that time, amplification was not recommended. Mr. Hall does not currently use amplification, but continues to report difficulties hearing in meetings, group conversations, and at restaurants.

Description of Activity Limitations and Participation Restrictions

Mr. Hall was asked to identify the possible causes for the difficulties experienced during meetings. Specifically, he was asked to consider (1) factors related to himself, (2) factors related to the people he communicates with, and (3) factors related to the environment in which the meetings are held. During discussions with the audiologist, several possible causes for the difficulties experienced were identified for each of the factors. The pertinent information related to Mr. Hall's rehabilitation needs and services are summarized in Table 3B–1, below.

Table 3B–1. Summary of Information Related to Mr. Hall's Rehabilitation Program

Background Information	▪ 58-year-old man; married ▪ Works as a Account Manager in a large bank ▪ Noticed difficulty hearing in business meetings and at restaurants approx. 3 years ago ▪ Results from hearing tests showed normal hearing up to 2000 Hz. Above this, a bilateral moderate hearing loss ▪ Amplification was not recommended at that time ▪ Not currently using amplification
Activity Limitations/ Participation Restrictions	▪ Reports difficulties hearing in meetings, group conversations, and at restaurants ▪ Work involves meeting with clients one-on-one and in groups, in his office, his clients' offices, and at restaurants (lunch and dinner)
Potential Factors that Contribute to the Problems	
Factors related to him:	▪ Difficulty concentrating and following conversations when meetings are held at night
Factors related to others:	▪ Difficulty following conversations that moved quickly from one talker to another. ▪ Difficulty tracking speakers when others speak quickly and when conversation moves quickly from one person to another

Table 3B–1. *continued*

Factors related to the environment:	▪ Attempts to seat himself so that he is able to see everyone at the table (both at office and in restaurants) ▪ The settings for meetings are often very noisy and distracting as they are at peak times. For example, at meetings held in the evening, the restaurants often turn lights down and music up
Negotiated Objective and Structure of the Intervention Program	▪ Intervention program to focus on identifying ways to deal with communication difficulties related to group meetings in the restaurant environment
Intervention Program	▪ Attend a four-session individual AR program that uses a problem-solving approach to deal with communication difficulties in the restaurant environment ▪ Learn to identify sources of difficulty related to the environment ▪ Learn strategies that can be used to counteract the effects of noise and of poor illumination. ▪ Activities include paper-and-pencil exercises, role-play, and discussion ▪ Learn how to optimally utilize personal FM system (prescribed and fitted) for use at meetings in office and restaurant environment
Outcome, Impact, and Consequences of Intervention	▪ Identifies sources of difficulty related to the environment; implements strategies to counteract the effects of noise and of poor illumination ▪ Applies communication strategies to deal with communication difficulties in group meetings at office and restaurants ▪ Schedules meetings in restaurants prior to peak hours ▪ At restaurants, attempts to reserve table in quiet area with good lighting away from music speakers; positions himself so that he had a good view of everyone at the table ▪ Limits groups meetings to a maximum of 4 persons ▪ Utilizes FM system with conference microphone with good success ▪ Now also uses FM system when watching television at home

4

The Psychological Effects of Social Stigma: Applications to People with an Acquired Hearing Loss

Jean-Pierre Gagné
Kenneth Southall
Mary Beth Jennings

In many societies, negative stereotypes and prejudices are attributed to people who have hearing loss. The general population perceives individuals with hearing loss as being "old," "cognitively diminished," "poor communication partners," and generally "uninteresting" (Blood, 1997; Doggett, Stein, & Gans, 1998; Erler & Garstecki, 2002; Franks & Beckmann, 1985; Hallberg & Jansson, 1996; Kochkin, 1993, 2007). Partly because of society's view of deafness,[1] many individuals who acquire hearing loss in adulthood are stigmatized. Often, individuals with hearing loss hold the same stereotypical and prejudicial views of deafness as does the general population. Hence, their social identity (how they perceive themselves) is altered due to society's perceptions and due to their own conscious (or unconscious) prejudicial views of hearing loss. This phenomenon, known as stigmatization, is very prominent in many western societies (and perhaps in others as well). The negative stereotypes and prejudices held by society and self-stigmatization that often develops within people who are the target of social stigmatization may have a negative effect on one's physical and psychological well-being as well as participation in activities of daily living.

[1]The general population does not readily recognize degrees of hearing impairment; mostly, people are thought to have normal hearing or no residual hearing. Hence, to members of the general population, people have "normal hearing" or they are "deaf."

Often, people who feel discriminated against by others, and who have a poor self-image are ashamed of themselves due to their discreditable attribute (e.g., hearing loss). Because the presence of hearing loss is not visible, some individuals may choose to conceal, deny, or minimize their hearing impairment. A variety of strategies are used to hide hearing impairment from others. One (maladaptive) coping strategy employed by some people who perceive themselves as being stigmatized due to hearing impairment is to isolate (and insulate) themselves from the world around them. As a result, individuals with hearing loss withdraw from family life and other social activities. By doing so, they can avoid responding inappropriately when someone interacts with them, and as a result they benefit by not disclosing to others that they have a personal attribute (hearing loss), that is discredited by themselves and by society (Vignette 4–1). In fact, concealing one's hearing loss prevents individuals from using communication strategies, as these strategies would inform and disclose the presence of their hearing loss. Moreover, significant cognitive and emotional resources are expended in attempts to conceal hearing loss and the effects of hearing loss on communication. The stress induced by this process may have a deleterious effect on psychological well-being as well as physical health. This may lead to a decrease in overall quality of life and may be the underlying cause of a number of health related problems (Leary, Tamlor, Terdaly, & Downs, 1995).

The stigma related to hearing loss constitutes a major obstacle to audiologic rehabilitation (AR). A person who denies having a hearing loss and conceals his or her hearing difficulties (and its effects) from others is not likely to seek services from an audiologist. Hence, the individual is deprived of rehabilitation services that are potentially helpful, such as obtaining hearing aids and other hearing assistive technologies (HATs), and

Vignette 4–1
Avoiding Social Interactions

Mr. A is a 55-year-old man who has worked in noisy industrial plants for more than 25 years. He and his wife have three daughters and six grandchildren. Mr. A's family, including the three sons-in-law and the grandchildren, has dinner together to celebrate special occasions. Over the past couple of years, Mr. A has noticed that he has more difficulty following the conversation when everyone is having dinner in the dining room. He suspects that his problems are due to hearing loss because his last hearing test at work indicated a significant hearing loss in the high frequencies. Mr. A wants to keep his hearing loss secret because he fears his sons-in-law will make fun of him. Recently, in order to avoid misunderstanding the others during the special family dinners, Mr. A finds an excuse to leave the table early after the meal. He goes to the living room to read his newspaper or he naps. By doing so, his chances of experiencing a communication breakdown are decreased and also he doesn't have to disclose his hearing loss to the members of his family. The avoidance strategy used by Mr. A has been very successful in concealing his hearing loss. However, he feels badly about not being honest with his family, and his concealment behavior induces some stress every time there is a family gathering. Lately, due to his unexplained "awkward behavior" and the tension that it brings about in the house, some family members have found excuses not to attend family dinners. As a result of these developments, some tension has been created between Mrs. and Mr. A. Mr. A feels terrible about the outcome of the situation. He has been moody, tends to isolate himself more and more from family interactions and activities.

learning to request and apply communication strategies that are known to be effective. These individuals deny themselves the opportunity to improve their communication skills and increase their level of participation in activities that are essential or considered important to them (Vignette 4–2).

Crocker, Major, and Steele (1998) have defined stigma as: the possession of, or the belief that one possesses, some attribute or characteristic that conveys a social identity that is devalued in a particular social context. Stigma is a social phenomenon that can be investigated from many different perspectives. For example, investigations may be conducted to explain why some people develop stereotypical (prejudicial) perceptions of subgroups of individuals who display certain characteristics. Or, investigations may attempt to understand how some discriminatory behaviors are formed and how they develop over time. Some examples of investigations from this area have focused on groups such as persons with mental illness, epilepsy, who are HIV positive, members of the gay and lesbian communities, and persons with visible stigmas such as women and African Americans. It is generally recognized that stigmatization involves a power relationship between a dominant group (the *outsiders*) and a minority group (the *insiders*; people who share some devalued characteristic that distinguishes them from the *outsiders*) (Link & Phelan, 2001, 2006; Oyserman & Swim, 2001). Many studies have focused on investigating the relationship that exists between *outsiders* and *insiders* relative to certain social phenomenon (e.g., American of European descendants vs. Americans of African descendants). Some investigations are designed to gain insights on the attitudes, beliefs, or behaviors of members of a specific *outsider* group towards members of a specific *insider* group (Hetu, Getty, & Waridel, 1994). For example, studies have described the perceptions of people with normal hearing toward people who wear hearing aids (the hearing aid effect: Blood, 1997; Doggett et al., 1998; Kochkin, 1993, 2007). Investigations involving *outsider* groups are useful to gain an understanding of the social determinants of stigma.

Studies of the perceptions, attitudes, beliefs, and behaviors of members of *insider* groups have revealed that there are similarities and differences in perceptions, behaviors, and attitudes across groups of individuals who are the target of stigmatization based on a specific set of attributes (e.g., the differences and similarities in the perceptions of educational opportunities by female college students who are American of African descent versus the employment opportunities of gay men

Vignette 4–2
Stigma as a Major Obstacle to Audiologic Rehabilitation

Ms. B who is in her mid-fifties suspects that she has a progressive hearing loss because of recently misheard information in conversations, and because of her family's history of progressive hearing loss. Mrs. B's impression of people who have hearing loss is not positive (she holds a stigmatizing view of people with hearing loss). She thought that her grandmother and her aunt who had hearing loss were social misfits because people always had to repeat things to them, and because they often replied inappropriately during conversations.

Because of her past experiences with people who have hearing loss, Ms. B decides that she will conceal her hearing loss from others. She will not consult a hearing health care professional because she does not want to use a hearing aid. She is unaware that rehabilitation services extend beyond the recommendation to use hearing aids. She also is unaware that, by not seeking services, she deprives herself from learning the communication strategies that can be effective to optimize speech understanding during conversations.

diagnosed as being HIV positive). A major finding of these studies was that large individual differences exist among members of the same *insider* group. Moreover, the results of investigations indicated that the perceptions and behaviors of individuals from the same group can change as a function of different variables. These findings led to studies that investigated the role of individual differences among people who were members of the same *insider* group (Brown & Pinel, 2003; Pinel, 1999). Investigators observed that several factors served to modulate the perceptions of people who were the target of stigmatization (Lightsey & Barnes, 2007; Vauth, Kleim, Wirtz, & Corrigan, 2007). The results of these investigations led to the development of conceptual models that describe the phenomenon of stigmatization from the perspective of people who are the target of prejudicial attitudes (Corrigan & Watson, 2002; Corrigan, Watson, & Barr, 2006).

The present chapter addresses issues relevant to describing and understanding the effects of social stigma on individual members of a specific *insider* group. Throughout the chapter an attempt is made to relate the information presented to adults who have an acquired hearing loss.[2] It is our view that a better knowledge of the factors that influence the social identity of people who have an acquired hearing loss, as well as a better understanding of the effects and consequences of being stigmatized, will be helpful to audiologists. Moreover, this knowledge should make it possible to develop intervention programs that will cater to the specific rehabilitation needs of people with hearing loss who are vulnerable to the negative effects social stigma. In the next section a definition and a description of social stigma is presented. Then, in the following section, the work of Hétu (1996) related to the stigmatization and normalization processes experienced by people with hearing loss is summarized. Later, we describe a generic model of stigma-induced identity threat and the possible effects of this threat on the persons who are stigmatized. Finally, based on the conceptual framework described, in the last section we discuss the types of intervention services that could be offered to individuals who show signs that their personal identity is diminished due to the fact that they have a hearing loss.

Definition of Stigma

Originally, individuals who were stigmatized were people who had a physical trait or characteristic that was considered "deviant" or "abnormal" relative to a reference group (i.e., the *outsider* group) in a given society (Goffman, 1963). The people who displayed these traits or characteristics were devalued as individuals and discredited as a member of their society. Any deviant trait or personal attribute (physical, behavioral, personality, psychological, etc.) that brings discredit to a person may be the source of stigma. Goffman (1963) suggested that stigma signified marks that designate the bearer of a spoiled identity and that this person was less valued in society. A wide variety of personal attributes may be the source of a social stigma. For example, in many western societies stigmatized individuals include people who have a history of psychiatric disorders as well as ex-convicts, pedophiles, and homosexuals. Stigmatized individuals may also include people who are obese, short, HIV positive, diagnosed with a genetic syndrome such as trisomy 21, who smoke tobacco, belong to a given ethnic or a specific religious group or sect, or who speak with a foreign accent. Stigmatized individuals are the target of prejudicial and discriminatory threats (Miller & Major, 2000). In most western societies (and perhaps in others as well), people who have

[2]In preparing the chapter it became apparent that, even among the population of people with hearing impairment, the specific factors that create an identity threat and the effects of perceiving oneself as being stigmatized would differ according to several factors, including: the degree of hearing loss (e.g., individuals with a moderate to moderately severe hearing loss vs. those with a profound hearing impairment), whether the hearing impairment was present at birth (or before the normal period for acquiring oral language) or whether it developed in adulthood; and, the age range of the population of interest (children vs. young adults vs. older adults). Consequently, a decision was made to focus the content of the present chapter to issues related to stigmatization among adults who acquire a hearing loss in adulthood.

hearing loss are stigmatized. It is interesting that Goffman (1963), a sociologist who authored a major treatise on social stigma, used hearing loss (he used the term deafness) to illustrate how an individual's distinguishing attribute could be generalized to other personal characteristics that carry a negative connotation. He noted that hearing loss is often misunderstood as an intellectual challenge or a deficiency in personality and character. The origins of stigmatizing persons who have congenital hearing loss can be traced back to Babylonian laws, pre-Christian laws, religious texts, and to the writings of Aristotle and Saint Augustine: persons who could not hear or speak were likened to animals that were not capable of having intelligence or faith in God (Roots, 1999).

Based on the above description, two characteristics of social stigma are worthy of discussion in relation to hearing loss. First, stigma is a social construction (a label attached by society; a phenomenon defined by society, Major & O'Brien, 2005). Within this context, the term "society" is defined from a sociological perspective, meaning: "a group of persons regarded as forming a single community" or "any organized group of people joined together because of some interest in common" (McKechnie, 1976). Personal attributes that are stigmatizing in one society may not be stigmatizing in another society. For example, being overweight may have a negative connotation in some societies but it may be a valued personal trait in another society. In a recent interview, Rihanna (a well known pop star) stated that in the United States of America being skinny was very much valued. She remarked, however, that in her country of origin (Barbados) it is women who have "curves" that are considered beautiful (*Allure Magazine*, 2008). A given personal attribute may be viewed as positive (or neutral) in one "micro" society (e.g., adults with hearing loss who are members of groups such as the Hearing Loss Association of America) whereas the same attribute may be viewed negatively in another "micro" society (an adult with a significant hearing loss who is a member of a highly competitive bridge club). Moreover, within a given society (e.g., North America) a given trait may be viewed as positive or neutral at one given point in time, and the source of stigmatization at another time. For example, only a few decades ago, smoking tobacco did not carry much of a negative connotation among most middle-class Americans of European descent. People smoked in a variety of social settings. Nowadays, in many respects, smokers are generally viewed negatively. To various extents, people who smoke are devalued as individuals and discredited as a member of society; they are stigmatized. The issue raised here is that stigmatizing attributes are defined by the collective perceptions and values that members of a society (*outsider* group members) hold at a given point in time. Related to hearing loss this is reassuring. It is possible (one would hope!) that the negative and prejudicial attitudes currently associated with hearing loss may change over time. Perhaps as baby-boomers get older and society's views become less conservative, the negative connotations associated with hearing loss will subside.

A second issue related to social stigma is especially noteworthy because it applies to hearing loss. In the social sciences, it is readily acknowledged that aspects of social stigma may differ depending on whether or not it is possible for the individual to conceal the personal characteristic that defines their stigma. Quinn (2006, p. 84) defined a concealed stigma as, "a stigmatized identity that is not immediately knowable in a social interaction." For example, a person with a history of mental illness or a person who is HIV positive may decide to conceal his or her stigmatizing attribute from some people with whom they interact. This option is not possible to someone who has a conspicuous stigma (e.g., skin color, visible physical deformity). Hearing loss is an invisible impairment that an individual can conceal from others. Social stigma research has shown that, relative to conspicuous stigmatizing attributes, having an invisible stigma has some advantages and some disadvantages.

People who have a concealable stigma may decide not to disclose their stigma and thus avoid being stigmatized. Alternatively, they may be able to decide if, when, and to whom they disclose their stigma. For example, an individual can decide if or when to reveal to another person that they have a hearing loss.

One drawback related to concealing a stigmatizing attribute is that there is always discomfort associated with the possibility of having the trait disclosed during a social interaction. Studies have shown that concealing one's stigmatizing trait increases the cognitive load required to take part in social interactions (Lane & Wegner, 1995; Smart & Wegner, 1999, 2000). For example, in addition to exerting the cognitive effort normally required to participate in a conversation, a person who is attempting to pass as normal will have to expend extra cognitive resources in order not to divulge any information, signal, or cues that would betray his or her attempt to conceal (Vignette 4–3). This may be particularly stressful for a person who has a hearing loss, given that due to the nature of the impairment, any normal conversation (even those where disclosing hearing loss is not an issue) invariably will require expending more cognitive resources than those typically required by persons with normal hearing who perform the same task.

It has been shown that the amount of stress associated with participating in a social interaction will vary according to the importance given to unwillingly disclosing the stigmatizing trait and the likelihood of that happening. For example, for someone who has an eating disorder that is not physically apparent to others, the stress associated with a conversation will be less when the topic of discussion does not center around food and eating whereas it will be more stressful when the discussion centers around food and eating. Hearing loss may represent a unique dimension of this situation. For people with hearing loss, in most social situations, they risk causing communication breakdowns due to their hearing impairment. Every time they converse, they risk revealing their stigmatizing attribute to others. This may explain why people with hearing loss often avoid social interactions altogether, as this is a safe strategy to ensure that they will not unwillingly disclose their stigma.

Results of investigations have also shown that the manner in which a stigma is disclosed and the timing of this disclosure will influence how well

Vignette 4–3
Additional Resources Required to Conceal Hearing Loss

Mr. C was recently diagnosed as having an acquired high-frequency, moderately severe hearing loss. Only immediate family members know about the hearing loss. He has chosen not to disclose this information to others. Since the hearing loss was diagnosed, Mr. C noticed that effective communication at work is much more effortful than it is at home. He finds that due to his hearing loss, taking part in work-related conversations requires a lot of concentration to limit the number of communication breakdowns that occur. In addition, unknowingly, Mr. C expends considerable resources making sure that he doesn't disclose his hearing loss to his work colleagues. Mr. C cannot understand why communicating in the workplace is more effortful than communicating at home and why more communication breakdowns occur in his work setting than at home.

Eventually, Mr. C consults an audiologist about the communication difficulties associated with many of his daily activities. He was surprised to learn that his communication difficulties at work may be associated to the additional cognitive resources he must expend to conceal his hearing loss in that setting. Specifically, he learned that, due to the nature of communication, persons with hearing loss must expend more effort to communicate effectively. He also learned that, due to the nature of communication, the risk of inadvertently disclosing his hearing loss is increased every time he interacts with colleagues at work. This makes him realize that the combination of work responsibilities, the stress associated with taking part in social interactions, and the effort expended to conceal his hearing loss left him depleted of resources to communicate effectively.

this information is received by others. For example, if someone's stigma is unwillingly disclosed by a third party, or if it is divulged only after a trusting relationship is formed, the stigmatized person may be seen as being dishonest or untrusting (Herek, 1996). If it is disclosed too soon after meeting someone, there is a danger that others will perceive that this disclosure was used as an excuse to explain some incompetence or social inaptitude (Bairan, Taylor, Blake, Akers, Sowell, & Mendolia, 2007; Corrigan & Matthews, 2003; Joachim & Acorn, 2000; Pachankis, 2007).

Studies also have shown that there is a direct relationship between the desire to conceal a stigma and the importance given to the stigmatizing trait. For example, Major and Gramzow (1999) showed that the more women felt that abortion was a stigmatizing attribute, the more they attempted to keep their own abortion secret from others. Extending this to hearing loss, one would presume that the greater the amount of negative stereotypes that someone attributes to having a hearing loss, the more effort that person will expend to try to conceal the hearing impairment from others.

Finally, a unique aspect of concealable stigmas is that the stigmatized person is more likely to know what family members, friends, and workmates think about that stigmatized trait. That is, because they are not aware that someone in their midst has a stigmatizing trait, close others are more likely to express their attitudes about that specific stigmatized attribute. This is different from a conspicuous stigma (e.g. obesity) because in the presence of a person with a visible stigma, others are likely to be more diplomatic (politically correct) about how they express their attitudes about the specific stigmatizing trait. This information may be of value for rehabilitation. Knowing the attitudes of significant others toward hearing loss should provide insights on how to proceed in disclosing the hearing loss to others. For example, the person with hearing loss may choose to first disclose the impairment to someone who is less prejudicial toward people with hearing loss. In addition, they may solicit their help in using repair strategies during conversations. This strategy will enable the person with hearing loss to improve his or her self-esteem and to gain confidence as a communication partner. When this occurs, it will become less stressful to employ the same strategies (disclosure and seeking help from communication partners) with people who have stronger stigmatizing views of hearing loss.

Self-Stigmatization and Persons with Hearing Loss

To our knowledge, Hétu (1996) was the first scholar to address the issue of stigma associated with hearing loss from the perspective of individuals with an acquired hearing loss. In his seminal article, "The stigma attached to hearing impairment" (Hétu, 1996), based on the generic literature available on stigma from the social sciences and on the results of interviews with adult males with an acquired hearing loss (and their spouses) he proposed two models: one that described the *stigmatization process* and another one that described the *normalization process*. According to Hétu (1996), people who are discredited (stigmatized) because of their hearing impairment experience shame. In this context, shame is the emotion that accompanies threats to one's sense of social belonging. It is a social control mechanism that serves to instill acceptable behavior and inhibit unacceptable behavior. According to Hétu (1996), the *stigmatization process* is the result of the communication breakdowns and other "deviant" behaviors that may occur when people with hearing loss interact with people who have normal hearing (Figure 4–1). The demeaning and discriminatory reactions of the communication partners to the "deviant behaviors" of the person who has a hearing loss leads the latter person to feel shame and guilt about themselves due to their hearing loss. As a consequence of the stress induced and the feelings of incompetency that develop, the person's self-esteem and social identity are diminished. The strategies often used to avoid the stress and the feelings of incompetency associated with unsatisfying social interactions (and the effect on their self-esteem), lead people with hearing impairment to conceal their hearing loss from their communication partners. In addition, many people decide to withdraw from social activities and isolate themselves (Vignette 4–4).

Hétu (1996) also described a two-step *normalization process* designed to help the person with

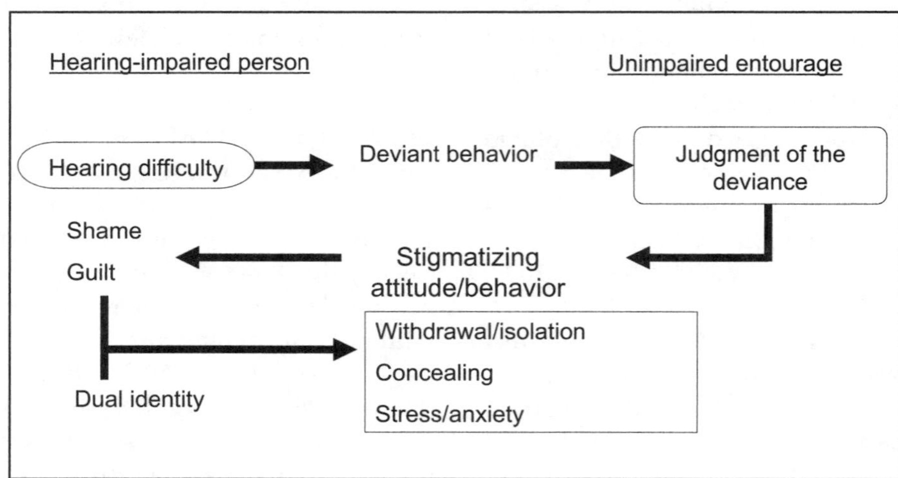

Figure 4–1. Stigma: Hétu's (1996) model of the stigmatization process (taken from Hétu, 1996).

Vignette 4–4
The Consequences of Hearing Loss on Self-Esteem and Social Identity

Mr. D is a retired person, and a devoted family person who held an important position as a corporate executive for many years. He has always prided himself for being a keen golfer and for being well informed about the professional golfing tour (PGA). For many years, Mr. D played several rounds of golf with his grandchildren every summer. However, he has found that the last few outings to be less satisfying. Often, because of his hearing loss, Mr. D is unable to follow the conversation when he plays golf with his grandchildren. When he makes inappropriate comments his grandchildren make fun of him and tease him for becoming a "deaf and senile old man." When he asks his grandchildren to repeat a comment they typically respond "Never mind. It wasn't important." More and more, the grandchildren tend to exclude Mr. D from their golf conversations. Although playing golf with his grandchildren used to be a very important activity for Mr. D, recently the golf outings have not been satisfying. These golf outings make Mr. D feel old, inadequate, and an uninteresting grandparent. His self-esteem is affected to the point where he decides to stop playing golf. Gradually, he even stops taking part in other activities with his grandchildren. He would rather stay at home and feel sorry for himself than to be devalued by his grandchildren.

hearing loss overcome feelings of shame and guilt associated with hearing impairment and regain a more favorable social identity (Figure 4–2, step 1). The first stage of the *normalization process* involves meeting and interacting with other people who have a hearing loss (members of the *insiders*), so that together they can share their experiences of hearing difficulties and the resulting unsatisfactory social interactions. This therapeutic activity helps the participants realize that unsatisfactory social interactions are the result of the hearing loss, rather than to other factors that may be unjustifiably attributed to them (e.g., being unwilling to communicate, or otherwise responsible for the communication breakdowns). Furthermore, the stigmatized person realizes that it is not unusual for people with hearing loss to feel denigrated, diminished or ashamed of themselves. They come to realize that other people with hearing loss have the same feelings of inaptitude and self-denigration. These realizations serve to trigger the *normalization process*. The individual realizes they are not alone in their feelings about their hearing loss and how they behave because of the hearing problems. They realize that other people experience the same feelings and that these feelings are "normal." As a result of this process, people with hearing loss start to feel better about themselves. The process of restoring a more positive social identity is initiated and they are more willing to engage in social activities and interactions. They may learn appropriate coping strategies and experience success in using these strategies when they interact in this favorable social environment (i.e., in the presence of others who have hearing loss).

In the second stage of the *normalization process* (Figure 4–2, step 2), people with hearing loss are encouraged to interact with people in their entourage who do not have a hearing loss. Moreover, they are taught and encouraged to inform their communication partners that they have a hearing loss, and to solicit the use of communication strategies that will optimize the exchange of information. Under these circumstances, communication partners are more likely to acquiesce to the requests of the persons with hearing loss. It is likely that communication will become more efficacious and more satisfying for both communication partners. The result of participating in more satisfying verbal conversations (social interactions) serves to further restore a more favorable social identity for the person with hearing loss. As the process of restoration continues, the person with hearing loss will gain more and more confidence in the ability to be a satisfying communication partner. As a consequence, they are more likely to participate in valued activities that include people who do not have a hearing impairment (members of the *outsiders*) and likely will regain a more positive image of themselves. Hétu's contribution of providing a conceptual model of stigmatization and guidelines for rehabilitative services that serve to restore a favorable social identity constituted an enormous contribution to audiological rehabilitation as well as to the social integration of adults with an acquired hearing loss.

In recent years, there have been significant breakthroughs in the conceptualization of social stigma from the perspective of the persons being stigmatized (i.e., self-stigma). In the next section, we describe one contemporary model of stigma. In our view, most of the concepts described in the model are applicable to the social stigma associated with hearing loss, and to the way that people with hearing loss feel and behave when their self-image is diminished because of the social stigma associated with their impairment. Moreover, we believe that audiologists will benefit from having a better understanding of the self-stigmatizing process and its effects on people who have a hearing loss. Integrating aspects of this model into the domain of AR will serve to complement and extend the current level of knowledge that is available to us, largely due to Hétu's work. Undoubtedly, a more comprehensive understanding of the self-stigmatizing process will lead to the development of more appropriate rehabilitation services for people who are stigmatized due to their hearing loss.

Model of Stigma-Induced Identity Threat

Major and her colleagues have proposed a model of stigma that is based on two premises. The first premise is that stigma puts a person at risk of experiencing threats to his or her social identity (Crocker et al., 1998; Major & O'Brien, 2005; Steele, Spencer, & Aronson, 2002). The second premise is that having one's social identity devalued leads to a potentially stressful situation. Furthermore,

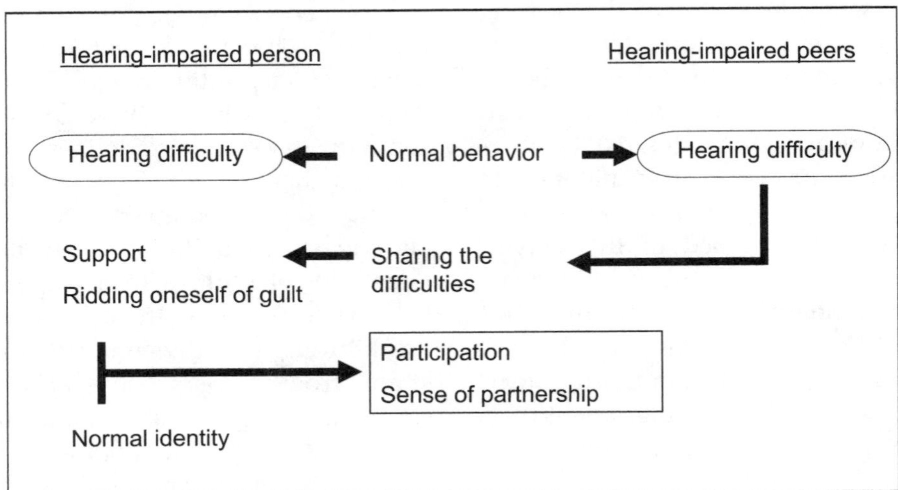

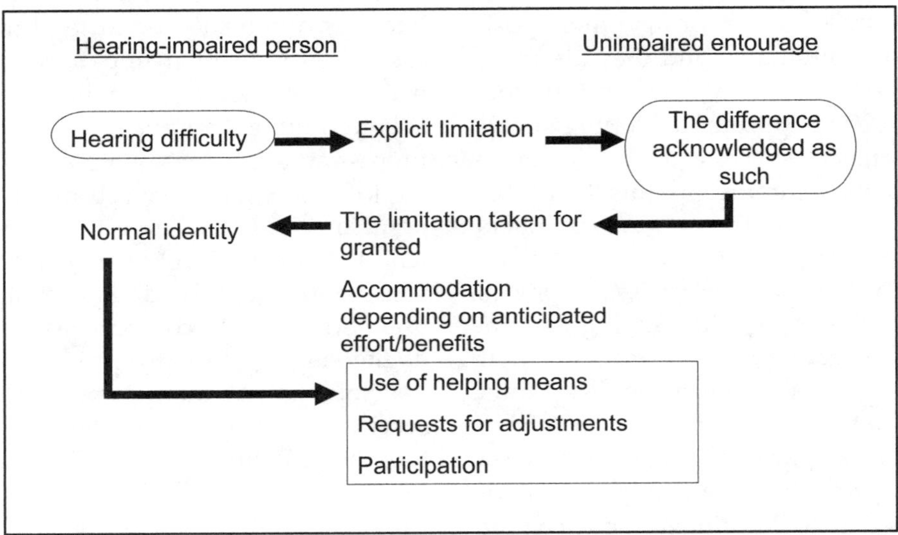

Figure 4–2. Hétu's (1996) two-step model of the stigma normalization process (taken from Hétu, 1996).

according to this model, responses to stigmatization may be similar to responses that may occur in any stressful situation. A diagram of the stigma-induced identity threat model proposed by Major and O'Brien (2005) is presented in Figure 4–3. In this model, responses to stigmatization are dependent on the stigmatized person's assessment of the demands of the situation. An event is deemed to be potentially stigmatizing (see box D) when the individual appraises the demands imposed by a stigma-relevant stressor as potentially harmful to his or her social identity, and when the stress induced by the situation is judged to exceed the resources available to cope with those demands.

Appraisals of one's identity threat (box D) are determined by the interaction of three constructs: collective representations (box A), situational cues (box B), and personal characteristics (box C). Responses to an identity threat can be involuntary (e.g., coping responses in the emotional, physiological, behavioral and cognitive domains: (box E) or voluntary (e.g., coping responses primarily in the behavioral and emotional domains) (box E). The outcomes of coping responses (box F) consist of attitudes (e.g., self-defeating, pessimistic), feelings (e.g., self-esteem, shame, fear, lack of confidence), or behaviors (e.g., academic achievement, communicative abilities, health) that emerge from the stigma-related experience that is taking place. Although not illustrated in the diagram, it is important to note that the model is recursive, in that the responses to an identity threat (box E) may feedback to the first level (boxes A, B, and C) and the second level (box D) of the model. These feedback processes may attenuate or exacerbate the effects of stigmatization.

In the following sections, we describe the components of the stigma-induced identity threat model and the process of self-stigmatization. Examples will be used to illustrate how the components of the model may be applied to understanding stigma associated with hearing loss from the perspective of the individual with hearing loss.

Collective Representations

Collective representations are the shared (societal) understandings and beliefs about stigmatizing conditions (Crocker, 1999). Based on prior experiences, as well as exposure to the dominant culture, members of stigmatized groups develop shared understandings of the dominant view of their stigmatized status in society. Importantly, even if they themselves do not endorse the dominant cultural representation of their stigma, it is assumed that members of the stigmatized group are aware of the dominant cultural stereotypes (Major, 2006; Steele, 1997). These collective representations include awareness that they are devalued in the eyes of others, a knowledge of the negative stereotypes held by the dominant society (the *outsiders*) concerning their stigmatized attribute, and the knowledge that they could be victims and targets of discrimination (Crocker et al., 1998). Collective representations influence how the stigmatized individual perceives and appraises stigma-relevant situations.

As mentioned in a previous section, several studies conducted in western societies have reported that hearing loss is a stigmatizing condition. People who have hearing loss are generally judged (by the members of the *outsiders*) as being, old, senile, cognitively diminished, poor, and uninteresting communication partners (see the descrip-

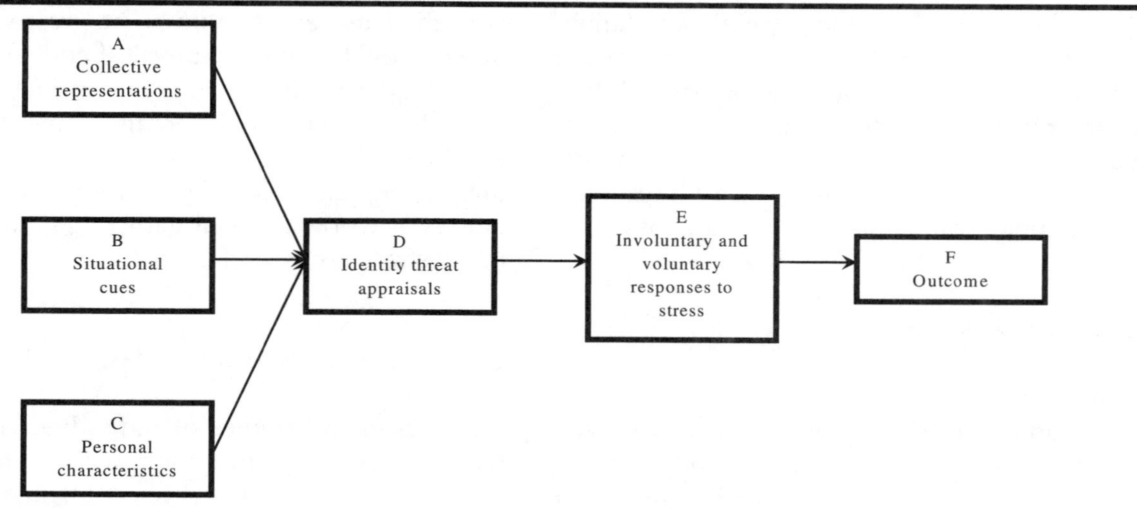

Figure 4–3. Conceptual framework displaying the elements of the stigma-induced identity threat described by Major and O'Brien (2005).

tion from Kochkin, 2007). Hétu, Getty, and Waridel (1994) reported that men with an acquired hearing loss were aware of the stereotypical representations that society holds concerning hearing loss. In fact, some individuals held the same prejudices before being informed (diagnosed) that they had a hearing impairment. Hétu, Riverin, Getty, Lalonde, and St-Cyr, (1990) reported that the cognitive dissonance (their general view of people with hearing loss versus the more positive view they have of themselves despite their hearing loss) was sometimes difficult to reconcile. Women with occupational hearing loss in Hallberg and Jansson's (1996) study reported that the attitudes of others negatively affected their self-image and social roles. The perceptions that people with hearing loss share with members of the *outsiders* will serve to denigrate and contribute to the appraisal their own devalued social identity.

According to the model, the strength of the collective representations held by society, as well as the stigmatized person's own view of the stigmatized trait will contribute to whether or not the person perceives an identity threat. It is interesting to note that in the first step of the normalization process described by Hétu (1996), it is proposed that individuals with hearing loss interact with other individuals with hearing loss. Relative to hearing loss, it is very likely that the collective representations of a group of adults with a hearing impairment will be less negative than the collective representations held by the general population. Thus, as described by Hétu (1996), when in the company of others with hearing loss, a strong identity threat is less likely to be triggered, thus making a supportive environment in which to initiate a rehabilitation process geared toward improving the social image of people with hearing loss.

Situational Cues

Situational cues are factors that are related to the physical and social environment in which a given activity takes place. However, it should be noted that one's perceptions of a situation does not always correspond to the reality of the situation. That is, one's "perception" of the level of threat associated with a given situation is more important than the actual objective level of threat present in that situation. Steele et al. (2002) reported that an identity threat is modulated as a function of the (perceived) situation in which the threat is appraised. For instance, Hallberg and Barrenas (1995) reported moderate identity threat appraisals by blue collar workers when they conversed with coworkers in the work area of the manufacturing plant (because it was very noisy so communication partners tended to speak more loudly and also because communication was difficult for everyone). However, in a previous study, Hallberg and Carlsson (1993) had reported that workers found the noise in the lunchroom particularly troublesome, presumably leading to more severe identity threat appraisals. Referring again to Hétu's (1996) work, recall that the first step of the normalization process involved interactions among people with hearing loss. In this physical and social context, the appraisal of one's identity likely will be less threatening than in a situation in which a person attempts to conceal his or her hearing loss from the others. The recognition that the physical and social situation in which an activity takes place influences the level of identity threat that a person with hearing loss perceives (relative to stigmatization) is a concept that can be used advantageously within the context of a rehabilitation program. For example, coping strategies used to overcome the involuntary responses (such as shallow breathing) to a threatening situation may be trained. First, these responses could be progressively practiced in less threatening physical and social environments (e.g., in the therapy room, at home, at a friend's home). Later, the same responses would be introduced in settings that are more threatening (e.g., at social gatherings with acquaintances, at work, at social gatherings attended by many strangers).

Personal Characteristics

The personal attributes of individuals may also modulate identity threat appraisals. These may include (but are not restricted to) age, gender, hearing impairment, educational level, occupation, aptitudes, attitudes, motivation, confidence level, importance given to one's self-esteem, level of optimism/pessimism, level of stigma-consciousness, and locus of control. Within the same stigmatized group, some individuals appear resilient to prejudice and display positive well-being, whereas other members of the same group do not (Friedman & Brownell, 1995). In addition, the research on stereotype threat demonstrated (Steele & Aronson, 1995) that the same individual may show different responses to prejudice as the context changes. Differential responses to stigma are observed between stigmatized groups, within stigmatized groups, and indeed within the same individuals across contexts. Several individual characteristics modulate the extent to which people appraise situations as relevant to their stigma. One is the extent to which an individual identifies with his or her stigmatized identity (Major, 2006). An example of how occupation modulates one's identity threat appraisal was provided in the Heiligenstadt testament that Beethoven wrote in 1802 (Appendix 4-A). In his testament, Beethoven mentioned that it was unconscionable that someone with his stature as a musician and composer have a hearing impairment. Because of his appraisal of the identity threat caused by his hearing loss, Beethoven tried to conceal his hearing loss from others. One strategy that Beethoven used to avoid having to reveal his hearing loss was to avoid unnecessary contact with others.

Results of investigations have shown that younger adults are more likely to reject hearing aids (presumably have their identity threatened) than older adults (Kochkin, 1993). For women, the stigma associated with hearing loss tends to decrease as they get older (Erler & Garstecki, 2002; Gilhome Herbst, Meredith, & Stephens, 1990). Differences in personality traits may explain (at least in part) variances in identity threat appraisals that are observed across individuals with similar degrees of hearing loss. Several individual characteristics modulate the extent to which people appraise situations as relevant to their stigma. For example, a person with a hearing impairment who is less conscious of the stigma associated with hearing loss, or someone who personally does not ascribe to the stereotypes concerning people with hearing loss, likely will have a higher threshold of identity threat than someone who holds strong prejudices toward people who have a hearing impairment.

A thorough summary of the effects of different personality traits on participation in rehabilitation programs has been reported by Kricos and colleagues (Kricos, 2000; Kricos, Erdman, Bratt, & Williams, 2007). In the future, it may be of interest to investigate the effects of specific personality traits on identity trait appraisal. This information may be useful in identifying the type of rehabilitation services that may be most appropriate for individuals with specific personality traits.

Identity Threat Appraisal

Identity threat appraisals are judgments made by the stigmatized person concerning a potentially stressful event. The person evaluates whether the present threat is relevant to personal goals or values, and determines if he or she has the necessary resources available to cope with this situation (Lazarus & Folkman, 1984). If the threat is perceived as taxing or exceeding one's personal resources, then the event is deemed to be a threat to one's identity. Contemporary perspectives on stigma emphasize that conscious and unconscious appraisals of a devalued social identity contribute to self-identity threat. Stigma-induced identity threat occurs when an individual appraises the demands imposed by a stigma-relevant stressor as potentially harmful to his or her social identity, and as exceeding his or her resources to cope with the demands. The appraisal process can be automatic, nonverbal, instantaneous, and occur outside of consciousness (Smith, 1991).

Major and O'Brien (2005) mention that, within the appraisals of stigma identity threat, there is the possibility that a given activity judged as potentially threatening and that a person assesses that he or she does have sufficient coping resources to meet the challenge of the demand (Vignette 4–5). Recently, Southall (one of the authors of this chapter) conducted personal interviews with people with hearing loss who were involved in activities designed to promote the well-being of people with hearing loss (e.g., they wrote books or plays that addressed the effects of hearing loss; they were members of the executive boards of self-help groups for people with hearing loss; they devoted hours as volunteers to provide services to people with hearing loss). In almost every case, it was reported that one of the reasons that prompted these individuals to get involved in such activities was the fact that at some point during their lives those individuals felt the deleterious effects of being stigmatized due to hearing loss. Perhaps, their pro-active involvement was due to the fact that, when they were confronted with an identity threat, these individuals determined that they had the resources required to undertake the challenge of defending the rights of people with hearing loss.

Audiologists should be aware that some people with hearing loss have the resources to overcome the potential identity threat challenges they may encounter. In designing rehabilitation programs to enable people with hearing loss to overcome identity threats, it may be worthwhile to gain an understanding of the characteristics of people who are able to meet (and even surpass) the demands of a situation. The information gained from their experiences may be helpful to people who perceive identity threats when taking part in the same (or similar) activities. Moreover, perhaps meeting, either individually or in a group, they could serve as models to other people who feel stigmatized.

Responses to an Identity Threat

One assumption of the proposed stigma-induced identity threat model is that experiencing a situation in which one's social identity is devalued is stressful. Women with occupational hearing loss in Hallberg and Jansson's (1996) study reported that most people in their surroundings were unwilling to adjust to their communication needs and that this caused emotional distress. According to Major and O'Brien (2005) the stress that accompanies a response to stigmatization has the same characteristics as the stress experienced in response to other instances. Major and O'Brien (2005) claim that the coping strategies used to deal with stress caused by an identity threat are the same as the coping strategies that an individual is likely to use in response to any other stressful

Vignette 4–5

Reacting Positively to Perceiving Oneself as the Target of Stigma

Notwithstanding the fact that she has a hearing loss, Ms. E, is determined that she wants to extend her yearly subscription to productions of the local theatre company. She is convinced that going to the theatre is a social activity that should be accessible to everyone, including those who have a hearing loss. Confronted with this self-imposed challenge, Mrs. E learns that some theatre companies make hearing assistive devices (HATS) accessible to persons who have difficulty hearing. Ms. E was disappointed to hear that her theatre company doesn't plan to purchase HATS because there has not been a great enough demand for those devices amongst the regular clients. Ms. E is convinced that the low demand is due to the fact that few people with hearing loss are aware that these types of devices exist and can be made available. Being distraught by the theatre company's response to her demand, Ms. E decides to take a very pro-active stand. First, she joins the local chapter of the self-help group for people with hearing loss. Furthermore, she agrees to be nominated to the executive board of the self-help group. Upon being named to the board, Ms. E convinces the other board members to organize an information campaign about the availability of HATS in public places, and encourages people with hearing loss to request HATS when they participate in activities that occur in public places (including the local theatre).

event. Accordingly, Major and O'Brien (2005) claim that generic transactional models of stress and coping (Lazarus & Folkman, 1984; Smith, 1991) may explain how individuals react when they perceive an identity threat due to a stigmatizing event. A discussion of the transactional model of stress and coping is beyond the scope of the present chapter. Readers interested in more information on coping and stress, as it relates to hearing loss should refer to the counseling chapter (Chapter 9) in this book, as well as the work of Andersson and Willebrand's (2003) and Trychin (1986).

Coping refers to the efforts that are deployed to regulate emotion, thought, behavior, physiology, and the environment in response to stressful events or circumstances (Miller & Kaiser, 2001). Responses to stressful events are assumed to be a function of two key processes: how individuals cognitively appraise the event, and the coping strategies used to deal with the events that are appraised as stressful. Coping responses may be classified as *problem-focused* or *emotion-focused*. For example, Vignette 4–5 illustrates an emotion-focused coping strategy whereby an individual with hearing loss joins a self-help group to ease the feelings of being disappointed and distraught. In the same vignette, the individual with hearing loss uses a problem-focused coping strategy when organizing a campaign to promote the installation and use of HATs.

The concept of coping is central to contemporary perspectives on stigma. In contrast to traditional views, these contemporary perspectives portray individuals who experience stigmatization not as passive victims, but as active agents attempting to make sense of their world by preserving their self-esteem (Major, 2006). Coping strategies may also be characterized as *engagement* versus *disengagement* strategies. Engagement coping strategies are often described as "approach or fight" responses, whereas disengagement strategies may be described as "avoid or flight" responses. An example of an engagement coping strategy is illustrated in Vignette 4–6. For an example of a

Vignette 4–6
Being Pro-Active Versus Being Negative

Mr. F has a noise-induced hearing loss but he is too proud to disclose his hearing loss to people other than the members of his immediate family. Although Mr. F refuses to use hearing aids (because they would disclose his hearing loss), he agrees to sign up for a communication strategies course in order to improve his speechreading skills, and to learn to apply communication strategies that do not require him to disclose his hearing loss. Following the completion of the course, Mr. F reports that the speechreading skills and the communication strategies he learned (and uses) are very helpful when he interacts with others on a one-to-one basis at work. When asked about other activity limitations he experiences, Mr. F reports that he stopped attending Bingo. When asked why, Mr. F replied that: 'The person calling the numbers at the Bingo hall was incomprehensible because he mumbled when calling the numbers. The embarrassment of not being able to participate became too much for him to handle, so he stopped going. During the session with the audiologist, Mr. F was surprised to learn that his approach to his communication difficulties at work constituted an excellent problem-focused coping response. On the other hand, his decision to stop going to Bingo was a very maladaptative emotion-focused coping response. Mr. F was invited to participate in a rehabilitation program that would focus on identifying a solution that would enable him to resume attending Bingo.

disengagement coping strategy see Vignette 4–7. Hallberg and Jansson (1996) reported that women with occupational hearing loss used controlling (engagement) and avoiding (disengagement) strategies alternatively to manage demanding situations. Avoiding strategies were used to minimize or hide the hearing loss from others. Controlling strategies were used by women who disclosed their hearing loss to others as they strived to maintain social relationships. Another coping strategy used by persons who are stigmatized is to adopt a blaming discrimination approach. Major and O'Brien (2005) report that when members of stigmatized groups encounter negative outcomes, one way they may cope with the threat to their self-esteem is by blaming the outcome on discrimination rather than on themselves (see Vignette 4–8).

According to Major and O'Brien (2005), the stress related responses and coping mechanisms that arise following an appraised identity threat may be *involuntary* or *voluntary*. An individual's involuntary responses to identity threats may include (but are not limited to) anxiety arousal, increased blood pressure, increase heart rate, increased (and shallower) breathing rate, and sweating. Not unlike any other stressful event, an individual's stress response due to an appraised identity threat can consume valuable resources. As illustrated in Vignette 4–3, the stress related to a person's preoccupation with being discriminated

Vignette 4–7
Disengaging Strategies

Due to her hearing loss, Ms. G has difficulty understanding others, especially in noisy settings. Because she is a very proud person, Ms. G does not want to disclose her hearing loss to others. Even more so, she can't fathom the thought of embarrassing herself by responding inappropriately to a question that might be addressed to her. Ms. G decides to stop attending the social events of the local 4-H club. When questioned by her daughter about this decision, Ms. G responds: "Those events are so noisy and everybody there speaks too softly, and too quickly. It gives me a headache!"

Vignette 4–8
A Blaming Discrimination Approach

Mr. H is a salesperson in an insurance company. He has a hearing loss. Although he has never disclosed this impairment to his colleagues, most of them know that he has difficulty hearing. Because of his difficulty hearing, his colleagues sometimes will unintentionally exclude him from their conversations at lunch (i.e., they don't naturally make any effort to accommodate Mr. H). Recently, having been left out of another conversation at lunch, Mr. H was angered and humiliated by being excluded (the incident had a very negative impact on his self-esteem). As a result of this experience, Mr. H decided to no longer interact socially with colleagues at work. When asked by his wife to explain his decision, Mr. H replied, "The young sales representatives think they know everything and they have no respect for older, more experienced salespersons."

against, and the coping responses employed to address one's threatened identity in a given social interaction will require the use of cognitive resources. The cognitive resources deployed reacting to a perceived identity threat will limit the resources available to engage in the social interaction. Therefore, events that are stigmatizing (or potentially stigmatizing) invariantly increase the probability of displaying observable signs and behaviors that will reinforce the prejudices associated with hearing loss (including, unsatisfactory communication exchange). Thus, almost all acts of communication with others will induce multiple sources of stress (i.e., the stress associated to identity threats, the stress related to the fear of not being an adequate communication partner).

Another example of an involuntary coping response to a stressful event is *righteous anger*. Righteous anger is an adaptive and positive response to situations of stigma that may trigger self-advocacy work and attempts to improve systemic failings for other people who are experiencing similar problems (Corrigan & Watson, 2002). An example of a person displaying righteous anger is presented in Vignette 4–9. Another common coping response may be unconscious avoidance (see Vignette 4–10).

Vignette 4–9
Righteous Anger

Ms. I, who has a hearing loss, is on a train on her way to DeKalb, Illinois. The train is so noisy that she missed the conductor's call on the public address system stating that the next stop was her destination. When she realized that she missed her stop, she requested help from a train employee. Again, because of the noise level on the train, she couldn't hear the explanation given to her. Finally, she gave up, smiled politely at the attendant, and walked away. She got off the train at the next stop and had to buy another ticket to get back home. Needless to say, the whole incident was quite stressful for Ms. I. When she finally got home later that day, she wrote a nasty letter to the complaints department of the train company. The letter provided some suggestions on how the train company could improve their services for older adults who have difficulty hearing in noisy settings.

Vignette 4–10
Unconscious Avoidance

Mr. J has difficulty hearing, but does not use a hearing aid. He has been a member of a bowling team for several years. Over the past year, he often responded inappropriately when his teammates spoke to him. This happened so often that his teammates started to call him Mr. "Outerspace." Although his teammates intended this to be a joke, Mr. J did not appreciate being teased. Being teased made him feel sad and this resulted in him becoming more guarded and withdrawn with the group. Mr. J had not realized that the teasing was the cause of this emotional state. This fall, Mr. J decided that he would forego bowling and not join his team this year. When his wife asked about this decision, Mr. J replied that bowling no longer provided him with as much pleasure as it once did.

It may be useful for audiologists who provide rehabilitation services to know and understand that individual responses (voluntary and involuntary) to situations of perceived identity threat will be basically the same as their responses to any other stressful situations. The professional may question the person with hearing loss about the coping strategies he or she typically uses in response to stressful situations (including both stressful situations related to the hearing loss and situations that do not involve hearing loss). An evaluation of typical coping strategies employed may make it possible to identify appropriate strategies (adaptive and effective), and those that are maladaptive. This information may be used as a starting point for the development of preferred coping strategies, and for reinforcing the use of well-established appropriate coping strategies already in their repertoire.

Finally, it is noteworthy that every stigma-coping strategy has costs and benefits (Corrigan & Matthews, 2003; Swim & Thomas, 2006). People tend to adopt the coping strategies that they judge to be effective. However, in doing so, they may overlook or minimize the costs of employing the selected strategies. For example, as mentioned previously, by deciding to conceal their stigmatized trait in a given situation, an individual may reap the benefits of being considered unmarked in a social interaction. However, there is a heavy cognitive burden associated with using this coping strategy. First, throughout the activity the person must be careful not to unwillingly disclose the hearing loss. Alternatively, there is the possibility that someone else participating in the activity may disclose the fact that they have a hearing loss. Finally, due to the nature of the impairment (hearing loss), and because of the cognitive resources deployed to conceal their hearing impairment, the likelihood that communication breakdowns or inappropriate responses will occur are maximized. Hence, after considering both the benefits and the costs, concealing one's hearing loss may not constitute an effective coping strategy to avoid hearing loss identity threat (refer to Vignettes 4–1 and 4–2).

To eliminate the risk of being stigmatized, an individual may decide to completely avoid taking part in social activities, and thus avoid having to deploy resources that may be required by choosing coping strategies other than avoidance. On the one hand, avoidance is an effective coping strategy because there is no risk of having one's stigma disclosed and the concomitant social identity threat. However, the cost of using this coping strategy is very high. First, the person with hearing loss may deprive him- or herself of participating in activities that are deemed interesting and important for the person (e.g., playing cards, golfing, bowling, and theatre). Second, in the long term, eliminating participation in all social activities, leads to social isolation, which in turn may have serious repercussions on physical and mental health. When discussing coping strategies with clients, audiologists should ensure that the client is aware of the costs as well as the benefits associated with a given coping strategy (Vignette 4–11).

Outcomes of Stigmatization

As mentioned in the previous section, coping strategies are used in reaction to the stress brought about by an identity threat. The goal of using coping strategies is to return the body, emotions, and behaviors into a state of equilibrium. The extent to which this goal is achieved will vary according to the effectiveness of the selected coping strategies used in a given situation. Some coping strategies may not be successful. In fact, they may lead to negative outcomes (Vignette 4–12). Other coping strategies may be well adapted and have successful outcomes (Vignette 4–13). Whenever coping strategies are used (consciously or unconsciously) to deal with a stressful situation, the outcome may be positive, negative or neutral. The outcomes of coping efforts may have repercussions for the individual at many different levels including physiological, psychological, emotional, and behavioral. Moreover, one coping strategy may have several outcomes at different levels. For example, in an attempt to conceal one's hearing loss by not responding appropriately in a given situation, one coping strategy may be to occupy all the conversational space by not giving the others the opportunity to express themselves. This strategy may be successful in relieving the potential stress of

Vignette 4–11
Long- and Short-Term Effects of Coping Strategies

Ms. K is a retired business executive who is a very proud person. She has a hearing loss, however, she denies this and refuses all rehabilitation services, including wearing hearing aids. Nonetheless, Ms. K experiences much difficulty communicating with others, especially in noisy environments. Because she fears that these communication problems will reveal her hearing loss to others, she gradually stops attending social events that take place in noisy settings. Mainly she stays at home, where she reads and plays bridge on the Internet. She finds her new activities less stressful because she doesn't have to worry about not being able to follow verbal conversations. At home there is little risk that she will unwillingly disclose her hearing loss to her friends and acquaintances. However, when she takes the time to really think about it, Ms. K does acknowledge that she is now a lonely person, and that she misses many of the social activities she used to participate in and enjoy. Her loneliness has led her to be somewhat depressed, and physically, she is not well; she has digestive problems attributable to acid-reflux. Both of those health problems are sufficiently important that Ms. K required medical care.

Vignette 4–12
Coping Strategies May Lead to Negative Outcomes

Mr. L is a middle-aged man who has a hearing loss attributable to noise exposure caused by his leisure activities (cutting trees with his chainsaw on his farmland). Mr. L is a sales representative in a large motorcycle store. Because his clients are mostly young adults, Mr. L refuses to use hearing aids. He feels it is important for him to portray the image of a young adult, like his clients. All of the other sales representatives in the store are younger than Mr. L. Recently, because of the stress associated with his desire to portray an image of a young, normal-hearing adult, Mr. L lost his temper and used very aggressive and abusive verbal language during an argument with another sale representative. As a consequence of his extreme reaction to the stressful event, Mr. L was transferred to another department. Although it was not stated implicitly, this lateral move within the company essentially eliminated any possibility that he had for a promotion within that firm. Mr. L is very unhappy in his new position.

inadvertently disclosing one's hearing loss. However, it may have a negative consequence in that many potential communication partners will shun the person with hearing loss because their social interactions are not particularly satisfying (Vignette 4–14).

Six issues are noteworthy concerning the outcomes of using coping strategies to deal with the stress created when one's social identity is threatened by stigmatization. First, as described by Major and O'Brien (2005), one must consider the feedback loops that may occur at different levels of the

Vignette 4–13
Coping Strategies May Lead to Positive Outcomes

Ms. M is a blue collar worker at a tire manufacturing plant. She has had a hearing loss for many years and she wears her hearing aids at work. Because she possesses innate leadership skills, she recently was elected to be the union representative on the health and safety committee for her company. Many plant managers sit on this committee. Their presence on the committee is a bit intimidating to Ms. M. She feels shy and ashamed of having a hearing loss. Also, she is disappointed because she thinks that company managers should be more aware of the communication difficulties that many employees experience due to the fact that they have a noise-induced hearing loss. To express her feelings/reactions concerning this issue, Ms. M decides that she will use her membership on the health and safety committee in the hope that she can convince the other committee members that the company should organize a symposium on the effects of hearing loss on communication and the use of effective communication strategies. In her proposal to the committee members, Ms. M promotes the idea that the symposium should be attended by both the blue collar workers and the people holding management positions within the firm.

Vignette 4–14
Maladaptive Coping Strategies

Mr. N is a retired industrial plant worker who has a hearing loss. He denies having a loss by stating: "It is normal that at my age I don't hear as well as when I was 20 years old. But I'm not deaf!" Mr. N and his wife have five older children who have all left home. Whenever there is a family gathering, it is very difficult for Mr. N to follow the conversation around the dining room table because it noisy and because everybody speaks at the same time. Unable to follow the conversation, Mr. N has reverted to simply staying at the table with the others and not even trying to understand what is going on. Often he looks disinterested and distracted ("in his bubble"). When someone asks him a question, he pretends that he doesn't remember, that he doesn't know the answer, or he answers inappropriately. Regardless of the topic of conversation (even when it deals with issues for which he once had a passion), he doesn't show any interest in participating in the discussion. Most of the family members are a little concerned about their father. They consider his behavior as being very antisocial and somewhat disrespectful. They think that he has aged significantly over the past few years and they wonder whether or not he is showing signs of senility. When his wife mentions this to him, Mr. N simply accepts the labels attributed to him rather than explaining that his behavior is due to the fact that he has trouble taking part in social activities because of his hearing loss.

model. For example, the coping strategies used in a given situation may have an impact on the level of stress induced due to the identity threat. They may also have an effect on the collective representations (e.g., the reactions of others involved in that situation) and the personal characteristics (e.g., changing one's attitude, positively or negatively, concerning identity threat in that situation). Depending on the outcome that results from using a coping strategy, the feedback may be positive (a successful approach to dealing with the identity threat and the stress) negative, or neutral. Second, because of these feedback mechanisms, it is likely that over time the effect of using a given coping strategy will influence the level of identity threat perceived in a given situation. Thereby, this feedback mechanism will also alter the level of identity threat required to trigger the coping response. Third, because identity threat appraisals vary as a function of time, it is important to monitor regularly and evaluate the outcome (consequences) of the coping strategies used in a given situation. Fourth, in evaluating outcomes, it is important to consider both the short-term as well as the long-term consequences using those strategies. Some coping strategies may result in positive short-term outcomes but be appraised negatively when considered from a long-term perspective. For example, avoiding social interactions by staying home alone (watching television or reading) may constitute a successful short-term strategy to reduce the stress of concealing one's hearing loss from others; however, in the long term, avoiding social interactions and isolating oneself from others may have negative outcomes on one's physical and mental health status (see Vignette 4–1 as well as Beethoven's testament in Appendix 4-A). Considered from a short-term perspective, disclosing one's hearing loss to others may increase the stress level associated with a given identity threatening event/situation. However, in the long term, this strategy may turn out to be positive because it will make it possible for the person with hearing loss to employ adaptive communication strategies that will minimize the number of communication breakdowns that occur, and thus become a better and more satisfying communication partner. Furthermore, the feedback given by the communication partners likely will enable the person with hearing loss to develop a more favorable social identity as well as more positive self-esteem. Fifth, coping strategies may act on various dimensions of the individual including at the physiologic, psychological, personality, communication, social, occupational, and economic levels. When evaluating the outcome of using a coping strategy to deal with identity threat, it is important to consider the outcome from a broad perspective. The consequences of using appropriate (or inappropriate) coping strategies may have far reaching consequences on several aspects of life. Finally, many issues related to the coping strategies used to respond to the stress induced due to an identity threat may be successfully incorporated into rehabilitation services for people with hearing loss.

Implications for Practice

The stigma-induced identity threat model may be useful for audiologists who work with clients who are susceptible to the effects of social stigma. Without describing a specific approach to the type of rehabilitation services that could be provided, the conceptual model developed by Major and O'Brien (2005), offers many insights concerning the content of, and techniques used in rehabilitation programs that might provide benefit to people with hearing loss who are (or who perceive themselves) as being stigmatized. In this section we provide some guidelines for rehabilitation services that may be helpful for managing and overcoming the effects of identity threat due to hearing loss.

According to Major and O'Brien (2005), the coping strategies that people use to deal with the stress induced by an identity threat are not different from other coping strategies that people use to deal with stress induced by any other source. This observation implies that components of any rehabilitation program that addresses issues related to coping with stress may be useful for addressing issues related to social stigma. Several researchers and clinicians have described AR programs that incorporate coping strategies intended to attenuate the stress related to specific aspects of having a hearing loss (Jennings, 1993; Trychin, 1986; 2003a-e; Wayner & Abrahamson, 1996). Components of such an AR program are outlined in Table 4–1.

In our view, the stigma-induced identity threat model itself constitutes a helpful tool for

Table 4–1. Components of an Audiologic Rehabilitation Program That Incorporate the Use of Coping Strategies to Alternate Stress

1. Persons with hearing loss are led in a group discussion that focuses on common situations where persons with hearing loss may experience stress related to communication difficulties, and instructed on how to recognize situations in which they personally experience stress due to hearing loss.
2. Typical psychological and physical reactions to stressful situations are described, and discussion focuses on how to recognize personal, psychological, and physical reactions to the situations.
3. Within the group setting, participants are oriented to, and role-play the use of specific strategies to manage stressful situations.
4. Relaxation techniques for coping with psychological and physical reactions to stressful situations are described and practiced.

rehabilitation as it provides a view of how stigma may occur from the perspective of the person who is stigmatized. Audiologists are likely to benefit from having a comprehensive description of the stigma creation process, as well as an outline of the reactions that people may have as a result of the stress induced from an identity threat. This model constitutes a valuable component of a cognitive approach to information counseling that addresses stigma with clients who perceive themselves as being stigmatized in some situations. A description of the model may even be included in general information courses (e.g., group communication strategies programs) designed to increase the awareness of the effects of hearing loss. People who may not be conscious of (or who deny) that they experience identity threat may benefit from this information by being able to identify the source of stress they experience in specific situations. Furthermore, this information may provide the impetus to reflect upon the types of coping strategies (and the effectiveness of the strategies) used in those situations. Similarly, a description of the model could be incorporated into individual intervention programs for people who are susceptible to experience identity threats when participating in certain activities. The model would also be a valuable component of information courses designed for family members and health care professionals.

A close examination of the stigma-induced identity threat model also provides useful guidelines for the design of intervention programs. The heart of this model (conceptually as well as physically as represented by the block diagram in Figure 4–3) is characterized by the stress that is induced by an identity threat. Logically, an intervention program would be considered successful if it managed to reduce the stress level experienced by the client. Thus, any rehabilitation program component designed to reduce stress would be useful for people who perceive an identity threat associated with their hearing loss. Trychin's (1986, 2003e), "Relaxation Training for Hard of Hearing People" manual and videotape provide useful examples of physical responses to distressing situations, how to identify distressing situations and reactions, the effects of muscle tension and anxiety on understanding, and training in the use of proper breathing and in the relaxation of various muscle groups.

Using the stigma-induced identity threat model as a guide, stress reduction can be achieved in two primary ways. First, a person's level of stress will be reduced if the identity threat is diminished. According to the model, the level of identity threat perceived is determined by an interaction of the three major constructs depicted at the front-end of the model, namely: collective representations, situational cues, and personal characteristics. Consequently, intervention programs that address one (or a combination) of those constructs may have an impact on the level of identity threat perceived. It is possible to address all three constructs. For instance, the intensity of the prejudicial attitudes or discriminatory behaviors associated with hearing loss may vary across subgroups of societies. For example, friends or acquaintances that one meets regularly at the local bar may hold stronger prejudicial views of hearing loss ('deafness') than would colleagues at work. Or, a spouse may be more sensitive to the effects of stigma than the regular clients at the local bar. Disclosing hearing loss or attempting to use new coping strategies may be a more effective approach in the presence of some people than others. Trychin's workbooks provide a variety of activities that can be used in training strategies for disclosing hearing loss (Trychin, 2003a, 2003b, 2003c, 2003d). Similarly, personal identity threat will vary according to the situation (e.g., the physical setting or the social context). Again, some situations may offer a more secure environment to apply newly learned coping strategies. Given that the level of identity threat perceived by a person will be influenced by the situation and the other people involved in that situation, it is likely that a solution-centered problem solving approach to rehabilitation (Gagné & Jennings, 2008) could be successfully used as an intervention strategy to overcome appraised identity threats.

According to the stigma-induced identity threat model, the characteristics of the person with hearing loss will also influence the level of identity threat perceived. From that perspective it is likely that a cognitive-behavioral approach to intervention as described above could be used to reduce the level of identity threat perceived. Recently, intervention programs based on the principles of Perceived Self-Efficacy (PSE) have been promoted as an approach to the rehabilitation of people with hearing loss (Jennings, 2005; Smith & West, 2006). A priori it would appear that the underlying principles of Perceived Self-Efficacy (PSE) are consistent with rehabilitation services designed to reduce perceived identity threat. Human functioning is viewed as the result of behavioral, cognitive, and other personal factors, and events in the environment. Each of these factors works together, but has different levels of influence depending on the specific situation, the specific environment, and the individuals themselves (Bandura, 1986). PSE refers to a person's belief in his or her ability to organize and execute courses of action that are required to manage prospective situations (Bandura, 1995). The aim of a PSE-based rehabilitation program is to increase participants' levels of PSE, using specifically designed approaches including: enactive mastery, vicarious experiences, verbal persuasion, and somatic and emotional states. Related to the model of stigma-induced identity threat, if the person has high levels of PSE, it is likely that the perceived demands of a relevant situation will not be appraised as exceeding his or her resources. On the other hand, for persons with low levels of PSE, it is likely that perceived demands of a relevant situation will be appraised as exceeding their resources, and a stigma-induced identity threat will result. PSE level will have an impact on volitional responses (i.e., problem-focused and emotion-focused coping strategies) as well as nonvolitional responses (i.e., arousal and increased blood pressure). For example, people with high PSE who have learned to identify their nonvolitional responses such as arousal and increased blood pressure are better able to interpret these responses as a "call to action." Thus, they are better prepared to use coping techniques to control the escalation of nonvolitional responses

Our interpretation of the stigma-induced identity threat model suggests that a person's level of stress will be reduced with carefully selected coping strategies. As outlined above, several rehabilitation programs are designed to teach clients how to use effective coping strategies (e.g., Jennings, 1993; Trychin, 1986; Tye-Murray, 2002; Wayner & Abrahamson, 1996). Communication training programs that promote and teach the use of anticipatory strategies, that emphasize assertive behaviors and the use of effective conversational strategies should also serve to reduce an individual's stress level (Heydebrand, Mauze, Tye-Murray, Binzer, & Skinner, 2005). Obviously, if someone who has a hearing loss learns appropriate conversational skills, the likelihood of communication breakdowns will decrease. If so, the stigma related stress associated with being an inadequate communication partner should also diminish. Similarly, the use of hearing aids (when appropriate) as well as other HATs (when called for) should reduce the probability of communication breakdowns and improve one's ability to participate in social activities (see Vignette 4–5).

The challenge for the audiologist is to persuade the person with hearing loss (whose self-esteem may be low, and whose social identity may be threatened) to actively participate in a rehabilitation program that calls for overt behavior change, such as the use of amplification devices, behavioral coping strategies, and expressive communication strategies. In our experience, it may be difficult to convince people who perceive themselves as being stigmatized, to use any strategy that entails the disclosure of hearing loss. However, people are more likely to agree to freely disclose their hearing loss if the strategies are believed to be effective in reducing the level of stress they experience in a given situation. It is our contention that it may be beneficial to adopt a cognitive-behavioral approach when designing rehabilitation programs that address social identity threats. The components of such an AR program are outlined in Table 4–2.

Table 4–2. Components of an Audiologic Rehabilitation Program Designed to Address Identity Threat

1. Describe and discuss the stigma-induced identity threat model to explain to the client the causes, consequences and the potential costs of the stress related to identity threat.
2. Establish a hierarchy of situations in which identity threat occurs.
3. Discuss, in parallel, the effectiveness of the client's typical coping strategies. Retain the strategies that are most appropriate or promising, and introduce new adaptive strategies.
4. Implement a problem-solving approach to address a situation of stigma-inducing identity threat identified by the client.
5. Train and encourage the client to apply the selected coping strategies in a secure environment (initially, implementing the strategies may be practiced during the therapy session).
6. Meet with the client to discuss the process of implementing and the consequences of applying the strategies (perhaps using the diagram of the model to identify the key elements).
7. Attempt a similar experience in a slightly more threatening situation/environment.
8. Increase the number of situations in which the client discloses his or her hearing loss and applies appropriate coping strategies, accompanied by reinforcing feedback rehabilitation sessions.

The use of appropriate strategies and the reinforcement obtained from the successful outcomes experienced should reduce the identity threat stress perceived in different settings. If this occurs, we would consider the rehabilitation program to be successful.

The stigma-induced identity threat model is consistent with the normalization process described by Hétu (1996). In the initial stage of Hétu's model (see Figure 4–2A), meeting other individuals who have a hearing loss serves to reduce the client's level of perceived identity threat by providing the participants opportunities to use and discuss coping strategies in a highly secure/protective environment. First, the client is invited to use the coping strategies in a secure situation (a therapeutic setting, in the company of a hearing health care professional). Second, the collective representation of that environment (i.e., other people who have a hearing loss) is encouraging and supportive to the individual group members. In this situation, the level of perceived identity threat and the level of stress induced by the identity threat would be reduced. Relative to the stigma-induced identity threat model, the feedback mechanisms involved at this level of the stigma normalization process will serve to alter aspects of the personal characteristics of the client (i.e., more confidence, less shame, higher self-esteem, improved social image, better communication skills). In turn, this will favorably influence the level of identity threat that the client will perceive when the second stage of the stigma normalization process is implemented (i.e., when the client moves forward to real-world situation and when interactions occur with people who do not have hearing loss). In addition, any appropriate coping strategies learned during the first stage of the normalization process (e.g. communication strategies, assertive behaviors) increase the level of resources the person will have at his or her disposal. Thus, later during the second phase of the normalization process and beyond, when the client is placed in a situation in which an identity threat is perceived, there is an increased likelihood that self-evaluation of the situation will lead to the conclusion that he or she has sufficient resources to confront the stigmatizing situation.

Conclusion

Anecdotal clinical reports and research investigations have clearly demonstrated that the stigma associated with hearing loss constitutes a significant obstacle to rehabilitation for many individuals who have a hearing loss. Until now, little was known about the social stigma associated with hearing loss from the perspective of the people who are being stigmatized. During the last decade, mainly in the social sciences, significant inroads have been made to broaden our understanding of the processes involved in creating a threatened social identity. The goal of the present chapter was to describe one generic model of self-stigma, the stigma-induced identity threat model proposed by Major and O'Brien (2005), and to discuss its applications to hearing loss. As a first approximation, the model appears to provide a framework that can be used to understand the manifestation of stigma among people who have hearing loss. Furthermore, the model offers a conceptual framework concerning the types of AR services that could be provided to people with hearing loss who perceive an identity threat. Our goal was to introduce the stigma-induced identity threat model to the field of AR. Hopefully, the contents of the chapter will serve as an impetus for further discussions and research on the topic of stigma associated with hearing loss.

References

Allure Magazine. (January 2008) [online]. Retrieved January 2nd, 2008, from http://www.allure.com.

Andersson, G., & Willebrand, M. (2003). What is coping? A critical review of the construct and its application to audiology. *International Journal of Audiology, 42,* S97–S103.

Bandura, A. (1986). *Social foundations of thought and action: A social cognitive theory.* Englewood Cliffs, NJ: Prentice-Hall.

Bandura, A. (1995). *Self-efficacy in changing societies.* Cambridge, UK: Cambridge University Press.

Blood, I. M. (1997). The hearing aid effect: Challenges for counseling. *Journal of Rehabilitation, 63*(4), 59–62.

Brown, R. P., & Pinel, E. C. (2003). Stigma on my mind: Individual differences in the experience of stereotype threat. *Journal of Experimental Social Psychology, 39,* 626–633.

Corrigan, P. W., & Matthews, A. K. (2003). Stigma and disclosure: Implications for coming out of the closet. *Journal of Mental Health. Special Issue: Stigma, 12*(3), 235–248.

Corrigan, P. W., & Watson, A. C. (2002). The paradox of self-stigma and mental illness. *Clinical Psychology: Science and Practice, 9*(1), 35–53.

Corrigan, P. W., Watson, A. C., & Barr, L. (2006). The self-stigma of mental illness: Implications for self-esteem and self-efficacy. *Journal of Social and Clinical Psychology, 25*(9), 875–884.

Crocker, J. (1999). Social stigma and self-esteem: Situational construction of self-worth. *Journal of Experimental Social Psychology, 35*(1), 89–107.

Crocker, J., Major, B., & Steele, C. (1998). Social stigma. In D. T. Gilbert, S. T. Fiske, & G. Lindzey (Eds.), *The handbook of social psychology* (Vol. 2, 4th ed., pp. 504–553). New York: McGraw-Hill.

Doggett, S., Stein, R. L., & Gans, D. (1998). Hearing aid effect in older females. *Journal of the American Academy of Audiology, 9*(5), 361–366.

Erler, S. F., & Garstecki, D. C. (2002). Hearing loss- and hearing aid-related stigma: Perceptions of women with age-normal hearing. *American Journal of Audiology, 11*(2), 83–91.

Franks, J. R., & Beckmann, N. J. (1985). Rejection of hearing aids: Attitudes of a geriatric sample. *Ear and Hearing, 6*(3), 161–166.

Friedman, M., & Brownell, K. (1995). Psychological correlates of obesity: Moving to the next research generation. *Psychological Bulletin, 117*(1), 3–20.

Gagné, J.-P., & Jennings, M. B. (2008). Audiological rehabilitation intervention services for adults with an acquired hearing impairment. In M. Valente, H. Hosford-Dunn & R. J. Roeser (Eds.), *Audiology: Diagnosis, treatment strategies, and practice management* (2nd ed., pp. 547–579). New York: Thieme.

Gilhome Herbst, K. R., Meredith, R., & Stephens, S. D. (1990). Implications of hearing impairment for elderly people in London and in Wales. *Acta Oto-Laryngologica Supplement, 476,* 209–214.

Goffman, E. (1963). *Stigma: Notes on the management of spoiled identity*. Englewood Cliffs, NJ: Prentice-Hall.

Hallberg, L., & Carlsson, S. G. (1993). A qualitative study of situations turning a hearing disability into a handicap. *Disability, Handicap and Society, 8*(1), 71–86.

Hallberg, L. R., & Barrenas, M. L. (1995). Coping with noise-induced hearing loss: Experiences from the perspective of middle-aged male victims. *British Journal Audiology, 29*(4), 219–230.

Hallberg, L. R., & Jansson, G. (1996). Women with noise-induced hearing loss: An invisible group? *British Journal of Audiology, 30*, 340–345.

Herek, G. M. (1996). Why tell if you're not asked? Self-disclosure, intergroup contact, and heterosexuals' attitudes toward lesbians and gay men. In G. M. Herek, J. Jobe, & R. Carney (Eds.), *Out in force: Sexual orientation and the military* (pp 197–225). Chicago: University of Chicago Press.

Hetu, R. (1996). The stigma attached to hearing impairment. *Scandinavian Audiology Supplement, 43*, 12–24.

Hetu, R., Getty, L., & Waridel, S. (1994). Attitudes towards co-workers affected by occupational hearing loss. II: Focus groups interviews. *British Journal of Audiology, 28*(6), 313–325.

Hetu, R., Riverin, L., Getty, L., Lalande, N. M., & St-Cyr, C. (1990). The reluctance to acknowledge hearing difficulties among hearing-impaired workers. *British Journal of Audiology, 24*(4), 265–276.

Heydebrand, G., Mauze, E., Tye-Murray, N., Binzer, S., & Skinner, M. (2005). The efficacy of a structured group therapy intervention in improving communication and coping skills for adult cochlear implant recipients. *International Journal of Audiology, 44*(5), 272–280.

Jennings, M. B. (1993). *Audiologic rehabilitation curriculum series: Hearing help class 2. Coping with hearing loss*. Toronto: Canadian Hearing Society.

Jennings, M. B. (2005). *Factors that influence outcomes from aural rehabilitation of older adults: The role of perceived self-efficacy*, Unpublished doctoral dissertation, University of Western Ontario, London.

Joachim, G., & Acorn, S. (2000). Stigma of visible and invisible chronic conditions. *Journal of Advanced Nursing, 32*(1), 243–248.

Kochkin, S. (1993). MarkeTrak III: Why 20 million in US don't use hearing aids for their hearing loss. *Hearing Journal, 46*(1), 20–27.

Kochkin, S. (2007). Marke Trak VII: Obstacles to adult non-user adoption of hearing aids. *Hearing Journal, 60*(4), 24.

Kricos, P. B. (2000). The influence of nonaudiological variables on audiological rehabilitation outcomes. *Ear and Hearing, 21*(4 Suppl.), 7S–14S.

Kricos, P. B., Erdman, S., Bratt, G. W., & Williams, D. W. (2007). Psychosocial correlates of hearing aid adjustment. *Journal of the American Academy of Audiology, 18*(4), 304–322.

Lane, J. D., & Wegner, D. M. (1995). The cognitive consequences of secrecy. *Journal of Personality and Social Psychology, 69*(2), 237–253.

Lazarus, R. S., & Folkman, S. (1984). *Stress, appraisal, and coping*. New York: Springer.

Leary, M. R., Tambor, E. S., Terdal, S. K., & Downs, D. L. (1995). Self-esteem as an interpersonal monitor: The sociometer hypothesis. *Journal of Personality and Social Psychology, 68*, 518–530.

Lightsey, O. R., & Barnes, P. W. (2007). Discrimination, attributional tendencies, generalized self-efficacy, and assertiveness as predictors of psychological distress among African Americans. *Journal of Black Psychology, 33*(1), 27–50.

Link, B. G., & Phelan, J. C. (2001). Conceptualizing stigma. *Annual Review of Sociology, 27*, 363–385.

Link, B. G., & Phelan, J. C. (2006). Stigma and its public health implications. *Lancet, 367*(9509), 528–529.

Major, B. (2006). New perspectives on stigma and psychological well-being. In S. Levin & C. Van Laar (Eds.), *Stigma and group inequality: Social psychological perspectives* (pp. 193–210). Mahwah, NJ: Lawrence Erlbaum Associates.

Major, B., & Gramzow, R. H. (1999). Abortion as Stigma: Cognitive and emotional implications of concealment. *Journal of Personality and Social Psychology, 77*(4), 735–745.

Major, B., & O'Brien, L. T. (2005). The social psychology of stigma. *Annual Review of Psychology, 56*, 393–421.

McKechnie, J. (Ed.). (1976). *Webster's new twentieth century dictionary of the English language, unabridged: Based upon the broad foundations laid down by Noah Webster* (2nd ed.). Cleveland, IL: Collins World.

Miller, C. T., & Kaiser, C. R. (2001). A theoretical perspective on coping with stigma. *Journal of Social Issues. Special Issue: Stigma: An insider's perspective, 57*(1), 73–92.

Miller, C. T., & Major, B. (2000). Coping with stigma and prejudice. In T. F. Heatherton, R. E. Kleck, M. R. Hebl, & J. G. Hull (Eds.), *The social psychology of stigma* (pp. 243–272). New York: Guilford Press.

Oyserman, D., & Swim, J. K. (2001). Stigma: An insider's view. *Journal of Social Issues, 57*(1), 1–14.

Pachankis, J. E. (2007). The psychological implications of concealing a stigma: A cognitive-affective-behavioral model. *Psychological Bulletin, 133*(2), 328–345.

Pinel, E. C. (1999). Stigma consciousness: The psychological legacy of social stereotypes. *Journal of Personality and Social Psychology, 76*(1), 114–128.

Quinn, D. M. (2006). Concealable versus conspicuous stigmatized identities. In S. Levin & C. van Laar (Eds.), *Stigma and group inequality: Social psychological perspectives. The Claremont Symposium on Applied Social Psychology* (pp. 83–103). Mahwah, NJ: Lawrence Erlbaum Associates.

Roots, J. (1999). *The politics of visual language: Deafness, language choice, and political socialization*. Ottawa, Canada: Carleton University Press.

Smart, L., & Wegner, D. M. (1999). Covering up what can't be seen: Concealable stigma and mental control. *Journal of Personality and Social Psychology, 77*(3), 474–486.

Smart, L., & Wegner, D. M. (2000). The hidden costs of hidden stigma. In T. F. Heatherton, R. E. Kleck, M. R. Hebl, & J. G. Hull (Eds.), *The social psychology of stigma* (pp. 2220–2242). New York: Guilford Press.

Smith, C. (1991). The self, appraisal, and coping. In C. Snyder & D. Forsyth (Eds.), *Handbook of social and clinical psychology: The health perspective* (pp. 116–137). Elmsford, NY: Pergamon.

Smith, S. L., & West, R. L. (2006). The application of self-efficacy principles to audiologic rehabilitation: A tutorial. *American Journal of Audiology, 15*, 46–56.

Steele, C., & Aronson, J. (1995). Stereotype threat and the intellectual test performance of African Americans. *Journal of Personality and Social Psychology, 69*(5), 797–811.

Steele, C. M. (1997). A threat in the air: How stereotypes shape intellectual identity and performance. *American Psychologist, 52*(6), 613–629.

Steele, C. M., Spencer, S. J., & Aronson, J. (2002). Contending with group image: The psychology of stereotype and social identity threat. In M. P. Zanna (Ed.), *Advances in experimental social psychology* (Vol. 34, pp. 379–440). San Diego, CA: Academic Press.

Swim, J. K., & Thomas, M. A. (2006). Responding to everyday discrimination: A synthesis of research on goal-directed, self-regulatory coping behaviors. In S. Levin & C. van Laar (Eds.), *Stigma and group inequality: Social psychological perspectives* (pp. 105–126). Mahwah, NJ: Lawrence Erlbaum Associates.

Trychin, S. (1986). Relaxation training for hard of hearing people. *SHHH Journal, 7*(1), 12–13.

Trychin, S. (2003a). *Communication rules* (Rev. ed.). Erie, PA: Author.

Trychin, S. (2003b). *Did I do that?* (Rev ed.). Erie, PA: Author.

Trychin, S. (2003c). *Is that what you think?* (Rev. ed.). Erie, PA: Author.

Trychin, S. (2003d). *Living with hearing loss workbook* (2nd Rev. ed.). Erie, PA: Author.

Trychin, S. (2003e). *Relaxation training workbook* (Rev. ed.). Erie, PA: Author.

Tye-Murray, N. (2002). *Conversation made easy: Speechreading and conversation training for individuals who have hearing loss (adults and teenagers)*. St. Louis, MO: Central Institute for the Deaf.

Vauth, R., Kleim, B., Wirtz, M., & Corrigan, P. W. (2007). Self-efficacy and empowerment as outcomes of self-stigmatizing and coping in schizophrenia. *Psychiatry Research, 150*, 71–80.

Wayner, D. S., & Abrahamson, J. A. (1996). *Learning to hear again: An audiologic rehabilitation curriculum guide*. Austin, TX: Hearing Again.

Appendix 4-A
Beethoven's Heiligenstadt Testament (1802)

For my brothers Carl and [Johann] Beethoven

O you men who think or say that I am malevolent, stubborn or misanthropic, how greatly do you wrong me, you do not know the secret causes of my seeming, from childhood my heart and mind were disposed to the gentle feelings of good will, I was even ever eager to accomplish great deeds, but reflect now that for six years I have been a hopeless case, aggravated by senseless physicians, cheated year after year in the hope of improvement, finally compelled to face the prospect of a lasting malady (whose cure will take years or, perhaps, be impossible), born with an ardent and lively temperament, even susceptible to the diversions of society, *I was compelled early to isolate myself, to live in loneliness, when I at times tried to forget all this, O how harshly was I repulsed by the doubly sad experience of my bad hearing, and yet it was impossible for me to say to men speak louder, shout, for I am* deaf. *Ah how could I possibly admit such an infirmity in the one sense which should have been more perfect in me than in others,* a sense which I once possessed in highest perfection, a perfection such as few surely in my profession enjoy or have enjoyed—*O I cannot do it, therefore forgive me when you see me draw back when I would gladly mingle with you, my misfortune is doubly painful because it must lead to my being misunderstood, for me there can be no recreations in society of my fellows, refined intercourse, mutual exchange of thought, only just as little as the greatest needs command disposition, although I sometimes ran counter to it yielding to my inclination for society, but what a humiliation when one stood beside me and heard a flute in the distance and I heard nothing, or someone heard the shepherd singing and again I heard nothing, such incidents brought me to the verge of despair, but little more and I would have put an end to my life*—only art it was that withheld me, ah it seemed impossible to leave the world until I had produced all that I felt called upon me to produce, and so I endured this wretched existence—truly wretched, an excitable body which a sudden change can throw from the best into the worst state—Patience—it is said that I must now choose for my guide, I have done so, I hope my determination will remain firm to endure until it please the inexorable parcae to break the thread, perhaps I shall get better, perhaps not, I am prepared. Forced already in my 28th year to become a philosopher, O it is not easy, less easy for the artist than for anyone else—Divine One thou lookest into my inmost soul, thou knowest it, thou knowest that love of man and desire to do good live therein. O men, when some day you read these words, reflect that you did me wrong and let the unfortunate one comfort himself and find one of his kind who despite all obstacles of nature yet did all that was in his power to be accepted among worthy artists and men. *You my brothers Carl and [Johann] as soon as I am dead if Dr. Schmid is still alive ask him in my name to describe my malady and attach this document to the history of my illness so that so far as possible at least the world may become reconciled with me after my death.* At the same time I declare you two to be the heirs to my small fortune (if so it can be called), divide it fairly, bear with and help each other, what injury you have done me you know was long ago forgiven. To you brother Carl I give special thanks for the attachment you have displayed towards me of late. It is my wish that your lives be better and freer from care than I have had, recommend virtue to your children, it alone can give happiness, not money, I speak from experience, it was virtue that upheld me in misery, to it next to my art I owe the fact that I did not end my life with suicide.—Farewell and love each other—I thank all my friends, particularly Prince Lichnowsky and Professor Schmid—I desire that the instruments from Prince L. be preserved by one of you but let no quarrel result from this, so soon as they can serve you better purpose sell them, how glad will I be if I can still be helpful to you in my grave—with joy I hasten towards death—if it comes before I shall have had an opportunity to show all my artistic capacities it will still come too early for me despite my hard fate and I shall probably wish it had come later—but even then I am satisfied, will it not free me from my state of endless suffering? Come when thou will I shall meet thee bravely.—Farewell and do not wholly forget me when I am dead, I deserve this of you in having often in life thought of you how to make you happy, be so—

Heiligenstadt, October 6, 1802,
Ludwig van Beethoven

N.B.: The sections in italics were selected by the authors of the chapter. In their view, these sections illustrate well some key issues addressed in the chapter including: identity threat appraisals (i.e., self-stigma), concealment of hearing loss, and the effect of stigma on self-esteem, social isolation, and general health.

Source: Taken from http://www.lvbeethoven.com/Bio/BiographyHeiligenstadtTestament.html (with permission, 16-02-2008).

Part II

Building the AR Plan: Assessment and Verification

5

Self-Assessment in Adult Audiologic Rehabilitation

William Noble

Introduction

The inclusion of self-assessment in clinical research on hearing impairment has been in evidence since the time of a pioneering study by Thomas Barr, reported in a paper to the Philosophical Society of Glasgow in 1886, under the main title: *Enquiry into the Effects of Loud Sounds upon the Hearing of Boilermakers* (Barr, 1886). Barr was a physician who became increasingly interested in and concerned about the hearing problems he observed in those of his patients who worked in one of the noisiest trades then extant: ship's boilermaking. This trade involves hammers and red hot rivets banged flat to secure heavy metal plates to each other in the construction of part of a steamship's engine. The noise generated by this activity is excruciatingly loud, and the incidence of severe hearing impairment among people engaged in boilermaking and similar metalworking has been found to be high (cf. Atherley, Noble, & Sugden, 1967).

In addition to functional testing, Barr's *Enquiry* included a question to the workers about their ability to hear the speaker at a public meeting such as in a church or hall. This was a highly salient context, socially and politically, given that such public gatherings would be an important source of education and information at that time, before the advent of electronic media. Asking questions of patients, of course, springs naturally from the clinical interview. There are several other significant features about Barr's study, but including direct inquiry of these workers about their hearing ability in the everyday context of hearing in a public meeting probably represents the first time such self-reporting was systematically recorded. Barr documented the frequency of responses indicating the range of severity of effect due to hearing difficulty in that setting. Of 100 boilermakers he tested and interviewed, 21 said their difficulty in public meetings was so great they had stopped attending (these are men of average age 35 years); only 25 of the 100 said they did not have difficulty in this kind of listening situation.

Barr's study illustrates well the point that it is the responses of people at the level of what something means in their lives that is most telling about the significance of what is being investigated. Once stated, the foregoing sort of observation is self-evident. A phenomenon like hearing impairment would not *be* the subject of investigation if it did not have consequences in everyday life that people were aware of; however, scientific motives and efforts go beyond people's reports of problems to try to discover the causes of what has led to those problems. Such pursuit must look to measurable signs of dysfunction, with the goal of linking those signs (for example, reflected in diagnostic and performance tests of various kinds) to sites of physical injury, and a deepening of understanding of the mechanism that explains the problem. Thus, the reason for the common report of particular difficulty hearing in background noise, in the case of cochlear hearing injury, can be better understood when the mechanics of cochlear tuning and de-tuning are appreciated (Moore, 1995).

One consequence of investigation into mechanism is that it necessarily yields results independent of any report by the person affected. This sets up a contrast between such results and the record of the original complaint, with the person's own report understood as the "subjective" element; the diagnostic and physical signs as "objective." The terms "subjective" and "objective" carry value loadings in many areas of inquiry, with the first connoting "belief," "opinion," "bias"; the second connoting "evidence," "fact," "truth." Self-assessment, which is necessarily a key starting point in the study of any human ailment, is ever in the position of being perceived as a poor cousin in the family of measurement techniques.

These points are made simply to allow a reader to appreciate some of the conceptual baggage that the category of "self-assessment" carries. We return later to certain practicalities related to the subjectivity question. Enough to claim here that, at least in the context of adult audiologic rehabilitation (AR), it is as legitimate to maintain clinical and research attention to the features of what the person reports as it is to understand the mechanisms giving rise to the impairments that generate those reports. If it were the case that physical means to address impaired hearing, such as hearing aids, implants, or surgery, offered seamless restoration of normal listening, then the role of self-assessment probably would be slight. As that is often far from the case, appraisal of the experience of initial and residual hearing difficulties, and the effectiveness of interventions, is an integral part of rehabilitation planning and management. In the case of tinnitus, self-assessment can be argued to be at the core of such management, just because tinnitus is essentially a subjective phenomenon.

An overall point is that public and private health care providers are increasingly engaged in cost-benefit analysis; the subdiscipline of *health economics* has burgeoned in recent years (cf. Drummond, 2005). Whatever debates may continue about appropriate methodology, self-assessment is a necessary component of benefit estimation.

In the sections that follow, several topics are addressed, starting with general background issues, then going to practical and measurement questions, and a brief consideration of forms of self-assessment. The remainder of the chapter describes the several areas of adult AR in which self-assessment has been and continues to be applied.

Philosophical Issues

Self-Knowledge

A classic paper in psychology (Ericsson & Simon, 1980) argues for the appropriateness of what is often referred to in that discipline as "verbal reports." The issue is to do with what can be relied on from answers or statements respondents provide, in coming to scientific conclusions about some state of affairs. It would take this chapter too far astray to examine the issue in any detail. Nonetheless, given the point made in the preceding section about the "questioned" status of self-assessment, it is worth noting that the debate in psychology has stemmed from a larger one, broadly characterized as that between the behavioral versus cognitive traditions.

The behavioral approach relies on study of "objective" events (behaviors, performances). Part of the cognitive tradition is to extend study to more subjective conditions, such as thoughts and images, memories and narratives (Leahey, 2004). Self-assessment sits readily in the cognitive camp, and the point Ericsson and Simon make is that when people are asked to report about their actions or behavior, what they have to say is at least approximately as valid as what they are observed to do. Increased validity comes from obtaining a good sample of such reports. It is only if people are asked to speculate about *causes* of behavior (their own or other people's), that the ground shifts to what lawyers in a courtroom might describe as "leading the witness."

If validity is improved by increasing the sample of reports from a respondent, then one way to increase the validity of self-assessment of abilities is to pose questions covering a range of contexts, thus sampling a spectrum of conditions and allowing aggregate estimates of capacity. The question of this sort of sampling relates to the topic of "representativeness," and is considered in the section on *measurement issues*.

Definitions

As a way to instill standardization of nomenclature in relation to human disease and injury, the World Health Organization published a scheme for distinguishing *disorder*, *impairment*, *disability*, and *handicap* (1980). As regards loss of hearing, the categories *disorder* and *impairment* are very much in the province of physical and objective assessment—diagnostics, electroacoustic, electrophysiologic, and performance measures. The categories *disability* and *handicap* entail assessment of the person's experience, hence necessarily include self-assessment.

In the 1980 WHO scheme, the term *disability* referred to everyday consequences of impairments. Applied to hearing loss, this means that an *impairment*, as measured with a performance or electrophysiologic test, may give rise to reduced ability (*disability*), such as, to detect warning sounds in the everyday world, to follow spoken speech, or to distinguish the whereabouts of surrounding objects. These disabilities, in turn, contribute to *handicaps*—effects on the person's occupational, social, family and emotional life. As a taxonomy, WHO (1980) definitions apply very effectively to the experience of hearing impairment. *Note:* For additional information on the WHO Classifications, the reader is referred to Chapter 3 of this text.

WHO produced a later classification scheme (*International Classification of Functioning, Disability and Health*, 2001) in which the distinction is drawn between *activity limitation* and *participation restriction*. The first of these terms covers the same sort of ground as *disability*, but the second has the effect of removing focus on *personal-emotional* handicapping consequences of disability. In addition, whereas *disability* and *handicap* are distinct as definitional nodes, the new phrases, in English at least, are difficult to contrast. Hearing impairment can cause powerful emotional as well as social handicaps due to the disruption to ongoing interpersonal communication and environmental connection (Eriksson-Mangold & Carlsson, 1991). The argument following from this point (Noble, Tyler, Dunn, & Bhullar, 2008a) is that the new WHO scheme does not serve hearing impairment, as a form of disorder, as effectively as the original one. The categories of *disability* and *handicap*, as defined by WHO (1980), are relied on in this chapter.

Practical Issues

Literacy

The literacy level of respondents needs to be appreciated and questions designed to match. This point is almost self-evident, but it needs to be attended to in devising or selecting content and method of presentation of self-assessment material. For example, does the vocabulary of one's questions match general levels of understanding in the population of interest, or does it reflect specialist jargon? Is it safe to assume that respondents will be able enough in reading skill to handle questions in written form, versus being interviewed? Matters like these become more prominent if inquiry is directed to special populations (very young people, people with known cognitive deficits, people with limited formal education).

Relevance

Can respondents relate to what you are talking about? This is different from whether they can understand your questions in a semantic-expressive sense, and goes to whether the questions are meaningful in relation to the world at large. The matter of relevance relates to but is not the same as "representativeness" (next section) and is more to do with the authenticity of what's being asked. Does the question ring true, or does it seem contrived?

Reliability

Reliability is a central issue for all forms of assessment; in the self-assessment arena it relates to the *subjective-objective* contrast mentioned above. How much reliance can be placed on the answers people provide to the questions they are asked? As noted in the next section, on "measurement issues," there has developed a quasitechnical vocabulary in the area of psychological assessment, and the term *reliability*, in this technical sense, refers to aspects of the performance of the assessment device itself. But it is straightforward to also use the word to talk about the "performance" of respondents (it is, after all, their responses that go into any appraisal of the assessment tool). Reliability can be thought of in two senses: (1) Are people being wayward versus consistent in how they respond to questions; and (2) are they being accurate?

Consistency

Assuming people are motivated to respond to one's inquiries, it may be expected they will attend to the task of providing coherent answers. Inconsistency by an individual respondent (compared with the rest of a sample) possibly indicates this person's attention has strayed. Even so, it could be worth further inquiry of such an individual in case there are particular conditions that might explain the eccentric result. Inconsistency observed across a group of respondents does implicate the assessment device being used, suggesting the questions are not well designed, leading to lack of coherence in responses. This is where reliability in the technical sense comes into the picture.

Accuracy

This issue covers a spectrum, from reluctance/minimisation (Hétu, Riverin, Getty, Lalande, & St.-Cyr, 1990), to exaggeration (Trier & Levy, 1965), with the former more likely to be observed as a response in the context of rehabilitation. This is because not everyone who shows up at an audiology clinic is there willingly (Goldstein & Stephens, 1981); many (perhaps most) will be attending due to prompting by family members (van den Brink, Wit, Kempen, & Heuvelen, 1996; O'Mahoney, Stephens, & Cadge, 1996), peers, or supervisors, and some may not (or not yet) be prepared to acknowledge that there is a problem with their hearing sufficiently serious to disrupt family or other communication. Thus, they may rate their levels of disability lower than other family members or peers would, and there is likely to be a greater proportion of males in this sort of category (Garstecki & Erler, 1999). A question that might suggest itself in these circumstances is the weight to put on such self-assessment. This is imponderable unless it is somehow shown that the respondent knows they are providing too high an assessment of their ability.

This chapter is not the context for discussion of approaches to rehabilitation that may help accommodate the needs of people who are reluctant to acknowledge the problem, hence who are also unlikely to want to display signs of hearing impairment, such as through use of hearing aids. Alternative strategies to help overcome difficulties include programs like *Active Communication Education* (ACE) (Hickson, Worrall, & Scarinci, 2006, 2007). Such a program may be useful with the reluctant client, besides its usefulness across a range of other contexts. (*Note*: For additional information on the ACE, the reader is referred to Chapter 18 of this text.)

Awareness

Matters to consider under this heading are not unconnected with the foregoing point. If someone is not (yet) ready to acknowledge they have a hearing problem is this due to lack of awareness of the extent of their difficulty, or due to unwillingness to say they have a problem? The path from beginning signs of hearing impairment to ready acknowledgement of that circumstance is not straightforward, nor is it trodden without backtracks (Jones, Kyle, & Wood, 1987).

Awareness of experienced problems can also be influenced by the context of inquiry. As an example (Noble, 2008) the *Glasgow Hearing Aid Benefit Profile* (GHABP) (Gatehouse, 1999) is a self-assessment protocol derived from a set of listening contexts almost all of which are to do with hearing speech. The Profile was developed from responses made by hearing clinic clients at the time of consultation. From the point made above about family prompting to attend for rehabilitation, it is not improbable that speech communication would be at the forefront of everyone's consciousness in coming up with problem scenarios, since breakdown in such communication is chief among the handicaps experienced and reported by family members (Hétu, Lalonde, & Getty, 1987).

From the viewpoint of the individual, speech hearing may not be so predominant as an issue in the world at large. Eriksson-Mangold and Carlsson (1991) observed a link between self-rated spatial localization ability and indicators of somatic distress. Gatehouse and Noble (2004) found that critical links with social and emotional handicap lay in the domain of dynamic spatial hearing as well as that of complex conversational settings. These connections are observed when people are probed using questions about everyday spatial hearing ability, a somewhat obscure auditory function. Hence, compared with the self-evidently prominent place of conversational interaction, it remains moot whether people would be spontaneously aware of difficulties in locating and discriminating the movement of objects and people around them, though Barcham and Stephens (1980) found a nontrivial minority of people noted localization as a problem in response to an open-ended question about hearing difficulties.

All this leaves the issue of awareness as a genuinely interesting issue for proponents of self-assessment, and one of the grounds critics may use to maintain a "poor cousin" attitude to the methodology. Whether or not such an attitude prevails is, however, irrelevant; it is just the case that self-assessment is firmly part of the assessment spectrum, its utility is demonstrable in a number of clinical contexts, as the "areas of application" section demonstrates.

Measurement Issues

There is a large literature on technical matters in the area of *psychometrics*; interested readers can browse accessible texts such as by Shum and colleagues (Shum, O'Gorman, & Myors, 2006). A recent paper (Hyde, 2000) illustrates the application of the principles of psychometrics to the audiological rehabilitation field. Mention was made earlier about the centrality of *reliability* to self-assessment test construction. Another central concept is *validity*, which refers to ways of determining what a given measure claims to be assessing. Here, two different matters are considered, bearing on the broader question of the appropriateness (hence, the value) of what is being assessed, both to the person providing the self-assessment and to the clinical or research endeavor.

Representativeness

Auditory reality (Noble, 2008) represents the gamut of circumstances that constitute anyone's auditory life. It incorporates the typical environments an individual creates, occupies and is otherwise exposed to, but goes beyond that to include the condition and changing condition of the receptor system the individual operates with. As noted before, the matter of the relevance of a self-assessment protocol is linked to the representativeness of what is being appraised. If what you are assessing is not representative of respondents' "auditory reality" then it will not be relevant to them either; equally, not all of what is representative of auditory reality, in the clinical or research sense, may be immediately relevant in the judgement of the respondent. But as long as it is representative, they will be able to make a coherent response.

The interplay between representativeness and relevance may be seen in the observation of increased level of hearing impairment with increasing age but accompanied by reduced self-rating of disability (Gatehouse, 1991, 1994). This, at first, counter-intuitive pattern of connection, is plausibly explained by the prospect that as people get older and their hearing ability progressively declines, they are increasingly likely to shrink their circle of personal and social activity, and hence reduce the typical range of auditory challenges they face. This picture is supported by findings of Erdman and Demorest (1998), based on responses to the Communication Environment subscales of the *Communication Profile for the Hearing Impaired* (CPHI) (Demorest & Erdman, 1987). Thus, the range of questions that may be representative of the auditory reality of someone younger may not fit that of someone much older. This would not be to argue, a priori, therefore, that disability level declines with increasing age, but that more representative forms of inquiry are needed to determine what may be the significant areas of hearing disability as age increases.

Usefulness

Not unrelated, then, is the question: Are your assessments providing you with information that is valuable for your clinical and/or research concerns? And will these assessments be of value, ultimately, for respondents? Do inquiries about disabilities and handicaps get to significant issues in the lives of people with impaired hearing, such that useful directions are opened up for improved service provision? Some of this sort of theme comes through in considering the "areas of application" of self-assessment.

Forms of Self-Assessment

A fairly natural progression suggests itself from a baseline of the clinical interview, through to open-ended inquiry among members of populations of research or clinical interest. Group sessions may be valuable in prompting people to respond in the light of others' reported experiences. This step is worthwhile when inquiry is going to areas previously unexplored, but with likely personal or social salience for people in the target population. Interviews with individuals, leading to successive iterations of how questionnaire items are expressed, is essential in order to maximize the chance that items will be intelligible across the spectrum of intended respondents. With due regard to the known characteristics of target populations, self-administered assessment can be relied on once the forms of items have been proven in the interview setting.

Areas of Application

The primary area of application of self-assessment, not unnaturally, is in appraisal of the efficacy of hearing prosthetics. A broader survey of self-assessment (Noble, 1998) analysed the range of assessment devices available to that date and described the main areas of application, including that of hearing devices. Subsequent, briefer reviews (Cox, 2003; Noble, 2004) have focused on the hearing aid domain. Following is an outline of areas in which self-assessment has been employed in recent years, with particular findings noted as considered appropriate. This does not aim to be an exhaustive review; rather, its purpose is to inform the reader about what is happening in the self-assessment sector of the rehabilitation field, and to give an appreciation of the range of applications of the method.

Acoustic Hearing Aids

Residual Disability and Handicap

The efficacy of hearing aid provision has been the subject of longitudinal investigation (Humes & Wilson, 2003; Humes, Wilson, Barlow, & Garner, 2002), with very clear signs of immediate benefit in performance and self-assessed terms, but with no sign of further benefit in the long term. Indeed, indications were mainly of a stable outcome over a 2 to 3-year period, postfit, with signs of increasing self-rated difficulty after 6 months of use. One measure included in these studies, the *Hearing Handicap Inventory for the Elderly* (Ventry & Weinstein, 1982), has been found independently (Taylor, 1993) to exhibit the above pattern over time. In a long-term (5–6 years) follow-up study (Kricos, Erdman, Bratt, & Williams, 2007), among VA clients, positive changes in (CPHI) ratings were reported among continuing users of hearing aids. Whereas the sample in the Humes et al. studies was managed in ways typically found in a hearing clinic, the VA clients were exposed ongoingly to advice and clinical supervision. This difference might account for the stronger long-term outcome in that study.

The above studies were conducted among relatively economically advantaged groups in the United States. Effective outcomes have also been reported among elderly Hong Kong Chinese residents (McPherson & Wong, 2005) fit with a single low-cost over-the-counter hearing aid, and followed up after three months in terms of real-ear gain and a range of self-assessment scales—the *Profile of Hearing Aid Performance* (PHAP) (Cox & Gilmore, 1990); the *Client-Oriented Scale of Improvement* (COSI) (Dillon, James, & Ginis, 1997), and the *International Outcome Inventory for Hearing Aids* (IOI-HA) (Cox et al., 2000).

Comparative Device/Fitting Performance

Linear/Nonlinear

Several major studies have compared linear versus nonlinear hearing aids. Humes et al. (1999) confirmed that both types of device offered significant benefit, assessed in both performance and self-rated terms, the latter assessment using the *Hearing Aid Performance Inventory* (HAPI) (Walden, Demorest, & Hepler, 1984). The nonlinear devices showed greater performance advantage, and better rated quality, but not in terms of self-assessed performance. A somewhat similar outcome is reported by Wood and Lutman (2004), using the *Abbreviated Profile of Hearing Aid Benefit* (APHAB) (Cox & Alexander, 1995), and the GHABP.

A project by Gatehouse and colleagues (Gatehouse, Naylor, & Elberling, 2006a, 2006b) used a mixture of performance and self-assessment methods, and throws useful light on the circumstances that might lead to linear versus nonlinear profiles being preferred and/or advantageous. This work demonstrates interactions between type of fitting (including varieties of nonlinear fittings), cognitive function, and the nature of different listening environments, showing that no one fitting style wins out across listeners and contexts.

Prefit Testing

One contrast in fitting included protocols that did or did not involve speech-in-noise and LDL testing at the time of initial fit (Shi, Doherty, Kordas, & Pellegrino, 2007), and outcome assessment using the APHAB as well as the *Satisfaction with Amplification in Daily Life* scale (SADL) (Cox & Alexander, 1999). Fewer postfit adjustments were needed in the group in whom loudness and speech-in-noise testing had been conducted, and SADL scores declined after a few months in the group that had not been exposed to such testing.

Microphone Directionality

Self-assessment has featured in comparisons of directional versus omnidirectional microphone technology (Kühnel, Margolf-Hacki, & Kiessling, 2001; Ricketts, Henry, & Gnewikow, 2003). Kühnel and colleagues included the *Oldenburg Inventory* in their assessment protocol (Holube & Kollmeier, 1991), and Ricketts and colleagues used the *Profile of Hearing Aid Benefit* (Cox, Gilmore, & Alexander, 1991). Kühnel and colleagues reported better speech-in-noise test performance and greater rated sound quality with the directional program (signal at 0°, noise at 180°). Ricketts et al. compared three listening conditions and found that the condition in which wearers could toggle between omnidirectional and directional (as against listening in only one or the other mode) was rated as more beneficial. They concluded that directionality may be advantageous in some everyday contexts, not in others. In a study involving a similar sort of design (Ruscetta, Palmer, Durrant, Grayhack, & Ryan, 2007), no differences were found in self-assessed localization disability and handicap, using a customized scale (Ruscetta, Palmer, Durrant, Grayhack, & Ryan, 2005), across the three listening conditions: directional, omnidirectional, and toggle between the two.

Unilateral/Bilateral

There have been several studies of the relative benefit of one versus two hearing aids that included self-assessment among the outcome measures, and these have been reviewed (Noble, 2006). The general conclusion is that two aids are likely to be preferred if the person has to function in complex listening environments, and/or as their hearing impairment becomes more noticeable. Noble and Gatehouse (2006) used the *Speech, Spatial, and Qualities of Hearing* scale (SSQ) (Gatehouse & Noble, 2004) to compare disability ratings in a sample not yet fit with hearing aids and in samples fit with one versus two aids. Substantial reductions in disability were observable with one hearing aid, largely in the conversational speech and hearing qualities domains. Bilateral fitting showed advantage especially over unaided or unilaterally aided conditions for monitoring dynamic spatial signals and for challenging (e.g., multiple speech stream) listening situations.

Moderators and Other Features of Outcomes

Aspects of personality (locus of control; extraversion) have been found to have a minor bearing on benefit as assessed with the APHAB (Cox, Alexander, & Gray, 1999). A comparison of two groups of clinic clients (Humes, Wilson, & Humes, 2003), who respectively retained or subsequently returned their hearing aids showed no difference in HHIE and CPHI scores; but the *retain* group tended to have better finger dexterity and higher LDLs than the *return* group. Somewhat similarly, a comparison of younger versus older clinic clients (Meister & von Wedel, 2003), controlling for hearing level, and including use of the *Gothenburg Profile* (Ringdahl, Eriksson-Mangold, & Andersson, 1998), found no differences between the two age groups, but the attribute of *handling* of the aid was significantly more important for the older group.

Bess (2000) drew attention to the fact that standard measures of overall *quality of life* (QoL) were insensitive to the often strongly beneficial effect of being fit with hearing aids. Standard QoL scales typically go to issues of self-care and mobility, and overlook interpersonal communication as providing quality in everyday living. Bess's point is confirmed in principle in a study (Joore, Brunenberg, Chenault, & Anteunis, 2003) that found no effect of first time hearing aid fitting on a generic QoL measure, but substantial effects in terms of disability reduction, using the *Amsterdam Inventory for Auditory Disability and Handicap* (Kramer, Kapteyn, Festen, & Tobi, 1995), and improvement in clients' prospects for paid employment. (*Note*: For further information on health-related quality of life, the reader is referred to Chapter 6 of this text.)

Implantable Hearing Devices

Cochlear Implants (CIs)

The major focus of attention over the last 20 to 30 years, in which multichannel cochlear implantation has become increasingly practiced, has been on speech test performance. With the emergence of bilateral implantation, and increasing incidence of a bimodal profile (CI with acoustic aid in the nonimplanted ear), clinical research interest has also extended to binaural function, including localization ability.

Robinson, Gatehouse, and Browning (1996) devised the *Glasgow Benefit Inventory* (GBI), which includes questions on such topics as self-confidence, embarrassment in company, future employment opportunities, and social restrictedness (what these authors called a *general* factor). As well there are questions about social/family support, and physical health, forming two separate factors. Robinson and colleagues applied the GBI to patients who had undergone a variety of otorhinolaryngologic procedures, including cochlear implantation, and observed very substantial improvements in the general factor, with no change in the health factor. This result was confirmed in a study (Vermeire et al., 2005) that included the *Hearing Handicap Inventory for Adults* (HHIA) (Newman, Weinstein, Jacobson, & Hug, 1990) as well as the GBI.

A related study (Mo, Lindbaek, & Harris, 2005) found that only one of eight subscales in a generic QoL measure showed significant change postimplantation, but that almost all of a range of more condition-specific benefit measures demonstrated evident improvement in patient QoL and in the QoL of family members. This outcome echoes that observed by Joore et al. (2003) in the case of hearing aids.

A longitudinal study of unilateral followed by bilateral implantation (Summerfield et al., 2006) used a generic and several, more condition-specific benefit measures. In line with the outcomes noted above, the generic QoL measure showed only modest beneficial change following unilateral implantation, whereas measures more closely oriented to QoL outcomes expected to flow from communication improvement showed much more substantial increases. Prior to and following the second implant, patients completed the SSQ (Gatehouse & Noble, 2004) and it was found that self-assessed spatial hearing showed particular further benefit from the second implant, with other qualities, speech scores and a condition-specific QoL measure showing lesser incremental benefit.

Two studies compared self-assessed handicap and disability in patients with one implant, those with two, and those with a bimodal profile, that is, a hearing aid in the nonimplanted ear (Noble, Tyler, Dunn, & Bhullar, 2008a, 2008b). Handicap was assessed with the HHIE and the *Hearing Handicap Questionnaire* (Gatehouse & Noble, 2004); disability was assessed using the SSQ. All three fitting profiles showed significant reductions in handicap, with the bilateral CI group having significantly greater reduction in social restriction. The bilateral group also showed consistently greater improvement in self-rated disabilities than the other profiles, significantly so for spatial hearing and aspects of other qualities. The bimodal profile showed less postimplant improvement than expected.

One study has reported comparative outcomes among implant versus acoustic hearing aid users (Mo, Lindbaek, Harris, & Rasmussen, 2004), applying the *Performance Inventory for Profound and Severe Loss* (PIPSL) (Owens & Raggio, 1988); both groups had severe-to-profound hearing impairment. The implant group generally scored higher than the acoustically aided group, although the poorest of the implant group were worse than the poorest of the aided group.

Bone-Anchored Hearing Aids

Used to provide more effective signal delivery in the case of conductive hearing loss, these implants have been found to significantly improve QoL as reflected in responses on the GHABP (McDermott, Dutt, Tziambazis, Reid, & Proops, 2002) and the GBI (Gillett, Fairley, Chandrashaker, Bean, & Gonzalez, 2006). In common with findings for acoustic hearing aids and cochlear implants, benefits are observed using measures that appraise in domains where QoL improvement can be expected, and not when applying a generic QoL assessment (Hol et al., 2004).

Middle-Ear Implants

Devices partly or wholly implanted in the middle ear have been developed as a treatment option for more moderate-to-severe hearing impairment, usually with other complications, making an acoustic aid of limited benefit. Such devices enable stronger signals with less distortion to be delivered directly via middle ear ossicles or the labyrinth. Self-assessments indicate substantial benefit compared with acoustic aids (Luetje et al., 2002). Devices that couple to the incus body have been shown to offer substantial improvements in performance and in terms of self-assessments using the *Gothenburg Profile* (Zenner et al., 2003; Zenner et al., 2004).

Screening

Hearing screening may be undertaken to identify general or particular (for example, at risk) adult population members who may benefit from service or hearing aid provision. Self-assessment has potential to make a useful contribution in this arena because it may provide adequate, highly cost-effective initial screen outcomes, leading to more thorough assessment of cases that fail such an initial screen. This has certainly been the experience over a number of different population-based investigations (Choi et al., 2005; Davis, Smith, Ferguson, Stephens, & Gianopoulos, 2007; Gomez, Hwang, Sobotova, Stark, & May, 2001). The American Speech-Language-Hearing Association guidelines (1997) for hearing screening recommend the use of self-assessment, specifically the HHIE-S (Ventry & Weinstein, 1983) or the Self-Assessment of Communication (SAC) (Schow & Nerbonne, 1982), in conjunction with pure-tone measurement for older adults.

Surgery

Various procedures have been practiced for decades with little or no involvement of patients, postoperatively, in appraisal of the outcome from the point of view of their ongoing abilities and QoL. In a retrospective study of unilateral stapedectomy cases (Lundman, Mendel, Bagger-Sjöbäck, & Rosenhall, 1999) it was found that the procedure had been successful in functional terms (closure of air-bone gap to within 20 dB), but that a high proportion of patients were left with poor outcomes in terms of imbalanced hearing, dizziness and unpleasant quality of hearing. Aspects of this finding were confirmed in a study that nonetheless also showed reasonable correlation between improved hearing level and reduction of handicap (Tan, Grolman, Tange, & Wytske, 2007).

Postoperative outcomes following reconstructive surgery (tympanoplasty) have been examined in terms of audiometric thresholds and a modified form of the *Amsterdam Inventory*. The results of this study (Korsten-Meijer, Wit, & Albers, 2006) showed that the major driver of improved self-assessment was the degree of contrast between pre and post-operative threshold, rather than post-operative threshold as such. Even small residual impairment levels (less than 25 dB HTL) were associated with self-assessment scores substantially below normal hearing standard.

Tinnitus

Tinnitus and self-assessment are very closely connected. This is because, by its nature as a phenomenon, tinnitus is personally and privately experienced. By way of contrast, the effect of hearing impairment is often first experienced by others, in the form of not getting a response or getting an erroneous one from the person whose hearing is declining (see the discussion earlier about the family experience of handicap due to a member having impaired hearing). Hearing impairment can thus be characterized as "socially distributed." Tinnitus is experienced by others only as complained of by the person suffering with it (Noble & Tyler, 2007); it is essentially subjective.

Three phases of investigation of tinnitus can be distinguished, as reflected in different topics for self-assessment (Noble, 2001). In the first phase, the direct effects of the disorder were studied—the disabilities and handicaps due to chronic tinnitus: cognitive and emotional distress; sleep disturbance (see also Hébert & Carrier, 2007); bodily distress; intrusiveness; effects on hearing. Two scales remain as standards of this era: the *Tinnitus Effects Questionnaire* (TEQ) (Jakes, Rachman, & Hinchcliffe, 1986b), and the *Tinnitus Handicap Questionnaire* (THQ) (Kuk, Tyler, Russell, & Jordan, 1990), the measurement properties of which have been broadly confirmed by independent research (Henry & Wilson, 1998).

This initial phase of self-assessment addressed the direct effects of tinnitus, the expectation being that one or more physical intervention (for example, use of masking noise, or a drug regime) could work to reduce the severity of the condition. As it has become clearer that most cases of tinnitus are not susceptible to physical cure, the second phase can be described as giving focus to the individual's reactions to tinnitus. Thus, if tinnitus cannot be cured, perhaps suffering can be reduced with appropriate forms of counselling or psychotherapy. The *Tinnitus Reaction Questionnaire* (TRQ) (Wilson, Henry, Bowen, & Haralambous, 1991) was devised specifically to assess individual responses to the experience of tinnitus, as a step on the path to developing ways to help people cope more effectively with the condition. This questionnaire remains the standard for assessment of distress, avoidant behaviors, and level of occupational/social intrusion due to tinnitus. Similar in content to the TRQ and aspects of the THQ is the *Tinnitus Handicap Inventory* (Newman, Jacobson, & Spitzer, 1996).

The third self-assessment phase focuses specifically on coping styles, with the development of two scales: the *Tinnitus Coping Style Questionnaire* (TCSQ) (Budd & Pugh, 1996a, 1996b) and the *Tinnitus Cognitions Questionnaire* (TCQ) (Wilson & Henry, 1998). These were independently derived and the studies undertaken to develop the respective assessment devices converge on the conclusion that a maladaptive coping style correlates with degree of annoyance and intrusiveness of tinnitus.

In the final analysis, it is probably the case that tinnitus is in a substantially different category from the other rehabilitation arenas considered in this chapter. Although tinnitus is evidently a disorder of hearing, and can cause problems directly for listening to wanted signals, such as speech or music (Tyler & Baker, 1983), the principal issues are more in the realm of psychological distress (heightened anxiety and depression, for example), and disturbances to sleep, concentration, and relaxation. Thus, tinnitus is probably best thought of as a somatopsychic as much as a hearing disorder (McKenna, 2004)—a physical phenomenon with potential to cause (or exacerbate) psychological problems. In this sort of situation, for more intractable cases of distress due to chronic tinnitus suffering, rehabilitation requires combining the skills of clinical audiology and clinical psychology (Noble & Tyler, 2007; Wilson, Henry, Andersson, Hallam, & Lindberg, 1998). This entails extending the range of self-assessments to include measures of psychological well-being in addition to measures specific to tinnitus distress or coping.

Summary and Conclusions

Self-assessment is used across a wide range of rehabilitation contexts, from acoustic hearing aid provision to any of several implant devices and profiles. Self-assessment appears to be a very valuable tool for special or general population screening purposes. It is now routinely relied on, along with appropriate performance measures, to appraise the outcome of different surgical and medical procedures, and it is central to management of tinnitus distress.

There is an evident problem regarding the position of generic Quality of Life assessments and the benefits of clinical hearing management. Generic measures appear to be insensitive to the beneficial impacts on QoL that flow from effective prosthesis fitting, implanting, surgery or psychotherapy. Improved societal recognition of the significant contribution of effective impaired hearing management and treatment will follow from development of a QoL measure that is recognized as valid within the community at large, and which properly reflects the value added to QoL of improved communication ability. Such a development, in turn, will increase the use made of hearing services within the community.

References

American Speech-Language-Hearing Association. (1997). *Guidelines for Audiologic Screening* [Guidelines]. Available from www.asha.org/policy.

Atherley, G. R. C., Noble, W., & Sugden, D. B. (1967). Foundry noise and hearing in foundrymen. *Annals of Occupational Hygiene, 10*, 255–261.

Barcham, L. J., & Stephens, S. D. G. (1980). The use of an open-ended problems questionnaire in auditory rehabilitation. *British Journal of Audiology, 14*(2), 49–54.

Barr, T. (1886). Enquiry into the effects of loud sounds upon the hearing of boilermakers and others who work amid noisy surroundings. *Proceedings of the Philosophical Society of Glasgow, 17*, 223–239.

Bess, F. H. (2000). The role of generic health-related quality of life measures in establishing audiological rehabilitation outcomes. *Ear and Hearing, 21*(Suppl. 4), 74S–79S.

Budd, R. J., & Pugh, R. (1996a). The relationship between coping style, tinnitus severity and emotional distress in a group of tinnitus sufferers. *British Journal of Health Psychology, 1*, 219–229.

Budd, R. J., & Pugh, R. (1996b). Tinnitus coping style and its relationship to tinnitus severity and emotional distress. *Journal of Psychosomatic Research, 41*(4), 327–335.

Choi, S.-W., Peek-Asa, C., Zwerling, C., Sprince, N. L., Rautiainen, R. H., Whitten, P. S., et al. (2005). A comparison of self-reported and pure tone threshold average in the Iowa Farm Family Health and Hazard study. *Journal of Agromedicine, 10*(3), 31–39.

Cox, R. M. (2003). Assessment of subjective outcome of hearing aid fitting: Getting the client's point of view. *International Journal of Audiology, 42*(Suppl. 1), 90S–96S.

Cox, R. M., & Alexander, G. C. (1995). The abbreviated profile of hearing aid benefit. *Ear and Hearing, 16*(2), 176–186.

Cox, R. M., & Alexander, G. C. (1999). Measuring satisfaction with amplification in daily life: The SADL scale. *Ear and Hearing, 20*(4), 306–320.

Cox, R. M., Alexander, G. C., & Gray, G. (1999). Personality and the subjective assessment of hearing aids. *Journal of the American Academy of Audiology, 10*, 1–13.

Cox, R. M., & Gilmore, C. (1990). Development of the profile of hearing aid performance (PHAP). *Journal of Speech and Hearing Research, 33*, 343–355.

Cox, R. M., Gilmore, C., & Alexander, G. C. (1991). Comparison of two questionnaires for patient-assessed hearing aid benefit. *Journal of the American Academy of Audiology, 2*, 134–145.

Cox, R. M., Hyde, M., Gatehouse, S., Noble, W., Dillon, H., Bentler, R., et al. (2000). Optimal outcome measures, research priorities, and international cooperation. *Ear and Hearing, 21*, 106S–115S.

Davis, A., Smith, P., Ferguson, M., Stephens, D., & Gianopoulos, I. (2007). Acceptability, benefit and costs of early screening for hearing disability: A study of potential. *Health Technology Assessment, 11*(42), 1–294.

Demorest, M. E., & Erdman, S. A. (1987). Development of the Communication Profile for the Hearing Impaired. *Journal of Speech and Hearing Disorders, 52*, 129–143.

Dillon, H., James, A., & Ginis, J. (1997). Client-Oriented Scale of Improvement (COSI) and its relationship to several other measures of benefit and satisfaction provided by hearing aids. *Journal of the American Academy of Audiology, 8*(1), 27–43.

Drummond, M. F. (2005). *Methods for the economic evaluation of health care programmes*. Oxford: Oxford University Press.

Erdman, S. A., & Demorest, M. E. (1998). Adjustment to hearing impairment II: Audiological and demographic correlates. *Journal of Speech, Language, and Hearing Research, 41*(1), 123–136.

Ericsson, K. A., & Simon, H. A. (1980). Verbal reports as data. *Psychological Review, 87*(3), 215–251.

Eriksson-Mangold, M., & Carlsson, S. G. (1991). Psychological and somatic distress in relation to perceived hearing disability, hearing handicap, and hearing measurements. *Journal of Psychosomatic Research, 35*(6), 729–740.

Garstecki, D. C., & Erler, S. F. (1999). Older adult performance on the Communication Profile for the Hearing Impaired: Gender difference. *Journal of Speech, Language, and Hearing Research, 42*(4), 785–796.

Gatehouse, S. (1991). The role of non-auditory factors in measured and self-reported disability. *Acta Oto-laryngologica*, (Suppl. 476), 249–256.

Gatehouse, S. (1994). Components and determinants of hearing aid benefit. *Ear and Hearing, 15*(1), 30–49.

Gatehouse, S. (1999). Glasgow Hearing Aid Benefit Profile: Derivation and validation of a client-centered outcome measure for hearing aid services. *Journal of the American Academy of Audiology, 10*, 80–103.

Gatehouse, S., Naylor, G., & Elberling, C. (2006a). Linear and nonlinear hearing aid fittings—1. Patterns of benefit. *International Journal of Audiology, 45*, 130–152.

Gatehouse, S., Naylor, G., & Elberling, C. (2006b). Linear and nonlinear hearing aid fittings—2. Patterns of candidature. *International Journal of Audiology, 45*, 153–171.

Gatehouse, S., & Noble, W. (2004). The Speech, Spatial and Qualities of Hearing Scale (SSQ). *International Journal of Audiology, 43*(1), 85–99.

Gillett, D., Fairley, J. W., Chandrashaker, T. S., Bean, A., & Gonzalez, J. (2006). Bone-anchored hearing aids: Results of the first eight years of a programme in a district general hospital, assessed by the Glasgow benefit inventory. *Journal of Laryngology and Otology, 120*(7), 537–542.

Goldstein, D. P., & Stephens, S. D. G. (1981). Audiological rehabilitation: Management model I. *Audiology, 20*, 432–452.

Gomez, M. I., Hwang, S.-A., Sobotova, L., Stark, A. D., & May, J. J. (2001). A comparison of self-reported hearing loss and audiometry in a cohort of New York farmers. *Journal of Speech, Language, and Hearing Research, 44*(6), 1201–1207.

Hébert, S., & Carrier, J. (2007). Sleep complaints in elderly tinnitus patients: A controlled study. *Ear and Hearing, 28*(5), 649–655.

Henry, J. L., & Wilson, P. H. (1998). The psychometric properties of two measures of tinnitus complaint and handicap. *International Tinnitus Journal, 4*(2), 114–121.

Hétu, R., Lalonde, M., & Getty, L. (1987). Psychosocial disadvantages associated with occupational hearing loss as experienced in the family. *Audiology, 26*, 141–152.

Hétu, R., Riverin, L., Getty, L., Lalande, N., & St.-Cyr, C. (1990). The reluctance to acknowledge hearing problems among noise exposed workers. *British Journal of Audiology, 24*, 265–276.

Hickson, L., Worrall, L., & Scarinci, N. (2006). Measuring outcomes of a communication program for older people with hearing impairment using the International Outcome Inventory. *International Journal of Audiology, 45*(4), 238–246.

Hickson, L., Worrall, L., & Scarinci, N. (2007). A randomized controlled trial evaluating the active communication education program for older people with hearing impairment. *Ear and Hearing, 28*(2), 212–230.

Hol, M. K. S., Spath, M. A., Krabbe, P. F. M., van der Pouw, C. T. M., Snik, A. F. M., Cremers, C. W. R. J., et al. (2004). The bone-anchored hearing aid—Quality-of-life assessment. *Archives of Otolaryngology-Head and Neck Surgery, 130*(4), 394–399.

Holube, I., & Kollmeier, B. (1991). Ein fragebogen zur erfassung des subjectiven hörvermögens: Erstellung der fragen und beziehung zum tonschwellen-audiogramm. *Audiologische Akustik, 2*, 48–64.

Humes, L. E., Christensen, L., Thomas, T., Bess, F. H., Hedley-Williams, A., & Bentler, R. (1999). A comparison of the aided performance and benefit provided by a linear and a two-channel wide dynamic range compression hearing aid. *Journal of Speech, Language, and Hearing Research, 42*(1), 65–79.

Humes, L. E., & Wilson, D. L. (2003). An examination of changes in hearing-aid performance and benefit in the elderly over a 3-year period of hearing-aid use. *Journal of Speech, Language, and Hearing Research, 46*(1), 137–145.

Humes, L. E., Wilson, D. L., Barlow, N. N., & Garner, C. B. (2002). Changes in hearing-aid benefit following 1 or 2 years of hearing-aid use by older adults. *Journal of Speech, Language, and Hearing Research, 45*(4), 772–782.

Humes, L. E., Wilson, D. L., & Humes, A. C. (2003). Examination of differences between successful and unsuccessful elderly hearing aid candidates matched for age, hearing loss and gender. *International Journal of Audiology, 42*(7), 432–441.

Hyde, M. L. (2000). Reasonable psychometric standards for self-report outcome measures in audiological rehabilitation. *Ear and Hearing, 21*(4), 24S–36S.

International Classification of Impairments, Disabilities, and Handicaps. (1980). Geneva: World Health Organization.

International Classification of Functioning, Disability, and Health. (2001). Geneva, Switzerland: World Health Organization.

Jakes, S. C., Hallam, R. S., Rachman, S., & Hinchcliffe, R. (1986b). The effects of reassurance, relaxation training and distraction on chronic tinnitus sufferers. *Behavioral Research and Therapy*, *24*(5), 497–507.

Jones, L., Kyle, J., & Wood, P. (1987). *Words apart: Losing your hearing as an adult*. London: Tavistock.

Joore, M. A., Brunenberg, D. E. M., Chenault, M. N., & Anteunis, L. J. C. (2003). Societal effects of hearing aid fitting among the moderately hearing impaired. *International Journal of Audiology*, *42*(3), 152–160.

Korsten-Meijer, A. G. W., Wit, H. P., & Albers, F. W. J. (2006). Evaluation of the relation between audiometric and psychometric measures of hearing after tympanoplasty. *European Archives of Otorhinolaryngology*, *263*, 256–262.

Kramer, S. E., Kapteyn, T. S., Festen, J. M., & Tobi, H. (1995). Factors in subjective hearing disability. *Audiology*, *34*, 311–320.

Kricos, P. B., Erdman, S. A., Bratt, G. W., & Williams, D. W. (2007). Psychosocial correlates of hearing aid adjustment. *Journal of the American Academy of Audiology*, *18*, 304–322.

Kühnel, V., Margolf-Hacki, S., & Kiessling, J. (2001). Multi-microphone technology for severe-to-profound hearing loss. *Scandinavian Audiology*, *52*(Suppl.), 65–68.

Kuk, F. K., Tyler, R. S., Russell, D., & Jordan, H. (1990). The psychometric properties of a tinnitus handicap questionnaire. *Ear and Hearing*, *11*(6), 434–445.

Leahey, T. H. (2004). *A history of psychology: Main currents in psychological thought* (6th ed.). Upper Saddle River, NJ: Prentice-Hall.

Luetje, C. M., Brackman, D., Balkany, T. J., Maw, J., Baker, R. S., Kelsall, D., et al. (2002). Phase III clinical trial results with the Vibrant Soundbridge implantable middle ear hearing device: A prospective controlled multicenter study. *Otolaryngology-Head and Neck Surgery*, *126*(2), 97–107.

Lundman, L., Mendel, L., Bagger-Sjöbäck, D., & Rosenhall, U. (1999). Hearing in patients operated unilaterally for otosclerosis: Self-assessment of hearing and audiometric results. *Acta Oto-Laryngologica*, *119*(4), 453–458.

McDermott, A.-L., Dutt, S. N., Tziambazis, E., Reid, A. P., & Proops, D. W. (2002). Disability, handicap and benefit analysis with the bone-anchored hearing aid: The Glasgow Hearing Aid Benefit and Difference Profiles. *Journal of Laryngology and Otology*, *116*(Suppl. 28), 29–36.

McKenna, L. (2004). Models of tinnitus suffering and treatment compared and contrasted. *Audiological Medicine*, *2*, 1–14.

McPherson, B., & Wong, E. T. L. (2005). Effectiveness of an affordable hearing aid with elderly persons. *Disability and Rehabilitation*, *27*(11), 601–609.

Meister, H., & von Wedel, H. (2003). Demands on hearing aid features—special signal processin for elderly users? *International Journal of Audiology*, *42*(Suppl. 2), S58–S62.

Mo, B., Lindbaek, M., & Harris, S. (2005). Cochlear implants and quality of life: A prospective study. *Ear and Hearing*, *26*(2), 186–194.

Mo, B., Lindbaek, M., Harris, S., & Rasmussen, K. (2004). Social hearing measured with the Performance Inventory for Profound and Severe Loss: A comparison between adult multichannel cochlear implant patients and users of acoustical hearing aids. *International Journal of Audiology*, *43*(10), 572–578.

Moore, B. C. J. (1995). *Perceptual consequences of cochlear damage*. Oxford: Oxford University Press.

Newman, C. W., Jacobson, G. P., & Spitzer, J. B. (1996). Development of the tinnitus handicap inventory. *Archives of Otolaryngology-Head and Neck Surgery*, *122*, 143–148.

Newman, C. W., Weinstein, B. E., Jacobson, G. P., & Hug, G. A. (1990). The hearing handicap inventory for adults: Psychometric adequacy and audiometric correlates. *Ear and Hearing*, *11*(6), 430–433.

Noble, W. (1998). *Self-assessment of hearing and related functions*. London: Whurr.

Noble, W. (2001). Tinnitus self-assessment scales: Domains of coverage and psychometric properties. *Hearing Journal*, *54*(11), 20–25.

Noble, W. (2004). Hearing aid outcome measurement: Design issues and options in the self-assessment domain. *Zeitschrift für Audiologie*, *43*(1), 22–28.

Noble, W. (2006). Bilateral hearing aids: A review of self-reports of benefit in comparison with unilateral fitting. *International Journal of Audiology*, *45* (Suppl. 1), S63–S71.

Noble, W. (2008). Auditory reality and self-assessment of hearing. *Trends in Amplification, 12*, 113–120.

Noble, W., & Gatehouse, S. (2006). Effects of unilateral versus bilateral hearing aid fitting on disabilities as measured using the Speech, Spatial and Qualities of Hearing Scale (SSQ). *International Journal of Audiology, 45*, 172–181.

Noble, W., & Tyler, R. (2007). Physiology and phenomenology of tinnitus: Implications for treatment. *International Journal of Audiology, 46*, 569–574

Noble, W., Tyler, R. S., Dunn, C., & Bhullar, N. (2008a). Hearing handicap ratings among different profiles of adult cochlear implant users. *Ear and Hearing, 29*(1), 112–120.

Noble, W., Tyler, R. S., Dunn, C., & Bhullar, N. (2008b). Unilateral and bilateral cochlear implants and the implant-plus-hearing-aid profile: Comparing self-assessed and measured abilities. *International Journal of Audiology, 47*, 505–514.

O'Mahoney, C. F., Stephens, S. D. G., & Cadge, B. A. (1996). Who prompts patients to consult about hearing loss? *British Journal of Audiology, 30*, 153–158.

Owens, E., & Raggio, M. (1988). Performance inventory for profound and severe loss (PIPSL). *Journal of Speech and Hearing Disorders, 53*, 42–56.

Ricketts, T., Henry, P., & Gnewikow, D. (2003). Full time directional versus user selectable microphone modes in hearing aids. *Ear and Hearing, 24*(5), 424–439.

Ringdahl, A., Eriksson-Mangold, M., & Andersson, G. (1998). Psychometric evaluation of the Gothenburg Profile for measurement of experienced hearing disability and handicap: Applications with new hearing aid candidates and experienced hearing aid users. *British Journal of Audiology, 32*, 375–385.

Robinson, K., Gatehouse, S., & Browning, G. G. (1996). Measuring patient benefit from otorhinolaryngological surgery and therapy. *Annals of Otology, Rhinology, and Laryngology, 106*(6), 415–422.

Ruscetta, M. N., Palmer, C. V., Durrant, J. D., Grayhack, J., & Ryan, C. (2005). Validity, internal consistency, and test/retest reliability of a localization disabilities and handicaps questionnaire. *Journal of the American Academy of Audiology, 16*(8), 585–595.

Ruscetta, M. N., Palmer, C. V., Durrant, J. D., Grayhack, J., & Ryan, C. (2007). The impact of listening with directional microphone technology on self-perceived localization disabilities and handicaps. *Journal of the American Academy of Audiology, 18*(9), 794–808.

Schow, R. L., & Nerbonne, M. A. (1982). Communication Screening Profile: Use with elderly clients. *Ear and Hearing, 3*, 134–147.

Shi, L.-F., Doherty, K. A., Kordas, T. M., & Pellegrino, J. T. (2007). Short-term and long-term hearing aid benefit and user satisfaction: A comparison between two fitting profiles. *Journal of the American Academy of Audiology*, (18), 6.

Shum, D., O'Gorman, J., & Myors, B. (2006). *Psychological testing and assessment*. South Melbourne: Oxford University Press.

Summerfield, A. Q., Barton, G. R., Toner, J., McAnallen, C., Proops, D., Harries, C., et al. (2006). Self-reported benefits from successive bilateral cochlear implantation in postlingually deafened adults: Randomised controlled trial. *International Journal of Audiology, 45*(Suppl. 1), S99–S107.

Tan, F. M. L., Grolman, W., Tange, R. A., & Wytske, J. (2007). Quality of perceived sound after stapedectomy. *Otolaryngology-Head and Neck Surgery, 137*(3), 443–449.

Taylor, K. S. (1993). Self-perceived and audiometric evaluations of hearing aid benefit in the elderly. *Ear and Hearing, 14*(6), 390–393.

Trier, T. R., & Levy, R. (1965). Social and psychological characteristics of veterans with functional hearing loss. *Journal of Auditory Research, 5*, 241–256.

Tyler, R. S., & Baker, L. J. (1983). Difficulties experienced by tinnitus sufferers. *Journal of Speech and Hearing Disorders, 48*, 150–154.

van den Brink, R. H. S., Wit, H. P., Kempen, G. I. J. M., & van Heuvelen, M. J. G. (1996). Attitude and help-seeking for hearing impairment. *British Journal of Audiology, 30*, 313–324.

Ventry, I. M., & Weinstein, B. E. (1982). The Hearing Handicap Inventory for the Elderly: A new tool. *Ear and Hearing, 3*(3), 128–134.

Ventry, I., & Weinstein, B. (1983). Identification of elderly people with hearing problems. *Asha, 25*, 37–42.

Vermeire, K., Brokx, J. P. L., Wuyts, F. L., Cochet, E., Hofkens, A., & Van de Heyning, P. H. (2005). Quality-of-life benefit from cochlear implantation in the elderly. *Otology and Neurotology, 26*(2), 188–195.

Walden, B. E., Demorest, M. E., & Hepler, E. L. (1984). Self-report approach to assessing benefit derived from amplification. *Journal of Speech and Hearing Research, 27*(1), 49–56.

Wilson, P. H., Henry, J., Bowen, M., & Haralambous, G. (1991). Tinnitus reaction questionnaire: Psychometric properties of a measure of distress associated with tinnitus. *Journal of Speech and Hearing Research, 34*, 197–201.

Wilson, P. H., & Henry, J. L. (1998). Tinnitus cognitions questionnaire: Development and psychometric properties of a measure of dysfunctional cognitions associated with tinnitus. *International Tinnitus Journal, 4*(1), 1–7.

Wilson, P. H., Henry, J. L., Andersson, G., Hallam, R. S., & Lindberg, P. (1998). A critical analysis of directive counselling as a component of tinnitus retraining therapy. *British Journal of Audiology, 32*, 273–286.

Wood, S. A., & Lutman, M. E. (2004). Relative benefits of linear analogue and advanced digital hearing aids. *International Journal of Audiology, 43*(3), 144–155.

Zenner, H. P., Baumann, J. W., Reischl, G., Plinkert, P., Zimmermann, R., Mauz, P. S., et al. (2003). Patient selection for incus body coupling of a totally implantable middle ear implant. *Acta Oto-Laryngologica, 123*(6), 683–696.

Zenner, H. P., Limberger, A., Baumann, J. W., Reischl, G., Zalaman, I. M., Mauz, P. S., et al. (2004). Phase III results with a totally implantable piezoelectric middle ear implant: Speech audiometry, spatial hearing and psychosocial adjustment. *Acta Oto-Laryngologica, 124*(2), 155–164.

6

Measuring Health-Related Quality of Life in Audiologic Rehabilitation

Harvey B. Abrams
Theresa Hnath Chisolm

As our current health care system finds cures for diseases and extends life, society is turning its focus from length of life to quality of life. The advances in medicine come at a great economic cost. As we continue to spend more of our nation's financial resources on health care, can we demonstrate that our expenditures have translated into an improved quality of life for our citizens? This question has emerged as an important health care policy and research issue. For example, the United States Federal Drug Administration (FDA) is encouraging pharmaceutical companies to include health-related quality of life (HRQoL) outcome measures as part of their clinical trials investigating new drugs (George, 2006). Within the field of audiology, it is important to determine whether advances in hearing-related technology (e.g., cochlear implants, middle ear implants, bone anchored and conventional hearing aids) and other aspects of audiologic rehabilitation (AR) (e.g. individual counseling, group sessions, auditory and speech reading training) result in concomitant improvements in the quality of life of our patients. This chapter reviews issues associated with the measurement of HRQoL with an emphasis on techniques appropriate for the assessment of AR outcomes.

In our discussion of quality of life assessment and AR, we are utilizing the definition proposed in the Preferred Practice Patterns of Audiology (15.0), Audiologic Rehabilitation for Adults (ASHA, 2006) and, for simplicity; we are focusing on the adult population. ASHA (2006) defines AR as a " . . . facilitative process that provides intervention to address the impairments, activity limitations, participation restrictions, and possible environmental and personal factors that may affect communication, functional health, and well-being of persons with hearing impairment or by others who participate with them in those activities." The clinical processes involved in AR include, but are not limited to, counseling, selection and fitting of hearing instruments and other hearing assistive technologies, individual and group training, and other forms of follow-up care. One of the expected outcomes of AR is the enhancement of *well-being and quality of life* of those individuals with hearing impairment, as well as their family members and/or care givers. The challenge to the clinician is measuring the extent to which an improvement in HRQoL has been achieved. In order to make such a measurement, we first need to determine what we mean by HRQoL.

Defining Health-Related Quality of Life

"Quality of Life," in its simplest form, can be thought of as "how good or bad you feel your life to be" (Bradley, Todd, Gorton, Symonds, Martin, & Plowright, 1999) and, of course, many factors can influence quality of life. According to the National Institutes of Health (NIH), factors influencing quality of life include cultural, psychological, interpersonal, spiritual, financial, political, temporal, and philosophical domains, as well as health status (NIH, 1993). Although health status may or may not affect other aspects of quality of life, nonhealth domains also can influence the impact of a disease or disorder and a person's response to treatment. Indeed, as early as 1948, the World Health Organization's (WHO) defined health as a "state of complete physical, mental and social well-being and not merely the absence of infirmity and disease" (WHO, 1948).

Although numerous definitions of HRQoL are proposed in the literature, there is general agreement that HRQoL is a multidimensional concept that focuses on the impact of diseases and disorders, as well as their treatments, on the well-being of individuals (Fairclough, 2002). It is not only the immediate impact of disease or disorder that must be considered but also the length of time an individual must deal with the consequences of the health condition. A definition of HRQoL that considers quantity as well as quality of life is suggested by Patrick (1993): "Health-related quality of life is the value assigned to duration of life as modified by the impairments, functional states, perceptions and social opportunities influenced by disease, injury, treatment or policy" (p. 82).

Measuring HRQoL

HRQoL assessment involves examining the extent to which one's usual or expected physical, emotional, and social well-being are affected by a health condition and its treatments. HRQoL cannot be measured objectively, but rather reflects the subjective assessment of an individual's perception of health status and well-being. As illustrated in Figure 6–1, there are two general types of HRQoL measures, health status and patient preference. Health status assessment is based on psychometric principles and involves the posing of a question or questions about a patient's well-being, with scores being derived from their responses. Patient preference assessment is derived from econometrics and is influenced by the concept of *utility*, or the making of decisions under known or assumed probabilities of outcomes (i.e., under risk or uncertainty). Scores reflect tradeoffs between quality and quantity of life.

As shown in Figure 6–1, both health status and preference-based HRQoL assessments can be classified as being either disease-specific or generic (NIH, 1993). Disease-specific measurement focuses on the effects of a single disease or disorder (heart disease, depression, hearing loss) and its treatments (surgery, medication, hearing aids). Disease-specific instruments serve an important function for the clinician because they are very responsive to intervention (pre- vs. post-treatment). Although audiologists can use a variety of disease-specific instruments to measure the impact of hearing loss and validate the benefits of AR, the results do not allow for comparison to the impact other diseases and disorders and their treatments. For example, with a disease-specific instrument we cannot compare the impact of depression to the impact of

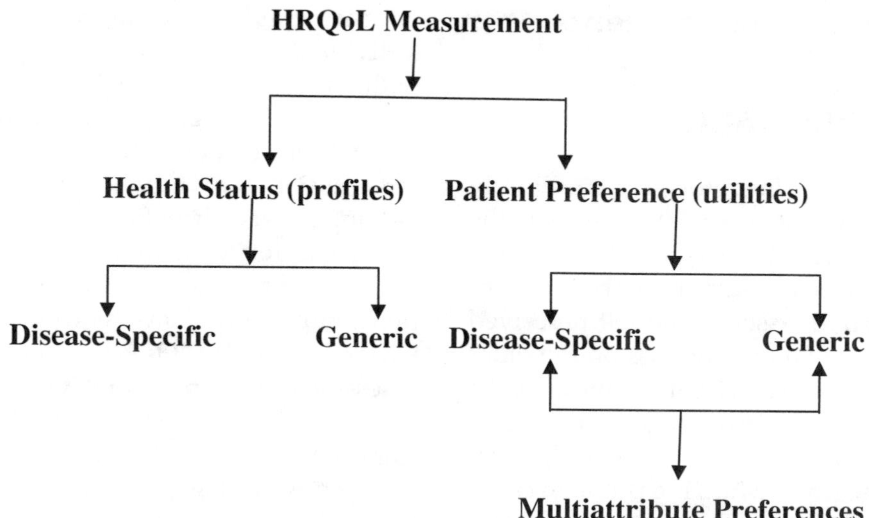

Figure 6–1. Schematic of types of health-related quality of life measurements.

hearing loss on HRQoL. Likewise, the effects of hearing aids on the HRQoL of an adult with hearing impairment cannot be compared to the effects of surgery for a patient with heart disease or medication for a patient suffering from depression. The ability to compare the effects of different diseases and disorders and their treatments is taking on increasing importance as society struggles with the question of which health conditions and interventions are worthy of third-party reimbursement and public funding for research.

To determine if depression is worse than hearing loss or whether we should be spending more money to find a cure for hearing loss vs. a cure for atherosclerosis, generic HRQoL measures are required. Generic measures do not focus on any particular disorder or treatment, but rather on the self-perceived overall health of the individual. Although generic measures have demonstrated negative impacts of hearing loss on HRQoL (e.g., Bess, Lichtenstein, & Logan, 1991; Chia, Want, Rochtchina, Cummig, Newall, & Mitchell, 2007; Mulrow, Aguilar, Endicott, Velez, Charlip, & Hill, 1990), most generic measures are not sensitive to the effects of treatment for hearing loss (Abrams, Chisolm, McArdle, & Wilson, 2005; Bess, 2000). The reason is a simple one. Although most generic profiles include items related to major health domains such as physical, social, and mental health, with few exceptions generic measurement instruments do not include questions that specifically address problems with communication or hearing.

As noted above, HRQoL also can be assessed by measuring the "preference" an individual or community expresses for a particular health state. These measures are referred to as "utilities" and can be considered as a cardinal measure of the strength of one's preference and is expressed as a value ranging from 0.0 (least desirable health state) to 1.0 (most desirable health state). The techniques associated with utilities emerged from von Neumann's and Morgenstern's (1944) decision-making theory and are increasingly being used by health care researchers to compare HRQoL across and within conditions and interventions.

What follows is a brief description of measuring instruments that have been used to assess the impact of hearing impairment on self-perceived HRQoL. The measures are categorized according to the model presented in Figure 6–1.

Health Status Instruments

Disease-Specific Profiles

The Hearing Handicap Inventory for the Elderly (HHIE; Ventry & Weinstein, 1982) is perhaps the most widely known disease-specific HRQoL instrument used in the assessment of the effects of AR. The 25-item HHIE assesses the self-perceived psychosocial effects of a hearing loss on the older individual. Thirteen of the HHIE items measure the emotional impact of the hearing loss and 12 items measure the effect of hearing loss on social/situational functioning. "Does a hearing problem cause you to feel embarrassed when meeting new people" is an example of an emotional-domain item; and, "Does a hearing problem cause you difficulty when listening to radio or TV?" is a social/situational domain item. For each item, the respondent answers "yes" (4 points), "sometimes" (2 points), and "no" (0 points) responses. The scores for each item are summed to provide a total score (range 0–100), as well as the emotional (0–52) and social/situational subscale scores. The higher each of these values the greater the self-perception of hearing handicap. The questionnaire can be administered pre- and post-AR to assess the change in HRQoL. When administered in a face-to-face format, a reduction in score of 18.7 points is needed for the clinician to conclude that real benefit has been attained. If a paper-and-pencil format is used, however, test-retest reliability diminishes and the 95% confidence interval for a true change in score becomes 36 points (Weinstein, Spitzer, & Ventry, 1988). Variations of the HHIE include a 10-item screening version, the HHIE-S (Ventry & Weinstein, 1983); a 25-item version for younger, working adults, the Hearing Handicap Inventory for Adults (and its shortened version, HHIA-S) (Newman, Weinstein, Jacobson, & Hug, 1991); and a Spanish version (Lopez-Vazques, Orozco, Jimenez, & Berruecos, 2002).

Another example of an audiology-specific instrument that assesses HRQoL is the International Outcomes Inventory-Hearing Aids (IOI-HA; Cox & Alexander, 2002). One of the 7 items on the inventory asks individuals how much the use of hearing aids has changed "enjoyment of life." Individuals respond on a 5-point Likert scale, with 1 indicating "worse" and 5 indicating "very much better." Originally designed for assessment of a variety of outcome domains of hearing aid intervention (i.e., number of hours per day of hearing aid use; benefit in terms of improvement in hearing-related activities; residual activity limitations; satisfaction; residual participation restrictions; impact on others; as well as quality of life), variations of the IOI have been developed for assessing other aspects of AR intervention and the perception of intervention effectiveness by significant others (Noble, 2002).

The Audiological Disabilities Presence Index (ADPI; Joore, Brunenberg, Zank, Boas, Anteunis, & Peters, 2002) was developed to measure hearing-related quality of life and differs from other disease-specific instruments by inclusion of a preference-based item. The ADPI was adapted from the Amsterdam Inventory for Auditory Disability and Handicap scale (AIADH; Kramer, Kapteyn, Festen, & Tobi, 1995). Although the AIADH is a 30-item questionnaire designed to assess the impact of hearing loss in daily life, the ADPI includes only five items. The questions in both the AIADH and ADPI assess sound distinction, intelligibility in quiet, intelligibility in noise, auditory localization, and sound detection. For the ADPI, each item has three possible answers "no problems," "moderate problems," and "severe problems," with higher numeric scores indicative of fewer problems. In addition to the five descriptive questions, the ADPI includes a "preference" measure, a horizontal visual analogue scale (VAS) of 10 centimeters length, with zero equal to "deaf" and 100 equal to "perfect hearing" (Joore et al., 2002). The inclusion of the hearing-specific VAS is an important innovation, as the scores can be compared to those obtained with the generic visual analogue scales described below.

Generic Profiles

As previously noted, although generic instruments can be sensitive to the effects of hearing loss in adults, they tend to be relatively insensitive to audiologic rehabilitation. Nonetheless, several generic measures have been used to study the impact of hearing loss and audiologic interventions on self-perceived HRQoL.

The Sickness Impact Profile (SIP; Bergner, Bobbitt, Carter, & Gilson, 1981) is a 136-item, self-administered questionnaire designed to access the impact of a disease or disorder on an individual's HRQoL across 12 activities of daily living categories, including: emotional behavior, body and movement, social behavior, sleep and rest, home management, mobility, work, recreation, ambulation, alertness behavior, communication, and eating. In addition to providing 12 subscale scores, scores can be combined to provide a physical score, a psychosocial score, and an overall or total score. The higher the SIP scores, the greater the negative impact on HRQoL. Bess and colleagues (1989) demonstrated that SIP scores increased as hearing loss increased in older adults. In addition, Crandall (1998) demonstrated statistically significant improvements in SIP total, physical, and psychosocial scores as a function of hearing aid intervention in 20 older adults. Although Crandall's data suggest that SIP might be a useful generic instrument for AR, because of its length, the SIP is time consuming and difficult to administer, thus limiting its clinical utility.

At only 36 self-recorded items, the MOS SF-36 Health Survey (SF-36; Ware & Sherbourne, 1992) is much shorter, and easier to administer than the SIP, and is popular among HRQoL researchers. The SF-36 measures several areas related to overall general health-related well-being, including: physical functioning, role limitations due to physical health problems, bodily pain, general health perceptions, vitality, social functioning, role limitations due to emotional problems, bodily pain, general health perceptions, vitality, social functioning, role limitations due to emotional problems, and mental health. In addition to providing eight subscale scores, the SF-36 yields two component scale scores: a Physical Component Summary (PCS) scale score and a Mental Component Summary (MCS) scale score. For the subscale and component scales, scores are standardized to a mean of 50 and a standard deviation of 10, with higher scores indicating more positive health status. Variations of the original SF-36 have been developed to include a screening version (SF-12), a health survey for children (SF-10), and a health survey designed to be used for very large population studies (SF-8) (Ware, Kosinski, Dewey, & Gandek, 2001).

Interestingly, in the aforementioned study by Crandall (1998), hearing aid intervention did not have a significant effect on the eight SF-36 subscale scores. Crandall's finding, however, may be due to a lack of power since there were only 20 participants. Support for a conclusion that the Crandall study was underpowered, comes from a study by Abrams and colleagues (2002) with a large number of participants (n = 105). Results demonstrated significant improvements for the MCS scale scores as a function of hearing aid intervention. As generic instruments tend to have few if any questions directly related to hearing and communication, it is likely that any treatment effects will be relatively small and the demonstration of statistical significance will require a relatively large number of subjects. (The interested reader is referred to Cohen [1988] for a discussion of effect size and power.)

A generic health-status instrument which includes questions about communication is the World Health Organization's Disability Assessment Schedule II (WHO-DAS II; World Health Organization, 1999). The WHO-DAS II is a 36-item questionnaire that assesses self-perceived functioning over an individual's past 30 days in six different life domains, including: communication (i.e., understanding and communicating with the world); mobility (i.e., moving and getting around); self-care (i.e., attending to one's hygiene, dressing, eating, and staying alone); interpersonal (i.e., getting along with people); life activities (i.e., domestic responsibilities, leisure, and work); and participation in society (i.e., joining in community activities). These six subscale scores map directly onto activity and participation domains of the World Health Organization's International Classification of Functioning, Disability and Health (WHO-ICF; World Health Organization, 2001). In addition to providing six subscale scores, the WHO-DAS II provides a total score. Scoring for the WHO-DAS II is based on averaging responses and then transforming scores into a standard scale, with higher scores indicating better HRQoL. The psychometric properties of the WHO-DAS II for the measurement of functional health status in adults with acquired hearing loss were evaluated by Chisolm and colleagues (2005). Results indicated that the communication and participation domains as well as the total score were psychometrically sound in an adult hearing-impaired population in terms of convergent validity, internal consistency, and test-retest stability.

Patient Preference Instruments

Generic Utilities

As previously described, a *utility* is a cardinal measure of the strength of one's preference and range from 0.0 (death) to 1.0 (perfect health). A cardinal utility is an economic concept which assumes that people are able to assign meaningful numbers (i.e., utils) to their satisfaction in one situation as compared to their satisfaction in an alternative situation. Utils are assumed to be similar to temperature or distance—that is, the incremental units are reasonably constant and objective. Although it is generally accepted that in practice the measurement of utilities is only roughly measurable, utility assessment has taken on an important role in health care economics. Utilities are particularly useful in making comparisons across diseases and interventions and are often used to calculate the cost of treatment outcomes in terms of improved HRQoL. Such economic evaluations are known as cost-utility analyses (CUA), the result of which is expressed as a cost per quality adjusted life year (QALY) gained (Drummond, Sculpher, Torrance, O'Brien, & Stoddart, 2005). The most common direct methods used to measure utility include the standard gamble, time tradeoff, and visual analogue scale techniques (Bennett & Torrance, 1996). Each is described briefly below.

Standard Gamble

The classic method of measuring health preference is the standard gamble (SG) approach. In a standard gamble, a person is offered a choice between two alternatives: living with health state "B" with certainty (which in a clinical population is presumably a patient's present health state); or, gambling on treatment "A." The result of treatment "A" is either perfect health or immediate death. The probabilities of perfect health and death in choice "A" are manipulated until a person is indifferent between his present health state ("B") and choice "A." An assumption of the technique is that the higher the probability of death a person is willing to consider, the lower is the health state (or quality of life) inherent in remaining with choice "B." Utility is calculated as 1.0 (perfect health) minus p (the probability of death in condition "A" when a person is unable to choose between "A" and "B").

Time Tradeoff

Another approach commonly used to measure health-state preferences is the time trade-off (TTO) technique. In TTO, a person is offered a choice between living a normal life span in the present health state or a shortened life span in perfect health. The number of years spent in perfect health is manipulated until a person is indifferent between the shorter period of perfect health and the longer period in the less desirable state. An individual who is willing to "trade off" years of life for a shorter life in perfect health (or perfect hearing) is assumed to be revealing a great deal about his or her perceived quality of life as imposed by a disease or a disorder.

Visual Analogue Scale

The use of a visual analogue scale (VAS) was briefly described above in the description of the ADPI (Joore et al., 2002). Measuring utility with a VAS or a "feeling thermometer" has the advantage of simplicity. A person or patient is simply required to rate his or her perceived health state on a scale marked with 0 at one end representing death or some least desirable state, and 100 at the other end representing perfect health or a most desirable state.

Disease-Specific Utilities

Disease-specific utilities are a relatively new approach to measuring HRQoL (Drummond et al., 2005). They combine the benefits of a generic utility measurement, that is, the ability to generate a single preference rating, with the advantage of a disease-specific measure which is more responsive to the disorder or intervention under study. The techniques used to measure utilities for specific diseases are no different than those described above (SG, TTO, VAS) with the exception that the choices or "anchors" describe the extreme of a specific disorder rather than "perfect health" or "death." For example, instead of asking the patient to choose between living a normal life span in his or her "present health state" or a shortened life span in "perfect health" the TTO may be worded in such a way to require the patient to choose between living a normal life span with his or her current hearing loss or living a shortened life span with perfect hearing. Examples of disease-specific utility studies include those examining the HRQoL impact of prostate cancer (Saigal, Gornbein, Reid & Litwin, 2002), schizophrenia (Lenert, Rupnow, & Elnitsky, 2005), and hearing aid use (Kenworthy, 2002; Piccirillo, Merritt, Valente, Littenberg, & Nease, 1997).

In our own work, we have developed a software program, Utility Measures for Audiological Applications (UMAA) and have obtained preliminary disease-specific utilities for tinnitus, benign paroxysmal positional vertigo, and hearing loss (Abrams, Roberts, Lister, & Hnath Chisolm, 2006). Figures 6–2, 6–3, and 6–4 demonstrate UMAA screen shot for hearing-specific utility assessment

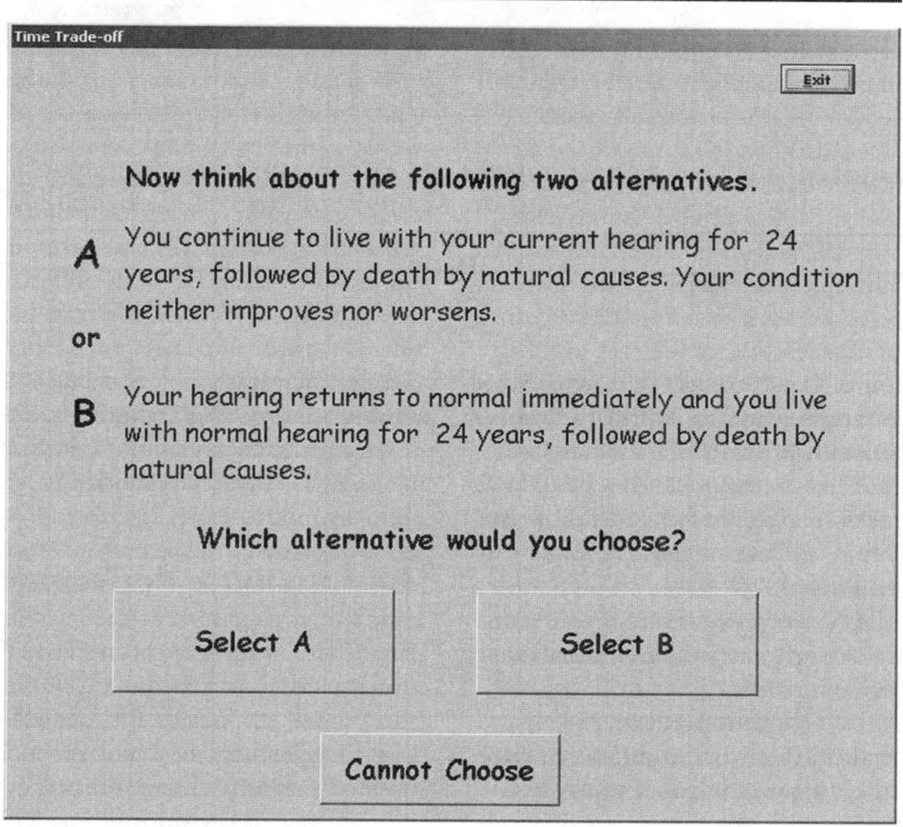

Figure 6–2. Screenshot from the Utility Measures for Audiological Applications (UMAA) showing an example of the time tradeoff technique for hearing.

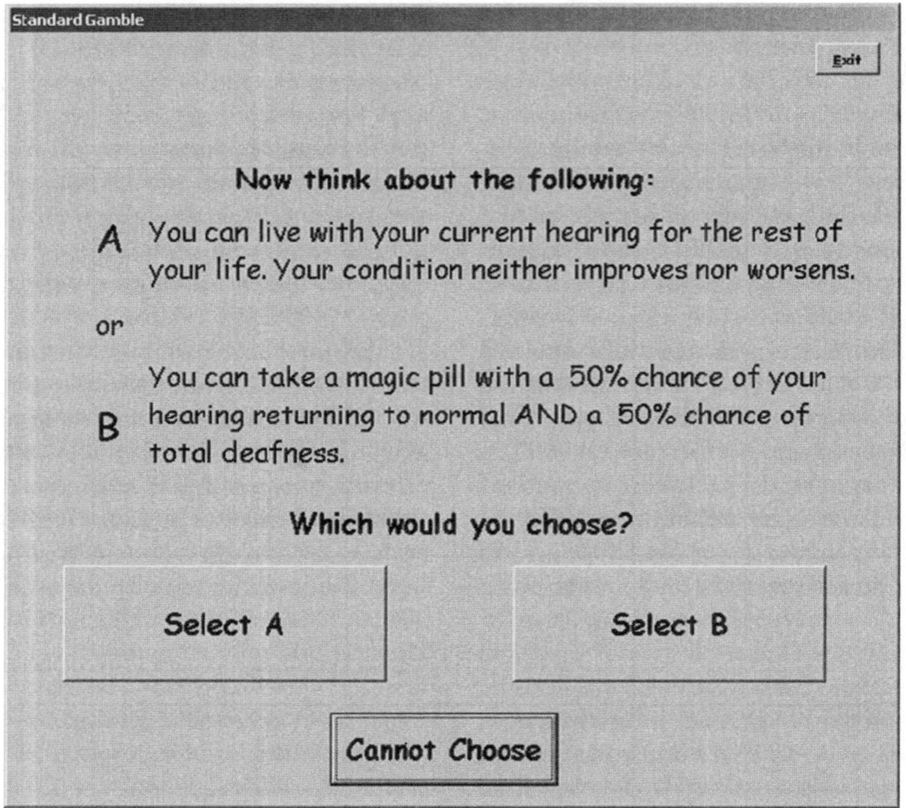

Figure 6–3. Screenshot from the Utility Measures for Audiological Applications (UMAA) showing an example of the standard gamble technique for hearing.

using time tradeoff, standard gamble, and VAS techniques, respectively. Significant correlations were obtained between utilities as measured with all three techniques and responses to the HHIE from 48 adults with hearing loss (Condill, 2006); as well as between utilities measured with all three techniques and responses to the Dizziness Handicap Scale (Jacobsen & Newman, 1990) from 52 patients with benign paroxysmal positional vertigo (BPPV) (Kirsch, 2006).

As described by Drummond et al. (2005) the use of disease-specific and generic utilities in a two-stage approach may allow for more appropriate resource allocation within disorders (as disease-specific utilities will be responsive to the effects of different interventions within the same disorder) and across disorders (as generic utilities provide data for making CUA comparisons across different disorders). An alternative to performing a two stage approach is using a multiattribute health status classification system.

Multiattribute Preferences

Direct measurement of utilities for health outcomes using the standard gamble, time tradeoff, and visual analogue approaches can be a very time-consuming and complex task. To overcome some of the difficulties with direct assessment of utilities in clinical populations, researchers have developed prescored multiattribute health status classification systems. Within each system, several dimensions or attributes of health are assessed

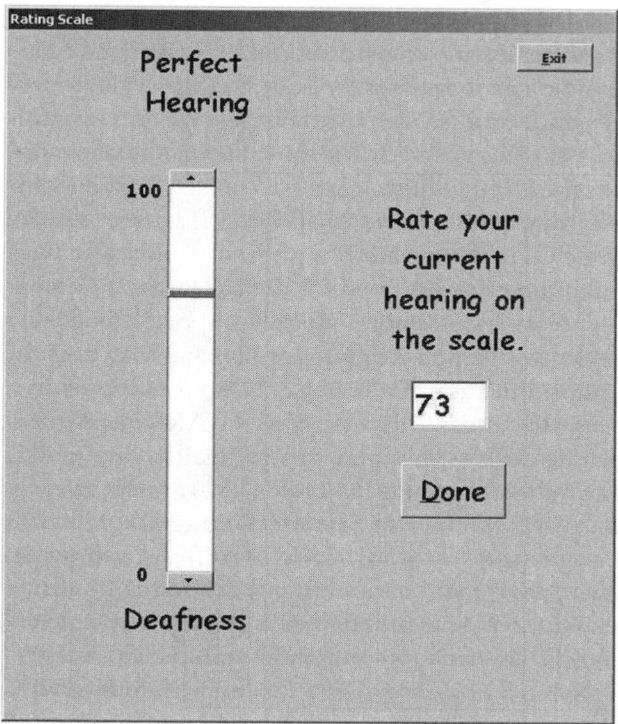

Figure 6–4. Screenshot from the Utility Measures for Audiological Applications (UMAA) showing an example of the visual analogue scale for hearing.

with a number of levels of functioning defined for each dimension. For example, the Health Utilities Index Mark 3 (HUI3) (Feeny, Furlong, Boyle, & Torrance, 1995; Furlong, Feeny, Torrance, et al., 1998) measures six health attributes—sensation, mobility, emotion, cognition, self-care, and pain. The sensation attribute is subdivided into vision, hearing, and speech. Each of these sub-attributes contain a list of level descriptors where level 1 (single attribute utility factor = 1.0) describes the highest health state or preference and level 6 (single attribute utility factor = 0.0) describes the lowest health state or preference. With regard to hearing, for example, Level 1 is associated with the statement "*Able to hear what is said in a group conversation with at least three other people without a hearing aid*" whereas the Level 6 statement indicates that the person is "*Unable to hear at all.*" In the HUI3 the scores of the six attributes are weighted and combined in a complex formula to create a single utility estimate. The multiplicative formulas used to determine the utility estimates for the HUI3, and for a related instrument, the Health Utilities Index Mark II (HUI2), are based on the direct assessments of utility using standard gamble and visual analogue scale techniques in Canadian adults.

Another commonly used multiattribute instrument is the EQ-5D (EuroQoL Group, 1990). At five questions, the EQ-5D provides a simple descriptive profile and a single index value. Each of the five questions relates to a different attribute of the respondent's self-perceived health status regarding mobility, self care, usual activities, pain/discomfort, and anxiety/depression. For each attribute, there are three levels—no problem, some problems, and major problems. Taken together, the questions can classify a person into one of 243 different health states. Initial preferences for the health states were based on a population study in the United Kingdom utilizing the time tradeoff technique. The EQ-5D was originally designed to complement other instruments such as the aforementioned generic profiles, the SIP and SF-36, but is now increasingly used as a stand-alone measure (http://www.euroquol.org).

In addition to the HUI3 and the EQ-5D, other commonly used multiattribute preference instruments include the Quality of Well-Being scale (QWB, Kaplan & Anderson, 1988) and the SF-6D (Brazier, Roberts, & Deverill, 2002). The QWB is a preference-weighted measure that combines three scales of functioning (i.e., mobility, physical activity and social activity) with a measure of symptoms and problems. Scoring functions for the QWB were obtained from a sample of the general public in San Diego, California. The SF-6D (Brazier et al., 2002) is based on the generic quality of life measure, the SF-36, and was developed as a means of converting SF-36 results to utilities. The SF-6D consists of six attributes: physical functioning, role limitations, social functioning, pain, mental health, and vitality; with four to six levels associated with the various attributes. The scoring model for the SF-6D was developed using standard gamble utilities obtained in the general population in the United Kingdom. The SF-6D can only be used in combination with the SF-36 or the SF-12.

Does Audiologic Rehabilitation Improve HRQoL?

Given that the definition utilized in this chapter for AR includes *counseling, selection and fitting of hearing instruments and other hearing assistive technologies, individual and group training, and other forms of follow-up care*, evidence related to hearing technologies as well as other forms of training are briefly reviewed.

Hearing Aids and HRQoL

In an extensive systematic review of the literature, in which the data from individual studies were combined in meta-analyses, Chisolm, Johnson, Danhauer, et al. (2007) concluded that hearing aids do, in fact, improve adults' HRQoL by reducing psychological, social, and emotional effects of sensorineural hearing loss as measured by some of the generic and disease-specific HRQoL profiles described above (e.g., MOS SF-36, HHIE). An important finding from the meta-analyses relates to the differences in effect size estimates obtained for the generic and disease-specific instruments. Effect sizes are considered measures of practical significance, and are independent of sample size (Cohen, 1988). In interpreting effect sizes, medium to large effect sizes are often considered indicative of robust clinical changes, whereas small effect sizes, although not to be ignored, are suggestive of a more subtle clinical change. The effect sizes calculated for the generic outcome measures by Chisolm et al. (2007) were small, whereas those calculated for disease-specific outcome measures were medium to large. These results highlight, as previously discussed by Bess (2000), the difficulty of demonstrating the positive effects of hearing aid intervention utilizing generic HRQoL instruments.

The importance of the inclusion of questions about hearing and/or communication in generic instruments used in assessing changes in HRQoL as a function of hearing aid intervention was highlighted in a study by McArdle and colleagues (2005). In this large, multisite, randomized, controlled trial examining the outcomes of hearing aid intervention in adults, the researchers found statistically significant HRQoL benefit from hearing aids as measured by both generic (WHO-DAS II) and disease-specific (HHIE) HRQoL instruments. As expected, a large effect size was found for the HHIE. Although the effect size reported for the total score on the WHO-DAS II was small, the effect size associated with the communication subscale of the WHO-DAS II was large.

Further support for the importance of the inclusion of questions regarding hearing and/or communication in generic HRQoL instruments used to assess the outcomes of AR comes from studies examining changes in health state utility from the use of hearing aids. For example, Barton, Bankart, Davis, and Summerfield (2004) failed to demonstrate a statistically significant improvement as a result of hearing aid fitting in 609 adults using the EQ-5D or the SF-6D. Significant improvements, however, were demonstrated on the HUI3. These findings highlight the importance of considering the descriptive system used to elicit generic HRQoL utilities. Indeed, the HUI3 is the only multiattribute preference instrument which includes a question about hearing. A similar finding was reported by Grutters et al. (2007) who found statistically significant changes on the HUI3 but not the EQ-5D in 70 adults fit with hearing aids. As a result, Grutters and colleagues concluded that the HUI3 should be the instrument of first choice when assessing utilities in populations with hearing impairment.

Cochlear Implants and HRQoL

Perhaps the area where HRQoL measures have been most extensively and successfully used as it relates to AR has been associated with cochlear implant research (e.g. Cheng, Rubin, Powe, Mellon, Francis, & Niparko, 2000; Francis, Nelson, Yeagle, Cheng, & Niparko, 2002; Summerfield, Marshall, & Archbold, 1997; Wyatt, Niparko, Rothman, & deLissovoy, 1996). An interesting example of a study that incorporated a cost-utility analysis to demonstrate the cost-effectiveness of cochlear implants was that by Evans, Seeger, and Lehnhardt, (1995) who used utilities to compare the cost per QALY gained among cochlear implant users ($15,590) against previously published costs per QALY gained for recipients of coronary angioplasties ($11,490), implantable defibrillators ($29,220), and knee replacements ($49,700).

Auditory Training and HRQoL

The issue remains however, as to whether or not noninstrument based intervention (e.g., auditory training or counseling-based AR) provides any HRQoL benefits separate from those obtained through the use of hearing aids or cochlear implants. Few studies have addressed this question with regard to auditory training. For example, in a recent systematic review of auditory training in adults, Sweetow and Palmer (2005) found only two studies which incorporated what has been identified in this chapter as a HRQoL instrument. Both studies were by Kricos and colleagues (1992, 1996) and the HHIE was used. Whereas Kricos and colleagues (1992) found a significant change in HHIE scores as a function of auditory training, Kricos and Holmes (1996) did not. More recently, in a study examining the efficacy of a home-based, interactive adaptive computer program, Sweetow and Sabes (2006) demonstrated statistically significant improvements on the HHIE or HHIA following 4 weeks of auditory training at 30 minutes a day for 5 days per week.

Group AR and HRQoL

The HHIE/A has also been used in several studies examining the effects of post-hearing aid fitting group audiologic rehabilitation. In a systematic review of group AR programs, Hawkins (2005) concluded that there was good evidence for the efficacy of the programs, with two studies which used the HHIE showing significant changes as a function of AR treatment. One of the studies demonstrating positive benefits was conducted by Abrams, Hnath-Chisolm, Guerreiro, and Ritterman (1992) who demonstrated significant improvement in HHIE scores among a group of adults who received hearing aids plus counseling-based AR compared to two other groups who received either hearing aids alone or no treatment. Positive results from group AR were also reported by Preminger (2003) who showed improvements among participants in a group counseling based AR program, as measured by the HHIE and the HHIA. Interestingly, the greatest reduction in hearing handicap was measured among those who participated in the AR program with their significant others.

Additional evidence supporting the importance of post-hearing aid fitting AR programs for improving disease-specific HRQoL outcomes is provided through a recent randomized trial by Kramer and colleagues (2005). Kramer and colleagues examined short- and long-term effects of an at-home, videotape/DVD-based, education program for older adults with hearing loss and their significant others. The outcome measure used in this study was the IOI. Recall that one of the items on the IOI was designed to assess quality-of-life by asking about enjoyment in life. Immediately postintervention, results revealed that those hearing impaired individuals who participated in the home education program had statistically significantly higher scores than those who did not on the HRQoL item. Interestingly, when long-term outcomes were assessed, the quality-of-life scores for the control group decreased while remaining relatively stable for the home-based education participants.

Although there is good evidence that post-hearing-aid fitting AR improves HRQoL when measured with disease-specific instruments, there are few studies which have examined the effects of post-hearing aid fitting AR using generic measures. One of the first studies to utilize a generic HRQoL instrument in assessing the outcomes of group AR was conducted by Abrams, Hnath Chisolm, and McArdle (2002) who administered the MOS-SF36V (a slightly modified version of the MOS-SF36 designed for the veteran population) to veterans receiving treatment by hearing aids alone and those receiving treatment by hearing aids plus participation in a posthearing-aids fitting group AR program. Overall, intervention resulted in a statistically significant improvement on the Mental Component Summary (MCS) scale, with a mean change of approximately 2 points. Although those who participated in group AR showed a mean change in the MCS scale of 3 points and those who received hearing aids alone had a mean change of only about 1.4 points, there was not a statistically significant difference in the pre- vs. postintervention change scores between the two groups. Despite the lack of a statistically significant differential treatment effect, Abrams and colleagues (2002) argued that the change in scores needed to be considered relative to the costs of treatments. When a cost-effectiveness analysis was conducted, it was found that hearing aids alone intervention cost $60.00 per QALY-gained, whereas the addition of group AR reduced costs to only $31.91 per QALY-gained.

Although it is encouraging that Abrams et al. (2002) concluded group AR was cost-effective based on the MCS scores of the SF-36, it is important to consider recent findings of a randomized controlled trial reported by Hickson, Worrall, and Scarinci (2007). In this study, participants were randomly assigned to a placebo, control social interaction group, or to an AR group focused on communication training. Interestingly, the control social group demonstrated a significant change on the MCS scores of the SF-36, whereas the AR group participants did not. These results suggested that it might simply have been the social interaction and not the communication-specific training that influenced changes in self-perceived HRQoL as measured by the SF-36. Given that SF-36 does not contain any questions regarding hearing and communication, but does contain questions regarding social functioning, this may be a very plausible conclusion. (For additional information on this study and evidence-based research, see Chapter 18 of this text.)

Conclusions

In this chapter, we reviewed the principle concepts of HRQoL, including its definitions, measurements, and AR-related research. The measurement of HRQoL will remain a critical determinant of the impact of disease and injury and the extent to which interventions are successful. The potential of HRQoL measures to allow comparisons within and across diseases and interventions make quality of life measures a powerful tool among clinicians, third-party payers, and health care policy makers. Although the research findings appear to be mixed, evidence is beginning to emerge that AR, to include both sensory aids and non- device based interventions, have a positive impact on the self-perceived HRQoL among those with hearing loss. Clearly more research in this area is needed. Future studies examining the efficacy of AR will require careful and thoughtful design to include a HRQoL measurement component if the profession of audiology hopes to claim that what we do makes a difference in the quality of life of the patients for whom we provide care.

Acknowledgements. This material is based upon work supported by the Department of Veterans Affairs, Veterans Health Administration, Office of Research and Development, Rehabilitation Research and Development. The contents do not represent the views of the Department of Veterans Affairs or the United States Government.

References

Abrams, H., Hnath Chisolm, T., Guerreiro, S., & Ritterman, S. (1992). The effects of intervention strategy on self-perception of hearing handicap. *Ear and Hearing*, *13*, 371–377.

Abrams, H., Hnath Chisolm, T., & McArdle, R. (2002). A cost utility analysis of adult group audiologic rehabilitation: Are the benefits worth the cost? *Journal of Rehabilitation Research and Development*, *39*(5), 549–558.

Abrams H., Chisolm, T. Hnath., McArdle, R., & Wilson, R. (2005). Health-related quality of life and hearing aids: A tutorial. *Trends in Amplification*, *9*, 99–109.

Abrams, H., Roberts, R., Lister, J., & Hnath Chisolm, T. (2006). *The Utility Measures for Audiology Applications (UMAA): Assessing audiologic HRQoL*. Presented at the annual meeting of the American Auditory Society, Scottsdale, AZ.

ASHA. (2006). Preferred practice patterns for the profession of audiology. 15.0 Audiologic rehabilitation for Adults. Retrieved October 10, 2007 from: http://www.asha.org/docs/html/PP2006-00274.html

Barton, G. R., Bankart, J., Davis, A. C., & Summerfield, Q. A. (2004). Comparing utility scores before and after hearing-aid provision: Results according to the EQ-5D, HUI3 and SF-6D. *Applied Health Economics and Health Policy, 3*, 103–105.

Bennett, K. J., & Torrance, G. W. (1996). Measuring health state preferences and utilities: Rating scale, time tradeoff, and standard gamble techniques. In B. Spilker (Ed.), *Quality of life and pharmacoeconomics in clinical trials* (2nd ed., pp. 253–265). Philadelphia: Lippincott-Raven.

Bergner, M., Bobbitt, R. A., Carter, W. B., & Gilson, B. S. (1981). The Sickness Impact Profile: Development and final revision of a health status measure. *Medical Care, 19*, 787–805.

Bess, F. H. (2000). The role of generic health-related quality of life measures in establishing audiological rehabilitation outcomes. *Ear and Hearing, 21*, 74S–79S.

Bess, F. H., Lichtenstein, M. J., & Logan, S. A. (1991). Making hearing impairment functionally relevant: Linkages with hearing disability and handicap. *Acta Otolaryngologica Supplementum (Stockholm), 476*, 226–231.

Bess, F. H., Lichtenstein, M. J., Logan, S. A., Burger, M. C., & Nelson, E. (1989). Hearing impairment as a determinant of function in the elderly. *Journal of the American Geriatrics Society, 37*, 123–128.

Bradley, C., Todd, C., Gorton, T., Symonds, E., Martin, A., & Plowright, R. (1999). The development of an individualized questionnaire measure of perceived impact of diabetes on quality of life: The ADDQoL. *Quality of Life Research, 8*, 79–91.

Brazier, J., Roberts, J., & Deverill, M. (2002). The estimation of a preference-based measure of health from the SF-36. *Journal of Health Economics, 21*, 271–292.

Cheng, A. K., Rubin, H. R., Powe, N. R., Mellon, N. K., Francis, H. W., & Niparko, J. K. (2000). Cost-utility analysis of the cochlear implant in children. *Journal of the American Medical Association, 284*, 850–856.

Chia, E. M., Wang, J. J., Rochtchina, E., Cumming, R. R., Newall, P., & Mitchell, P. (2007). Hearing impairment and health-related quality of life: The Blue Mountains Hearing Study. *Ear and Hearing, 28*, 187–195.

Chisolm, T., Johnson, C., Danhauer, J., Portz, L., Abrams, H., Lesner, S., et al. (2007). A systematic review of health-related quality of life and hearing aids: Final report of the American Academy of Audiology Task Force on the Health-Related Quality of Life Benefits of Amplification in Adults. *Journal of the American Academy of Audiology, 18*, 151–183.

Chisolm, T. H., Abrams, H., McArdle, R., Wilson, R., & Doyle, P. (2005). The WHO-DAS II: Psychometric properties in the measurement of functional health status in adults with acquired hearing loss. *Trends in Amplification, 9*, 111–126.

Cohen, J. (1988). *Statistical power for the social sciences* (2nd ed.). Hillsdale, NJ: Lawrence Erbaum Associates.

Condill, S. (2006). *Utility measures in patients with hearing loss*. Unpublished Doctor of Audiology project, University of South Florida.

Cox, R. M., & Alexander, G. C. (2002). The International Outcome Inventory for Hearing Aids (IOI-HA): Psychometric properties of the English version. *International Journal of Audiology, 41*, 30–35.

Crandall, C. C. (1998). Hearing aids: Their effects on functional health status. *Hearing Journal, 52*, 22–32.

Drummond, M., Sculpher, M., Torrance, G., O'Brien, B., & Stoddart, G. (2005). Cost-utility analysis. In *Methods for the economic evaluation of health care programmes* (3rd ed., pp. 137–210). Oxford: Oxford University Press.

EuroQoL Group. (1990). EuroQoL—a new facility for the measurement of health-related quality of life. *Health Policy, 16*, 199–208.

Evans, A. R., Seeger, T., & Lehnhardt, M. (1995). Cost-utility analysis of cochlear implants. *The Annals of Otology, Rhinology, and Laryngology*, (Suppl. 166), 239–240.

Fairclough, D. (2002). Introduction. In *Design and analysis of quality of life studies in clinical trials* (pp. 1–18). Boca Raton, FL: Chapman & Hall.

Feeny, D., Furlong, W., Boyle, M., & Torrance, G. (1995). Multi-attribute health status classification systems: Health Utilities Index. *PharmacoEconomics, 7*, 490–502.

Francis, H. W., Nelson, C., Yeagle, J., Cheng, A., & Niparko, J. K. (2002). Impact of cochlear implant on the functional health status of adults. *Laryngoscope, 112*, 1482–1488.

Furlong, W., Feeny, D., Torrance, G. W., Goldsmith, C. H., DePauw, S., Zhu, Z., et al. (1998). Multiplicative multi-attribute utility function for the Health Utilities Index Mark 3 (HUI3) System: A technical report. *McMaster University Centre for Health Economics and Policy Analysis Working Paper*, 98–111.

George, L. K. (2006). Perceived quality of life. In R. H. Binstock, & L. K. George (Eds.), *Handbook of aging and the social sciences* (6th ed., pp. 320–336). Burlington, MA: Academic Press.

Grutters, J. P., Joore, M. A., van der Horst, F., Verschuure, H., Dreschler, W. A., & Anteunis, L. J. (2007). Choosing between measures: Comparison of EQ-5D, HUI2 and HUI3 in persons with hearing complaints. *Quality of Life Research, 16*, 1439–1449.

Hawkins, D. (2005). Effectiveness of counseling-based adult group aural rehabilitation programs: A systematic review of the evidence. *Journal of the American Academy of Audiology, 16*, 485–493.

Hickson, L., Worrall, L., & Scarinci, N. (2007). A randomized controlled trial evaluating the active communication education program for older people with hearing impairment. *Ear and Hearing, 28*, 212–230.

Jacobson, G. P., & Newman, C. W. (1990). The development of the dizziness handicap inventory. *Archives of Otolaryngology-Head and Neck Surgery, 116*, 424–427.

Joore, M., Brunenberg, D., Zank, H., van der Stel, H., Anteunis, L., Boas, G., et al. (2002). Development of a questionnaire to measure hearing-related health state preferences framed in an overall health perspective. *International Journal of Technology Assessment in Health Care, 18*, 528–539.

Kaplan, R. M., & Anderson, J. (1988). A general health policy model: Update and applications. *Health Services Research, 23*, 203–235.

Kenworthy, M. K. (2002). *An examination of the relationship between the U-Titer II and hearing aid benefit.* Unpublished Doctor of Audiology project, University of South Florida.

Kirsch, M. (2006). *Utility measures in patients with benign paroxysmal positional vertigo.* Unpublished Doctor of Audiology project, University of South Florida.

Kramer, S., Kapteyn, T., Festen, J., & Tobi, H. (1995). Factors in subjective hearing disability. *Audiology, 34*, 311–320.

Kramer, S. E., Allessie, G. H., Dondorp, A. W., Zekveld, A. A., & Kapteyn, T. S. (2005). A home education program for older adults with hearing impairment and their significant others: A randomized trial evaluating short- and long-term effects. *International Journal of Audiology, 44*, 255–264.

Kricos, P., Homes, A., & Doyle, D. (1992). Efficacy of a communication training program for hearing impaired elderly adults. *Journal of the Academy of Rehabilitative Audiology, 25*, 69–80.

Kricos, P., & Holmes, A. (1996). Efficacy of audiologic rehabilitation for older adults. *Journal of the American Academy of Audiology, 7*, 219–229.

Lenert, L., Rupnow, M., & Elnitsky, C. (2005). Application of a disease-specific mapping function to estimate utility gains with effective treatment of schizophrenia. *Health and Quality of Life Outcomes, 3*, 57.

Lopez-Vazquez, M., Orozco, J., Jimenez, G., & Berruecos, P. (2002). Spanish Hearing Handicap Inventory for the Elderly. *International Journal of Audiology, 41*, 221–230.

McArdle, R., Chisolm, T. H., Abrams, H., Wilson, R., & Doyle, P. (2005). The WHO-DAS II: Measuring outcomes of hearing aid intervention for adults. *Trends in Amplification, 9*, 127–143.

Mulrow, C. D., Aguilar, C., Endicott, J. E., Velez, R., Tuley, M. R., Charlip, W. S., et al. (1990). Association between hearing impairment and quality of life of older individuals. *Journal of the American Geriatrics Society, 38*, 45–50.

National Institutes of Health. (1993). Quality of life assessment: Practice, problems, and promise. *Proceedings of a Workshop*, October, 1990. National Institutes of Health, Bethesda, MD.

Newman, C. W., Weinstein, B. E., Jacobson, G. P., & Hug, G. A. (1991). Test-retest reliability of the hearing handicap inventory for adults. *Ear and Hearing, 12*, 355–357.

Noble, W. (2002). Extending the IOI to significant others and to non-hearing-aid-based interventions. *International Journal of Audiology, 41*, 27–29.

Patrick, D. L. (1993). Reactions and recommendations: Quality of life in NIH-sponsored studies.

In National Institutes of Health (1993). Quality of Life Assessment: Practice, problems, and promise. *Proceedings of a Workshop*, October, 1990 National Institutes of Health, Bethesda, MD.

Piccirillo, J. F., Merritt, M. G., Valente, M., Littenberg, B., & Nease, R. F. (1997). U-Titer: A new tool for measuring preferences for hearing. *Second Biennial Hearing Aid Research and Development Conference; Program and Abstracts*, p. 38.

Preminger, J. E. (2003). Should significant others be encouraged to join adult group audiologic rehabilitation classes? *Journal of the American Academy of Audiology, 14*, 545–555.

Saigal, C., Gornbein, J., Reid, K., & Litwin, M. (2002). Stability of time tradeoff utilities for health states associated with the treatment of prostate cancer. *Quality of Life Research, 11*, 404–414.

Summerfield, A. Q., Marshall, D. H., & Archbold, S. (1997). Cost-effectiveness considerations in pediatric cochlear implantation. *American Journal of Otology, 18*, S166–S168.

Sweetow, R., & Palmer, C. (2005). Efficacy of individual auditory training in adults: A systematic review of the evidence. *Journal of the American Academy of Audiology, 16*, 494–504.

Sweetow, R., & Sabes, J. (2006). The need for and development of an adaptive listening and communication enhancement (LACE™) program. *Journal of the American Academy of Audiology, 17*, 538–558.

Ventry, I., & Weinstein, B. (1982). The Hearing Handicap Inventory for the Elderly: A new tool. *Ear and Hearing, 3*, 128–133.

Ventry, I., & Weinstein, B. (1983). Identification of elderly people with hearing problems. *Asha, 25*, 37–42.

von Neumann, J., & Morgenstern, O. (1944). *Theory of games and economic behaviour*. Princeton, NJ: Princeton University Press.

Ware, J. E., Kosinski, M., Dewey, J. E., & Gandek, B. (2001). *How to score and interpret single-item health status measures: A manual for users of the SF-8™ Health Survey*. Lincoln, RI: QualityMetric.

Ware, J. E., & Sherbourne, C. D. (1992). The MOS 36-item Short-Form Health Survey (SF-36): I. Conceptual framework and item selection. *Medical Care, 30*, 473–483.

Weinstein, B., Spitzer, J., & Ventry, I. M. (1986). Test-re-test reliability of the Hearing Handicap Inventory for the Elderly. *Ear and Hearing, 7*, 295–299.

World Health Organization. (1948). Preamble to the Constitution of the World Health Organization as adopted by the International Health Conference, New York, 19–22 June, 1946; signed on 22 July 1946 by the representatives of 61 States (Official Records of the World Health Organization, No. 2, p. 100) and entered into force on 7 April 1948.

World Health Organization. (1999). *The World Health Organization Health Disability Assessment Schedule II Field Trial Instrument*. Geneva, Switzerland: Author.

World Health Organization. (2001). *International Classification of Functioning, Disability and Health*. Geneva, Switzerland: Author.

Wyatt, J. R., Niparko, J. K., Rothman, M., & deLissovoy, G. (1996). Cost utility of the multichannel cochlear implant in 258 deaf individuals. *Laryngoscope, 106*, 816–821.

7

Assessment for Implantable Technologies

Jaclyn B. Spitzer
Dean M. Mancuso

Introduction

At the time of writing this chapter, our field is faced with a diversity of implantable hearing devices (IHDs) in varying stages of approval by the Food and Drug Administration (FDA), clinical trials, and off-label applications. In this chapter, "IHD" will refer to the full range of implantable hearing devices, ranging from bone-anchored to middle ear implants to cochlear and brainstem implants. Audiologists must determine how we contribute to the evaluation of potential candidates for these devices and what methods are to be applied in an ongoing assessment of their safety and efficacy.

The first, and most obvious, question to be asked is "What is the purpose of assessment?" This seemingly simple question has several answers. The most direct objective in performing assessments for IHDs is to identify candidates that meet selection criteria. In this way, we can undertake proper counseling regarding the range of appropriate options. Based on finding that a candidate does, in fact, meet the selection criteria for a class of IHDs, we still have an ethical obligation (Berg, Herb, & Hurst, 2005; Hyde & Power, 2006) to provide information about competing technology and communication methods, including nonsurgical options. Alternative rehabilitation and educational paths are overtly discussed with parents of infants and children being evaluated for cochlear implants (CIs), but such discussion must also take place when the candidate is an adult. It is widely acknowledged that we have this obligation while we are engaged in a clinical trial, but the requirement to present alternatives continues beyond an IHD's approval by the FDA for clinical use. Even when the audiologist is an advocate for treatment with a specific IHD, accepting that that class of device is the current "standard of care," there is still an obligation to present information about the possible benefits and limitations of alternatives.

The second objective of assessment for IHDs is to identify non-candidates and to counsel them and their families regarding alternatives. As the audiologic rehabilitation specialist on an implant team, the audiologist should formulate the alternative recommendations, guided by knowledge of competing technology, counseling options, and rehabilitative planning. Periodic re-examination, review of needs, changes in selection criteria, and emerging technologies may eventually move a current non-candidate into the range of qualifying for an IHD when followed longitudinally.

Another important purpose in carrying out a comprehensive evaluation for IHDs is to prepare the candidate and the implant team for postimplantation needs. Through thorough assessment, rehabilitative planning or support services can be made available in anticipation of the implantee's needs or anticipated limitations. For example, in an implant candidate whose pre-operative evaluation demonstrated active caloric responses in the ear to be implanted, the team could formulate tentative plans for vestibular rehabilitation in an extended recovery period.

Assessment in the Historical Context

Assessment has been at the heart of demonstrating to governmental agencies (especially the Food and Drug Administration, FDA), the professional community, and the Deaf and general public that IHDs are safe and provide substantial benefit that outweighs the risks. Beginning in the 1970s, clinical trials with CIs received considerable media attention. Early work with the single channel CI was criticized as having excessive reliance on anecdotal reporting of benefit. Thus, later studies needed to be more fastidious in producing tight, pre-/post-designs to document safety and efficacy.

Multichannel CI devices have undergone a stepwise progression in hardware and software design. With each iteration, the clinical trials have had rigorous, structured baseline testing with contemporary hearing aids and postoperative examination using reliable measures in controlled test environments. Many of the procedures that were used in the clinical trials of the 1980s and 1990s continue in use in the post-FDA approval clinical milieu. As new IHDs are developed, with differing target patient populations and divergent capabilities, it is reasonable to project that the clinical protocols in use today will require modification in order to demonstrate that advanced features make a significant difference in patient outcomes.

Selection Criteria: Influence on Assessment Methods

In designing an evaluation protocol, documentation of preintervention function is needed to serve as a baseline. The assessment methods should be clearly related to determining whether the selection criteria are met. The dimensions to be assessed should address areas known to be affected by the intervention with an IHD, as well as parameters that may have an indirect impact. The Bone-Anchored Hearing Assistive (Baha®) device (also known as a bone-anchored cochlear stimulator and formerly known as a bone-anchored hearing aid) will be used as an illustration of how the evaluation components need to address selection criteria and form a relevant baseline against which comparisons can be made effectively.

As illustrated in Table 7–1, outlining the evaluation protocol for Baha®, multiple dimensions of patient characteristics and performance are examined. The medical criteria relate to factors intrinsic to the patient, such as age or diagnosis (e.g., congenital aural atresia), or historical information, such as prior surgery for cholesteatoma, in addition to physical findings. The otologist will initiate the requests for computed axial tomography (CAT or CT scan) or magnetic resonance imaging (MRI), dependent on the underlying pathology and device option being explored, in order to visualize the anatomy to determine if a condition exists which precludes implantation or may alter the surgical approach.

At various points during the evaluation protocol, the otologist may seek input or clearance from the primary care physician or specialists, especially in regard to the candidate's ability to undergo surgery and the impact of health conditions on the healing process. For example, a patient with diabetes may pose a problem in terms of

Table 7–1. What Constitutes a Basic Baha® Selection Protocol?

Category of Assessment	Methods/Tests	Considerations
Medical/surgical evaluation	▪ History ▪ Physical examination ▪ Radiologic workup	▪ Anatomic appropriateness for IHD ▪ Determining contraindications to surgery, often in consultation with primary care physician and/or specialists
Unaided evaluation under headphones/insert earphones	▪ Basic comprehensive audiologic examination ▪ Tympanometry and acoustic reflexes	▪ Where there are limitations in administration level by air conduction testing, consider administration of speech stimuli via bone oscillator ▪ Importance of using recorded stimuli to assure ability to make pre-/post comparisons
Aided evaluation in sound field	▪ Warble tone thresholds ▪ Spondee thresholds ▪ Speech recognition in quiet ▪ Speech recognition noise with the location of noise source chosen based on side to be implanted ▪ Localization evaluation, if equipment is available	▪ Using personal amplification ▪ Using competitive technology ▫ Conventional hearing aid, if appropriate ▫ Baha® with headband for conductive or mixed HL, esp. atresia ▫ CROS or BICROS for SSD application
Nonaudiologic criteria	▪ Direct observation of manipulation of device and batteries	▪ Adequate manual dexterity or support system for management of device ▪ Assistance with visual inspection of the abutment and surrounding skin interface ▪ Support system and availability determined through interview of patient and/or significant other
	▪ Handicap assessment	▪ Examine motivation for surgery and for adjustment to novel devices or stimulation
	▪ Interview by both Otologist and Audiologist and/or other team members, with conference on impressions	▪ Realistic expectations
	▪ Interview with Baha® user	▪ Provides realistic feedback about life with a Baha®
	▪ Psychological screening if necessary	▪ May be able to address unrealistic expectations or barriers to proceeding with intervention
	▪ Visual information access	▪ May require consultation by optometry or ophthalmology
	▪ Communication effectiveness, as evaluated by Speech-Language Pathologist or Auditory-Verbal Therapist	▪ Ability to communicate preoperatively, including use of visual information via lipreading and gestures ▪ Utilization of repair strategies

healing of incisions, or in the case of the Baha®, in terms of healing of the skin around the abutment. In such a condition, the physician's monitoring of the patient may be more vigilant than in a less complex case.

Audiologically, the pictures that are appropriate for Baha® candidates may entail bilateral conductive or mixed hearing loss, unilateral conductive hearing loss, or unilateral profound sensorineural hearing loss, also called "single-sided deafness (SSD)" (Wazen, Spitzer, Ghossaini, et al., 2003). Attention is directed to the levels of bone-conducted responses, which cannot exceed 45 dB Hearing Level (HL) for the present generation of head-level Baha® devices. In terms of performance with a hearing aid or Baha® device on a headband, there are no explicit candidacy requirements for the extent of aided threshold improvement or speech recognition performance. Baha® is an example, albeit a rarity in the field of IHDs, of a situation in which we can evaluate the candidate with a simulator (Baha® on a headband) to obtain preoperative data; this also affords the patient an opportunity to listen to a sound which simulates the postoperative outcome. Although there may be some underestimation of the gain to be obtained, the candidate nonetheless can formulate an impression of the sound quality to be achieved with Baha®.

The audiologic procedures of interest for Baha® are to demonstrate improved auditory sensitivity, speech recognition in quiet and noise, and localization ability. Thus, the preoperative baseline can include conditions that pose communicative difficulty for the candidate's level and configuration of hearing loss. It is also generally accepted in evaluation of IHDs, particularly with middle ear implants and CIs, that evaluation should be accomplished after the candidate has had sufficient experience with competitive technology to permit the assessment to reflect maximal performance. Thus, a trial with a CROS hearing aid may precede an evaluation of a candidate for the SSD application of Baha®. The audiologist must ensure that the trial is with a device that truly is competitive technology, and neither outdated as some candidate's older personal hearing aids might be nor suboptimal as in an underpowered in-the-canal hearing aid for a severe to profound hearing loss.

It is worthwhile to explore responses to noise in differing juxtapositions to the listener. As in Figure 7–1A, unaided speech recognition testing or measurement with an adaptive procedure, such as the Hearing-in-Noise Test (HINT; Nilsson, Soli, & Sullivan, 1994) can document for both the SSD patient and the clinician the disadvantage experienced in conditions when speech originates on the poorer side and noise is on the better side. The results of this condition are then compared to those in the aided condition, as in Figure 7–1B, when the IHD is in place. Such testing can provide data which are very reinforcing to the potential IHD user, as an illustration of the advantage to be gained.

The audiologist also has a significant role in determining whether the candidate can contend with the IHD's practical application. Verification that the patient has adequate manual dexterity or support system for management of the day-to-day maintenance of the device can be accomplished by watching the patient handle a demonstration device and batteries. In the case of Baha®, the audiologist and/or otologist must determine how the patient will be able to care for the abutment site and surrounding skin interface, or whether assistance will be needed with visual inspection of the area.

Although involvement of a psychologist is highly variable in current implant team settings, some form of psychological screening or full evaluation is generally acknowledged as necessary to examine such intrinsic factors as psychological status and acceptance of implantation whenever questions arise. The general understanding is that a candidate must have realistic expectations about outcomes from the IHD. The method for determining that someone has realistic expectations is also highly variable, and may be based on a team consensus. Extrinsic factors that may have an impact on the candidate's success with an IHD should also be addressed, including family support, social network, vocational demands, and avocational interests. In some teams, the latter issues are addressed by a social worker, but these social dimensions often arise in counseling ses-

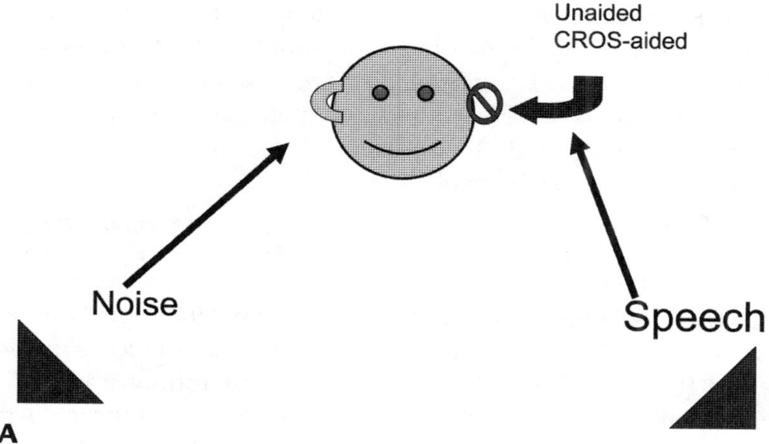
Listening in noise may be one of the key challenges for the unilateral hearer.
Unaided
CROS-aided
Noise
Speech
A

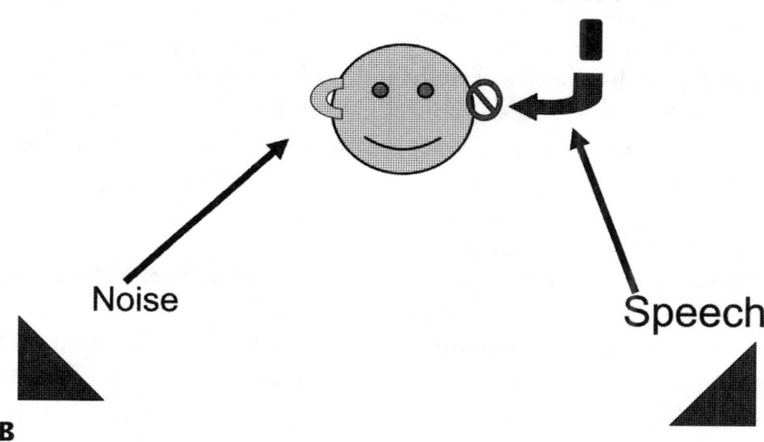
Speech perception testing in noise may reveal the advantage offered by implantation.
BAHA
Noise
Speech
B

Figure 7–1. Illustrates the use of speech in noise testing. In comparing speech recognition performance in the unaided (**A**) and aided (**B**) conditions with noise on the side of the better hearing ear, it is possible to demonstrate the advantage offered in the Single-Sided Deafness (SSD) scenario to a potential Baha® user. This arrangement of noise and speech may be useful in demonstrating benefit to users of other IHDs.

sions with the audiologist as well. When psychologists are involved in the initial assessment, it is reasonable for them also to follow the implantee over time to assess the impact of implantation (Knutson, Murray, Husarek, Westerhouse, Woodworth, Gantz, et al, 1998).

Adjustment to hearing loss and its impact on social, emotional, and vocational aspects can also be assessed formally using self-assessment/hearing handicap scales. Selecting the appropriate scale for the level of hearing loss is critical. Thus, using the Hearing Handicap Inventory for Adults (HHIA, Newman, Weinstein, Jacobson, & Hug, 1990, 1991) for adults under 60 years old, or the Hearing Handicap Inventory for the Elderly (HHIE; Weinstein & Ventry, 1983) for adults over 60 years old, would be reasonable for mild to moderate levels of hearing loss. When the loss is severe to profound, however, a scale should be selected that is aimed at the communicative challenges associated with that level of loss, such as the Performance Inventory for Severe and Profound Loss (PIPSL, Owens & Raggio, 1988). When selecting a handicap scale, it is important to keep test-retest reliability in mind, since high reliability is required (cf. Weinstein, Spitzer, & Ventry, 1986) if the measurement is to be repeated postintervention and periodically thereafter; in this way, changes measured can be attributed to the impact of intervention, rather than variability inherent to the handicap scale.

Reviewing the handicap scale responses with the candidate and significant other(s) is a suitable launch to discussions of adjustment to loss, coping mechanisms, need for changes in or implementation of repair strategies, and how the postoperative function may be significantly different on an auditory basis but still require use of strategies to maximize successful communication. These discussions in a family context can be very revealing about the level of support available to the potential implantee, and what obstacles must be addressed in the family milieu.

It is important to determine if there are any visual limitations that may impinge on the ability to access visual communication information. Sometimes, visual deficits become apparent during meetings with other team members. It is often in the formal assessment of baseline communication abilities, as carried out by the speech-language pathologist, audiologist, or auditory-verbal therapist, that limits in accessing visual communication are discovered. When such visual deficits are identified, it is necessary to obtain consultation with an optometrist to improve/correct refraction or with an ophthalmologist to address any remediable ocular problem. Although good vision is not a prerequisite for IHDs, and in fact persons with low vision or blindness have been implanted with Baha® or CIs (Daneshi & Hassanzadeh, 2007), maximization of communication skills through every available modality should be part of the preoperative phase.

Current Audiologic Methods

There is no universally-accepted test battery for IHDs. When a device is in clinical trials, its assessment must follow a rigorous protocol to document safety and efficacy. After FDA approval in the United States, considerable discretion is applied, with implant centers seeking to find an economical balance (Cheng & Niparko, 1999) between scientific rigor and clinical feasibility. The pressure to streamline assessment is a reality which each practitioner must face.

A test battery should be device-oriented so that assessment reflects areas in which a particular IHD will/may provide benefit. A brief summary of the current audiologic benefits of IHDs appears in Table 7–2.

Preoperative Assessment

Threshold improvement and improved speech recognition are documented in a straightforward manner, using measures with which audiologists are very familiar; however, the standard battery of tests should be "sharpened" by consistent use of recorded speech stimuli to control test-retest variability influences and routinely obtaining the maximum speech recognition scores (Phonetically Balanced maximum performance or PB_{max}). It is also worthwhile to remember that the preoperative examination is a medicolegal document, which substantiates the need for intervention, conformance with accepted selection criteria or, where there are deviations from such criteria, the rationales or aspects of performance that motivated a surgical treatment.

Table 7–2. Sample Audiologic Benefits with Current Generation of Implantable Hearing Devices (IHDs)

Device	Application	Sample Audiologic Benefit	Representative Citation Documenting Benefit
Baha®	Bilateral conductive or mixed HL[1]	Improved threshold sensitivity	Tjellstrom, Lindstrom, Hallen, et al. (1981); Wazen, Caruso, & Tjellstrom (1998);
		Speech recognition in quiet	Spitzer, Ghossaini, Wazen (2002); Hol, Snik, Mylanus, & et al. (2005)
	Unilateral conductive or mixed HL	Improved threshold sensitivity	Wazen, Spitzer, Ghossaini, et al. (2001); Snik, Mylanus, Cremers (2002)
		Speech recognition in quiet	
	Single-sided deafness	Improved speech recognition in noise	Wazen, Spitzer, Ghossaini, et al. (2003)
Middle ear implantable device (IMEHD)[2]	Mild to severe sloping SNHL[3]	Improved threshold sensitivity	Luetje, Brackman, Balkany, et al. (2002); Uziel, Mondain, Hagen, et al. (2003); Jenkins, Niparko, Slattery, et al. (2004)
	Conductive or mixed HL[4]	Improved speech recognition in quiet	Luetje, Brackman, Balkany, et al. (2002); Re: Conductive HL: Venail, Lavieille, Meller, et al. (2007)
		Reduction in occlusion effect	Luetje, Brackman, Balkany, et al. (2002)
Cochlear Implant	Severe to profound SNHL; Auditory Neuropathy	Improved threshold sensitivity	Connell & Balkany (2006); Re: Auditory neuropathy: Shallop, Peterson, Facer, et al. (2001); Peterson, Shallop, Driscoll, et al. (2003)
		Improved speech recognition in quiet	Balkany et al. (2007)
		Improved speech recognition in noise	
		Reduced hearing handicap	Spitzer, Kessler, & Bromberg (1992)
Auditory Brainstem Implant	In patients with neurofibromatosis II, neural HL or HL affecting eighth nerve and extracanicular space; In cases of failed cochlear implantation[4]	Improved threshold sensitivity	Otto, Brackmann, Hitselberger, et al. (2002) RE: Failed cochlear implant: Colletti, Fiorino, Carner, et al. (2004)
		Support to lipreading	Schwartz, Otto, Brackmann, et al. (2003)
		Limited open-set speech recognition	Otto, Brackmann, Hitselberger, et al. (2002)

[1]HL, hearing loss.

[2]Only FDA-approved devices at the time of writing is the Med-El Vibrant Soundbridge and Soundtec (inactive); publications cited also refer to Otologics MET, which is in clinical trials.

[3]SNHL, sensorineural hearing loss.

[4]Not an FDA-approved application at the time of writing.

In the selection protocol, there is a focus on speech perception performance that (1) establishes preoperative function; and (2) is used to determine conformance with published guidelines. For example, the current criterion for adult candidacy for a CI include speech recognition for sentence material no better than 50% in the ear to be implanted, and no better than 60% in the opposite ear. In the case of implantable middle ear hearing devices (IMEHDs), the criterion is stated as a range, often an extremely wide range, such as 20 to 80% correct for monosyllables, or may not be stated explicitly (Magnan, Manrique, Dillier, Snik, & Hausler, 2005).

The following case study demonstrates that a single test protocol, in this case to determine candidacy for a Baha®, may not be an appropriate approach. Both flexibility and creativity must be employed to demonstrate the potential benefit of an IHD to a given patient.

Case Study

Patient S.M., a 20-year-old male, was referred to our center for evaluation of candidacy for Baha® implantation.

Clinical History

The patient's mother reported that he was born full-term via forceps delivery. The patient presented with left congenital aural atresia and stenosis. The right pinna appeared normal; however, the patient's mother reported an unspecified abnormality of the ossicular chain in the right ear. The patient took synthroid for hypothyroidism. He was also a long time wearer of a digital behind-the-ear style hearing aid in the right ear.

Summary of Audiologic Findings

A Type A tympanogram was obtained in the right ear (–75 daPa peak pressure). Ipsilateral acoustic reflexes were absent in the right ear at equipment limits. Immittance testing could not be performed for the left ear due to the aforementioned stenosis. As seen in Figure 7–1, the results showed a moderate to profound mixed hearing loss, bilaterally. Due to the masking dilemma, it was not possible with currently available equipment to determine the exact, ear-specific bone-conduction thresholds for all test frequencies in each ear. However, unmasked bone conduction thresholds reveal that *at least one* ear has sufficient bone conduction thresholds to consider Baha® implantation. Additionally, though the *masked* air-conduction thresholds indicate a profound impairment, the *unmasked* thresholds were used in judging candidacy as this reflected his hearing status in the real world without the presence of masking noise. The speech recognition thresholds corroborated pure-tone averages, bilaterally.

Baha® Evaluation

Aided soundfield evaluation was completed. For the majority of the evaluation, the patient wore a Baha® Divino on the left side. The left side was chosen because the patient was unable to wear a conventional hearing aid on that side, due to the aforementioned stenosis/aural atresia. Pure tone thresholds were obtained, along with speech testing using a 50-word CNC list, and HINT sentences. All speech testing was performed using recorded materials, and stimuli were presented at 70 dB HL, with the patient seated in front of the loudspeaker at 90-degrees azimuth. Aided hearing was within normal limits for pure tones from 500 Hz to 2000 Hz. CNC phonemes correct score was 89%, and HINT sentences score was 98% in quiet, 0% in noise with the Baha® in "omni" mode, and 74% in noise (+10 dB S/N ratio) with the D-mic engaged. The patient also used his personal high-end digital power BTE. HINT score in quiet for the hearing aid only 98% phonemes correct, whereas the HINT in noise (+10 dB S/N ratio) with the hearing aid in directional mode was 18%. The combined performance of the Baha® and the hearing aid in noise (also +10 dB S/N ratio) was 73% of words correctly identified. The patient also expressed a favorable opinion of the sound quality of the Baha®.

Summary of Baha® Candidacy Findings

Results of this evaluation indicated that the patient was an excellent Baha® candidate. It was likely that the patient would continue to use a hearing aid on the side opposite the Baha®. Speculatively, this may yield improved sound localization relative to using the Baha® only. Additionally, due to the presence of bilateral conductive pathology, the patient was also a candidate for future evaluation to consider bilateral Baha® implantation.

Treatment Plan

Appropriate manufacturer's literature was provided to the patient, and he was referred back to his otologist to further discuss the medical and surgical considerations associated with Baha® implantation.

Discussion

This case illustrates that the clinician cannot be content with the utilization of a "cookie-cutter" approach when evaluating Baha® candidacy. Frequently, as in this case, the patient's individual needs and issues will provide the impetus to modify the typical evaluation protocol. In this case, assessment of the patient's performance using the hearing aid was added to the usual protocol, and the inability to determine ear-specific masked bone-conduction thresholds for the majority of frequencies tested was considered but not found to be an impediment to the patient's candidacy. Other possible scenarios that may require modification of the "standard" protocol include patients with unilateral deafness (Single-Sided Deafness, or SSD), patients with congenital versus acquired hearing loss, the patient's performance in noise, the patient's listening environments and lifestyle issues, the patient's ability to perform the whole test battery (i.e., younger children who may have reduced attention span). During the Baha® evaluation, as with virtually any other Audiological test battery, flexibility and insight on the part of the clinician are paramount to successful outcome.

In the past, assessment using nonspeech stimuli was common, especially in the evaluation of persons with profound hearing loss. The Minimal Auditory Capability (MAC) battery (Owens, Kessler, Raggio, & Schubert, 1985) included subtests with identification of environmental sounds and discrimination of voice versus noise. In present day evaluations, use of nonspeech stimuli has been given reduced importance based on the greater anticipated benefits of implantation. The thinking is that such measures provide too low a target for postimplant comparisons with the current, successful generation of devices. However, as the field of CIs has expanded to include prelinguistically impaired adult candidates (Waltzman & Cohen, 1999), potential implantees with limited auditory experience are expected to perform poorly pre- and postoperatively on open-set monosyllabic or sentence material despite some improvements that can be documented. In order to demonstrate that implantation improved some dimensions of auditory perception, tasks in addition to those focusing on open-set speech recognition, such as those included in the MAC battery, should be considered.

A number of electrophysiologic tests have a role in preoperative assessment. Auditory Brainstem Response (ABR) is used to verify the level of hearing loss (Spraggs, Burton, & Graham, 1994) and, in combination with otoacoustic emissions (OAEs), to identify the profile referred to as auditory neuropathy/auditory dyssynchrony (Shallop, Peterson, Facer, & Fabry, 2001). In an unselected sample of people with congenital hearing loss, Cross, Stephens, Francis, Hourihan, and Reardon (1999) demonstrated that a functional overlay or nonorganic hearing loss may be encountered. Thus, in the interest of ruling out a functional hearing loss in an adult IHD candidate, ABR continues to have a role.

When insertion of the IHD electrode entails invasion of the cochlea or round window (RW) or placement of a vibrating prosthesis in the RW, electronystagmography (ENG) or videonystagmography (VNG) is used by some implant teams to document pre- and postoperative vestibular function (Brey, Facer, Trine, Lynn, Peterson, & Suman, 1995) and provides insight as to anticipated postoperative dizziness. It has been suggested that performing ENG does not have any predictive value for CI speech perception performance outcomes (Chen, Shipp, Al-Abidi, Ng, & Nedzelski, 2001). In an effort to streamline IHD evaluations, ENG/VNG is, therefore, sometimes eliminated from the protocol, despite recent evidence that 32% of patients reported vestibular disturbance and had poorer Dizziness Handicap Inventory (DHI) and Activity Balance Confidence (ABC) after surgery. Fina et al. (2003) reported that 39% of patients experienced postoperative dizziness. The majority of cases had delayed, episodic vertigo. Dizziness was greater in those patients with preoperative dizziness, older at implantation, and older at onset of hearing loss. The latter report suggests that, if ENG/VNG is to be eliminated from the general IHD protocol, there may be value in retaining the test for older candidates or persons with a history of dizziness in order to have both baseline information on those candidates and insight into the mechanism for postimplantation recovery of function.

Self-Report in IHD Evaluation

A variety of self-report measures have been used in evaluation of candidates for IHDs. In CI candidates, assessment has employed questionnaires in hearing (Spitzer, Kessler, & Bromberg, 1992; Vermeire, Brokx, Wuyts, Cochet, Hofkens, De Bodt, & Van de Heyning, 2006), tinnitus (Tyler, 1995; see Noble (2000) for a review of self-report of tinnitus and CIs and Chapter 5 in this text) and dizziness (Enticott, Tari, Koh, Su, Dowell, & O'Leary, 2006) handicap scales, balance confidence (Enticott et al., 2006), quality of life assessment (Faber & Grøntved, 2000; Spitzer et al., 1995; Vermeire et al., 2006; Wanscher, Faber, & Grøntved, 2006), and employment and job satisfaction (Fazel & Gray, 2007). As is true in other applications, self-report measures may provide a starting point for counseling based on responses to the questionnaires.

In addition to handicap and quality of life assessments, other scales have been used extensively with Baha® and to a lesser extent with middle ear implants, such as the Med-El Vibrant Soundbridge and Otologics MET. These other scales include the Abbreviated Profile of Hearing

Aid Benefit (APHAB; Cox & Alexander, 1995), Glasgow Hearing Aid Benefit Profile (Kemper & Holmes, 2004), and a sound quality rating (Gabrielsson, Hagerman, Bech-Kristensen, & Lundberg, 1990). Table 7–3 summarizes the outline of audiologic methods for evaluation of IHDs in adults and illustrates the linkage with various dimensions of anticipated benefit.

A meeting or contact with a current IHD user is a step that many IHD teams include routinely. When a prospective implantee has the opportunity to meet with a current user, there are information and emotional exchanges that cannot be conveyed by the professionals on the team. Such a meeting can promote realistic expectations and reduce fears about implantation. The CI manufacturers, recognizing the potential benefit to persons undergoing evaluation, have facilitated meetings with CI users through associations of implantees, such as the Bionic Ear Association (Advanced Bionics) and online resources, such as The Nucleus Forum and the Cochlear™ Community (a Web site for CI and Baha® users by Cochlear Americas) and Hearing Companions (Med-El Corporation). These resources allow users to express their viewpoints and provide opinions, in much the same way as do self-help organizations.

Perioperative Testing

Assessment is also performed in the operating room. Testing of the integrity of the just inserted electrode is commonplace in surgery for cochlear implantation. It is also standard procedure to evaluate the responses of the eighth nerve using such techniques as Neural Response Telemetry [NRT; King, Polak, Hodges, Payne, & Telischi (2006); Potts, Skinner, Gotter, Strube, & Brenner, 2007] or Neural Response Imaging [NRI; Caner, Olgun, Gultekin, & Balaban, 2007]. These measures reflect neural responses which are electrically evoked, and permit an estimate of a comfortable listening level perceptually; clinicians may use these results to draft initial programs or starting points for electrical stimulation in subsequent programming sessions.

An appealing technique used in the operating room is observation of the electrically stimulated stapedial reflex (ESRT; Battmer, Laszig, & Lehnhardt, 1990; Buckler, Dawson, & Overstreet, 2003). Direct observation of contraction of the stapedial muscle and measurement by an immittance meter with a probe in the contralateral, nonsurgical ear are alternatives for obtaining the ESRT. As pointed out by Buckler et al., a systematic relationship is found between ESRT and behaviorally measured comfortable levels. The latter approach entails using bands of sound, rather than discrete frequency stimuli to evoke the reflex. The role of the audiologist in testing for IMEHDs is still evolving at this time.

Value of Pre-/Post-Testing

Although we may be treating a candidate with the IHD that is currently regarded as the "standard of care," as CIs are considered for profound SNHL,

Table 7–3. Outline of Audiologic Methods for Evaluation of Implantable Hearing Devices (IHDs) in Adults: Linkage with Dimensions of Anticipated Benefit

Test Phase	Dimension to Be Assessed	Relevant Devices	Tests in Current Usage
Preoperative baseline	Description of residual hearing sensitivity, nature of loss, speech recognition ability	All	Comprehensive audiologic evaluation under headphones/insert phones: ▪ pure-tone air- and bone-conduction thresholds ▪ speech recognition for NU-6 words
		Baha®	Speech recognition via bone-conduction oscillator if air-conduction headphones cannot deliver sufficient sensation level

continues

Table 7–3. *continued*

Test Phase	Dimension to Be Assessed	Relevant Devices	Tests in Current Usage
Preoperative baseline *continued*	Performance with competitive technology in sound field	All	Warble tone thresholds Speech recognition: ▪ NU-6 words ▪ Consonant-nucleus-consonant (CNC) monosyllables ▪ Hearing-In-Noise Test (HINT) sentences in quiet ▪ HINT sentences in S/N = +10 dB ▪ HINT sentences in S/N = +5 dB ▪ Handicap measurement ▪ Satisfaction/quality of life questionnaires
		Baha®	HINT paradigm to document dB advantage in noise (Nilsson, Soli, & Sullivan, 1994); Quik SIN (Snapp & Telischi, 2008)
		IMEHDs	Speech Perception-In-Noise (SPIN) sentences
Perioperative	Integrity of electrode	Cochlear implant (CI)	Electrical impedance test
	Estimate of comfort levels	CI	▪ Neural response telemetry or neural response imaging ▪ Electrically induced Stapedial Reflex Thresholds (ESRTs) ▪ Electrically evoked Auditory Brainstem Response (ABR)
	Confirmation of placement of electrode array/paddle	Auditory Brainstem Implant (ABI)	Electrically evoked Auditory Brainstem Response (ABR)
Postoperative, 3 months, 6 months, 12 months, annually thereafter	Description of residual hearing sensitivity, nature of loss, speech recognition ability[1]	All	Comprehensive audiologic evaluation under headphones/insert phones: ▪ pure-tone air- and bone-conduction thresholds ▪ speech recognition for NU-6 words
	Performance with implanted technology in sound field	All	Warble tone thresholds Speech recognition: ▪ NU-6 words ▪ Consonant-nucleus-consonant (CNC) monosyllables ▪ Hearing-In-Noise Test (HINT) sentences in quiet ▪ HINT sentences in S/N = +10 dB ▪ HINT sentences in S/N = +5 dB ▪ Handicap measurement ▪ Satisfaction/quality of life questionnaires
	Electroacoustic assessment	CI plus hearing aid	Comparable to above
	Localization	Bilateral applications of Baha®, CIs, EAS	Requires sound field array

[1]Postoperatively and at intervals required for confirmation of impact of surgery and standard of care.

continued evaluation in a time-structured protocol is important. Again, using Baha® as an exemplar, follow-up testing is necessary to: (1) document benefit of actual implant performance, which may exceed that with the headband simulation; (2) establish a baseline of implanted function, against which future assessments will be compared; (3) provide feedback to the IHD user about performance; and (4) follow-up annually, ideally, to detect alterations in the underlying condition and the impact use of Baha®.

Recognizing that upgrades in performance are to be anticipated with both hardware and software improvements in IHDs, we must establish a data reference that permits critical examination of advances in the field and alters our expectations of performance. For example, we can review outcomes recently reported regarding a new device, the Nucleus Freedom implant and processor. For this device, a recent study (Balkany, Hodges, Menapace, et al., 2007) reported mean scores for CNC words of 57%, HINT sentences in quiet, 78%, and HINT sentences in noise, 64%. Thus, our expectations increase for performance in both quiet and noise.

Assessment of Localization and IHDs

Evaluation of localization with Baha® has focused on post-implantation performance (Bosman, Snik, van der Pouw, & Mylanus, 2001; Wazen, Ghossaini, Spitzer, & Kuller, 2005). Bosman et al. (2001) demonstrated that bilateral Bahas® resulted in localization ability. In addition, Snik, Mylanus, & Cremers (2002) reported that, at least for patients with adventitious unilateral conductive hearing loss, Baha® permitted localization, whereas the performance of congenitally impaired persons was erratic or poor.

Wazen et al. (2005) pursued responses on questionnaires by several SSD patients that they believed their localization ability had improved while using Baha®. The study was undertaken to evaluate the impact of using a Baha® on localization performance and to quantify the deficit in localization encountered by persons with profound SNHL on one side and normal hearing in the better ear. The method entailed presentation of narrow bands at 500 Hz and 3000 Hz via speakers separated by 45 degrees of arc. Randomized trials of 5 presentations per speaker from each of 8 speakers yielded 40 stimuli per frequency band. The performance of normal hearing controls was compared to SSD subjects. An unaided trial preceded a Baha®-aided trial. Accuracy did not exceed chance for most SSD subjects unaided and accuracy did *not* improve when wearing the Baha®.

A number of authors have demonstrated that bilateral cochlear implantation improves the implantee's ability to determine the direction of a source (Grantham, Ashmead, Ricketts, Labadie, & Haynes, 2007; Neuman, Haravon, Sislian, & Waltzman, 2007). Grantham et al. demonstrated that subjects with CIs were able to localize sounds only in the bilateral implant condition. Participants were performing with excellent accuracy at 5-months poststimulation, and showed the ability to learn to apply cues so that poor performers improved in accuracy with additional listening experience.

At this time, counseling for bilateral implantation, for CI or Baha®, acknowledges that we anticipate improvement in localization and speech perception in noise, but we lack methods that can determine, for a particular candidate, that such abilities are likely. Based on both Baha® and CI experience, the person with an adventitious loss is more likely to develop good, or possibly, normal accuracy in localization tasks, and there is likelihood that experience with bilateral stimulation will result in further improvements in this ability.

Developing New Procedures

We are at a significant juncture in assessment of potential IHD candidates and in documentation of benefit postintervention. Several criticisms may be leveled at current tests and methods, including ceiling effects, lack of real-world challenges, and a need for assessments of sound quality, especially as it affects music perception.

Ceiling effects are reflected in reports of exceptionally high performance by each successive generation of IHDs. For example, Staller, Arndt, and

Brimacombe (2000) reported speech recognition performance in open-set sentences of 79.6% in quiet, in users of the Nucleus 24 Contour electrode and ear-level speech processor. Other investigators have reported similar outcomes for the other 2 FDA-approved cochlear implants (Hamzavi, Franz, Baumgartner, & Gstottner, 2001; Shapiro, Green, Bromberg, Gomolin, & Waltzman, 2000; Valimaa & Sorri, 2000). The range of scores includes high performers who achieve 100% or very high scores early in their CI experience, implying that we cannot assess accurately continued growth in perception as a consequence of experience and/or training. Thus, there is a need to develop materials that will present greater challenges in CI assessment. Real-world challenges might include introduction of highly variable, speech babble competition, simulation of reverberation or reverberation plus noise, and elevated level of linguistic sophistication. Such ecologically valid stimuli might be applicable for the "star" performers who find the current materials and methods insufficiently difficult.

When asked about listening habits and enjoyment of music, 52% of a sample of postlinguistically deaf adults stated that they enjoyed listening to music postimplantation, although music was less enjoyable than it was preimplantation (Lassaletta, Castro, Bastarrica, Perez-Mora, Madero, DeSarria, & Gavilan, 2007). This finding reinforces earlier reports by Gfeller and coworkers (Gfeller, Witt, Woodwarth, Mehr, & Knutson, 2000b; Gfeller, Christ, Knutson, Witt, Murray, & Tyler, 2000a), in which CI users indicated an overall decrease in musical enjoyment compared to the remembered preimplant condition. These findings have added impetus to development of processing strategies to increase naturalness of sound and improve music appreciation. (*Note:* For additional information on music perception and CIs, see Chapter 17 in this text.)

Despite the recognition of the importance of music enjoyment to IHD users (Buckler, Dawson, Lisbona, & Zimmerman-Phillips, 2006), including CI recipients, the development of new tests of musical appreciation (Spitzer & Mancuso, 2006; Spitzer, Mancuso, & Cheng, 2008) and perceptual skills (Nimmons, Kang, Drennan, Longnion, Ruffin, Worman, Yueh, & Rubinstein, 2008) is in their early phases. Questionnaires regarding musical appreciation have not yet been broadly utilized. Studies with these measures in CI recipients using advanced processing strategies, incorporating fine structure of signals, are currently under way.

Electrophysiologic measures show great promise for evaluation of the impact of intervention. Work in children (Bauer, Sharma, Martin, & Dorman, 2002; Sharma, Dorman, & Spahr, 2002) has revealed brain plasticity that relates to success with CI use. Ponton, Eggermont, Don, Waring, and Kwong (2002) suggested that mismatched negativity (MMN) is a means to study the effects of auditory deprivation and the impact of cochlear implantation. Clinical application of evoked potentials as a means of evaluating an IHD user's adjustment to his or her device may help us to understand the wide variety of outcomes we encounter in practice.

Another promising area for evaluation of the brain's accommodation to sensory deprivation is functional imaging, including functional Magnetic Resonance Imaging (fMRI) and activated Positron Emission Tomography (activated PET). Although fMRI may be an unsuitable evaluation post-some IHDs' implantation, as a preoperative measure, it may provide insight into how the auditory cortex is functioning in relation to various (nonauditory) stimulations. Activated PET has been used in a variety of studies (cf. Catalán-Ahumada, Deggouj, De Volder, Melin, Michel, & Veraart, 1993; Ito, Momse, Oku, Ishimoto, Yamasoba, Sugasawa, & Kaga, 2004; Lee, See, Oh, Kim, Kim, Chung, Lee, & Kim, 2001; Lee, Lee, Oh, Kim, Kim, H, Koo, Kang, Chung, & Lee, 2003; Roland, Tobey, & Devous, 2001) as an index of the impact of CI use. PET offers the possibility of studying the impact of reintroduction of stimulation after sensory deprivation, and observing brain changes in the auditory cortex and association areas. For example, Ito et al. (2004) evaluated 8 postlingually deafened CI users within the first 2 months post-CI initial stimulation. An abnormal pattern of activation was obtained in comparison to a normal listener control group. In the CI subjects, when stimulated by a 1000-Hz tone burst, strong and broad activation was obtained in the ipsilateral primary auditory cortex, with a weaker activation in the contralateral primary auditory cortex; in normals, activation was in the contralateral primary auditory cortex only. When stimulated by word stimuli, activation was observed in the superior frontomedian cortex [supplementary motor area and cingulated gyri] in the CI users, with no such finding in the normal listeners. Activation was also reduced in the immediate association areas. Evidence of plasticity was seen in activity in the periphery of association cortex. Thus, Ito et al. demonstrated both abnormal activation patterns and plasticity by mobilization of association cortex during the early phases of adjustment to electrical stimulation.

Tobey, Devous, Buckley, Overson, Harris, Ringe, and Martinez-Verhoff (2005) described the impact of drug therapy in conjunction with audiologic rehabilitation (AR) (2 months of auditory training) on cerebral blood flow. In their line of research, Single Photo Emitted Computed Tomography (SPECT) findings in auditory primary and association areas were diminished in CI users compared to normals. The authors evaluated the impact of pharmacological enhancement of rehabilitation using either amphetamine or placebo during intensive auditory training. An enhancement effect was documented in pharmacologically assisted therapy. These intriguing findings provoke the questions of how to maximize behavioral training methods in IHD users.

As is clear from this chapter, the clinician's creativity is an element that cannot be undervalued in the development of protocols and test materials for assessment of candidates for IHDs, and measurement of the impact of intervention. The continued evolution in technology must be accompanied by evolution in assessment to capture the dramatic changes experienced by the hearing-impaired patients making use of implantable devices.

References

Balkany, T., Hodges, A., Menapace, C., Hazard, L., Driscoll, C., Gantz, B., et al. (2007). Nucleus Freedom North American clinical trial. *Otolaryngology-Head and Neck Surgery, 136*(5), 757–762.

Battmer, R. D., Laszig, R., & Lehnhardt, E. (1990). Electrically elicited stapedius reflex in cochlear implant patients. Cochlear implants. *Ear and Hearing, 11*(5), 370–374.

Bauer, P. W. Sharma, A., Martin, K., & Dorman, M. (2006). Central auditory development in children with bilateral cochlear implants. *Archives of Otolaryngology-Head and Neck Surgery, 132*(10), 1133–1136.

Berg, A. L., Herb, A. & Hurst, M. (2005). Cochlear implants in children: Ethics, informed consent, and parental decision-making. *Journal of Clinical Ethics, 6*(3), 237–248.

Bosman, A. J., Snik, A. F., van der Pouw, C. T., & Mylanus, E. A. (2001). Audiometric evaluation of bilaterally fitted bone-anchored hearing aids. *Audiology, 40*(3), 158–167.

Brey, R. H., Facer, G. W., Trine, M. B., Lynn, S. G., Peterson, A. M., & Suman, V. J. (1995). Vestibular effects associated with implantation of a multiple channel cochlear prosthesis. *American Journal of Otology, 16*(4), 424–430.

Buckler, L., Dawson, K., Lisbona, K., & Zimmerman-Phillips, S. (2006) *Music benefits with HiRes 120 sound processing*. Presented at CI2006, Vienna, Austria.

Buckler, L., Dawson, M. A., & Overstreet, E. (2003). Relationship between electrical stapedial reflex thresholds and HiRes™ program settings: Potential too for pediatric cochlear-implant fitting. *Ear and Hearing, 21*, 164–174.

Caner, G., Olgun, L., Gultekin, G., & Balaban, M. (2007).Optimizing fitting in children using objective measures such as neural response imaging and electrically evoked stapedius reflex threshold. *Otology and Neurotology, 28*(5), 637–640.

Catalán-Ahumada, M., Deggouj, N., De Volder, A., Melin, J., Michel, C., & Veraart, C. (1993). High metabolic activity demonstrated by positron emission tomography in human auditory cortex in case of deafness of early onset. *Brain Research, 623*, 287–292.

Chen, J. M., Shipp, D. Al-Abidi, A., Ng, A., & Nedzelski, J. M. (2001). Does choosing the "worse" ear for cochlear implantation affect outcome? *Otology and Neurotology, 22*(3), 335–339.

Cheng, A.K., & Niparko, J.K. (1999). Cost-utility of the cochlear implant in adults: A meta-analysis. *Archives of Otolaryngology-Head and Neck Surgery, 125*(11), 1214–1218.

Colletti, V., Fiorino, F. G., Carner, M., Miorelli, V., Guida, M., & Colletti, L. (2005). Auditory brainstem implant as a salvage treatment after unsuccessful cochlear implantation. *Otology and Neurotology, 25*(4), 485–496.

Connell, S. S., & Balkany, T. J. (2006). Cochlear implants. *Clinics in Geriatric Medicine, 22*(3), 677–686.

Cox, R. M., & Alexander, G. C. (1995). The abbreviated profile of hearing aid benefit. *Ear and Hearing, 16,* 176–186.

Cross, N. C., Stephens, S. D. G., Francis, M., Hourihan, M. D., & Reardon, W. (1999) Computed tomography evaluation of the inner ear as a diagnostic, counselling and management strategy in patients with congenital sensorineural hearing impairment. *Clinical Otolaryngology, 24*(3), 235–238.

Daneshi, A., & Hassanzadeh, S. (2007). Cochlear implantation in prelingually deaf persons with additional disability. *Journal of Laryngology and Otology, 121*(7), 635–638.

Enticott, J. C., Tari, S., Koh, S. M., Dowell, R. C., & O'Leary, S. J. (2006). *Otology and Neurotology, 27*(6), 824–830.

Faber, C. E., & Grøntved, A. M. (2000). Cochlear implantation and change in quality of life. *Acta Otolaryngologica Supplement, 543,* 151–153.

Fazel, M. Z., & Gray, R. F. (2007). Patient employment status and satisfaction following cochlear implantation. *Cochlear Implants International, 8*(2), 87–91.

Fina, M., Skinner, J., Goebel, J. A., Piccirillo, J. F., & Neely, J. G. (2003). Vestibular dysfunction after cochlear implantation. *Otology and Neurotology, 24*(2), 234–242.

Gabrielsson, A., Hagerman, B., Bech-Kristensen, T., & Lundberg, G. (1990). Perceived sound quality of reproductions with different frequency responses and sound levels. *Journal of the Acoustical Society of America, 88*(3), 1359–1367.

Gfeller, K., Christ, A., Knutson, J. F., Witt, S., Murray, K. T., & Tyler, R. S. (2000a). Musical backgrounds, listening habits, and aesthetic enjoyment of adult cochlear implant recipients. *Journal of the American Academy of Audiology, 11*(7), 390–406.

Gfeller, K., Witt, S., Woodwarth, G., Mehr, M. A., & Knutson, J. (2002b). Effects of frequency, instrumental family, and cochlear implant type on timbre recognition and appraisal. *Annals of Otology, Rhinology, and Laryngology, 111,* 349–356.

Grantham, D. W., Ashmead, D. H., Ricketts, T. A., Labadie, R. F., & Haynes, D. S. (2007). Horizontal-plane localization of noise and speech signals by postlingually deafened adults fitted with bilateral cochlear implants. *Ear and Hearing, 28*(4), 524–541.

Hamzavi, J., Franz, P., Baumgartner, W. D, & Gstottner, W. (2001). Hearing performance in noise of cochlear implant patients versus severely profoundly hearing-impaired patients with hearing aids. *Audiology, 40,* 26–31.

Hol, M. K., Snik, A. F., Mylanus, E. A., & Cremers, C. W. (2005). Long-term results of bone-anchored hearing aid recipients who had previously used air-conduction hearing aids. *Archives of Otolaryngology-Head and Neck Surgury, 131,* 321–325.

Hyde, M., & Power, D. (2006) Ethics of cochlear implantation. *Journal of Deaf Studies and Deaf Education, 11*(1), 102–111.

Ito, K., Momse, T., Oku, S., Ishimoto, S., Yamasoba, T., Sugasawa, M., & Kaga, K. (2004). Cortical activation shortly after cochlear implantation. *Audiology and Neuro-Otology, 9*(5), 283–293.

Jenkins, H. A., Niparko, J. K., Slattery, W. H., & Neely, J. G. (2004). Otologics middle ear Transducer™ ossicular stimulator: Performance results with varying degrees of sensorineural hearing loss. *Acta Oto-Laryngologica, 124,* 391–394.

Kemker B. E., & Holmes A. E. (2004). Analysis of prefitting versus postfitting hearing aid orientation using the Glasgow Hearing Aid Benefit Profile (GHABP). *Journal of the American Academy of Audiology, 15*(4), 311–323.

King, J. E., Polak, M., Hodges, A. V., Payne, S., & Telischi, F. F. (2006). Use of neural response telemetry measures to objectively set the comfort levels in the Nucleus 24 cochlear implant. *Journal of the American Academy of Audiology, 17*(6), 413–431.

Knutson, J. F., Murray, K. T., Husarek, S., Westerhouse, K., Woodworth, G., Gantz, B. J., et al. (1998). Psychological change over 54 months of cochlear implant use. *Ear and Hearing, 19*(3), 191–201.

Lassaletta, L., Castro, A., Bastarrica, M., Perez-Mora, R., Madero, R., DeSarria, J., et al. (2007). Does music perception have an impact on quality of life following cochlear implantation? *Acta Otolaryngologica, 127*(7), 682–686.

Lee, D. S., See, J. S., Oh, S. H., Kim, S-K., Kim, J-W., Chung, J-K., et al. (2001). Cross modal plasticity and cochlear implants. *Nature, 409,* 149–150.

Lee, J. S., Lee, D. S., Oh, S. H., Kim, C. S., Kim, J-W., Hwang, C. H., et al. (2003). PET evidence of neuroplasticity in adult auditory cortex of postlingual deafness. *Journal of Nuclear Medicine, 44*, 1435–1439.

Luetje, C. M., Brackman, D., Balkany, T. J., Maw, J., Baker, R. S., Kelsall, D., et al. (2002). Arts A. Phase III clinical trial results with the Vibrant Soundbridge implantable middle ear hearing device: A prospective controlled multicenter study. *Otolaryngology-Head and Neck Surgery, 126*(2), 97–107.

Magnan, J., Manrique, M., Dillier, N., Snik, A., & Hausler, R. (2005). International consensus on middle ear implants. *Acta Oto-Laryngologica, 125*(9), 920–921.

Neuman, A. C., Haravon, A., Sislian, N., & Waltzman, S. B. (2007). Sound-direction identification with bilateral cochlear implants. *Ear and Hearing, 28*(1), 73–82.

Newman, C. W., Weinstein, B. E., Jacobson, G. P., & Hug, G. A. (1990). The Hearing Handicap Inventory for Adults: Psychometric adequacy and audiometric correlates. *Ear and Hearing, 11*(6), 430–433.

Newman, C. W., Weinstein, B. E., Jacobson, G. P., & Hug, G. A. (1991). Test-retest reliability of the Hearing Handicap Inventory for Adults. *Ear and Hearing, 12*(5), 355–357.

Nilsson, M., Soli, S. D., & Sullivan, J. A. (1994). Development of the Hearing-in-Noise Test for the measurement of speech reception thresholds in quiet and in noise. *Journal of the Acoustical Society of America, 95*(2), 1085–1099.

Nimmons, G. L., Kang, R. S., Drennan, W. R., Longnion, J., Ruffin, C., Worman, T., et al. (2008). Clinical assessment of music perception in cochlear implant listeners. *Otology and Neurotology, 29*, 149–155.

Noble, W. (2000). Self-reports about tinnitus and about cochlear implants. *Ear and Hearing, 21*(4 Suppl.), 50S–59S.

Otto, S. R., Brackmann, D. E., Hitselberger, W. E., Shannon, R. V., & Kuchta, J. (2002). Multichannel auditory brainstem implant: Update on performance in 61 patients. *Journal of Neurosurgery, 96*(6), 1063–1071.

Owens, E., Kessler, D. K., Raggio, M. W., & Schubert, E. D. (1985). Analysis and revision of the minimal auditory capabilities (MAC) battery. *Ear and Hearing, 6*(6), 280–290.

Owens, E., & Raggio, M. W. (1988). Performance inventory for profound and severe loss (PIPSL). *Journal of Speech and Hearing Disorders, 53*, 42–57.

Peterson, A., Shallop, J., Driscoll, C., Breneman, A., Babb, J., Stoeckel, R., et al. (2003). Outcomes of cochlear implantation in children with auditory neuropathy. *Journal of the American Academy of Audiology, 14*(4), 188–201.

Ponton, C. W., Eggermont, J. J., Don, M., Waring, M. D., Kwong, B., Cunningham, J., et al. (2000). Maturation of the mismatch negativity: Effects of profound deafness and cochlear implant use. *Audiology and Neuro-Otology, 5*(3–4), 167–185.

Potts, L. G., Skinner, M. W., Gotter, B. D. Strube, M. J., & Brenner, C. A. (2007). Relation between neural response telemetry thresholds, T- & C-levels, and loudness judgments in 12 adult Nucleus 24 cochlear implant recipients. *Ear and Hearing, 28*(4), 495–511.

Roland, P. S., Tobey, E. A., & Devous, M. D. (2001). Preoperative functional assessment of auditory cortex in adult cochlear implant users. *Laryngoscope, 111*(1), 77–83.

Schwartz, M. S., Otto, S. R., Brackmann, D. E., Hitselberger, W. E., & Shannon, R. V. (2003). Use of a multichannel auditory brainstem implant for neurofibromatosis type 2. *Stereo-tactic and Functional Neurosurgery, 81*(1–4), 110–114.

Shallop, J. K., Peterson, A., Facer, G. W., & Fabry, L. W. (2001). Cochlear implants in five cases of auditory neuropathy: postoperative findings and progress. *Laryngoscope, 111*(4 Pt. 1), 555–562.

Shapiro, W. H., Green, J., Bromberg, B., Gomolin, R., & Waltzman, S. W. (2000). The effect of varying stimulus repetition rate on speech perception abilities of adults using the Clarion cochlear implant: A pilot study. In S. B. Waltzman & N. L. Cohen (Eds.), *Cochlear implants* (pp. 347–348). New York: Thieme.

Sharma, A., Dorman, M. F., & Spahr, A. J. (2002). A sensitive period for the development of the central auditory system in children with cochlear implants: Implications for age of implantation. *Ear and Hearing, 23*(6), 532–539.

Snapp, H., & Telischi, F. (2008). A recommended protocol for BAHA assessment and verification for individuals with single-sided deafness. *Audiology Today, 20*, 20–27.

Snik, A. F., Mylanus, E. A., & Cremers, C. W. R. J. (2002). The bone-anchored hearing aid in patients with a unilateral air-bone gap. *Otology and Neurotology, 23*, 61–66.

Spitzer, J. B., Ghossaini, S. N., & Wazen, J. J. (2002). Evolving applications in the use of bone-anchored hearing aids. *American Journal of Audiology, 11*, 96–103.

Spitzer, J. B., Kessler, M. A., & Bromberg, B. (1992). Longitudinal findings in quality of life and perception of handicap following cochlear implantation. *Seminars in Hearing, 13*, 260–270.

Spitzer, J. B., & Mancuso, D. M. (2006). Appreciation of music in cochlear implantees [AMICI]. In W. D. Baumgartner (Ed.), *Wiener Medizinische Wochenshrift*, 9th International Conference on Cochlear Implants and Related Sciences (p. 103). Vienna.

Spitzer, J. B., Mancuso, D. M., & Cheng, M. Y. (2008). Development of a clinical test of musical perception: Appreciation of music by cochlear implantees (AMICI*) Journal of American Academy of Audiology, 19*(1), 56–81.

Spraggs, P. D., Burton, M. J., & Graham, J. M. (1994). Nonorganic hearing loss in cochlear implant candidates. *American Journal of Otology, 15*(5), 652–657.

Staller, S. J, Arndt, P., & Brimacombe, J. A. (2000). Nucleus 24 cochlear implant: Adult clinical trial results. In S. B. Waltzman & N. L. Cohen (Eds.), *Cochlear implants* (pp. 349–351). New York: Thieme.

Tjellström, A., Lindström, J., Hallén, O., Albrektsson, T., & Brånemark, P. I. (1981). Osseointegrated titanium implants in the temporal bone. *American Journal of Otology, 2*, 304–310.

Tobey, E. A. Devous, M. D., Sr., Buckley, K., Overson, G., Harris, T., Ringe, W., et al. (2005). Pharmacological enhancement of aural habilitation in adult cochlear implant users. *Ear and Hearing, 26*(Suppl. 4), 45S–56S.

Tyler, R. S. (1995). Tinnitus in the profoundly hearing-impaired & the effects of cochlear implants. *Annals of Otology, Rhinology, and Laryngology Supplement, 165*, 25–30.

Uziel, A., Mondain, M., Hagen, P., Dejean, F., & Doucet, G. (2003). Rehabilitation for high-frequency sensorineural hearing impairment in adults with the symphonix vibrant soundbridge: A comparative study. *Otology and Neurotology, 24*(5), 775–783.

Valimaa, T. T., & Sorri, M. J. (2002). Speech perception after multichannel cochlear implantation in Finnish-speaking postlingually deafened adults. *Scandinavian Audiology, 29*, 276–283.

Venail, F., Lavieille, J. P., Meller, R., Deveze, A., Tardivet, L., & Magnan, J. (2007). New perspectives for middle ear implants: First results in otosclerosis with mixed hearing loss. *Laryngoscope, 117*(3), 552–555.

Vermeire, K., Brokx, J. P., Wuyts, F. L., Cochet, E., Hofkens, A., De Bodt, M., et al. (2006). Good speech recognition and quality-of-life scores after cochlear implantation in patients with DFNA9. *Otology and Neurotology, 27*(1), 44–49.

Waltzman, S. B., & Cohen, N. L. (1999). Implantation of patients with prelingual long-term deafness. *Annals of Otology, Rhinology, and Laryngology Supplement, 177*, 84–87.

Wanscher, J. H., Faber, C. E., & Grøntved, A. M. (2006). Cochlear implantation in deaf adults: Effect on quality of life. [in Danish]. *Ugeskrift for Laeger, 168*(33), 2656–2659.

Wazen, J. J., Caruso, M., & Tjellstrom, A. (1998). Long-term results with the titanium bone-anchored hearing aid: The U.S. experience. *American Journal of Otology, 19*, 737–741.

Wazen, J. J., Ghossaini, S. N., Spitzer, J. B., & Kuller, M. (2005). Localization by unilateral BAHA users. *Otolaryngology-Head and Neck Surgery, 132*(6), 928–932.

Wazen, J. J., Spitzer, J. B., Ghossaini, S., Fayad, J. N., Niparko, J., Brackmann, D., et al. (2003). Transcranial contralateral cochlear stimulation in unilateral deafness. *Otolaryngology-Head and Neck Surgery, 129*(3), 248–254.

Wazen, J. J., Spitzer, J. B., Ghossaini, S. N., Kacker, A., & Zschommler, A. (2001). Results of the bone-anchored hearing aid (BAHA) for unilateral hearing loss. *Laryngoscope, 111*, 955–958.

Weinstein, B. E., Spitzer, J. B., & Ventry, I. M. (1986). Test-retest reliability of the Hearing Handicap Inventory for the Elderly. *Ear and Hearing, 7*(5), 295–259.

Weinstein, B. E., & Ventry, I. M. (1983) Audiometric correlates of the Hearing Handicap Inventory for the Elderly. *Journal of Speech and Hearing Disorders, 48*(4), 379–384.

8

Developments in Hearing Aid Technology and Verification Techniques

Ruth Bentler
Yu-Hsiang Wu

History of Hearing Aids

It has been surmised that the earliest man-made hearing aids were probably hollowed-out animal horns or broken sea shells, both used to collect sound and direct it into the ear canal (Berger, 1974). The earliest published description of hearing "aids" dates back to the early 1800s and suggests that trumpet-shaped devices either held and extended from the ear or discreetly housed in canes, vases and armchairs. Even pinna inserts (coated with a radioactive substance) and artificial eardrums (using a pig's bladder) saw a surge in popularity before the introduction of the first electronic hearing aids circa 1900.[1] The time line in Figure 8–1 shows the related discoveries and patents starting from the early vacuum tube options to the current digital hearing aids. The earliest carbon hearing aids consisted of a microphone, an earphone, and a battery. The amplifier (or "booster" as it was called) was added circa 1924, allowing for up to 47 dB of gain on some models. The frequency response was very narrow (~1000-Hz wide) and distortion prominent due, in part, to the carbon granules reaction to body movement and/or temperature and humidity fluctuation. The first vacuum tube hearing aid (circa 1921) was commercially distributed by the Western Electric Company. The leather covered carrying case was 7⅛" long, 7¼" high, and 3 15⁄16" wide. The price was $135. The original 45-volt battery was eventually reduced to 30 volts, then 22½ volts, and finally was powered by a mere 15 volts. By the early 1900s, almost 100,000 units were sold per year in the United States (Berger, 1974).

Modern Hearing Aids

Hearing aid technology has undergone tremendous change in the past 10 years. From smaller size

[1]The reader is referred to K. W. Berger's *The Hearing Aid: Its Operation and Development* (1974) and for a rich literary and pictorial history of the earlier nonelectronic options for persons with hearing loss.

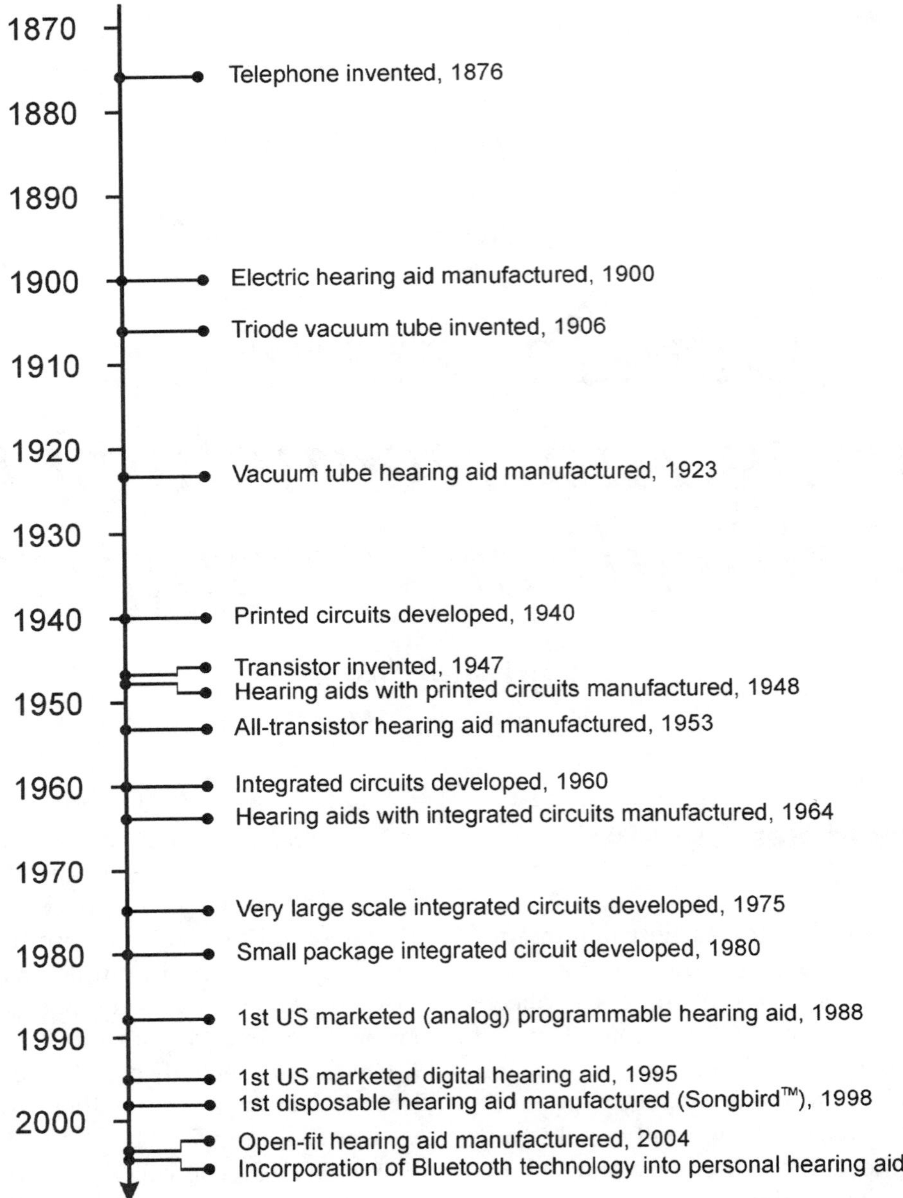

Figure 8–1. Time line of the history of hearing aids. Adapted from Berger, K. W. (1974). *The Hearing Aid: Its Operation and Development.*

to improved processing schemes, the outcome has been increased fidelity, decreased distortion, and (one hopes) improved satisfaction by the hearing impaired/hearing aid user.

Modern hearing aids are available in four basic styles: body, eyeglass, behind-the-ear (BTE), and in-the-ear (ITE). Included in the category of ITE hearing aids are in-the-canal (ITC) and completely-in-the-canal (CIC) styles (all shown in Figure 8–2). The four most common sizes of hearing aids are shown here. Each style has its application in today's market.

The BTE style hearing aid is housed in a small curved case which fits behind the ear and is

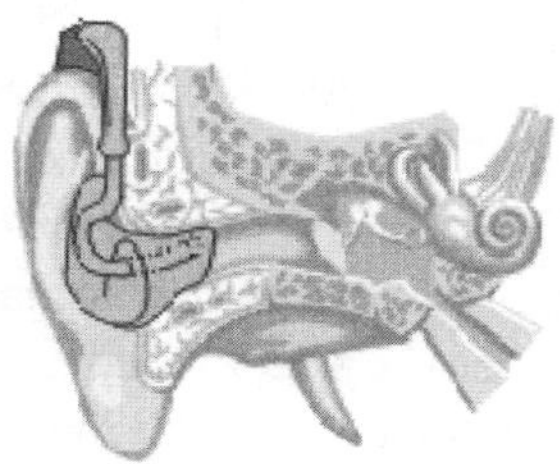

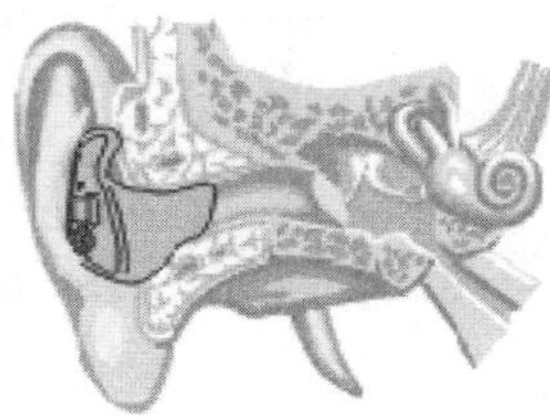

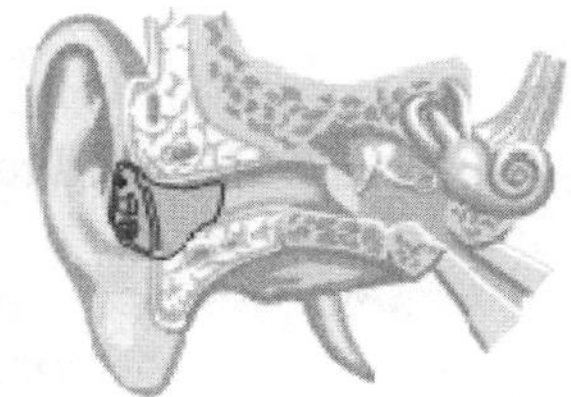

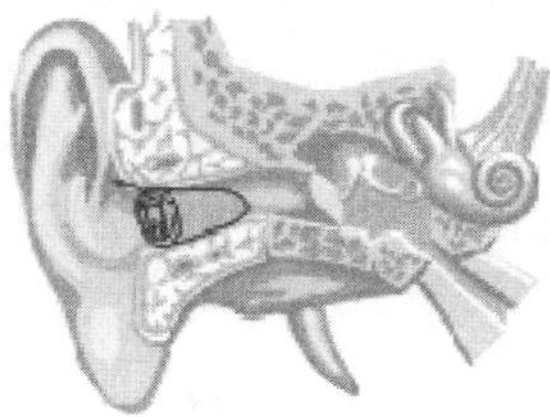

Figure 8–2. The most common styles in current hearing aid use: behind-the-ear (BTE), in-the-ear (ITE), in-the-canal (ITC), and completely-in-the-canal (CIC).

attached to a custom earpiece molded to the shape of the outer ear. Some BTE models do not use a custom earpiece; instead the rubber tubing is inserted directly into the ear. The case typically is flesh colored, but can be obtained in many colors and/or patterns. Other features include:

- BTEs may be the most appropriate choice for young children, as only the earmold needs to be replaced periodically as the child grows and the ear changes in dimension.
- Typically, BTEs are the most powerful hearing aid style available, and may be the best option for persons with severe-to-profound hearing loss.
- FM and direct auditory input are typically available as an optional or standard feature.
- Telecoil circuitry is often more powerful than with ITEs.
- Nonoccluding earmolds can be used with BTE hearing aids, if a medical condition exists or if the patient reports a "plugged" sensation when wearing other hearing aid styles.
- Larger battery sizes used in many BTEs may be easier to handle than smaller styles for those with limited manual dexterity or vision deficits.

The ITE style hearing aid fits directly into the external ear. The circuitry is housed primarily in the concha (external) portion of the ear. Due to the miniaturization of the component parts (including the microphone, receiver, and battery), it is possible to make hearing aids small enough to fill only a portion of the concha (ITC) or fit deeply into the ear canal (CIC). All three of these styles have typically been considered to be more modern and cosmetically appealing. Other features of in-the-ear instruments are as follows:

- Less wind noise in the smaller styles than with BTEs.
- Deep microphone and receiver placement with CICs may result in increased output at the eardrum compared with other styles.
- All components are integrated into a one-piece shell, which may be easier to handle and operate than for BTE styles.

Although body and eyeglass-style hearing aids were regularly used 40 to 50 years ago, they comprise only about 1% of all hearing aids marketed today. Instead, most individuals choose either ITE (approximately 45%) or BTE (approximately 55%) style hearing aids. This transition in style, use, and preference is occurring for a number of reasons, including the reduction in the size of the components, durability, and cosmetic concerns on the part of the consumer. Although the majority of hearing aids sold in the United States as recently as 2005 were ITE styles, a mini-BTE revolution has resulted in *total* sales increasing as well as a shift back to BTE accounting for the majority of the sales (Strom, 2007). This open-canal style (OC or open-fit, or mini-BTE) provides for sufficient gain without the annoyance of feedback or occlusion for the hearing aid user. Unlike its closed-mold counterpart, this hearing aid is not appropriate for the more severe losses.

Signal Processing in Digital Hearing Aids

Digital signal processing (*dsp*) hearing aids were first introduced to the U.S. market in the mid-1990s. They were limited in application and high in power consumption. Nowadays, digital hearing aids are the mainstream of the market. It is estimated about 95% of hearing aids sold in the United States are *digital* processors (Strom, 2007). In fact, many manufacturers have discontinued their analog products because (1) it is cheaper to produce digital circuits; and (2) it is cheaper to repair/replace digital circuits. Still, the cost of R & D (research and development) far exceeds the cost of component assembly, and the cost to consumers remains high.

How *dsp* Works

An analog signal is continuous in time and in amplitude. A digital signal, in contrast, consists of discrete steps (e.g., strings of ones and zeros) used to represent the magnitude of the signal over time. When a sound wave arrives at the microphone of a hearing aid, this acoustic signal is transformed to its electrical analog. The analog signal is then transformed to its digital equivalent by the analog-to-digital (A-to-D) converter. Following the digitization, the digital signal is processed by microprocessors (like the CPU in a computer). At this stage, digital values can be processed, using addition, subtraction, or more complicated mathematical operations. The ways of signal processing are governed by *algorithms*. An algorithm is step-by-step instructions determined by a set of mathematical formula or rules to perform a specific task. For example, the noise reduction algorithm may use a set of rules to judge if the input signal is speech or noise, and reacts to it accordingly. After signal processing, the digital signal has to be converted back to the analog form. This conversion is accomplished at the digital-to-analog (D-to-A) converter. The analog signal is transmited to the hearing aid receiver of the hearing aid, and is then transformed to an acoustic signal. A schematic of this digital signal processor is shown in Figure 8–3.

Advantages of Digital Signal Processing

Digital processors have several advantages over analog processors:

Physical Size. Thanks to advancements in chip technology, digital microprocessors are much smaller and faster than before. Complex tasks can be realized in extremely small processors. Because numerical computations, instead of resistors or capacitors, are used in digital signal processing, the size of the microprocessor is much smaller than the analog circuit that can perform the same task. The miniaturization of processors has enabled manufacturers to build digital hearing aids of styles, including CIC, ITE, BTE, and mini-BTE.

Power Consumption. Current digital devices have lower power consumption compared to their analog counterparts. Digital hearing aids with processing abilities comparable to those of analog aids may consume even less power. This advantage allows manufacturers to maintain the optimal balance between performance and power consumption.

Complexity. Complex tasks can be realized by small digital processors. With appropriate designs, algorithms can filter digital signals, extract frequency content of the signals, obtain statistical information of the signals, and so on. These complex tasks are critical in advanced hearing aid features

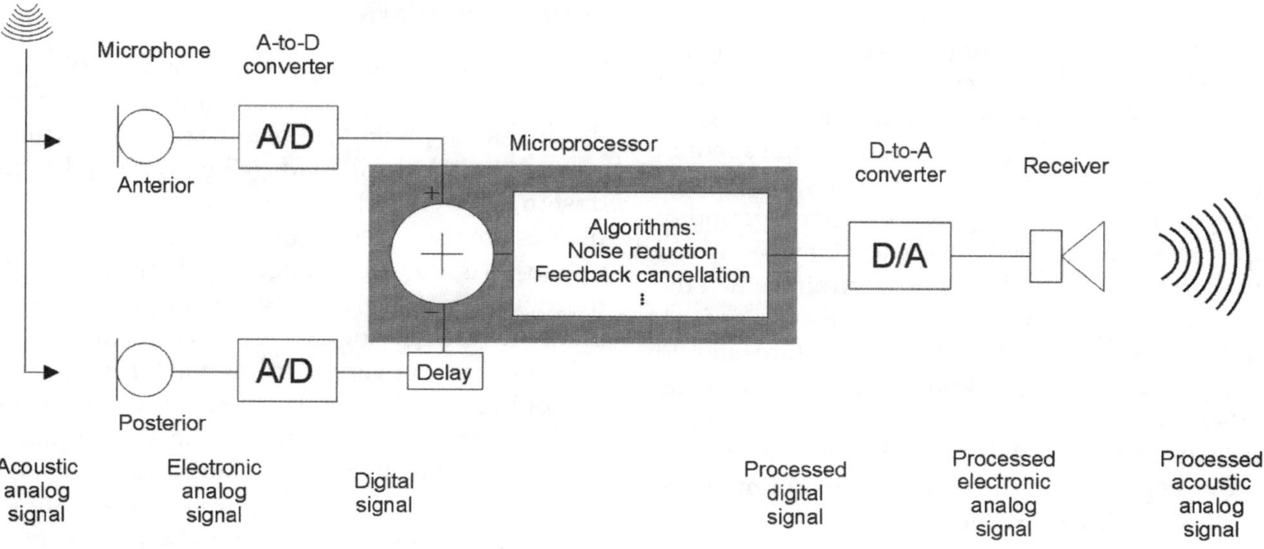

Figure 8–3. Schematics of a digital hearing aid and a directional microphone system.

(see below), and can only be accomplished, practically, by digital technology.

Flexibility. Digital systems can be extremely flexible. There are virtually unlimited ways in which the signals can be manipulated. A programmable digital system allows for hearing-aid algorithms/ features to be changed without changing the hardware. The programmability allows for digital hearing aids to be customized to a specific environment or hearing loss.

Data Storage. Digital data can be stored very easily on a variety of data carriers. With this advantage, modern hearing aids are capable of monitoring and storing information about hearing aid use and listening environments, such as hearing aid/ feature/program use time, the level of input signals, and the characteristics of input signals. These data may improve hearing aid fittings.

Although the arrival of digital technology in ear-level hearing aids has been met with great enthusiasm, early experimental comparisons between digital and analog hearing aids have shown that little efficacy in the digital aids is obtained with objective measures of speech recognition, whereas the subjective measures of benefit often suggested significant self-perceived improvement (Arlinger, Billermark, Oberg, Lunner, & Hellgren, 1998; Boymans, Dreschler, Schoneveld, & Verschuure, 1999; Walden, Surr, Cord, Edwards, & Olson, 2000). However, the importance of using blinded trials in the evaluation of new digital technologies was shown in a study addressing the bias of digital *labeling* (Bentler, Niebuhr, Johnson, & Flamme, 2003). That is, if a subject is led to believe a hearing aid to be better (usually based on marketing), the perceived benefit is greater. The real advantage of digital hearing aids is that more complex algorithms and features can be implemented in *real time*. These algorithms/features, such as the directional microphone, noise reduction algorithm, and feedback cancellation, show potential to improve benefit and satisfaction with hearing aids.

Features of Digital Hearing Aids

Classifiers and Data Logging

Implicit in modern digital hearing aid function is a stage in which incoming signals are analyzed and categorized in order that various automatic functions can occur. These are referred to *classifiers* or *classification schemes*. This information can be as simple as the amount of time the device has been on or as complex as the distribution of the types of auditory inputs based on classification algorithms. Different manufacturers implement this feature differently. The clinician may have access to the number of hours the user was wearing the hearing aid each day, the percent of time spent in quiet listening environments, or even the average level of the incoming signal for a given period of time. In addition, the information may be tapped by the different algorithms to determine when the directional microphone should activate or adapt, or whether the noise reduction feature should engage. In effect, the technology of digital hearing aids now offers the opportunity to obtain direct measures of input characteristics. The usefulness of that capability in the establishment of management strategies for the new (or experienced) hearing aid user is obvious.

Directional Microphones

The directional microphone is one feature of modern hearing aids that has been shown to improve signal-to-noise ratio (SNR) and speech intelligibility in noise for the hearing aid wearer. The rationale of directional microphone hearing aid design is based on different spatial properties of speech and noise. Typically, speech comes from a listener's front (i.e., on-axis), whereas competing noises come from directions other than the front (i.e., off-axis). Directional technology has the potential to improve speech intelligibility in noise because it maintains the on-axis sensitivity, while reducing the off-axis sensitivity. In contrast, hearing aids with omnidirectional microphones cannot improve SNRs because the microphones have the same sensitivity for sounds from all directions.

How They Work

There are several ways to construct a directional microphone system in a hearing aid. Among them, the dual-microphone system is the one used in most current digital hearing aids (Chung, 2004). In this design, two matched omnidirectional microphones are used (see Figure 8–3). The two microphone ports are placed anteriorly-posteriorly with the housing of the hearing aid on a horizontal plane (re: the hearing aid user). The acoustic signals are first converted to digital form by each microphone (and A-to-D converter), and then the output signal of one microphone is subtracted from that of the other. Before subtraction occurs, a delay (i.e., internal delay) is applied to the signal from the posterior microphone. Acoustic signals from different angles arrive at the two microphone ports at different times. If the internal delay is the same as the time it take for an acoustic signal to travel from one microphone port to the other (i.e., external delay), the output signals from the two microphones before subtraction will be exactly the same, resulting in no output from the microphone system after subtraction. With different internal delays, different directional patterns, also called *polar patterns*, can be generated. That is, the directional microphones will have better/poorer sensitivity to sound arriving from different azimuths. As shown in Figures 8–4 and 8–5, the common polar patterns have one or two *nulls* (reduced sensitivity) somewhere between 90 and 270° relative to the listener's forward face. The *goodness* of a directional microphone scheme is often measured and reported as its Directivity Index (DI)[2] and refers to the effectiveness of the design to reduce background inputs relative to the omnidirectional

[2]The mathematical formula for calculating the directivity index is:

$$DI(f) = 10 * Log_{10}\left[\frac{4\pi|p_{ax}|^2}{\int_0^{2\pi}\int_0^{\pi}|p(\phi,\theta)|^2|\sin\phi|\,d\phi\,d\theta}\right]$$

where,

$|p_{ax}|^2$ is the magnitude of the on-axis mean-square sound pressure microphone response to a plane-wave signal in free field. The theoretical DI for the various polar patterns is omnidirectional (0 dB), cardioid (4.6 dB), supercardioid (5.4 dB), and hypercardioid (6.0 dB).

$|p(\phi,\theta)|^2$ is the magnitude of the off-axis mean-square sound pressure microphone response to a diffuse sound field.

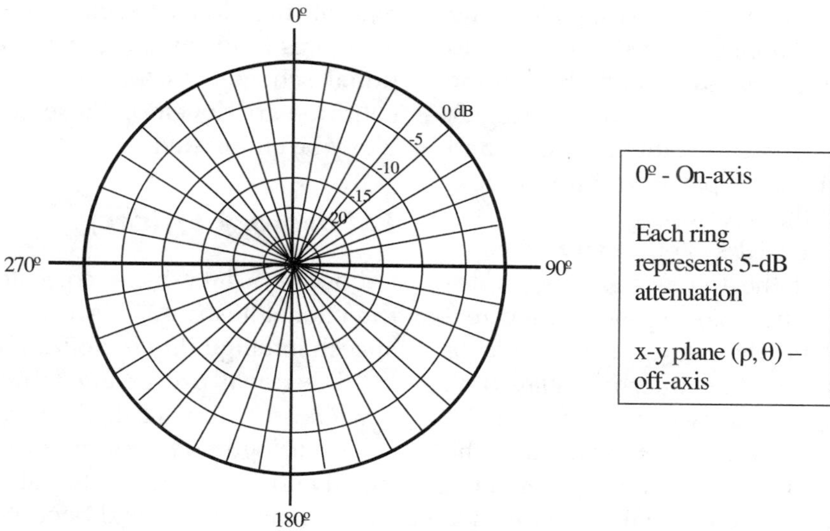

Figure 8–4. How to read a polar pattern: 0° azimuth represents the direction the listener is facing. Each concentric circle represents the reduction in gain (at a particular azimuth) as a result of the microphone's reduced sensitivity.

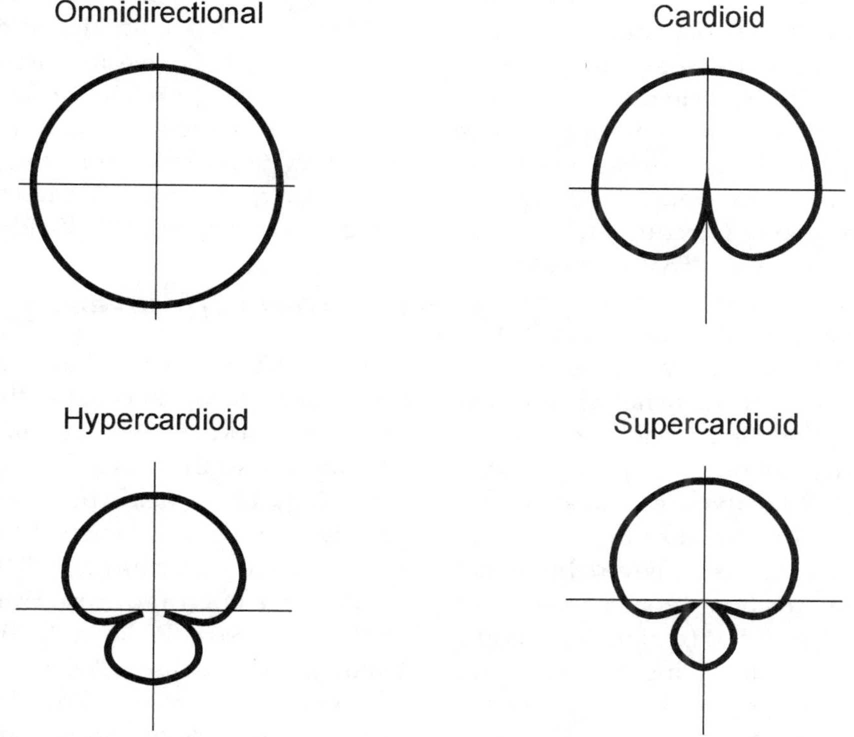

Figure 8–5. The typical polar patterns generated by directional microphone schemes.

mode. A directional microphone hearing aid using more than two microphones or ports is referred to as a *higher order* directional system. Although the calculated DI would be higher for such designs, issues of microphone matching, internal noise, and reduced incidental—and perhaps important—inputs have limited the development.

Currently, directional systems can be one or some combination of the following: fixed, automatic, and adaptive. In a *fixed* system, the directional pattern will be the same in all kinds of environments after a certain internal delay time has been programmed. This system usually can be switched between the omnidirectional and the directional modes manually by shutting down the posterior microphone. The manual switch means that hearing aid users have to identify the characteristics of listening environments and then switch to the appropriate microphone mode. In the *automatic* system, the algorithm detects and analyzes acoustic characteristics of environments, and then switches to the appropriate microphone mode automatically according to some decision rules. *Adaptive* refers to the capability of the directional system to change the directional pattern in different noise configurations. There are two ways of changing the pattern: (1) the system can "steer" the nulls of the directional pattern to the appropriate azimuths (e.g., the azimuth of the noise source) and achieve maximal SNR improvement; and (2) the system can apply addition gain reduction to sounds arriving from off-axis origins. That is, in addition to the reduced sensitivity of the microphone to sound arriving off axis, an additional gain reduction may be applied. Adaptivity can be realized independently in different frequency channels in a multichannel adaptive directional hearing aid.

Although directional microphone technology can improve the SNR for the user, there are several disadvantages. First, because the directivity of the directional system is achieved by signal subtraction, the subtraction process results in lower microphone sensitivity (re: omnidirectional processing) for low-frequency inputs. Extra gain compensation may be provided to equalize the frequency responses of the microphones. However, increasing gain results in higher internal electrical noise of the microphone system. Another disadvantage of directional technology is that it typically generates louder wind noise than the omnidirectional scheme. As technologies and algorithms continue to develop, these disadvantages will likely be eliminated.

Laboratory Efficacy

Laboratory data have consistently shown that directional hearing aids can improve SNR and speech intelligibility in noise. The benefit afforded by directional processing is referred to as *directional benefit*, and is calculated as the difference in speech recognition performance between the directional and the omnidirectional modes of the same hearing aid. Directional benefit obtained across a wide variety of experimental conditions ranges from –1 dB to 16 dB with an average of 3.4 dB (Amlani, 2001; Chung, 2004), or from 2% to 30% with an average of approximate 20 to 25% across studies (Bentler, Egge, Tubbs, Dittberner, & Flamme, 2004; Kuk, Kollofski, Brown, Melum, & Rosenthal, 1999; Ricketts, Henry, & Hornsby, 2005; Ricketts & Hornsby, 2006; Sandlin, 2000; Valente et al., 1995; Walden et al., 2000). Besides objective directional benefit, researchers have also demonstrated hearing aid users' strong preference for directional processing over omnidirectional processing in various laboratory noisy environments (Amlani, Rakerd, & Punch, 2006; Boymans & Dreschler, 2000; Preves, Sammeth, & Wynne, 1999; Walden et al., 2000).

Real-World Effectiveness

Although laboratory data have consistently shown significant directional benefit, directional processing is not always preferred in the real world. Among studies that have investigated directional technology using field trials, some have shown perceived functional benefit (Preves et al., 1999; Ricketts, Henry, & Gnewikow, 2003), whereas more studies have not (Cord, Surr, Walden, & Dyrlund, 2004; Cord, Surr, Walden, & Olson, 2002; Surr, Walden, Cord, & Olson, 2002; Walden et al., 2000). For example, in a recent blinded 4-week field trial using hearing aids configured with an omnidirectional/directional toggle switch, the DIR mode was preferred 24.5%, and the OMNI mode was preferred 47.0% of the time (Wu, 2007). The response of No Preference was selected 28.5% of the time. Contrarily, in the laboratory environments with similar speech/noise configurations, the prevalence of each response was 51.1% (DIR), 8.5% (OMNI), and 40.4% (No Preference). That is, the DIR mode was more preferred in the laboratory (51.1% of the time) and the OMNI mode was more preferred in the field (47% of the time). Furthermore, it has not been possible to predict real-world benefit of directional technology by data obtained in the laboratory. An example of this laboratory-field discrepancy was demonstrated by Cord et al. (2004), who investigated the extent to which a laboratory measurement can predict success with directional processing in everyday lives. They found that laboratory-measured directional benefit of successful and unsuccessful directional microphone users (defined by how often the subjects switched microphone modes) was the same statistically. That is, subjects who had large directional benefit in the laboratory were not necessarily able to tell the difference between microphone modes and switch between them.

Several variables have been suggested to explain the limited benefit of directional technology in the real world, including speech/noise configuration, SNR, and reverberation. The directional microphone can improve the SNR only when speech is presented in front of the listener and noise is presented in the rear hemisphere of the listener or is presented around the listener. However, this speech/noise configuration is not very common in the real world. It is estimated that these environments constitute only one-third to one-fourth of the total active listening time in everyday lives (Cord, Walden, Surr, & Dittberner, 2007; Walden & Walden, 2005). Even if the speech/noise configuration are appropriate for the directional microphone, directional technology only provides benefit within a certain SNR range. If the SNR is very favorable (e.g., not too noisy), both directional and omnidirectional aided performance may be good. On the other hand, if the SNR is too unfavorable (e.g., too noisy), neither microphone mode is good (Walden, Surr, Grant, Van Summers, Cord, & Dyrlund, 2005). Reverberation also reduces directional benefit (Hawkins & Yacullo, 1984; Ricketts & Hornsby, 2003). In a reverberant environment, directional benefit is decreased because the noise signal emitted from a source behind a listener will bounce off the wall and eventually arrive from the listener's front. The reflections make it difficult for the directional microphone to spatially separate speech and noise.

One additional variable that has been shown to decrease real-world directional benefit is the availability of visual cues (Wu, 2007), which has long been known to aid in speech intelligibility (Sumby & Pollack, 1954). In environments that favor directional processing (e.g., talker in front of the listener), visual cues are usually available and accessible. With the help of visual cues, the omnidirectional aided performance is typically good enough to approach the inherent limitation of the listener's speech recognition ability (i.e., ceiling). Switching to the directional mode only brings a small difference in performance that is too small to perceive. Therefore, a hearing aid user with excellent speechreading/lipreading ability may only obtain minimal benefit from directional technology.

Digital Noise Reduction (DNR)

Noise reduction schemes have been implemented in wearable hearing aids since the middle of the previous century (Bentler et al., 1993a, 1993b). The early analog schemes were primarily designed to reduce gain/output in the presence of high input levels. In most of the early designs, this modification occurred in the lower frequency region, presumably to keep higher energy, low-frequency sounds from either (1) triggering the compressor and thus reducing gain in the entire frequency range, or (2) increasing the likelihood of upward spread of masking. Although the efficacy or effectiveness of any of the early efforts was limited, some showed evidence of providing "listening ease" (Bentler et al., 1993a).

How They Work

Unlike the earlier analog schemes, current DNR schemes are manufacturer-specific algorithms developed to acoustically analyze the incoming signal and alter the gain/output characteristics according to predetermined rules. Although most are modulation- based schemes (i.e., differentiating speech from noise based on temporal characteristics), others include concurrent Wiener filter processing as well as impulse noise, wind-noise, and microphone noise reduction algorithms (refer to Bentler & Chiou, 2006). Because the digital signal processor is capable of analyzing the incoming signal in real time, the algorithms can be designed or written to alter gain/frequency depending on ever changing modulation rate, modulation depth, input level, and so on. Figure 8–6 shows and example of how seven different manufacturers implement their algorithms for different input stimuli. Each of the company's premiere hearing aids was set for a 50 dB HL flat hearing loss. DNR was set to maximum (where adjustable) and all other features were disengaged. In the top panel a 1.5 minute file of speech-in-noise (at –10dB SNR) was fed to the hearing aid in both the DNR-on and DNR-off modes. The gain change that occurred is shown for the seven hearing aids. In the bottom panel, the stimulus applied was a random (white) noise signal. The differences across products are evidence of each manufacturer's unique application of DNR.

The speed at which these schemes engage across manufacturers also differs. There are several time constants in current algorithms: an analysis time (5–15 seconds), an onset time (2 msec to 5 sec), a recovery time (which incorporates a second analysis time with recovery to previous gain levels). As with the gain effect, manufacturers implement their own rationales, these *time constants* are often the same as used by the manufacturer for the compression action, or other adaptive features.

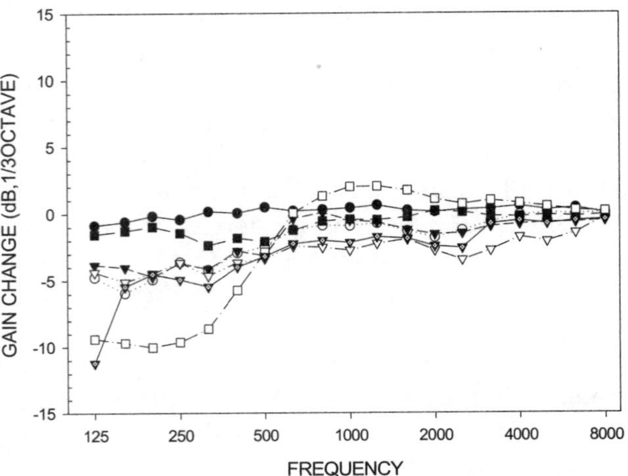

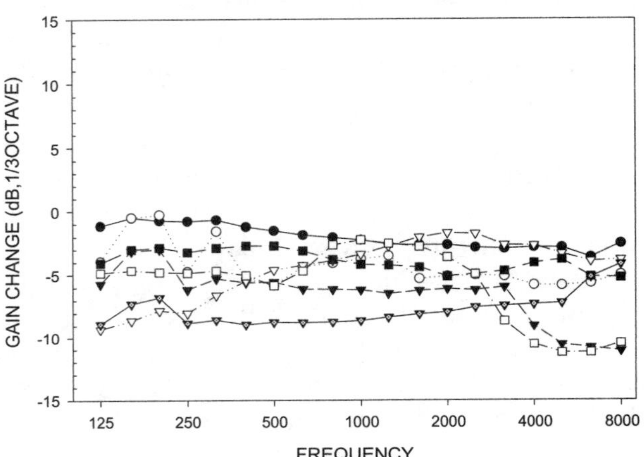

Figure 8–6. Examples of the impact of the DNR algorithms in seven different hearing aids. Each was programmed for a flat 50 dB hearing loss. The upper panel shows the resultant gain reduction for a speech-in-babble noise (–10 dB SNR) stimulus, and lower panel shows the resultant gain reduction for a white noise input.

Laboratory Efficacy

Laboratory data have consistently shown that digital noise reduction, regardless of the specific implementation, improved listening ease and comfort (e.g., Alcantara, Moore, Kuhnel, & Launer, 2003; Bentler, Wu, Kettel & Hurtig, 2008; Ricketts & Hornsby, 2005) with little effect on speech perception ability.

Real-World Effectiveness

There are few reports of noise reduction effectiveness in real world communication settings (Bentler et al., 2008; Boymans & Dreschler, 2000; Walden et al., 2000). In a study primarily aimed at assessing the effectiveness of directional microphones, Walden et al. (2000) found significantly better sound comfort ratings when DNR was used in conjunction with directional microphone technology than with directional microphone technology alone. And, although the Aversiveness subscale of the self-report inventory Abbreviated Profile of Hearing Aid Benefit (APHAB) (Cox & Alexander, 1995) showed poorer scores in the aided condition (versus pretesting) in one study (Palmer, Bentler & Mueller, 2006), several studies have confirmed that DNR-off versus DNR-on results in reduced self-reported Aversiveness during field trials, as well as reported of easier listening (Boymans & Dreschler, 2000; Bentler et al., 2008). None of these field or laboratory data indicate improved speech perception in noise with the current generation of DNR. At the same time, improved listening ease, comfort, and so on, are still a positive outcomes.

Feedback Management

Feedback occurs when output from a hearing aid receiver re-enters the microphone port. As a consequence, the signal received by the microphone consists of two components: the desired signal and undesired feedback signal, which is correlated with the output of the receiver. The feedback signal will be amplified along with incoming signals arriving at the input. When the combined acoustic energy exceeds a certain level, it will begin to oscillate. Leakage of the feedback signal can be (1) acoustic through the vent or poor mechanical coupling of earmolds with the external ear, or (2) electrical through the electronic components of the hearing aid.

There are several negative effects of feedback. First, hearing aid gain may be limited. Dyrlund and Lundh (1990) reported that approximately 10 dB gain reduction from the prescribed values was required in order to eliminate acoustic feedback in profoundly hearing-impaired children. The limitations were greatest for frequencies above 1000 Hz. Using computer simulation, Kates (1988) found that acoustic feedback limits the maximum possible gain to less than 40 dB. George, Wood, and Engebretson (1993) showed that the acoustic feedback restricted the volume control adjustments that hearing aid wearers could make to compensate for loss of audibility in soft speech environments. Secondly, feedback can cause distortion. Even when the hearing aid gain is set to a level below oscillation, the signal feeding back may still cause the output to increase or decrease at certain frequencies, which may result in extra peaks in the hearing aid frequency response. When the formant transitions of speech are near the frequencies of these peaks, speech signals may be severely distorted and detract from their perception by listeners with hearing impairment (Preves, 1988). It has been suggested that insertion gain should be 4 to 8 dB less than values at which audible feedback occurs to avoid the deleterious effects of this suboscillatory feedback (Skinner, 1988).

A number of approaches have been used to reduce the effects of acoustic feedback in order to permit the hearing aid user to obtain more usable gain. These approaches include decreasing the vent size, remaking or recoating the earmolds or shells so that there is less leakage between the mold/shell and the walls of the ear canal, turning the volume control or gain control down to the point below oscillation, rolling off the gain of the high frequencies, reducing the gain around the offending frequency, frequency shifting, varying the phase responses of the potential feedback frequencies, adaptive band gain reduction via notched filter, and adaptively estimating and canceling the acoustic feedback path (typically referred to as adaptive feedback pathway cancellation, or AFPC). Although these algorithms continue to be refined, audible consequences of the hearing aid mistaking an externally generated signal for an internally generated feedback signal are prone to occur. This misstep results in "entrainment," a term borrowed from 17th century physics. Defined as "the tendency for two oscillating bodies to lock into phase so that they vibrate in harmony,"[3] current

[3]www.soundfeelings.com/products/alternative_medicine/music_therapy/entrainment.htm

usage relative to feedback cancellation algorithms refers to the result of an AFPC algorithm attempting to eliminate the squeal of the hearing aid when the source is actually external to the hearing aid. The result is an audible "twirping" sound that can be heard by the hearing aid wearer.

Prescribing Gain/Output

Determining the appropriate gain and output for an individual has been the goal of much clinical and research effort over the past 60 years. From mirroring the audiogram (Knudsen & Jones, 1935), in which every decibel of hearing loss was compensated by a decibel of gain, to the most recent National Acoustic Laboratories (NAL-NL[4]) and Desired Sensation Level (DSL[5]) algorithms, where audibility, listening comfort, and age-related acoustical transforms are considered, the quest for the best fit may be over. Early philosophy supported a "one size fits all" approach to assigning gain to a given hearing loss. The Harvard Report (Davis et al., 1946) had profound influence on this practice. Generally, the report supported the use of hearing aids with frequency responses rising at a rate of +6 dB/octave for all potential hearing aid wearers, regardless of audiometric configuration. The popular approach of that era involved choosing two or three clinic stock hearing aids and evaluating them on the patient. Although this "comparative approach" to fitting hearing aids has often been credited to Raymond Carhart (Humes, 1996), his battery was actually quite more extensive. Other prescriptive attempts have included amplifying speech to the hearing aid user's Most Comfortable Listening Level (MCL) (Watson & Knudson, 1940), or bisecting the dynamic range between threshold and loudness discomfort level (LDL) to determine optimal hearing level (Wallenfels, 1967).

Today, although some manufacturers promote their own proprietary fitting algorithms, most clinicians use either the current version provided by the DSL (Canadian) or the NAL (Australian) groups. The DSL first introduced the concept of the SPL-ogram (upside-down representation of decibels, with the reference being the eardrum SPL), with the primary focus being on the audibility of the speech within the dynamic range of the potential hearing aid user. The NAL was introduced as a gain-based prescription, with the primary goal of making all bands contribute equally to the loudness of the speech input. Over the years, both camps have introduced age-appropriate corrections for gain and output considerations, correction factors for hearing aid style, venting effects, and binaural loudness summation. Both approaches have evolved following a number of studies addressing preference and performance by hearing impaired/hearing aid users. Either is a justifiable choice in current hearing aid fitting efforts.

Establishing Outcomes

Fitting Considerations

There have been reports in the literature for 30 years that hearing aid intervention *itself* can lead to improvements in social functioning (e.g., Joore, Brunenberg, Chenault, & Anteunis, 2003), quality of life (e.g., Crandell, 1998), handicap (e.g., Primeau, 1997), disability (e.g., McArdle et al., 2005), and psychosocial domains (e.g., Mulrow et al., 1990). Yet, extensive efforts to determine predictors of hearing aid success have been generally unsuccessful at relating any actual audiometric variables to any aided outcome (see Bentler, 2007, for a summary). Some of the more recent and most comprehensive undertakings relative to under-

[4]NAL-NL-1, which refers to National Acoustics Laboratory Non-Linear, Version 1, is the latest in a series of gain/frequency prescriptions from the researchers in that facility in Sydney Australia. Originally developed by Denis Byrne, the efforts are now coordinated by Harvey Dillon (Dillon, 2006).

[5]DSL refers to the Desired Sensation Level approach to fitting hearing aids. Originally developed by Richard Seewald and his colleagues at the University of Western Ontario, this fitting scheme has undergone a number of revisions in the past 20 years. The current version is referred to as DSLv5.0 (Scollie, 2006).

standing this relationship are attributable to Humes and his colleagues (Humes, 1999, 2001; Humes et al., 2002a, 2002b; Humes et al., 2003). In the absence of any published large-scale studies aimed at modeling hearing aid "success" and identifying those factors that influence this success, Humes (2003) has undertaken several factor-analysis efforts in an attempt to determine the number and nature of the dimensions of successful hearing aid outcome. The primary finding of those efforts indicated:

1. Aided speech perception was best predicted by degree of hearing loss, cognitive performance, and age;
2. Hearing aid use was best predicted by previous hearing aid use;
3. Hearing aid satisfaction was best predicted by aided sound quality measures.

In the current evidence-based practice (EBP) milieu, both research and clinical settings are challenged to document outcomes of both the fitting itself (verification) as well as the longer term outcomes of the fitting and the rehabilitative process (validation). In this chapter we focus on the verification outcomes only.

Verification

Guidelines for fitting of hearing aids have been published and adopted as "best practice" in audiology (AAA, 2006; ASHA, 1998). *Verification* begins once the amplification goals have been established. This component of the process refers to measurement-taking to ensure that the hearing aids meet standards of electroacoustic performance, cosmetic appeal, comfortable fit, and real-ear acoustical performance.

Electroacoustic standards refer to the ANSI S3.2-2003 measures to ensure that the hearing aids are working as intended by the manufacturer. With current digital hearing aids, obtaining those measures can be a challenge. With the cascading algorithms currently marketed, obtaining baseline performance measures can be difficult. The steps towards electroacoustic verification that the hearing aid is functioning as intended by the manufacturer are provided in Appendix 8–A. Although it has been often assumed by clinicians that the computer monitor reflection of the manufacturer's fitting scheme provides sufficient evidence of electroacoustic performance, such is often not the case. Hawkins and Cook (2003) found evidence of large discrepancies amongst manufacturers for coupler gain and insertion gain estimates. Although most manufacturers incorporate some fitting algorithm similar to NAL-NL-1 (Dillon, 1999) or DSL (DSLv5.0, Seewald et al. 2005), the clinician must verify that the goal of improving audibility (reducing the disability) has been achieved. That verification is best accomplished *in situ* (in-the-ear). In the early 1980s computerized *real-ear* measurement tools were finding their way onto the U.S. market. By attaching a microphone to a small silicone tube that could be inserted into the ear canal for direct measures of hearing aid performance, a new era was sprung. Yet despite being touted as *best practice* (AAA, 2006; ASHA, 1998), fewer than one-third of current practicing clinicians routinely use the technology (Mueller, 2005). Excuses aside, there is no better—or more direct—manner of establishing the *goodness* of a fitting effort re: audibility. Measures of gain and output are easily achievable and standard procedures readily available. Terminology and methodology have been standardized for these real-ear measures of hearing aid performance (ANSI 3.45, 2003). Real-Ear Unaided Response (REUR) measures provide an indication of the natural resonance characteristics of the ear canal. Real-Ear Aided Response (REAR) measures indicate the SPL at the eardrum with the hearing aid and earmold in place. The difference between the two has been termed Real-Ear Insertion Gain (REIG), whereas the maximum output in the ear canal (or real-ear equivalent to OSPL90) has been termed Real-Ear Saturation Response (RESR). A clear understanding of the calibration procedures, including insertion depth of the probe tube, and placement of the loudspeaker, are critical to obtaining both valid and reliable measures of gain and output in the aided ear.

More recently, *speech mapping* has found its way into the probe-measure repertoire. Speech mapping refers to the visual representation impact of the gain on a typical long-term average speech spectrum (LTASS). Since providing audibility of speech is our primary objective with most hearing aid fittings, looking at the impact of our decision-making in terms of that spectrum seems logical and desirable. Different manufacturers of hearing aid test and probe microphone equipment have implemented this speech mapping in different ways. As shown in Figure 8–7, the audibility of the soft and loud components (peaks) of speech are easily discernable for two different input levels. Should any of the speech peaks approach the upper end targets of the dynamic range (depicted by the asterisks) and thus approach an uncomfortable level, the levels can also be easily visualized for both clinician and client. Figure 8–8 shows the usefulness of speech mapping for the verification of directional microphones and DNR features.

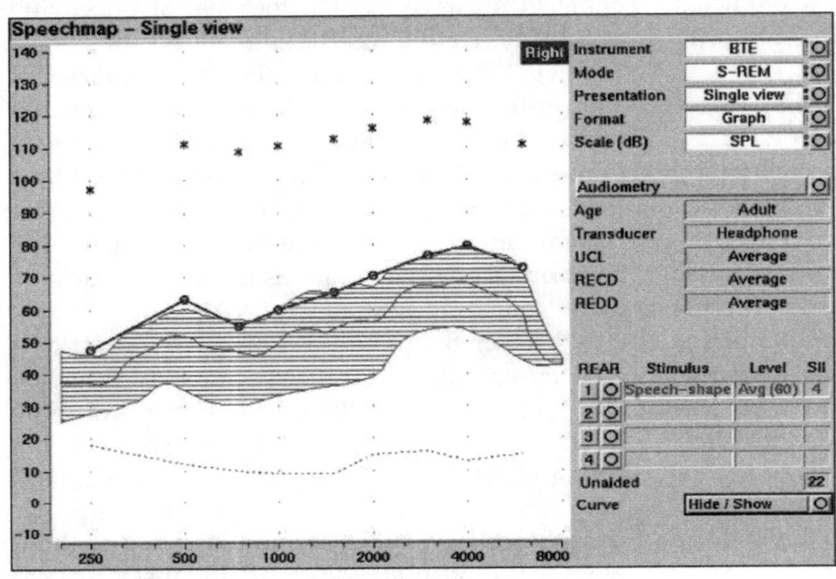

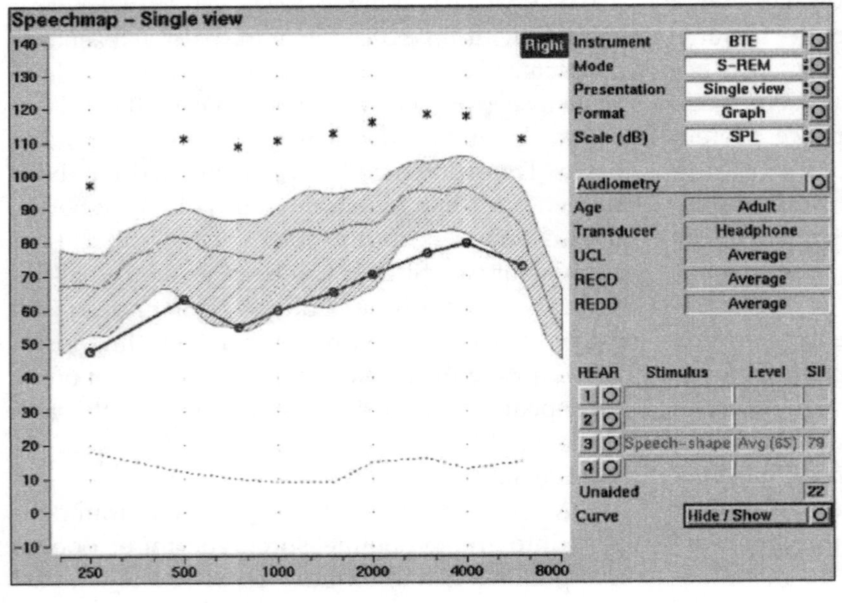

Figure 8–7. An example of speech mapping. The entire dynamic range of an average speech spectrum (sometimes referred to as the "speech banana") is shown for two different amplification schemes. In each figure, the open circles indicate the hearing thresholds and the asterisk symbols represent the maximum output targets. In the upper panel it is evident that the speech input is not audible to this listeners. The lower panel shows evidence of nearly all of the speech cues being audible, but not uncomfortable for the listener. (Courtesy of Bill Cole, Audioscan™)

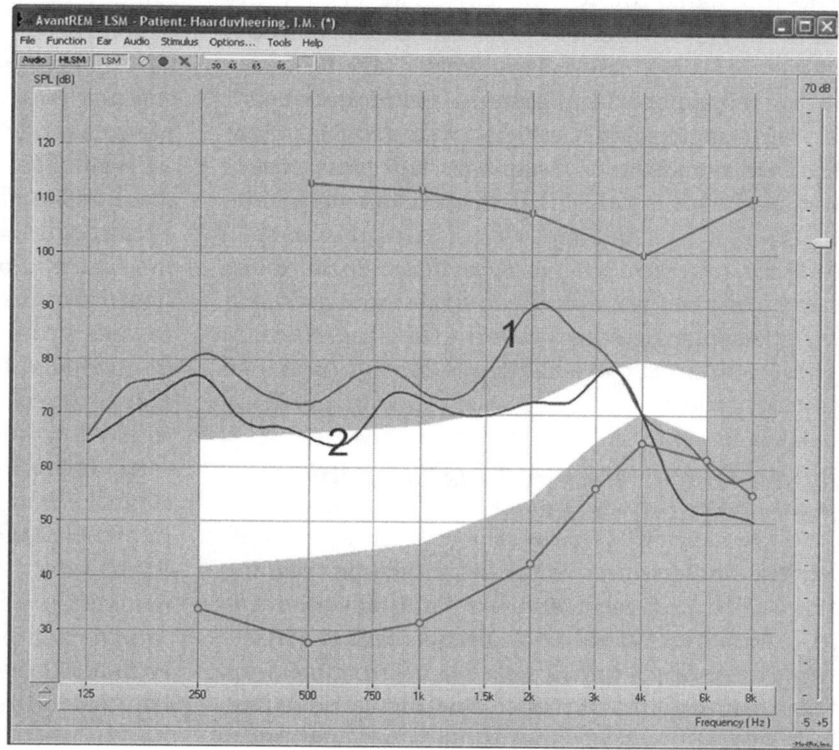

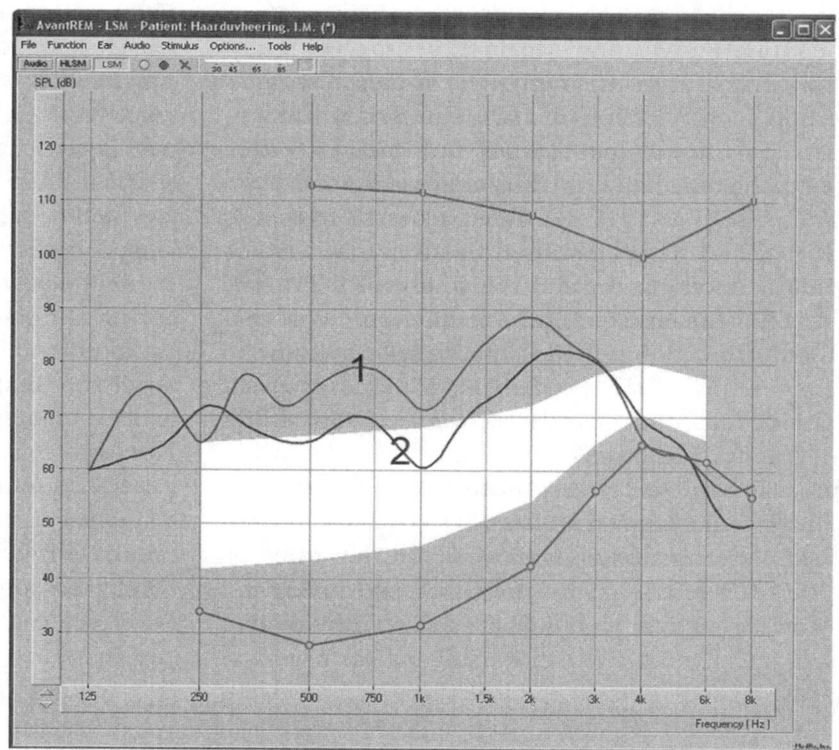

Figure 8–8. Speech mapping can also be used to verify the features on a hearing aid. In the top panel a directional microphone is being assessed. Curve 1 indicates the response for inputs to the front microphone. Curve 2 indicates the (reduced) response for inputs to the back microphone. In the bottom panel, the DNR feature is being assessed. Curve 1 indicates the measures response for an adult female in a quiet background. Curve 2 shows the (reduced) response from the hearing aid to cafeteria noise. Thresholds are shown by the open circles, and maximum output targets are indicated by the U (Uncomfortable) symbols. (Courtesy of Brad Ingrao, MedRX™)

The top panel shows the LTASS levels for the front-facing microphone in a directional scheme in Curve 1, and the LTASS levels for the back-facing microphone in Curve 2. It is apparent that the output from the hearing aid is reduced from the rear microphone, indicating a properly functioning hearing aid. The bottom panel shows the LTASS levels for a female talker in quiet (Curve 1) and for cafeteria noise (Curve 2). From these curves one can see that the output in the presence of noise is reduced relative to the single talker. These measures can be taken in situ or on a 2 cc coupler mode.

Does Verification Include Speech Perception Measures?

Speech audiometry had its inception during World War II in the military rehabilitation centers (e.g., Newby, 1972). The original speech materials were developed under government contract for the purpose of comparing communication systems in transmitting speech. Although the lists were originally developed and tested on normal hearing listeners (Davis, 1947), it became apparent that the same lists could be used for the differentiation of normal and hearing impaired ears as well. Today the debate is on as to whether speech testing is actually a verification (of audibility) or a validation (of the particular management scheme). However used, the outcome is only as good as the test used to obtain it. To that end, without normative data or critical difference[6] values to assist in the interpretation of the results, the time spent on this form of "outcome measure" is not time well spent. The most commonly used speech tests include:

The CID W-22 test (Hirsh et al., 1952) consists of four lists of 50 words each, for a total of 200 words. A male voice recites the test. Each word is preceded by the carrier phrase, "You will say . . . " The words included in the CID W-22 are among the 400 most common words of English writing of 1932. The test is considered to approximate the phonetic balance of spoken English. Although critical difference (CD) values are not available, tables of confidence levels for determining the probability of differences between speech-discrimination scores based on arc-sine transforms applied to a binomial distribution have been developed (Thornton & Raffin, 1978). In lieu of test-specific data, these tables allow for comparisons between ears, technologies, and even pre-post intervention.

The NU-6 test (Tillman & Carhart, 1966) consists of four lists of 50 words each, for a total of 200 words. A male voice recites the test. Each word is preceded by the carrier phrase, "Say the word . . . " The NU-6 is designed phonemically, with each word being a CVC monosyllable. The same issue exists relative to establishing true differences in a clinical setting.

The California Consonant Test (CCT; Owens & Schubert, 1977) consists of a single list of 100 words. The test was designed for analyzing consonant confusion in patients with hearing loss. For each presentation, the patient is given four options and is instructed to select the one matching the word heard. No norms or psychometric data are available.

The Speech-in-Noise (SIN) test (Fikret-Pasa, 1993) consists of nine lists of 40 sentences. The test was developed to investigate the effects of various compression ratios on speech intelligibility. A female voice recites the test in the presence of four-talker babble recorded on a single channel. The signal-to-noise ratio decreases as the test progresses. Normative data and critical difference values have been established (Bentler, 2000).

The Hearing-in-Noise Test (HINT; Nilsson, Soli, & Sullivan, 1994) consists of 25 phonemically balanced and equivalent 10-sentence lists. Speech-spectrum shaped noise is presented at a fixed level, and the sentence level changes adaptively. Normative data and critical difference values are published within the manual.

The Connected Speech Test (CST; Cox, Alexander, & Gilmore, 1987) consists of 48 passages of connected speech. A female voice recites the test. Subjects are expected to repeat each sentence of the

[6]Critical difference (CD) refers to the score change for an individual that would be statistically significant (refer to Hyde, 2000). Without CD values, it is not possible to tell whether two hearing aids result in different speech perception outcomes for a given listener, or whether the aided performance is better than the unaided performance, and so on.

passage, and are scored on 25 key words in each passage. Normative data and critical difference values have been established and are published in the original article.

In summary, *verification* refers to ensuring that the hearing aid is the style, fit, appearance, and comfort that the client intended it to be (AAA, 2006; ASHA, 1998). The clinician must verify that the microphone is not hidden behind the tragus, the hearing aid and its battery can be inserted and extracted with relative ease, and that controls are manageable for the user. In addition, the verification stage confirms that the hearing aid works as the manufacturer intended, and that the gain and output goals of the fitting have been achieved such that speech is audible and comfortable. Verification should include assessment of the features (e.g., directional microphone, digital noise) that are intended to alter the gain/output in certain environments. Verification might also include tests of speech perception to better quantify the audibility afforded by the particular fitting. In short, verification is the stage during which all of those fitting efforts are checked to confirm that we got what we intended to get with this particular choice of amplification. Verification is done at the time of the fitting, or within the adjustment period. *Validation*, to be discussed in Chapter 14, is done to assess the eventual outcome of our management plan. Each is equally important to the success of the hearing impaired, hearing aid user.

References

Alcantara, J. I., Moore, B. C., Kuhnel, V., & Launer, S. (2003). Evaluation of the noise reduction system in a commercial digital hearing aid. *International Journal of Audiology, 42*, 34–42.

American Academy of Audiology. (2006). Guidelines for audiologic management of adult hearing impairment. *Audiology Today, 18*(5).

American Speech-Language-Hearing Association. (1998). Guidelines for hearing aid fitting for adults. *Asha, 40*(Suppl. 18).

Amlani, A. M. (2001). Efficacy of directional microphone hearing aids: A meta-analytic perspective. *Journal of the American Academy of Audiology, 12*(4), 202–214.

Amlani, A. M., Rakerd, B., & Punch, J. L. (2006). Speech-clarity judgments of hearing-aid-processed speech in noise: Differing polar patterns and acoustic environments. *International Journal of Audiology, 45*(6), 319–330.

ANSI. (2003). *Specification of hearing aid characteristics (ANSI S3.22)*. New York: Author.

ANSI. (2003). *Methods of measurement of real-ear performance of hearing aids (ANSI S3.45)*. New York: Author.

Arlinger, S., Billermark, E., Oberg, M., Lunner, T., & Hellgren, J. (1998). Clinical trial of a digital hearing aid. *Scandinavian Audiology, 27*(1), 51–61.

Bentler, R. A. (2000). List equivalency and test-retest reliability of the Speech in Noise (SIN) test. *American Journal of Audiology: A Journal of Clinical Practice, 9*, 3–10.

Bentler, R. A. (2007) Audiometric considerations for hearing aid fitting (and success). *Proceedings of Hearing Care for Adults: An International Conference*. Chicago.

Bentler, R. A., Anderson, C. V., Niebuhr, D., & Getta, J. (1993a). A longitudinal study of noise reduction circuits. Part I: Objective measures. *Journal of Speech and Hearing Research, 36*, 808–819.

Bentler, R. A., Anderson, C. V., Niebuhr, D., & Getta, J. (1993b). A longitudinal study of noise reduction circuits. Part II: Subjective measures. *Journal of Speech and Hearing Research, 36*, 820–831.

Bentler, R. A., & Chiou, L-K. (2006). Digital noise reduction: An overview. *Trends in Amplification, 10*(2), 71–82.

Bentler, R. A., Egge, J. L., Tubbs, J. L., Dittberner, A. B., & Flamme, G. A. (2004). Quantification of directional benefit across different polar response patterns. *Journal of the American Academy of Audiology, 15*(9), 649–659.

Bentler, R. A., Niebuhr, D. P., Johnson, T. A., & Flamme, G. A. (2003). Impact of digital labeling on outcome measures. *Ear and Hearing, 24*(3), 215–224.

Bentler, R., Wu, Y-H., Kettel, J., & Hurtig, R. (2008). Digital noise reduction: Outcomes from field and lab studies. *International Journal of Audiology, 47*(8), 447–460.

Berger, K. W. (1974). *The hearing aid: Its operation and development* (2nd ed.). Livonia, MI: National Hearing Aid Society.

Boymans, M., & Dreschler, W. A. (2000). Field trials using a digital hearing aid with active noise reduction and dual-microphone directionality. *Audiology, 39*(5), 260–268.

Boymans, M., Dreschler, W. A., Schoneveld, P., & Verschuure, H. (1999). Clinical evaluation of a full-digital in-the-ear hearing instrument. *Audiology, 38*(2), 99–108.

Chung, K. (2004). Challenges and recent developments in hearing aids. Part I. Speech understanding in noise, microphone technologies and noise reduction algorithms. *Trends in Amplification, 8*(3), 83–124.

Cord, M. T., Surr, R. K., Walden, B. E., & Dyrlund, O. (2004). Relationship between laboratory measures of directional advantage and everyday success with directional microphone hearing aids. *Journal of the American Academy of Audiology, 15*(5), 353–364.

Cord, M. T., Surr, R. K., Walden, B. E., & Olson, L. (2002). Performance of directional microphone hearing aids in everyday life. *Journal of the American Academy of Audiology, 13*(6), 295–307.

Cord, M. T., Walden, B. E., Surr, R. K., & Dittberner, A. (2007). Field evaluation of an asymmetric directional microphone fitting. *Journal of the American Academy of Audiology, 18*(3), 245–256.

Cox, R. M., & Alexander, G. C. (1995). The abbreviated profile of hearing aid benefit. *Ear and Hearing, 16,* 176–186.

Cox, R. M., Alexander, G. C., & Gilmore, C. (1987). Development of the Connected Speech Test (CST). *Ear and Hearing, 8*(5), 119S.

Crandell, C. C. (1998). Hearing aids: Their effects on functional health status. *Hearing Journal, 52,* 22–32.

Davis, H. (1947). *Hearing and deafness: A guide for laymen.* New York: Murray Hill Books.

Davis, H., Hudgins, C. V., Marquis, R. J., Nichols, R. H., Peterson, G. E., Ross, D. A., et al. (1946). The selection of hearing aids. *Laryngoscope, 56,* 85–115, 135–163.

Dillon, H. (1999). NAL-NL1: A new prescriptive fitting procedure for nonlinear hearing aids. *Hearing Journal, 52*(10), 10–16.

Dillon, H. (2006). What's new from NAL in hearing aid prescriptions? *Hearing Journal, 59*(10), 10–16.

Dyrlund, O., & Lundh, P. (1990). Gain and feedback problems when fitting behind-the-ear hearing aids to profoundly hearing-impaired children. *Scandinavian Audiology, 19,* 89–95.

Fikret-Pasa, S. (1993). *The effects of compression ratio on speech intelligibility and quality.* Unpublished doctoral dissertation, Northwestern University, Ann Arbor, MI.

George, M. F. S., Wood, D. J., & Engebretson, A. M. (1993). Behavioral assessment of adaptive feedback cancellation in a digital hearing aid. *Journal of Rehabilitation Research and Development, 30,* 17–25.

Hawkins, D., & Cook, J. (2003). Hearing aid software predictive gain values: How accurate are they? *Hearing Journal, 56*(7), 26, 28, 32, 34.

Hawkins, D. B., & Yacullo, W. S. (1984). Signal-to-noise ratio advantage of binaural hearing aids and directional microphones under different levels of reverberation. *Journal of Speech and Hearing Disorders, 49*(3), 278–286.

Hirsh, I. J., Davis, H., Silverman, S. R., Reynolds, E. G., Eldert, E., & Benson, R. W. (1952). Development of materials for speech audiometry. *Journal of Speech and Hearing Disorders, 17,* 321–337.

Humes, L. E. (1996). Evolution of prescriptive fitting approaches. *American Journal of Audiology, 5,* 19–23.

Humes, L. E. (1999). Dimensions of hearing aid outcome. *Journal of the American Academy of Audiology, 10,* 26–39.

Humes, L. E. (2001). Issues in evaluating the effectiveness of hearing aids in the elderly: What to measure and when. *Seminars in Hearing, 22,* 303–314.

Humes, L. E., Wilson, D. L., Barlow, N. N., & Garner, C. B. (2002a). Measures of hearing aid benefit following one or two years of hearing aid use by the elderly. *Journal of Speech-Language-Hearing Research, 45,* 772–782.

Humes, L. E., Wilson, D. L., Barlow, N. N., Garner, C. B., & Amos, N. (2002b). Longitudinal changes in hearing-aid satisfaction and usage in the elderly over a period of one or two years following hearing aid delivery. *Ear and Hearing, 23,* 428–438.

Humes, L. E., Wilson, D. L., & Humes, A. C. (2003). Examination of differences between successful and unsuccessful elderly hearing aid candidates matched for age, hearing loss, and gender. *International Journal of Audiology, 42,* 432–441.

Hyde, M. L. (2000). Reasonable psychometric standards for self-report outcome measures in audiological rehabilitation. *Ear and Hearing, 21*(Suppl.), 37S–49S.

Joore, M. A., Brunenberg, D., Chenault, M. N., & Anteunis, L. J. (2003). Societal effects of hearing aid fitting among the moderately hearing impaired. *International Journal of Audiology, 42*, 152–160.

Kates, J. M. (1988). A computer simulation of hearing aid response and the effects of ear canal size. *Journal of the Acoustical Society of America, 83*, 1952–1963.

Knudsen, V. O., & Jones, I. H. (1935). Artificial aids to hearing. *Laryngoscope, 45*, 48–69.

Kuk, F., Kollofski, C., Brown, S., Melum, A., & Rosenthal, A. (1999). Use of a digital hearing aid with directional microphones in school-aged children. *Journal of the American Academy of Audiology, 10*(10), 535–548.

McArdle, R., Chisolm, T. H., Abrams, H. B., Wilson, R. H., & Doyle, P. J. (2005). The WHO-DAS II: Measuring outcomes for hearing aid intervention for adults. *Trends in Amplification, 9*, 127–143.

Mulrow, C. D., Aguilar, C., Endicott, J. E., Tuley, M. R., Velez, R., Charlip, W. S., et al. (1990). Quality-of-life changes and hearing impairment: A randomized trial. *Annals of Internal Medicine, 113*, 188–194.

Mueller, H. G. (2005). Probe-mic measures: Hearing aid fitting's most neglected element. *Hearing Journal*, 58(10), 21–30.

Newby, H. A. (1972). Testing the hearing function: Speech audiometry. In *Audiology* (3rd ed., pp. 116–143). Englewood Cliffs, NJ: Prentice-Hall.

Nilsson, M., Soli, S. D., & Sullivan, J. A. (1994). Development of the Hearing in Noise Test for the measurement of speech reception thresholds in quiet and in noise. *Journal of the Acoustical Society of America, 95*(2), 1085–1099.

Owens, E., & Schubert, E. D. (1977). Development of the California Consonant Test. *Journal of Speech and Hearing Research, 20*(3), 463–474.

Palmer, C., Bentler, R., & Mueller, H. G. (2006). Amplification and the perception of annoying and aversive sounds. *Trends in Amplification, 10*, 83–94.

Preves, D. A. (1988). Principles of signal processing. In R. E. Sandlin (Ed.), *Handbook of hearing aid amplification, Vol. I: Theoretical and technical considerations* (pp. 91–120). Boston: College-Hill Press.

Preves, D. A., Sammeth, C. A., & Wynne, M. K. (1999). Field trial evaluations of a switched directional/omnidirectional in-the-ear hearing instrument. *Journal of the American Academy of Audiology, 10*(5), 273–284.

Primeau, R. L. (1997). Hearing aid benefit in adults and older adults. *Seminars in Hearing, 18*, 29–36.

Ricketts, T., Henry, P., & Gnewikow, D. (2003). Full-time directional versus user selectable microphone modes in hearing aids. *Ear and Hearing, 24*(5), 424–439.

Ricketts, T., Henry, P. P., & Hornsby, B. W. (2005). Application of frequency importance functions to directivity for prediction of benefit in uniform fields. *Ear and Hearing, 26*(5), 473–486.

Ricketts, T., & Hornsby, B. W. (2003). Distance and reverberation effects on directional benefit. *Ear and Hearing, 24*(6), 472–484.

Ricketts, T., & Hornsby, B. (2005). Sound quality measures for speech in noise through a commercial hearing aid implementing digital noise reduction. *Journal of the American Academy of Audiology, 16*, 270–277.

Ricketts, T., & Hornsby, B. W. (2006). Directional hearing aid benefit in listeners with severe hearing loss. *International Journal of Audiology, 45*(3), 190–197.

Sandlin, R. E. (2000). *Textbook of Hearing Aid Amplification* (2nd ed.). San Diego, CA: Singular.

Scollie, S. (2006). The DSL method: Improving with age. *Hearing Journal, 59*(9), 10–16.

Seewald, R., Moodie, S., Scollie, S., & Bagatto, M. (2005). The DSL method for pediatric hearing instrument fitting: Historical perspective and current issues. *Trends in Amplification, 9*(4), 145–157.

Skinner, M. W. (1988). *Hearing aid evaluation*. Englewood Cliffs, NJ: Prentice-Hall.

Strom, K. (2007). Hearing aids are not only for old people. *Hearing Review, 14*(11), 8.

Sumby, W. H., & Pollack, I. (1954). Visual contribution to speech intelligibility in noise. *Journal of the Acoustical Society of America, 26*(2), 212–215.

Surr, R. K., Walden, B. E., Cord, M. T., & Olson, L. (2002). Influence of environmental factors on hearing aid microphone preference. *Journal of the American Academy of Audiology, 13*(6), 308–322.

Thornton, A. R., & Raffin, M. J. M. (1978). Binomial characteristics of speech discrimination scores. *Journal of Speech and Hearing Research, 21*, 507–518.

Tillman, T. W., & Carhart, R. (1966). An expanded test for speech discrimination using CNC monosyllabic words, Northwestern University Auditory Test No. 6. *USAF School of Aerospace Technical Report*.

Valente, M., Fabry, D., & Potts, L. (1995). Recognition of speech in noise with hearing aids using dual microphones, *Journal of the American Academy of Audiology, 6*, 440–449.

Walden, B. E., Surr, R. K., Cord, M. T., Edwards, B., & Olson, L. (2000). Comparisons of benefits provided by different hearing aid technologies. *Journal of the American Academy of Audiology, 11*, 540–560.

Walden, B. E., Surr, R. K., Grant, K. W., Van Summers, W., Cord, M. T., & Dyrlund, O. (2005). Effect of signal-to-noise ratio on directional microphone benefit and preference. *Journal of the American Academy of Audiology, 16*(9), 662–676.

Walden, T. C., & Walden, B. E. (2005.) Unilateral versus bilateral amplification for adults with impaired hearing. *Journal of the American Academy of Audiology, 16*, 574–584.

Wallenfels, H. G. (1967). *Hearing aids on prescription*. Springfield, IL: Charles C. Thomas.

Watson, N. A., & Knudson, V. O. (1940). Selective amplification in hearing aids. *Journal of the Acoustical Society of America, 11*, 406–419.

Wu, Y. H. (2007). *Impact of visual cues on directional benefit and preference*. Doctoral thesis. University of Iowa, Iowa City.

Appendix 8-A
ANSI S3.22 Tests Used to Measure the Electroacoustic Performance of Hearing Aids

Test	Explanation of Test Result	Gain Setting	AGC	Input (dB SPL)	Frequency	Measure or Calculate	Tolerance
OSPL90 curve	Coupler SPL as a function of frequency for a 90 dB input SPL	Full on	Min	90	200–5000 Hz	Coupler SPL	unspecified
Maximum OSPL90	The maximum value of the OSPL90 curve	Full on	Min	90	Frequency of maximum	Maximum of OSPL90 curve	+3 dB
HFA-OSPL90	Average of the OSPL90 values	Full on	Min	90	HFA	Average coupler SPL at HFA frequencies	±4 dB
HFA full-on gain (HFA-FOG)	Average of the full-on gain at the HFA frequencies	Full on	Min	50	HFA	Average gain at HFA frequencies	±5 dB
Reference test gain (RTG)	Average of the gain at the HFA frequencies for a 60 dB input SPL, with gain control at RTS	RTS	Min	60	HFA	Average gain at HFA frequencies	unspecified
Frequency range	Range between the lowest and the highest frequency at which the frequency response curve is 20 dB below its HFA value	RTS	Min	60	From the lowest frequency (f1) to the highest frequency (f2) at which the frequency response curve is 20 dB below its HFA average		unspecified
Frequency response curve	Coupler SPL as a function of frequency for a 60 dB input SPL, with gain control at RTS	RTS	Min	60	From the higher of f1 or 200 Hz to the lower of f2 or 5000 Hz. Wider range may be shown.	Coupler SPL or Gain	±4 dB from the lesser of 1.25 f1 or 200 Hz to 2 kHz. ±6 dB from 2 kHz to the lesser of 4 kHz or 0.8 f2.

continues

Appendix 8–A. *continued*

Test	Explanation of Test Result	Gain Setting	AGC	Input (dB SPL)	Frequency	Measure or Calculate	Tolerance
Total harmonic distortion (THD)	Ratio of sum of the powers of all the harmonics to the power of the fundamental	RTS	Min	70 except 65 @ highest frequency	500, 800, 1600 Hz (HFA) or ½ the SPA frequencies		+3%
Equivalent input noise (EIN)	SPL of an external noise source at the input that would result in the same coupler SPL as that caused by all the internal noise sources in the hearing aid	RTS	Min	OFF and 50	(Coupler SPL with no input)—(HFA gain with a 50 dB input SPL)		+3 dB
Battery current	Electrical current drawn from the battery when the input SPL is 65 dB at 1000 Hz and the gain control is at RTS	RTS	Min	65	1000 Hz	Battery current	+20%
SPL for an inductive telephone simulator (SPLITS)	For hearing aids with an inductive input coil (T-coil), the coupler SPL as a function of frequency when the hearing aid, with gain control at RTS, is oriented for maximum output on a telephone magnetic field simulator (TMFS). BTE is as flat as possible on test surface. ITE or ITC with faceplate as close as possible and parallel to test surface.	RTS	Min	Telephone magnetic field simulator (TMFS)	200–5000 Hz	Coupler SPL	unspecified
HFA-SPLITS	Average of the SPLITS at the HFA frequencies	RTS	Min	TMFS	HFA	Average SPLITS values at the HFA frequencies	±6 dB
RSETS	Relative simulated equivalent telephone sensitivity	RTS	Min	TMFS	HFA	HFA-SPLITS minus (RTG + 60)	unspecified
Input-output curves	For hearing aids with AGC, the coupler SPL as a function of the input SPL, at one or more of 250, 500, 1000, 2000, 4000 Hz, with the gain control at RTS	RTS	Max	50–90 in 5 dB steps	One or more of 250, 500, 1000, 2000, 4000 Hz	Coupler SPL vs. Input SPL	±5 dB at 50 and 90 dB input SPL when matched at 70 dB input SPL

Test	Explanation of Test Result	Gain Setting	AGC	Input (dB SPL)	Frequency	Measure or Calculate	Tolerance
Attack time	For hearing aids with AGC, the time between an abrupt change from 55 to 90 dB input SPL and the time when the coupler SPL has stabilized to within 3 dB of the steady value for a 90-dB input SPL, at one or more of 250, 500, 1000, 2000, 4000 Hz, with the gain control at RTS	RTS	Max	Step from 55 to 90	Same frequencies used for input-output curves.	Time from input step until coupler SPL settles within 3 dB of its steady value for 90 dB input SPL	±5 ms or 50%, whichever is greater
Release time	For hearing aids with AGC, the time between an abrupt change from 90 to 55 dB input SPL and the time when the coupler SPL has stabilized to within 4 dB of the steady value for a 55 dB input SPL, at one or more of 250, 500, 1000, 2000, 4000 Hz, with the gain control at RTS	RTS	Max	Step from 90 to 55	Same frequencies used for input-output curves.	Time from input step until coupler SPL settles within 4 dB of its steady value for 55 dB input SPL	±5 ms or 50%, whichever is greater
Abbreviations	▪ HFA: High-Frequency Average—the average of values at 1000, 1600, and 2500 Hz. In all tests, HFA may be replaced by SPA: Special Purpose Average—the average of values at three frequencies specified by the hearing aid manufacturer that are at 1/3 octave frequencies separated by 2/3 octave. ▪ RTS: Reference Test Setting—setting of the gain control (i.e. volume control, master or overall gain control) required to produce an HFA-gain within ± 1.5 dB of the HFA-OSPL90 minus 77 dB for a 60 dB input SPL or, if the full-on HFA gain for a 60 dB input SPL is less than the HFA OSPL90 minus 77 dB, the full-on setting of the gain control. ▪ AGC: Automatic Gain Control—means for controlling gain as a function of signal level. It includes expansion and various forms of compression.						

Source: Courtesy of Bill Cole, Etymonic Research.

Part III

The Rehabilitative Toolbox: Therapeutic Management

9

Audiologic Counseling: A Biopsychosocial Approach

Sue Ann Erdman

Introduction

The obvious isn't obvious, until it's obvious.
Beatrice Wright

The ideal outcome of rehabilitation is the successful management of a chronic illness or disability by the individual who has such a condition. To say that audiologists manage hearing impairment, or, that we manage patients with hearing impairment, in reality, misses the mark. The audiologist's responsibility is to establish a therapeutic relationship and facilitate adjustment to hearing impairment by engaging patients in the actual management of their hearing problems. Although the semantic differences may seem minor, they are, in fact, focal to the rehabilitation process. Acute health problems can often be resolved by specific and immediate medical treatments; chronic conditions, however, persist—often for the rest of the individual's life. Life-long adaptations are required to adjust to the changes imposed by chronic conditions to minimize the impact on quality of life. Incurring a chronic condition, even one as insidious as hearing impairment, alters one's self-perception. It detracts from one's being "the picture of health" or "whole." Our goal is to ensure that our patients[1] assimilate this "loss" or altered self-image and that they can manage the challenges that hearing impairment imposes on their daily lives. They must adjust to the loss of hearing, make adaptations, and develop the skills to cope with the communication and adjustment issues they experience. Obviously, unless they are able to do so, the outcome of audiologic rehabilitation (AR) will not be successful. Counseling is the means by which we facilitate patients' realization of the confidence and skills they need to manage their hearing problems effectively.

[1]The terms patient and client are used interchangeably in audiology. Audiologists in hospital settings tend to use patient whereas those in private practice often use client. The term patient once suggested a passive role in health care. This connotation has abated in view of current emphasis on patients' rights, patient self-management, and the patient's focal role in the biopsychosocial model and the therapeutic alliance. Both terms are used herein.

Traditionally, counseling in rehabilitation has been viewed as a specific *clinical activity*, which it is; but it is also more than that. Counseling is the ongoing *facilitative process* in which the practitioner/patient relationship evolves and functions thereby creating opportunities to enhance patients' self-efficacy (Bandura, 1977, 2004), the key to successful management of a chronic condition. Above all else, however, counseling is the *therapeutic context* in which all aspects of audiologic services occur. The context is biopsychosocial, patient-centered, empathic, interactive, and facilitative in nature. It is within this philosophical context that the direction and goals of the counseling process, and the audiologist's role and responsibilities in it, are established for each individual patient. As the counseling process unfolds, individualized interactive and facilitative activities promote the patient's capability to manage his or her chronic condition successfully.

The implications of counseling in audiology are myriad. Counseling influences adherence to treatment recommendations and the realization of treatment goals. It enhances benefit from and satisfaction with all aspects of intervention. It empowers. It instills hope and the belief that one can cope. It enables patients to eliminate or reduce the limitations and restrictions experienced secondary to hearing impairment. It establishes the audiologist as a credible and valued ally in minimizing the effects of hearing impairment on communication, psychosocial functioning, and quality of life. More than any other factors, the effectiveness of our counseling influences the opinion patients have of our competence, professionalism, and commitment to their well-being. This chapter consists of an examination of the need to shift audiologic service delivery from the traditional biomedical model to a biopsychosocial model to better meet the needs of our hearing-impaired patients and their families. Within such a model, the patient's experience of hearing impairment rather than the hearing impairment per se becomes the clinical focus. Audiologic counseling defines the rehabilitative context, process, and activities. This realignment of our philosophical underpinnings will maximize the benefits of audiologic intervention, enhance outcomes and improve patient satisfaction.

Health Care: Crisis and Change

I sometimes feel as though we are so caught up in the demands of day-to-day practice that we have lost sight of where we came from and what our work is primarily about.

Michael J. Mahoney (2005)

There is reason to view counseling in audiology from a somewhat different perspective than we may have in the past. Periodically, we all pause and take a step back from the thoughts and activities in which we are busily immersed, and suddenly see the world and ourselves in a different light. Doing this often results in one of those astonishing moments of awareness. The revelations (in truth, nothing more than the present reality), constitute crystal-clear cognizance of things we have failed to notice or appreciate from within our own insular worlds. This moment of awareness may just be serendipitous happenstance. It could also result from a necessary, perhaps even painful, reappraisal following a sudden or impending change in our lives. If audiology were to pause and take stock of all that is going on around it, reality could pack a major punch. The punch could be at once humbling, worrisome, and exciting. At the very minimum, it would be thought provoking. The current convergence of exigent circumstances, paradigm shifts, emergent theories, and advances in techniques and technologies warrants a new look at audiology's philosophical underpinnings, our purpose, and the extent of our success as a profession. (*Note:* For further information regarding defining audiologic rehabilitation, the reader is referred to Chapter 2 of this text.)

Throughout health care, consumers are frustrated with the quality of care, the cost of care, and decreases in access to care. As Seaburn (2005) succinctly puts it, the system is "fragmented, overburdened, and under-responsive" (p. 398). Resources and attention are disproportionately focused on advances in medical technology. At the same time, there are glaring shortages in preventive and primary medical care, and woeful inadequacies in how chronic illness and disability are addressed. These shortages and inadequacies are largely responsible for patients' failure to adhere to treatment recommendations. Nonadherence contributes to a vicious cycle that includes:

1. treatment failures,
2. spurious effects on outcome studies,
3. deteriorations in health, functioning, and quality of life,
4. increased demands on limited resources, and
5. continued escalations in health care costs.

Annual health care costs in the United States have surpassed $2.3 trillion (Rooney & Perrin, 2008) over 80% of which is attributable to chronic illness and disability (Nuovo, 2006). It is projected that by 2020, half of the U.S. population will have a chronic health condition (Anderson & Horvath, 2004). A health care system that is not set up to address chronic illness and disability efficiently or adequately is being drained by those very problems.

The aging population and advances in acute care portend increasing numbers of patients with chronic conditions. Why then is health care so ill prepared to address chronic illness and disability? The answer is, quite literally, centuries old. The parameters of medical science and practice have long been anchored in the biomedical model, a product of *dualism and reductionism*. In philosophy of mind, dualism posits the view that mind and body are separate and independent entities. This view was adamantly upheld by the Church through the 16th and 17th centuries because the mind was perceived to be soul-related and, therefore, strictly in God's purview. The Church, however, did permit study and dissection of the body. Ever since that time, the sole focus of medical science and practice in western medicine has been on the human body. From the perspective of reductionism, all matter and phenomena are reduced to their parts, and those parts, in turn, are reduced to their parts. This explains how molecular biology has emerged as the science underlying modern medicine.

Fueled by the Industrial Revolution, medicine made and has continued to make rapid advances. Not surprisingly, high-tech, cutting-edge medical care has come to involve increasingly sophisticated treatment, repair, or removal of diseased, malfunctioning, or impaired parts. Physicians have been trained to disregard patients' subjective accounts of illness, and to use only "reliable" technical procedures and laboratory measurements. Observable, objective phenomena alone are relevant in medicine, which helps explain how patients became "cases." The biomedical model can also be held responsible for the fact that the medical profession has not adequately addressed chronic conditions. Inescapably, chronic illness and disability include subjective, psychosocial, and behavioral phenomena. Symptoms that do not fit the biomedical model, quite literally, have been disregarded because they are not "medical" issues. Consequently, the biomedical model offers no mechanisms to address critical issues such as lifestyle, health beliefs, hypochondriasis, illness behaviors, disablement, coping skills, defense mechanisms, nonadherence to treatment recommendations, or any of the myriad societal factors that impinge upon health such as illiteracy and poverty. The effectiveness of medicine based on the biomedical model has also not been particularly successful in preventing or managing hypertension, asthma, chronic obstructive pulmonary disease (COPD), diabetes mellitus, eating disorders, addictions, or chronic pain—all of which are influenced by cognition, affect, and behavior, distinctly human variables, but definitely not body parts. Not surprisingly, psychiatry which, ironically, could actually provide valuable insights into many of these issues, has often been viewed disparagingly by other medical specialties who question whether or not psychiatry actually constitutes medicine (Engel, 1977a).

The Biopsychosocial Model

George Engel's most enduring contribution was to broaden the scope of the clinician's gaze.
Borrell-Carrió, Suchman, and Epstein (2004)

George L. Engel (1913–1999), an internist and psychiatrist, argued passionately that health care has long outgrown the utility of the biomedical model. He faulted the scientific limitations of reductionism and dualism in understanding health and illness, and he deplored the objectification and disempowerment of the patient inherent in the biomedical approach. Engel also viewed the model as inherently flawed because it cannot account for individual differences in perceived "illness," the subjective experience of disease. As Engel (1977a) repeatedly pointed out, illness cannot be understood without knowing why this particular patient, is presenting in this particular way, at this particular time. The issue of individual differences is also important when it comes to patients' experience of disability, that is, the subjective experience of impairment and its associated limitations and restrictions. Research in audiology has demonstrated the effects of individual differences in a number of ways. Consistent findings indicate that although audiometric measures and self-reported hearing problems are correlated, one cannot predict a patient's communication and adjustment difficulties from the audiogram (e.g., Brainerd & Frankel, 1985; Erdman & Demorest, 1998b; Hawes & Niswander, 1985; Hideki, Kyoko, & Eiji, 2004; Kielinen & Nerbonne, 1990; Kramer, Kapteyn, Festen, & Tobi, 1996; Rowland, Dirks, Dubno, & Bell, 1985; Speaks, Jerger, & Trammel, 1970; Weinstein & Ventry, 1983a, 1983b). Furthermore, the decision to seek audiologic services is correlated more strongly with self-reports of hearing problems than it is with the audiogram (e.g., van den Brink, Wit, Kempen, & van Heuvelen, 1996; Swan & Gatehouse, 1990).

Engel's alternative to the biomedical model is the *biopsychosocial model*, a patient-centered approach based on systems theory rather than dualism and reductionism. Some consider it one of the most significant contributions to health care of the 20th century (Smith & Strain, 2002). In fact, according to Fava and Sonino (2008), Engel's seminal article, *The Need for a New Medical Model: A Challenge for Biomedicine* (1977a) has been cited close to 1,900 times. In Engel's mind, he was presenting a scientific model that simply takes into account the dimensions left out of the biomedical model. That it does. It includes the patient, a person—a human being. In the biopsychosocial model, biological, psychological, and social systems are integral and interactive elements of health and illness. The patient's "humanness" influences and is influenced by his or her biological and social systems. The importance of changing service delivery models and engaging patients in the management of their health needs resulted in a comparison of delivery models in audiology that is shown in Table 9–1. The comparisons included in the table were originally labeled "medical" model and "rehabilitative" model (Erdman, Wark,

Table 9–1. Comparison of Characteristics of Biomedical and Biopsychosocial Models

Biomedical Model	Biopsychosocial Model
Top-down communication	Horizontal communication
Authoritarian	Interactive, facilitative
Clinician determines diagnosis and treatment of patients	Patient identifies problems and decides treatment with clinician
Clinician does something "to" patients	Clinician does something "with" patients
Disease focused	Patient focused
Clinician knows what is right and best for patients	Patients' needs and perceptions determine goals and strategies
May be appropriate and necessary in acute, emergency situations	Ideal for chronic illness and disabilities requiring adherence to treatment regime
"Curative"	Empowering, self-actualizing

Source: Based on Erdman, Wark, & Montano (1994).

& Montano, 1994). Without modifying the characteristics of either model, "biomedical" and "biopsychosocial" are now apt descriptors. Elements of the biopsychosocial model have been worthy goals in audiology for some time now.

The key aspects of the biopsychosocial approach as proposed by Engel (1977a, 1977b), include the following:

1. a view of the patient as a "whole," a person whose fundamental nature is at once biological, psychological, and social;
2. a triadic process of observation, introspection, and dialogue through which the patient's subjective experiences become scientific data;
3. a clinical interview in which the patient's narrative is allowed to unfold without interruptions and with minimal prompting or interrogation;
4. a practitioner-patient relationship that fosters shared and complementary communication and responsibilities;
5. a mutual understanding of the patient's narrative that ensures inclusion of his or her perceptions and experiences in the assessment and diagnostic process;
6. patient engagement in the treatment process and plans that are intended to alleviate or resolve perceived illness or disability; and
7. systems theory rather than reductionism as the approach to analyzing and understanding health and illness.

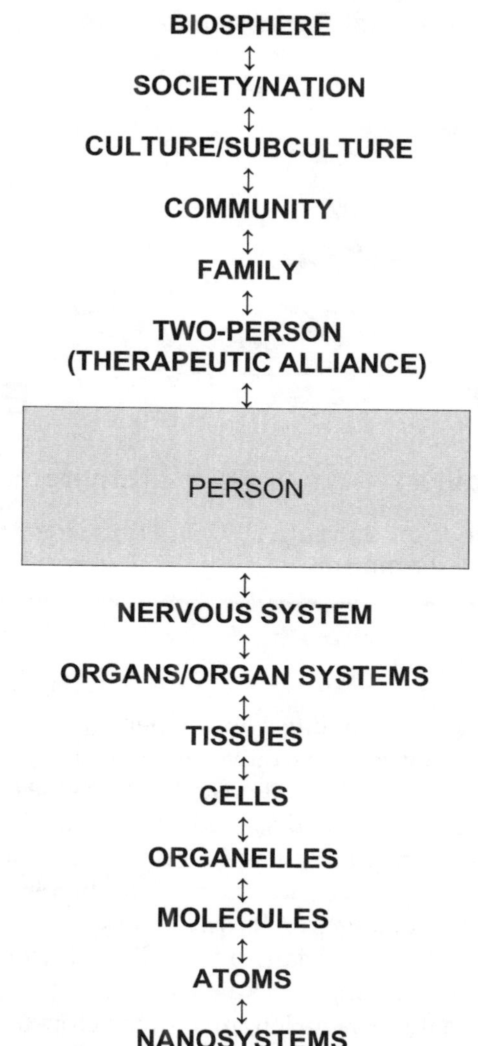

Figure 9–1. Hierarchy of levels of natural systems organization. Adapted from Engel (1980).

Systems theory facilitates understanding of illness and disease through a hierarchical ordering of systems along a continuum as shown in Figure 9–1. Engel's model includes systems from molecular levels to societal levels. This framework allows both intra- and inter-system study. The person who is the focus, can be viewed as the end of the "organism/biologic" continuum, and the beginning of the societal/social continuum. These systems can also be represented as a nested, concentric progression from the molecule at the center, to the biosphere as the outermost layer. Viewed as a nested continuum, it is evident that each system is both a whole and a part of a larger system. How a person idiosyncratically *experiences* the effects of these internal and external systems, governs the way in which those internal and external systems are affected in return. Bandura's (1978) principle of reciprocal determinism is strikingly similar; psychological functioning includes reciprocal interaction of behavioral, personal inner experiential (e.g., cognitions, perceptions, and affect), and environmental variables as shown in Figure 9–2. Bandura's and Engel's models both feature bidirectional effects and influences from and on the external world, that is, the environment/society.

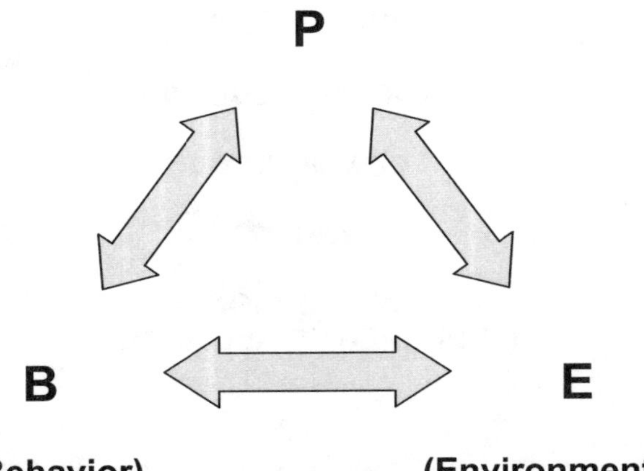

Figure 9–2. Bandura (1978). Principle of reciprocal determinism.

The clinical interview, when appropriately executed, elicits a "narrative" in which the patient's experience and the systems relevant to the experience are "naturally" disclosed. Seaburn (2005), who worked with Engel, has found that by listening attentively to patients' stories, the biopsychosocial model emerges on its own. The key is truly listening. Many clinicians find it difficult to refrain from interrupting. Beckman and Frankel (1984) found that the mean length of time before a physician interrupts a patient is 18 seconds. There are also those who believe that interrogating patients saves time, particularly when using a pre-established format to "cover all the bases." In a study comparing biomedical versus patient-centered interviewing, investigators found that the patient-centered interview took one minute longer (Stewart, Brown, & Weston, 1989). Important also is the fact that intake forms and routine questions often fail to tap the specifics of an individual patient's experience of illness. In a narrative that unfolds as a patient's story, however, the critical details are revealed quite readily. Not having specific necessary information can impede or derail diagnoses, interfere with the patient's ability to feel understood, and, ultimately, negatively affect outcome. The Institute of Medicine (IOM, 2000) affirms that communication lapses and relationship obstacles can contribute to preventable harm, even death. On the positive side, studies indicate that the patient-centered interview is associated with positive psychosocial and medical outcomes and patient satisfaction (Stewart, Brown, Donner, McWhinney, Oates, Weston, & Jordan, 2000; Stewart, Belle-Brown, Weston, & McWhinney, 2003).

Engel's model evolved as a function of his own life experiences (see Engel, 1996). Nonetheless, he insisted that the model simply reflects good medical practice. Others insist his practice simply epitomized the good doctor (Smith & Strain, 2002). Engel's influence has been widespread. Skeptics, who initially thought the model was too complex, have come to value the more complex ways in which disease and health can be examined. Herman (1989/2005) suggested the need for a transitional model, but an encouraging letter from Engel and continued experience with the model convinced him and his colleagues otherwise. As Biderman, Yeheskel, and Herman have since observed " . . . we did our learning and our teaching simultaneously" (2005). A copy of Engel's gracious and helpful 1989 letter (2005) accompanied their article.

A Biopsychosocial Exemplar: A New Understanding of Pain

The number of medical residents from other countries who came to the United States and trained or worked with Engel has contributed to a worldwide appreciation of the biopsychosocial model. Smith and Strain (2002), for example, indicate that health care in Australia became biopsychosocial without even knowing it. An entire generation of Australian medical students has learned the interviewing skills necessary to elicit patients' narratives and elucidate their experience of illness. Dunstan and Covic (2006) recommend a psychosocial approach to understand and manage work-related injuries thereby reducing Australia's disability costs. In Canada, Truchon and Fillion (2000) have investigated biopsychosocial determinants of chronic disability related to low back pain, and a biopsychosocial approach has been evaluated and recommended to manage osteoarthritis of the knee (Hunt, Birmingham, Skarakis-Doyle, & Vandervoort, 2008). Research by Belgian and Dutch investigators (e.g., Crombez, Vlaeyen, Heuts, & Lysens; 1999; Goubert, Crombez, & Van Damme, 2004; Peters, Vlaeyen, & Weber, 2005; and Vlaeyen & Morley, 2005) has demonstrated the role of pain-related fear, hypervigilance, and catastrophizing in the transition of acute and subacute pain to chronic pain. Turk and Okifuji (2002) identify patients' appraisals of their pain (i.e., the meaning they ascribe to their pain) and their capacity to manage fears of reinjury or exacerbation of pain as critical variables in the development of chronic pain.

Moving from the biomedical model to the biopsychosocial model to advance the understanding of the vicissitudes of pain has resulted in an explosion of research. Findings have already led to changes in treatment that will benefit millions of patients and evidence suggests these advancements will result in cost-savings (Gatchel & Okifuji, 2006). Researchers hope to gain greater insight into treatment methods and etiologic variables that can lead to the prevention of chronic pain. Congress has designated 2001 to 2010 as "The Decade of Pain Control and Research." A comprehensive review of major breakthroughs in pain research demonstrates clearly that viewing old problems in a new light can yield information that was heretofore unknowable (Gatchel, Peng, Fuchs, Peters, & Turk, 2007). The biopsychosocial model can account for the variability in the relationship between tissue damage and pain; moreover, it can provide explanations for the variability in the relationship between the experience of pain and perceived disablement. Whereas the perception of pain and the feelings and behaviors associated with it are normal, adaptive psychological processes in an acute or subacute stage of pain, they are dysfunctional in the experience of chronic pain. Physical, emotional, cognitive, and behavioral problems can become a vicious cycle through which the patient becomes entrapped in chronic pain (Vlaeyen, Crombez, & Goubert, 2007). In short, pain puts patients at high risk for emotional problems (e.g., depression, anxiety), maladaptive cognitions, and ineffective coping behaviors including reduced movement. Reduced activity levels lead to declines in functional ability and physical fitness, which exacerbate cognitive, affective, and behavioral reactions. Turk and Okifuji (2002) cite several studies of chronic pain in which self-efficacy is related to activity levels, medication use, and return to work.

The interdependencies and interactions among multiple systems that are implicated in pain cannot be examined or studied within the biomedical framework. Advances in the evaluation and management of pain have had effects beyond the level of the individual patient. The practice of withholding medications unless pain became intolerable has been replaced by an emphasis on controlling pain before it becomes intolerable. Pain is now the fifth vital sign that practitioners are required to assess along with blood pressure, pulse, core temperature, and respiration. The entire philosophy of pain treatment has been changed because of a new approach to understanding it. It is reasonable to hope for fewer medical appointments, prescription medications, and sick days, as well as fewer compensation claims, as progress is made in reducing the incidence of chronic pain and facilitating patients' ability to manage it successfully through whatever medical or rehabilitative means are deemed effective.

This discussion of pain has been included to illustrate how extensively and rapidly research and practice in one area can be transformed by viewing the problem from a different perspective. Research and developments in pain medications and in surgical techniques including ablations—logical consequences of a biomedical approach to pain—have had only minimal, and not always positive, effects. A biopsychosocial perspective has brought cognitive, affective, and behavioral variables into play, which has elucidated the path to chronic pain and identified a wide range of intervention options. If we pause and assimilate this dramatic evolution, our next question is likely to be, "Has it made major differences in other areas?" In fact, it has. Hypertension, coronary disease, asthma, stroke, chronic obstructive pulmonary disease, diabetes mellitus, cancer, organ transplants, palliative care, alcohol and substance abuse, dermatological disorders and chronic itching, eating disorders, obesity, bruxism, and even toilet training are but some of the health issues that are benefiting from a biopsychosocial approach.

Audiology: Biomedical or Biopsychosocial

It should be emphasized that two principles remain fundamental, that auditory impairment is primarily a medical problem and that an otologist must always be in overall charge of the plan.

Leslie E. Morrissett, M.D. (1957)

Our logical next question is, of course, "Has the biopsychosocial approach made a difference in audiology?" An appropriate answer to this question involves an understanding of where we started, where we have been, and where we are going, as well as an appreciation of how firmly entrenched the biomedical model remains in society. In light of the above quotation, let us consider the latter first.

After hundreds of years as the model for medical science and practice, the biomedical model has so deeply infiltrated the western mindset that it has become dogma (Engel, 1977a). On an institutional level, the dogmatic effects of the biomedical model can be seen in resistance to change. Holman (1976) goes so far as to claim that the medical establishment is not primarily interested in the pursuit of knowledge to inform medical science and practice but "in special interest advocacy and pursuing and preserving social power" (p. 11). He also argues that the dominance of professionals has "perpetuated prevailing practices, deflected criticisms, and insulated the profession from alternate views and social relations that would illuminate and improve healthcare" (p. 21). Wampold, Ahn, and Coleman (2001) maintain that there is no empirical support for the medical model in the counseling professions. They argue persuasively in favor of a contextual model within which the person can be understood in relation to his or her particular circumstances. Sensitivity to individual and cultural differences in counseling is contingent upon a model that espouses a person in context approach.

Hewa and Hetherington (1995) suggest that the biomedical model's survival can be attributed to the fact that adoption of a broader model could erode the authority of medical practitioners. Resistance to the addition of social and behavioral sciences into medical school curricula is yet another sign of vested interest in perpetuating a professional hierarchy that precludes a team approach to the management of illness and disability (Carr, Emory, Errichetti, Johnson, & Reyes, 2007; Dobie, 2007).

Whatever self-importance or self-serving factors might be implicated in maintaining the biomedical model, there are more formidable factors. Health care has become an impersonal, industrial behemoth that is more and more concerned with the bottom line than with patients' welfare. Managed care has so depersonalized patient care that it is now considered a major plus if a plan permits patients to select their own physicians. Even more insidious is the extent to which expenditures in medical technology and the drug industry perpetrate a biomedical approach upon the health care system. The underlying premise is still a mechanistic approach to fixing whatever is broken. From microsurgery to drugs that alter neurochemical transmitters, the health care industry has the technologies to diagnose and treat whatever ails us. Moreover, many are of the belief that if there is a problem the biomedical model has not yet solved, it will certainly be able to do so in the future. This mechanistic approach tends to be more prevalent in some medical specialties than in others. Family practice, pediatrics, rehabilitation medicine, and psychiatry, for example, are more patient oriented than are pathology, surgery, or anesthesiology.

Which brings us back to our question: has the biopsychosocial model made a difference in audiology? A recent search of PubMed, PsychArticles, and CINAHL for the term "biopsychosocial" paired with "hearing impairment," "hearing loss" or "audiology," identified two publications[2]: *Psychosocial Adaptations to Dual Sensory Loss in Middle and Late Adulthood*, by Brennan and Bally (2007) and *An Approach to Rehabilitation with Amplification*,

[2]Three additional articles were retrieved that pertained to deafness. The articles, however, did not relate to issues in which audiology, as a profession, would be involved; hence, they are not included.

by Hardick and Gans (1982). In the first article, the authors discuss the application of different models to the understanding of dual sensory impairment, one of which is described as a "biopsychosocial—spiritual model." In the second article, the "unique biopsychosocial characteristics" of an elderly population are considered in relation to a long-standing AR program in which they were enrolled. The appearance of two articles in 25 years does not appear to constitute an emerging trend.

Biomedical thinking is found in many aspects of audiology. Diagnostics rule. From the days of the tuning fork, our armamentarium of diagnostic technologies has come to include computerized and automated audiometers, tympanometers, ABR equipment, ENG equipment, OAE systems, real-ear measurement and hearing aid test systems, computer administered self-assessments, and video-otoscopy and microscopy. Treatment wise the list is equally hi-tech: remote-controlled hearing aids, in the ear hearing aids, behind the ear hearing aids, and CROS and BICROS hearing aids; Bahas®, cochlear implants, and middle ear implants; FM, infrared, and wireless technologies; video and computer-administered training; and an increasing array of assistive technologies. A true assembly line of technologies awaits the patient who comes to see an audiologist.

The importance of patients' perceptions of their hearing difficulties is not something to which audiologists' have been completely oblivious. During the 1980s and 1990s there was considerable research in the area of self-report measures to assess patients' perceptions of their hearing problems. Some of the instruments were for screening purposes; others were designed to provide a global perspective of the individual's experience of communication problems and associated adjustment difficulties. A wide range of studies continue to demonstrate that although correlations between audiometric and self-report measures are statistically significant, they are not very strong (Brainerd & Frankel, 1985; Erdman & Demorest, 1998b; Hallberg & Carlsson, 1991; Hawes & Niswander, 1985; Hétu, Lalonde, & Getty, 1987; High, Fairbanks, & Glorig, 1964; Kielinen & Nerbonne, 1990; Kramer, Kapteyn, Festen, & Tobi, 1996; Marcus-Bernstein, 1986; McCartney, Maurer, & Sorenson, 1976; Newman, Weinstein, Jacobson, & Hug, 1990; Rowland, Dirks, Dubno, & Bell, 1985; Schow & Nerbonne, 1980; Speaks, Jerger, & Trammel, 1970; Swan & Gatehouse, 1990; Weinstein & Ventry, 1983a, 1983b). The following conclusions (Erdman, 1994) can be made from these findings.

1. The activity limitations, participation restrictions, and psychosocial fallout revealed in the results of self-assessment are related to hearing impairment.
2. This relationship, however, does not permit the difficulties experienced secondary to hearing impairment to be predicted from the audiogram.
3. The variability in the experience of hearing impairment suggests that other factors determine the extent to which it does or does not become a disabling condition.
4. Assessment of hearing impairment is an inadequate means of assessing clients' rehabilitative needs.

It was anticipated that audiologists would use the results of patients' self-report measures to help identify relevant issues for each patient, to guide the development of intervention goals, to counsel their patients, and to evaluate treatment outcome (Erdman, 1993b). Unfortunately, to date, the extent to which that has occurred is minimal.

Many audiologists say they simply do not know what to do with the results of self-report measures. In the interests of evidence-based practice, however, they administer the measures so treatment benefit can be documented. There is a strong preference for short instruments and ones that are computer administered, neither of which facilitates development of a practitioner-patient relationship founded on rapport and mutual goals. The amount of time required to complete an audiogram, even with a difficult patient, is never questioned. If complications develop during the course of an ABR, there is always time to complete it. The same commitment to assessing the impact hearing impairment has on daily living and quality of life is missing. In actuality, it is not a matter of time; it is a matter of interest and focus. The patient's experience of hearing impairment does not fit into the biomedical model. The fact that audiologists are not sure how to use the results of self-report measures suggests insufficient emphasis on the disabling aspects of hearing impairment in curriculum and practicum experiences. Consequently, clinicians do not feel adequately prepared to discuss these issues with their patients. It would follow that they are also not providing their patients with the necessary assistance to minimize communication and adjustment difficulties. Because the psychosocial and behavioral implications of hearing impairment are not integral to the audiologic evaluation, this information is all too often avoided and ignored. Not only is there little evidence of a biopsychosocial approach in audiology, there is considerable evidence of the biomedical one.

Of course, many audiologists do focus on how hearing impairment affects their patients and they provide counseling to ensure that patients adjust to their hearing problems and manage them successfully. Many more audiologists would do so if institutional resistance did not exist on several different levels. Professional training in audiology is not approached from a biopsychosocial perspective. Physical sciences dominate the curriculum with minimal emphasis on social and behavioral science. This mirrors the situation that has existed in medical schools. In practicum settings, skill and speed in administering the battery of audiologic measures and determining a diagnosis from those findings is emphasized. Service delivery is based on a top-down model in which the clinician provides the diagnosis and recommends the treatment. Third-party payers dictate which procedures are covered and which are not. Audiology is a system that mirrors the health care system of which it is a part.

AR—The Military Experience

Audiology has its roots in the AR programs that were implemented during World War II to care for military personnel who incurred deafness or hearing impairment secondary to their military service (Gaeth, 1979; Morrissett, 1957). At the time, the AR programs actually approximated a biopsychosocial approach. The programs were situated at three medical facilities: Borden General Hospital in Chickasha, OK; Hoff General Hospital in Santa Barbara, CA; and Deshon General Hospital in Butler, PA. An Army Captain who served at Deshon as an acoustic physicist came from Northwestern University. Captain Raymond Carhart later returned to Northwestern where he started the first educational program in audiology. (*Note:* For further information on the history of AR, the reader is referred to Chapter 1 of this text)

Otolaryngologic and psychiatric evaluations were conducted on an in-patient basis as part of the admission process. Following the in-patient medical exams, the soldiers resided in convalescent centers for the duration of the three-month AR program. Once accepted into the program, a Red Cross caseworker was assigned to each patient to handle any concerns he might have and to facilitate contact and communication with family members. Lipreading teachers, speech therapists, and social workers were involved in the daily training. Dr. Walter Hughson, an otologist serving as a civilian consultant, urged the inclusion of evaluations of mental ability and educational achievement to ensure that the patients could be expected to benefit from the program and, subsequently, to realize successful vocational rehabilitation. Hughson praised the realistic approach to the total problem of hearing loss with its recognition of the psychologic implications. According to Morrissett, who became chief of the Otolaryngology Branch in the Surgical Consultants Division in the Army Surgeon General's Office in 1944, the programs gave specific attention to:

1. social and psychiatric treatment to overcome possible trauma associated with combat related hearing loss and to rule out "hysterical" deafness,
2. medical and surgical treatment as necessary,
3. hearing aid fittings for those who were anticipated to accrue benefit from them, and
4. "education for social living" p. 449.

Education for social living included a program of recreational and educational activities, training in lipreading and speech correction, and "indoctrination of the soldier's family" (Morrissett, 1957). Absent the technologic advances in diagnostic audiology and hearing aids, the emphasis on rehabilitation focused directly on the patient.

> *A special effort was always made to make clear to each patient precisely what he could expect from the rehabilitation course. It was explained unequivocally that a . . . person could not expect to regain his full hearing but that he could be taught methods of compensating for his disability. It was emphasized that nothing could be accomplished without his own full cooperation; and it was only in the exceptional case that such cooperation was not given.* (p. 469)

In 1945, Truex (1957) conducted a follow-up survey of 468 patients from the AR program at Deshon General Hospital at least six months following their hospital stay. Thirty-three of the surveys were undeliverable, 261 of the remaining 435 were completed and returned. Inasmuch as these patients were already discharged from military service, there should have been no concerns about possible negative ramifications. Nonetheless, respondents were told that a signature was not necessary and that there would be no repercussions whatsoever from participation. The results of this study sparked an interest in establishing similar programs in the civilian sector after the war. Of the 261 respondents, only two did not consider the time spent in the program worthwhile. Of even greater significance is the fact that 91.6% indicated that they were using their hearing aids. Among those who were not wearing their hearing aids, the primary reasons given included headaches, difficulty obtaining batteries, hearing aid was in need of repair, did fine without aid, aid was too noisy, aid was too cumbersome, and external otitis. In terms of daily use, 23% indicated they wore their hearing aid 5 to 8 hours per day, 21% reported 9 to 12 hours of hearing aid use, and 22% said they wore their hearing aids more than 12 hours per day. Of those who only used their hearing aids 1 to 4 hours per day, the vast majority indicated that they did not wear their hearing aids at work in factories, or on farms, and so forth. Several respondents failed to indicate how many hours per day they wore their instruments.

Following the war, the military AR programs were consolidated and based at Walter Reed General Hospital, later designated Walter Reed Army Medical Center. In contrast to the statement from Morrisett quoted above, with the move to Walter Reed, audiologists rather than otolaryngologists managed the AR program. The vast majority of patients presented with bilateral high-frequency sensorineural hearing impairment secondary to long term noise exposure. Referrals for psychiatric evaluations were essentially nonexistent. Although changes in the program occurred over the years, an AR program was offered at Walter Reed for over 50 years. Demise of the program since the turn of the century can be attributed directly to the biomedical model as discussed below. Data from two follow-up surveys of Walter Reed program's patients are available. Northern, Ciliax, Roth, and Johnson (1969) conducted a follow-up study of patients who had attended a three-week AR program. The return rate was 77% yielding 199 usable questionnaires. The results indicate that 93.5% of the respondents wore their hearing aids "Always" or "Often." Only 4.5% said they "Never" wore their hearing aids and 2% indicated that they seldom wore them. When asked if they would refer a military colleague with hearing loss to the program, only one of 199 patients indicated that they would not.

By the 1980s, the AR program had been shortened to nine days. Spouses were frequently included and the number of female patients was increasing. Better hearing aid technology and milder hearing impairments contributed to improvements in acceptance of, and adjustment to, the use of amplification. As the degree of patients' average hearing loss became milder, less emphasis was placed on speechreading and auditory training. Instead, emphasis was placed on enhancing patients' awareness of the benefits of hearing aid use. Recorded exercises in varied listening environments were used to compare unaided and aided performance. These exercises were very effective in demonstrating the benefits of hearing aid use in terms of speech intelligibility and even more so perhaps, in terms of listening ease and the associated decrease in stress and anxiety. Patients were continuously amazed to realize how much they had been missing and how much more relaxed and confident they were when listening in the aided condition. The course of the program represented an opportunity for patients to adjust to the use of amplification while working closely with program audiologists. Adjustment difficulties, specific fitting problems, and perceived benefit and satisfaction were closely monitored throughout the program to ensure acceptance of and adjustment to the use of amplification. Patients were afforded the opportunity to try alternate fittings and to evaluate monaural vs. binaural amplification when appropriate. Their active engagement in this evaluation and decision-making process undoubtedly was implicated in the program's successfulness. Results of the long-term follow-up of patients who participated in the National Institutes on Deafness and Other Communication Disorders/Veterans Affairs (NIDCD/VA) Hearing Aid Clinical Trial also suggest that patients' active engagement in the selection of an optimal hearing aid fitting has positive effects on treatment outcome (Kricos, Erdman, Bratt, & Williams, 2007). The AR program at Walter Reed also featured individual and group counseling sessions that included assertiveness training, stress management techniques, and problem solving based on analysis of the patients' specific communication difficulties. The group format was invaluable. As one patient stated,

> *I really didn't think I needed to come to this course. But so many things were helpful, especially the feelings others expressed as to their personal problems with hearing loss and the suggestions everyone gave each other. I'm a bit of a loner, but I felt really comfortable being with others who are experiencing the same problems I've been having.*

A senior officer who completed the program with a group of 11 other patients including enlisted personnel and other officers made a statement to the group at the end of the program, *"This group has changed a lot of people since Day 1."*

Routine follow-up of the AR patients through the 1980's consistently revealed hearing aid use rates comparable to those reported by Truex's (1957) study of patients who attended the program in 1945 and Northern and colleagues survey of patients some 20 years later (1969). Erdman and Demorest (1987) compared pre- and post-program CPHI (Demorest & Erdman, 1986, 1987) results for former AR patients ($N = 70$) eight months to a year following their enrollment. Hearing aid use rates in the 90% range were reported. Moreover, significant improvements in scores were demonstrated in all areas of Communication Performance, Attitudes of Others, Maladaptive Strategies and Verbal Strategies, and all but one scale (Displacement of Responsibility) in the Personal Adjustment area (see Erdman & Demorest [1998a, 1998b] for a review of current CPHI scales and Erdman [2006] for CPHI interpretation guidelines). The results of the follow-up study indicate broad-based treatment effects for the hearing aid and counseling-based AR intervention.

For over half a century, the Army AR programs achieved successful hearing aid outcomes at a rate that has yet to be replicated elsewhere. It is ironic, of course, that the influence of the biomedical model on audiology triggered an end to this remarkable program just as efforts to improve treatment outcomes for chronic conditions are leading to an integration of psychosocial interventions throughout health care. Patients' belief in the program and support for it remained solid throughout its life span. Unfortunately, as audiologists who worked in the program moved on or retired, replacements became difficult to find. Failure to emphasize the human element in educational programs in audiology has led to fewer and fewer audiologists who are psychosocially or counseling oriented. Institutional variables also contributed to the program's demise. Unlike the convalescent centers that housed the AR programs during the war, Walter Reed is an acute care facility without the resources necessary for rehabilitative care. Active-duty personnel for whom hearing aids were being recommended for the first time, were referred to Walter Reed from across the eastern half of the United States. Transportation, meals, and housing were not systematically determined for the patients; varying procedures at the referring military installations resulted in disparate arrangements for the attendees. Some of the AR patients were admitted to their local military hospital and transferred to Walter Reed as inpatients.

Others were sent on "temporary duty" (TDY) to the program with funding allotted for travel and daily expenses. Service members stationed within the DC metropolitan area were placed on administrative leave and traveled to Walter Reed from their homes on a daily basis.

The lack of standard referral and funding procedures for out-patient rehabilitative care, in conjunction with scarce housing options, resulted in a recurring need to justify the AR program. A facility that was specifically designed to address acute care, not surprisingly, has experienced woeful inadequacies in restorative and rehabilitative care for active-duty service members. The biomedical model is directly responsible; it is to blame for indefensible failures in the provision of quality care for wounded soldiers returning from combat zones around the world. Widespread publicity of the bureaucratic nightmares and deplorable conditions faced by patients who require extended care secondary to amputations, traumatic brain injuries, and post-traumatic stress disorder has resulted in criticism of how Walter Reed Army Medical Center has been run. Clearly, criticism is warranted; nonetheless, this unacceptable situation is a symptom of a much larger problem: the health care system's intractable, dogmatic subservience to the scientifically challenged biomedical model. Effective mechanisms for managing chronic health conditions will not emerge until the fixated, narrow focus on one specific aspect of care—be it the disease or the impairment—is replaced by an all-encompassing recognition of the complexity inherent in human experience. A giant in the field of rehabilitation, Franklin Shontz (1977), eloquently summarized this point.

> *Of all the factors that affect the total life situation of a person with a disability, the disability itself is only one, and often its influence is relatively minor. This implies, in the final analysis, that the understanding of psychological reaction to physical disability requires the understanding of individual human beings in all of their complexity.*

The image of audiology as a microcosm of the health care system makes it easier to address how the limitations and inadequacies of the biomedical model affect our practice and research and, similarly, how the extended scope and flexibility of the biopsychosocial model changes that scenario. In addressing these questions, it helps to keep a couple of things in mind. The first is this: tackling these questions is not merely an option; it is an inevitable necessity on all levels ranging from the individual clinician, to clinical supervisors, to clinic directors, to the hearing aid industry, to faculty members and deans, to the governance of professional organizations, and to third-party payers. The second point is this: the fundamental change that is necessary is a shift in perspective, from the hearing impairment to the person with hearing impairment—a simple thought with myriad implications.

Just as some dispute the need for a biopsychosocial approach in medicine, some may debate the need to shift audiology's focus. As one colleague —a basic scientist at heart argues, "Fixing what's wrong, fixes everything." Still others will respond, "But that only makes things more complicated." Yes and no. Expanding the focus of practice to facilitate diagnosis and patient engagement entails looking at more factors, but it also means revealing more relevant variables that ultimately can facilitate adjustment and enhance outcomes.

The benefits of the biomedical model in medicine are mirrored in audiology. The diagnostic technologies available to us today were unfathomable in the early years of the profession. These advances and others throughout medicine have contributed to an unprecedented increase in our understanding of the anatomy and physiology of the auditory system down to its molecular bases. From body hearing aids to implantable devices, there is no question that innovations in amplification technology have improved the quality and sophistication of products available for the remediation of hearing impairment.

Nonetheless, there are signs of limitations to a biomedical focus in audiology. To what extent has progress in technology translated into improvements in the lives of those who live with hearing impairment? Has satisfaction with hearing aids increased significantly? Are those who wear hearing aids experiencing fewer residual problems than hearing aid users in the past? How are we addressing the problems of patients who are not achieving sufficient benefit or are simply not adjusting to hearing aid use? How are we addressing the needs of family members who are unavoidably affected by their loved one's hearing impairment? *Why* have we not seen improvements on the human level that correspond to improvements on the technological level? In short, how successful have we been in addressing hearing impairment as a chronic condition? These questions are not a matter of self-recrimination; they are representative of the crisis facing all of health care today.

The classic biomedical response to suggestions that patient variables are implicated in treatment failures has been, "That is not our problem." To the contrary—when advances in biomedical thinking do not result in comparable advances in health and well-being it is everyone's problem. Professionally, morally, and ethically, it is our responsibility to respond accordingly. Audiologists are faced with a multitude of situations in which the biomedical approach can pose limitations. From dissatisfaction with hearing aids, to residual communication difficulties, to nonadherence to treatment regimens, how are we addressing these limitations in audiology? Does the biomedical approach adequately serve our patients in terms of their specific communication needs and environments? Does it address the impact of hearing impairment on patients' personal adjustment and on the members of their families?

The focus of audiologic intervention must shift from the hearing impairment to the person with the hearing impairment. The reason is simple. Patient-centered approaches to health care result in greater patient satisfaction, enhanced treatment adherence, and better treatment outcomes than do services emanating from traditional biomedical or "disease" focused approaches (Bodenheimer, Wagner, & Grumbach, 2002; Carr, Emory, Errichetti, Johnson, & Reyes, 2007; Earp, French, & Gilkey, 2007; Falvo, 2004; Stewart, Belle-Brown, Weston, & McWhinney, 2003).

Ironically, in many ways, the shift for audiology is a return to our roots. In the early AR programs, the purpose was to "restore the person" rather than to "restore the hearing." Shifting our perspective allows us to undergo a fundamental realignment of our philosophical underpinnings that reflects more accurately audiology's identity as a rehabilitative profession. This shift in paradigm is a matter of priorities and a matter of focus; it is a matter of understanding what living with a hearing impairment means to each of our patients. The patient-centered focus, as Engel (2005) describes it, involves "learning how to embed the illness (disability) in the patient's life," (p. 377). It is by incorporating this philosophical reorientation into our clinical perspective and practice that the role of counseling emerges front and center.

Audiologic Counseling: The Obstacle Course

We need to see what can be changed so that it is easier for us to live with ourselves, so that the public can readily perceive how we contribute to the welfare of clients, and so that, at the same time, we do not compromise our ethical standards.

Heaton (1992)

Several years ago, the observation was made that "counseling has been slow to evolve into a systematic, well-defined process in rehabilitative audiology" (Erdman, 1993a, p. 374). In fact, the difficulty in integrating systematic counseling into audiologic practice may result from trying to insert psychosocial and behavioral variables into a biomedical service delivery model in which they simply do not fit. In their discussion of service delivery models, Erdman, Wark, and Montano (1994) concur with Heaton's observation and state:

> *The minimal emphasis on rehabilitation perpetuates the perception of audiology as a diagnostic profession with adherence to a medical model of service delivery. Failure to modify service delivery to better meet the needs of individuals with hearing impairment when we know change is needed and when we know we can do better, is unethical. To assume the position that change is not possible because of time constraints or reimbursement constraints when we know change is indicated is indefensible.*

Unfortunately, the thoughts expressed in each of the above statements have not led to change in audiologic service delivery. The obstacles that collaboratively reinforce the biomedical model's hold on audiology have not been overcome to date. Counseling remains ill defined and unsystematic in audiologic curricula, practice, and research. The reasons are not new.

The Pitfalls of Arbitrary Definitions

The persistent depiction of counseling as a dichotomy consisting of informational counseling and adjustment counseling continues to hamper effective integration of counseling into audiologic practice. This arbitrary conceptualization, aside from being unrelated to established counseling theory and methods, is flawed and unsustainable. It is unrelated to the areas of knowledge and skill required for audiologists who provide AR services (ASHA, 2001), (Table 9–2), and the Preferred Practice Patterns for counseling in audiology (ASHA, 2006), (Table 9–3). For over 20 years, Wylde (1987) and Erdman (1993a, 2000) have stressed the erroneous nature of the information-adjustment dichotomy pointing out that it ignores the relationship between cognition and affect. Information can have very powerful effects on adjustment; this is the very principle on which cognitive approaches to counseling are based. Neuroscience corroborates the extent to which cognition and affect are interconnected, if not interdependent phenomena. Functional brain imaging depicts the two separate but interacting processes mediated by separate but interacting brain systems (Greenberg, 2008).

On a practical level, consider a patient who believes incorrectly that his recent diagnosis of hearing impairment portends eventual deafness. Consequently, he is overwhelmed with feelings of despair, fear, anxiety, and sadness. The audiologist who voices understanding of his concern and reassures him that eventual deafness is highly unlikely, particularly given the etiology of his hearing problem, can resolve his emotional distress immediately. Correction of an erroneous belief through cognitive intervention can facilitate a change in affective state, i.e., emotional adjustment.

Affect, cognition, and behavior are interconnected phenomena, a concept covered in entry-level courses in psychology. It is important to couch our understanding of counseling theory and its methodologies in established psychological conceptualizations to ensure that our clinical practice and research is consistent with scientific knowledge. There is no rationale or justification for doing otherwise. Understanding the experience of hearing impairment, adjustment to hearing impairment, and the sources of individual differences inherent in each, requires that we do so.

Educational Implications

I have learned that people may forget what you said and people may forget what you did. But people will never forget how you made them feel.

Maya Angelou

The need for counseling is recognized by many audiologists and has been emphasized by professional organizations (e.g., AAA, 2004; ASHA, 2001, 2004, 2006, 2008). The absence of social and behavioral sciences in graduate programs in audiology is troubling. Virtually every course is rooted in the physical sciences (e.g., anatomy and physiology, hearing disorders, genetics, neuroscience, diagnostic procedures, acoustics, electroacoustics, instrumentation, evaluation of amplification systems, etc.). It is ironic indeed that, historically, the study of communication sciences and disorders has been categorized as a social and behavioral science. Numerous calls to add counseling coursework to the curriculum in education programs in audiology (Crandell, 1997; Crandell & Weiner, 2002; Culpepper, Mendel, & McCarthy, 1994; Erdman, 1993a, 2000; McCarthy, Culpepper & Lucks, 1986) have been met with slow and limited success. A review of curricula among Au.D. programs reveals variability in the extent to which counseling, and social and behavioral science in general, are emphasized. Some programs offer no counseling courses; others offer an elective counseling

Table 9–2. Excerpt from *Knowledge and Skills Required for the Provision of Audiologic Rehabilitation by Audiologists* (ASHA, 2001)

IX. Effects of Hearing Impairment on Psychosocial, Educational, and Occupational Functioning
Describe and evaluate the impact of hearing impairment on psychosocial development and psychosocial functioning;
Describe systems and methods of educational programming (e.g., mainstream, residential) and facilitate selection of appropriate educational options;
Describe systems and methods of educational programming (e.g., mainstream, residential) and facilitate selection of appropriate educational options;
Describe and evaluate the effects of hearing impairment on occupational status and performance (e.g., communication, localization, safety);
Describe and evaluate the effects of hearing impairment on occupational status and performance (e.g., communication, localization, safety);
Identify the effects of hearing problems on marital dyads, family dynamics, and other interpersonal communication functioning;
Identify the need and provide for psychosocial, educational, family, and occupational/vocational counseling in relation to hearing impairment and subsequent communication difficulties;
Provide assessment of family members' perception of and reactions to communication difficulties.
X. AR Case Management
Use effective interpersonal communication in interviewing and interacting with individuals with hearing impairment and their families;
Describe client-centered, behavioral, cognitive, and integrative theories and methods of counseling and their relevance in AR;
Provide appropriate individual and group adjustment counseling related to hearing loss for individuals with hearing impairment and their families;
Provide auditory, visual, and auditory-visual communication training (e.g., speech speech-reading, auditory training, listening skills) to enhance receptive communication;
Provide training in effective communication strategies to individuals with hearing impairment, family members, and other relevant individuals
Provide for appropriate expressive communication training
Provide appropriate technological and counseling intervention to facilitate adjustment to tinnitus;
Provide appropriate intervention for management of vestibular disorders;
Develop and implement an intervention plan based on the individual's situational/environmental communication needs and performance and related adjustment difficulties;
Develop and implement a system for measuring and monitoring outcomes and the appropriateness and efficacy of intervention.

Table 9–3. Preferred Practice Patterns in Audiology: Counseling (ASHA, 2006)

Expected Outcome(s)

- Counseling enhances patients' and their families' understanding of, acceptance of, and adjustment to auditory, vestibular, or related disorders.
- Counseling enhances acceptance of and adjustment to hearing aids and hearing assistive technology systems designed to maximize communication skills.
- Counseling engages patients in the management of their communication problems and enhances the physical and psychosocial well-being and quality of life for individuals with hearing impairment and other auditory disorders.
- Counseling increases awareness of the need for prevention of further damage to auditory, vestibular, or related systems.
- Counseling enhances compliance with treatment recommendations.
- Counseling enhances benefit from and satisfaction with treatment.

Clinical Indications

- Counseling is indicated for all patients and their family members/caregivers as an integral part of audiologic services.

Clinical Process

- Counseling goals are established based on assessment of patients' needs.
- Counseling goals and approaches are modified to facilitate patients' motivation, progress, and engagement in the management of auditory and nonauditory effects of hearing impairment and other auditory, vestibular, or related disorders.
- Counseling is individualized for each patient using culturally and linguistically appropriate language.
- Counseling approaches may be cognitive, affective, behavioral, or eclectic in nature based on the patient's specific needs and target goals.
- Counseling for patients and their families/caregivers may focus on one or more of the following:
  - evaluation procedures
  - diagnosis and results of evaluation
  - treatment options
  - communication problems experienced secondary to hearing disorders
  - effects of hearing and balance disorders on psychosocial and behavioral adjustment including interpersonal relationships, social activities, education, and occupational options and performance
  - affective/emotional reactions to auditory, vestibular, or other related disorders
  - development of problem-solving skills and compensatory behaviors
  - development and coordination of self-help and support groups
- Counseling should include referral to and consultation with appropriate professionals and nonprofessionals as appropriate.

course from another department. Still other programs feature one or two courses that cover self-awareness, loss and grieving, health psychology, rehabilitation theory, psychosocial adjustment to disability, and psychosocial adjustment to hearing loss. Faculty members with strong interests in rehabilitative audiology try to incorporate counseling as a fundamental ingredient throughout the audiology curriculum. This approach is consistent with a scenario in which counseling is a part of the very fabric of audiology. It is also consistent with demands throughout health care to infuse social and behavioral sciences into the education of health care professionals and into the health care process.

Despite increasing evidence of the role of psychosocial and behavioral variables in disease and health care, calls for inclusion of social and behavioral sciences in medical school curricula were essentially ignored for some 30 years. Institutional resistance persisted in the form of the "hidden curriculum" (Dobie, 2007; Wear, 1998) even when changes in curricula purportedly had been made. The current health care crisis, however, has prompted a series of events and directives that are finally leading to curriculum change. In 2002, the Institute of Medicine (IOM) convened a committee to review the status of behavioral and social sciences in medical school curricula, determine a priority list for such curricula, and identify barriers to incorporating new curricula into medical education (Carr, Emory, Errichetti, Johnson, & Reyes, 2007). Recommended priorities in subject matter include mind-body interactions, patient behavior, physician role and behavior, physician patient interactions, social and cultural issues in health care, and health policy and economics. Not surprisingly, these priorities reflect growing acceptance of the biopsychosocial model. The IOM and the Association of American Medical Colleges (AAMC) (Cuff & Vanselaw, 2004) have prompted modifications in how course content is monitored. Licensing exams now also include assessment of knowledge in the behavioral sciences. Similar curriculum changes are needed to expand audiology's focus on the psychosocial implications of hearing impairment. Moreover, communication and counseling skills need to be taught and evaluated systematically.

Professional Identity

Some audiologists have questioned whether they have the necessary qualifications to provide counseling. There are two important points to remember here. First, our qualifications to provide audiologic counseling consist of a recognized degree in the profession, the requisite certification or licensure, and having the necessary knowledge and skills. These areas of knowledge and skill (ASHA, 2001) appear in Table 9–1, shown earlier. Clinicians who are not comfortable that they possess the requisite knowledge and skills can consider enrolling in a counseling course, pursue continuing education in this area, or seek out a mentor. Second, counseling is included in audiologists' scope of practice. The Preferred Practice Patterns describe the wide range of relevant counseling responsibilities in audiology; they appear in Table 9–2, shown earlier. This is further evidence that audiologists are expected to provide counseling to help patients and their families resolve the communication problems and adjustment difficulties they experience because of hearing impairment.

Long-standing misperceptions regarding mental health among individuals with hearing impairment may contribute to the doubts some audiologists have about their qualifications to counsel. For hundreds of years, individuals with hearing impairment were institutionalized along with individuals manifesting every imaginable mental health problem because their behavior and strange vocalizations (unexplainable at the time) were viewed as aberrant. Even when hearing impairment became a diagnosable condition, the "suspiciousness" attributed to people with hearing problems led to a belief that they were paranoid. This lack of insight into hearing problems is, unfortunately, highly pervasive. Stika (1997) conducted a survey of members of the SHHH organization (now the Hearing Loss Association of America, HLAA) to obtain information regarding the use of mental health services by those who have hearing problems. The results show that, in general, respondents sought mental health services for many of the same reasons the general population does. Many, however, also indicated that they sought counseling for issues directly or indirectly related to their hearing problems. Their comments revealed mental health counselors' disconcerting lack of knowledge and understanding of hearing loss. Stika includes the following comments:

She had no understanding of hearing loss. I had to spend part of my session—that I was paying for—educating her.

She did not understand the stress and responsibility I feel to make the communication process successful. At times, she would say things like, "You're taking communication too seriously. Everyone misses part of what is being said anyway."

I understand well in one-on-one situations so they were unable to comprehend the problems I said I had. They were somewhat incredulous and disbelieving. They would argue as if they could convince me that my hearing loss didn't exist!

The psychiatrist could not differentiate between neurotic defenses and defensive behavior caused by the frustration of not hearing well, especially at parties, professional meetings, etc. One doctor, who is now becoming hard of hearing, recently admitted to me that he now realizes he was wrong to keep dismissing my complaints of how much I was missing.

Although many of the respondents had received satisfactory counseling services, the lack of awareness of the difficulties commonly associated with hearing loss among mental health professionals is disturbing. Some of the counselors appeared to be unaware of the special communicative needs of their patients (e.g., the importance of visual cues, good lighting, and a well-modulated voice). There was limited understanding of the effects of hearing loss and background noise on speech comprehension. Some of the mental health professionals were not cognizant of the vastly different needs of those with congenital versus acquired deafness and hearing impairment. A lack of insight into the psychosocial effects of hearing loss in terms of personal adjustment, relationships, family life, and occupation was especially hard to believe. Most alarming, however, is the apparent tendency for mental health professionals to discount or refute patients' complaints of hearing difficulty when such problems are not evidenced in the one-on-one counseling encounter. This introduces the very real possibility of potentially damaging misdiagnoses. Moreover, it precludes the possibility of a trusting relationship and the possibility for an empathic understanding of the patient's problems. Indeed, the single most important goal is to ensure that the individual *feels* understood. It is discouraging to see continuing evidence of what Meadow-Orlans (1985) refers to as the "persistent myth" regarding the mental health of people who have hearing problems. Stika stresses the need for change in meeting the mental health needs of those with hearing problems. Hallam, Ashton, Sherbourne, and Gailey (2006) echo this need for counseling services from professionals who are cognizant of the issues facing those with hearing impairment. Their investigation of individuals specifically with acquired profound hearing impairment suggests that although this is not a frequent clinical phenomenon, the counseling needs of these individuals pose a critical need for expanded service in this area.

Many of the individuals who participated in Stika's survey were seeking assistance for problems related to their hearing difficulties. The irony is, of course, that audiologists are exceptionally well qualified to be of assistance with such problems. A number of respondents stated that they realized later just how much hearing loss was implicated in their decision to seek counseling in the first place. The insidious nature of hearing impairment manifests itself in many different ways. Audiologic counseling can be and should be an option for patients with adjustment problems related to their hearing loss. For patients whose mental health status warrants actual psychologic or psychiatric intervention, audiologists should facilitate a team approach to ensure that both the patient's hearing and mental health needs are addressed optimally. The lack of appropriate counseling services for those with hearing impairment is a serious issue; mechanisms are needed to address this clinical deficiency.

Hearing Impairment and Psychological Adjustment

Thomas (1984) disputes the idea that suspiciousness and paranoid psychoses are more common among those with hearing impairment and maintains that hearing impairment does not affect basic personality structure. His findings are concordant with rehabilitation psychology which holds that disabilities are not associated with type or degree of personality traits, or with adjustment. Nonetheless, he stresses that people can experience significant psychological distress secondary to hearing impairment. Although controversy remains over the relationship between hearing impairment and mental health, there is general concurrence that individual differences play a major role and that the experience of hearing impairment is highly idiosyncratic. Consequently, audiologists should be prepared to meet the individual needs of each patient. Counseling is the primary means of doing so. Thomas' work represents a marked departure from the psychoanalytic thought that dominated the "psychology of hearing loss" for a number of years. Knapp (1953) suggested the possibility that "unconscious attitudes centered in the ear may actually alter its physiology" (p. 107) and cites a review with evidence that emotional factors may serve as an activating agent in otosclerosis. Knapp contended that the ear has a definite role in psychic life. Many of those trained in Freudian theory believed that the sexual symbolism associated with the ear and with hearing allows an understanding of the psychological reactions seen in patients with hearing loss (Rousey, 1971). Psychoanalytic writings such as *The Madonna's Conception Through the Ear* (Jones, 1951) reveal some interesting, if not improbable, conceptualizations.

Freud was a significant figure in psychotherapy throughout the 20th century and, in all probability, will remain so for many years to come. His psychoanalytic theory is the most comprehensive ever developed. It covers personality development, a philosophy of human nature, and psychotherapeutic methodology. Freud was not particularly fond of those who disagreed with him and some of the greatest minds in psychology broke with him rather than compromise their own beliefs. Psychoanalysts who came later, immersed themselves in Freud's theories and further developed his ideas. Consequently, psychoanalysis is a less obscure endeavor with a broader range of applications today.

The intensity and duration of psychoanalysis preclude its utility in most rehabilitation situations. However, knowledge of psychoanalytic theory is invaluable to counselors in many areas of rehabilitation counseling. Ego defenses first described by Freud are often implicated in adjustment to disability. Descriptions of such defenses are included in Table 9–4. Counselors can gain a better understanding of patients' coping behaviors by understanding the role such defenses can play in the adjustment process. In addition to the importance of defense mechanisms in rehabilitation, other psychoanalytic applications pointed out by Livneh and Siller (2004) include the effect of disability on self-perception and body image; the study of reactions to loss, trauma, and disability (e.g., anger, denial, depression, mourning); and the implications of attitudes toward people with disabilities.

Freud was a complicated man who is widely reported to have suffered from phobias and psychosomatic disorders himself. He was a proponent and user of cocaine, which led some to speculate as to the influence that may have had on the development of his theories. In the final analysis, Freud's own fixation—clearly oral—ultimately led to his demise. He was an incessant cigar smoker and developed oral/mandibular cancer for which he had 33 surgical procedures over a period of two decades. He was a prolific writer—his writings comprise 24 volumes—until the intractable pain led him to beseech his friend and physician to assist him in finding final peace. Freud and his "talking cure" have had a profound impact on the mental health field. Familiarity with the underpinnings of psychoanalysis is of significant value for anyone in the helping professions.

What Is Counseling?

It is a process, a thing-in-itself, an experience, a relationship, a dynamic.

Carl Rogers (1951)

The chronic nature of hearing impairment, in and of itself, indicates the need for a biopsychosocial approach in audiology. By shifting the focus to our patients and attending to the actual reasons

Table 9–4. Examples of Psychoanalytic Ego Defenses Manifested in Reactions to Disability

Defense Mechanism	Definition	Example
Repression	Forcing intrapsychic conflicts, painful experiences, and disturbing memories out of conscious awareness	Person with a visible congenital disability repressing feelings of shame and embarrassment triggered by early life reactions of others
Projection	Externalizing unconscious forbidden ideas, needs, and impulses and attributing them to other people or environmental conditions	Blaming others for onset of disability, or attributing lack of progress in rehabilitation to staff incompetence rather than own lack of effort
Rationalization	Using after the fact, false reasons to offset negative emotional or consequences.	Person who gradually loses hearing and attributes lack of participation to boredom, lack of interest, or fatigue
Sublimation	Adopting useful, socially acceptable behaviors to express forbidden and socially unacceptable wishes and impulses	Anger and desire to retaliate against an uncaring society channeled into artistic endeavors
Reaction formation	Substituting and expressing responses and feelings that are exact opposites of those that are deemed verboten or unacceptable	Replacing initial feelings of aversion and rejection toward a child born with a severe disfigurement with overly demonstrative affection and protectiveness
Regression	Reverting to childlike behaviors first exhibited during an earlier developmental stage	A recently disabled person whose temper tantrums are activated when needs are not immediately gratified or who daydreams rather than pursue treatment
Compensation	Seeking to excel in functionally related activities or behaviors to make up for disability-generated loss	Person who lost sight at an early age and has achieved success as a musician
Denial	Resolution of emotional conflict and reduction of anxiety by refusing to perceive, accept or acknowledge threatening aspects of external reality	Failure to perceive or acknowledge effects of hearing impairment on job performance
Displacement	Shifting energy toward a less intimidating or more accessible object or person to reduce anxiety	Blaming others for not speaking clearly rather than admit to having a hearing problem

Source: Adapted from Cubbage & Thomas (1989), Livneh & Siller (2004), and Livneh & Cook (2005).

they seek audiologic intervention, the foundation on which to base relevant counseling emerges. Perceived impediments to incorporating counseling in audiology practice are not insurmountable. The first step is to acknowledge the unacceptable limitations that the biomedical model places on the provision of audiologic care. That simple acknowledgement, a change in mindset, will significantly enhance our ability to overcome any remaining obstacles. Undoubtedly, systemic difficulties will need to be confronted and resolved. Awareness of the limitations of the current model, however, is a critical move in the right direction.

Professionals' effectiveness in health and rehabilitation involves many factors. Berven, Thomas, and Chan (2004) identify several key ingredients:

1. establishing a therapeutic relationship with patients,
2. communicating with patients and their families in facilitative ways,
3. obtaining information from individuals in a thorough, attentive manner,
4. helping patients identify their problems and explain their needs,
5. conceptualizing problems in ways that will facilitate an appropriate treatment plan, and
6. facilitating adherence to plans that patients have decided to pursue.

These responsibilities mirror key elements of the biopsychosocial approach (Frankel, Quill, & McDaniel, 2003; Sarafino, 2005) and are considered focal areas throughout rehabilitation literature (Chan, Berven, & Thomas, 2004; Dell Orto & Powers, 2007; Falvo, 2005; Livneh & Antonak, 1997; Martz & Livneh, 2007; Parker, Szymanski, & Patterson; 2004) and patient education (Christensen, 2004; Falvo, 2004; O'Donahue & Levensky, 2006). Each of these responsibilities is among the commonalities that exist across a wide range of counseling approaches (Corey, 2008; Mahoney, 2003; Norcross & Goldfried, 2005; Wampold, 2001; Wampold & Brown, 2005; Welfel & Patterson, 2004).

The terms counseling and psychotherapy, more often than not, are used interchangeably in the literature. The titles and content of current textbooks reflect the fact that the conceptual foundations, theories, and methodologies for counseling and psychotherapy are not just similar, they are the same. Consider, for example, *The Theory and Practice of Counseling and Psychotherapy* (Corey, 2008), *Ethics in Psychotherapy and Counseling: A Practical Guide* (Pope & Vasquez, 2007), and *Theories of Psychotherapy and Counseling: Concepts and Cases* (Sharf, 2007) to name but a few. Carl Rogers summed it up well in his book *Counseling and Psychotherapy—Newer Concepts in Practice* (1942).

> *... Most frequently, (these processes) are termed counseling, a word in increasingly common use, particularly in educational circles. Or such contacts, with their curative and remedial aim, may be classed as psychotherapy, the term most frequently used by social workers, psychologists, and psychiatrists in clinics. These terms will be used more or less interchangeably in these chapters, and will be so used because they all seem to refer to the same basic method—a series of direct contacts with the individual, which aims to offer him assistance in changing his attitudes and behavior . . . It is also plain that the most intensive and successful counseling is indistinguishable from intensive and successful psychotherapy. Consequently, both terms will be employed, as they are in common use by workers in the field.* (pp. 3–4)

Interestingly, Rogers also noted that a "great many professionals" provide these services and that regardless of how such individuals might refer to themselves, their approach was the relevant consideration. Consistent with its inception in psychiatry and a traditional focus on pathology, psychotherapy tends to connote long-term treatment of psychologic and personality disorders. Counseling, on the other hand, which evolved from education, suggests a problem-focused learning process that is adjustment oriented. Within the profession, there appears to be universal agreement that the latter more appropriately describes the process involved in AR.

The number of different approaches in counseling has grown exponentially in the past 40 years. The major approaches (humanistic/affective, cognitive, and behavioral) and recent integrative movements have been described previously (Erdman 1993a, 2000). There are specific counseling variables and conceptualizations that are central to the biopsychosocial approach. Included among these are the patient's story, patient centeredness, counselor characteristics, the practitioner-patient/clinician-client relationship, the therapeutic alliance, engagement of the patient, and self-efficacy. These key elements of a biopsychosocial approach to chronic illness and disability are discussed in more detail below. The significance of the practitioner-patient relationship and the critical need to engage patients in their own health care are recurrent areas of emphasis in the medical, nursing, counseling and rehabilitation literatures pertaining to chronic illness and disability.

Evidence of Counseling Effectiveness in AR

There is evidence that counseling in audiology is effective and warranted. In a study based in Finland (Vuorialho, Karinen, & Sorri, 2006), in-home counseling was provided to first time hearing aid users six months after their hearing aid fitting and initial counseling. The counseling was focused primarily on hearing aid use. At a 12-month visit, over half of those who had only been using their hearing aids "occasionally" at the six-month point had since become regular users. Even more remarkably, a third of the non-users had become regular users. At the 12-month point, patients felt less of a need for counseling than they had at six months. They demonstrated greater skill in managing hearing aids in terms of maintenance and telephone use and in inserting or positioning their hearing aids. Their analyses showed the counseling sessions to be highly cost-effective. The authors acknowledge that the problem is finding the resources to provide the counseling. They point out, however, that studies have demonstrated that increased expenditures in one budget can result in corresponding or greater savings elsewhere. The focus of this study, albeit narrow, addresses weaknesses in the hearing aid delivery process. Despite initial counseling, a significant portion of these new hearing-aid users were not successfully "oriented" to their hearing aids. It indicates a critical need to evaluate carefully what follow-up care entails. Moreover, it suggests a need to examine specifically what is entailed in adjusting to a new hearing aid.

Hawkins (2005) conducted a review of counseling-based group programs in AR and concludes that such programs provide at least short-term reduction in perceived hearing handicap and quality of life, potential benefits in the use of communication strategies and hearing aids, and possible improvements in personal adjustment. Hawkins recommends that future research include heterogeneous populations of individuals with hearing impairment, randomized controlled trials, adequate numbers of subjects, multiple outcome measures, evaluation of the effects of including significant others, and assessment of short- and long-term benefits. Studies by Abrams, Chisolm, and McCardle (2002); Beynon, Thornton, and Poole (1997); and Chisolm, Abrams, and McCardle (2004) are well designed and provide excellent examples of evaluations of audiologic counseling benefits.

Psychosocial Influences

There is an international body of audiologic literature with a psychosocial focus. Audiologists and psychologists in Australia, Canada, Denmark, England, New Zealand, Norway, Scotland, and Sweden have made innumerable contributions to the literature on hearing impairment as it relates to coping, well-being, family, marriage, occupation, psychological adjustment, and stigma. This invaluable body of work is noteworthy in many respects. Much of the work stems from systematic dedicated research that has advanced our understanding of the experience of hearing impairment and produced ongoing learning threads for the audiology community and beyond. A second point worth noting is the extent to which this work consistently draws on knowledge from other disciplines. It reflects an awareness of what the social and behavioral sciences can offer to a more holistic understanding of the wide-ranging effects of hearing impairment on the human condition.

The work of the late Raymond Hétu and his colleagues, for example, provides a systematic examination of occupational hearing loss (OHL). A qualitative analysis of hearing handicap among individuals with OHL (Hétu, Riverin, Getty, Lalande, & St-Cyr, 1988) and an investigation of the psychosocial disadvantages experienced by family members of individuals with OHL (Hétu, Lalonde, & Getty, 1987) was followed by a study of workers' reluctance to admit to hearing problems (Hétu, Riverin, Getty, Lalande, & St-Cyr, 1990). These investigations led to the development of a rehabilitation program for individuals with OHL (Getty & Hétu; 1991; Hétu & Getty, 1991), an examination of how workers overcome difficulties in the workplace (Hétu & Getty, 1993), and an evaluation of coworkers attitudes towards individuals with OHL (Hétu, Getty, Beaudry, & Philipert, 1994; Hétu, Getty, & Waridel, 1994). The culmination of Hétu's research is his seminal article on the stigma related to hearing impairment (Hétu, 1996). This critical work has been continued by Gagné, Jennings, and Southall (2009; see Chapter 3).

The effects of hearing impairment on significant others cannot be overemphasized. A survey conducted by Hétu, Lalonde, and Getty (1987) indicates that family members experience several consequences from the hearing impairment of workers' with OHL as well as from their actual noise exposure. Their conclusions indicate that spontaneous coping efforts do not achieve effective resolution of communication difficulties; moreover, immediate family members do not automatically seek mutually acceptable solutions to hearing problems. This highlights the importance of including family members in audiologic counseling. More recently, Anderson and Noble (2005) investigated couples' attributions regarding the behaviors associated with hearing difficulties. Their findings suggest a relationship between such attributions and marital satisfaction. Scarinci, Worrall and Hickson (2008) conducted a qualitative analysis of interviews with older couples to (a) describe the experience of living with a person who has hearing impairment, (b) describe the effect of hearing impairment on their communication and relationship, and (c) identify the coping strategies adopted by their spouses with hearing impairment. Their analysis indicates that the range of effects hearing impairment has on spouses lives is very broad. The results also emphasize the spouses' continual need to adapt to their partners' hearing problems. Another important variable influencing the impact on spouses is acceptance of the hearing impairment by the hearing-impaired partner. Specifically, the greater the extent to which the individual appears to have accepted hearing impairment, the less effect it has on the spouse. Aging and retirement issues also emerged as a consistent theme. Not surprisingly, hearing problems became more evident following retirement when couples spent more time together. Retirement, although typically viewed as the gateway to more leisurely experiences, frequently triggers a stressful period of adjustment. Retirees are initially somewhat lost with so much free time on their hands and expect time and attention from their partners. Conversely, partners who had already retired or who were not working outside the home find their daily routines disrupted by the presence and demands of those who are newly retired. Frustration and irritation are not uncommon. Superimposing hearing problems on this stressful adjustment period can easily exacerbate the situation. Spouses do, however, perceive hearing loss to be an inevitable part of aging about which nothing can be done. Scarinci and colleagues also report that spouses believe age has a limiting effect on the extent to which their partners can adapt or learn coping skills. The results of this analysis are being investigated further by the authors.

Correlations between patients' self-assessments and their spouses' corresponding measures using the Denver Scale (McCarthy & Alpiner, 1983), the HHIE (Newman & Weinstein, 1986), and the CPHI (Erdman, 1995) consistently indicate disparities in couples' perceptions of the communication difficulties experienced as a result of one partner's hearing impairment. Mean scores are similar for individuals with hearing impairment and their spouses/significant others. Nonetheless, correlations, although significant, are not strong. The low correlations are indicative of disparate views within dyads. Simply stated, couples view hearing problems from different perspectives, a fact that has important implications for couple and family counseling. It is not surprising that couples do not come to agreement on solutions when perceptions of the problem differ markedly. Common complaints such as "My wife mumbles all the time," and "He can hear just fine when he wants to," illustrate the lack of shared understanding of the problems hearing impairment creates. The spousal assessments of their partner's hearing problems are not intended to corroborate the patient's difficulties. Rather, they provide valuable insight into the nature of communication difficulties that develop subsequent to those caused by the hearing impairment. For example, when spouses come to believe that their partners simply "do not care enough to listen," the nature of the communication problems becomes significantly more complicated. When counseling couples, it is important to retain a neutral position while explaining the reasons for the differences in their perceptions. Specifically, couples need to recognize that there are as many perspectives as there are people, that there are no right or wrong answers, and that, for continuing difficulties, mutually acceptable solutions can be found. It is highly rewarding to witness the relief and increased togetherness experienced by couples when they grasp the logical reasons for their disparate views. Audiologic counseling can literally wipe away years of frustration and hurt feelings by increasing couples understanding of the communication problems they have experienced.

The relationship between hearing impairment and psychological state has been the subject of considerable debate over the years. A number of studies have been reported in which investigators specifically examined the effects of hearing impairment on psychological well-being. Scherer and Frisina (1998) found that even marginal hearing impairment has an impact on the well-being of older adults. The authors recommend identifying the personal and interpersonal concerns of these individuals to inform treatment planning and achieve a higher rate of adherence to rehabilitation efforts. Consistent with the literature relating audiologic and self-report data, Helvik, Jacobsen, and Hallberg (2006) found that well-being (defined as health-related quality of life) among adults with acquired hearing impairment is associated with activity limitations and participation restrictions, but not with degree of hearing impairment. Their results indicate that the well-being of older adults is less likely to be affected in comparison to younger adults. Erdman and Demorest (1998b) report similar results with the possible exception of poorer adjustment among the oldest old. A survey of cochlear implant users in the United States and in Sweden indicates that their psychological well-being is influenced by age, perceived social support, participation restrictions in social life, and the attitudes of other people (Hallberg, Ringdahl, Holmes, & Carver, 2005).

A review of the literature pertaining to hearing impairment and depression reveals disparate findings (Erdman, 2007). Hallberg, Hallberg, and Kramer (2008) have concluded that the psychosocial impact of hearing impairment cannot be predicted from audiometric data. Lee and Gomez-Marin (1997) conducted a study of Puerto Ricans, American-Cubans, and Mexicans with hearing impairment and found no increased risk for depression. Thomas (1984) refuted the notion that hearing impairment results in some specific psychologic disturbance or that it alters personality. He was also the first to suggest that psychological disturbance may be the independent rather than the dependent variable. Yueh, Collins, and Souza (2007) examined over 100 veterans and concluded that depressive symptoms may influence responses on self-report measures of hearing difficulties. Similarly, correlations between scales from the Personal Adjustment section of the CPHI and selected psychological measures, (Erdman & Demorest, 1996; Erdman, 2001) suggest that psychological distress exacerbates adjustment to hearing impairment and not vice versa. Some studies suggest that hearing impairment plays a role in the onset of depression. Results of a survey by the National Council on the Aging (NCOA, 1999), for example, have been interpreted as evidence that hearing loss is associated with depression among older adults and that such depression is attenuated by hearing aid use. Respondents were asked if they had felt sad, blue, or depressed for two weeks or longer during the past year. Although hearing problems can certainly be "depressing," and an individual may feel "depressed" about hearing problems, such feelings do not constitute a diagnosis of depression. The DSM-IV criteria for a diagnosis of depression are shown in Table 9–5. Depression is a complex disorder that has psychological, physiologic, and behavioral symptoms that can be manifested in different ways. Although hearing problems can be depressing, upsetting, and stressful, the preponderance of evidence indicates that hearing impairment does not affect personality, nor does it "cause" depression. In fact, the best predictor of depression is a prior episode; hence, individuals with hearing loss who have a predisposition for depression, may be more likely

Table 9–5. Diagnostic Criteria for Depression (DSM-IV, 2000)

Five or more of the following symptoms nearly every day in a 2-week period:

- Depressed mood most of the day
- Markedly diminished interest or pleasure in all or most activities
- Significant weight loss or gain, or decrease or increase in appetite
- Insomnia or hypersomnia
- Observable psychomotor agitation or retardation
- Fatigue or loss of energy
- Feelings of worthlessness or excessive or inappropriate guilt (which may be delusional)

Additional Criteria

- Symptoms do not meet criteria for mixed episode
- Symptoms cause clinically significant distress or impairment in social, occupational, or other functioning
- Symptoms are not due to the direct physiological effects of a substance, drug, or disease
- Symptoms are not better accounted for by bereavement
- Symptoms persist more than 2 months or are characterized by marked functional impairment, morbid preoccupation with worthlessness, suicidal ideation, psychotic symptoms, or psychomotor retardation

to have a recurrence. Depression is known to have a negative impact on motivation and is often characterized by a withdrawal from interactions. Depressed individuals also experience considerable difficulty adjusting to daily challenges. As such, depression is believed to have deleterious effects on adjustment to hearing loss also. Intervention in the form of HA's and CI's can often alleviate feelings of stress, loneliness, and sadness. Nonetheless, it cannot be said that they constitute treatment for depression or anxiety per se.

Poor research design, disparate measures and populations, and investigators' lack of understanding of the effects of hearing impairment or conversely, the effects of psychological variables, have contributed to equivocal findings regarding the relationship between psychological status and hearing impairment. A study by Mahapatra (1974), for example, involved testing patients while they were hospitalized and about to undergo surgery for otosclerosis. It goes without saying that those awaiting imminent surgery, which, theoretically, could result in total deafness or even facial paralysis, would be in a heightened state of anxiety. Further investigation is warranted to elucidate the emotional impact of hearing impairment. Particular attention should be paid to differentiating between affective states and traits. Moreover, the use of psychological screening measures, or worse yet, single item assessments, is inadequate in studies intended to clarify the relationship between personal adjustment and hearing impairment. Danermark (1998) argues persuasively that rehabilitation must focus on the emotional aspects of hearing difficulties for the person and significant others. Service delivery that brings the psychosocial consequences of hearing impairment to the forefront is, therefore, especially important.

The psychosocial impact of hearing impairment is a matter of concern in other professions as well. Nursing, social work, and vocational rehabilitation are addressing the implications of hearing impairment in clinical programs and research. The Kooser Program, for example, is an "aural rehabilitation" program developed by social worker Cathy Kooser, who has a severe hearing impairment (Sharp, 2007). Her disillusionment with the lack of counseling she received from audiologists over the years motivated her to develop a course that addresses issues related to living with hearing loss. The program receives referrals from vocational rehabilitation counselors, ENT clinics, and audiologists. The Kooser Program is now being marketed to audiologists. Ironically, by virtue of our scope of practice, we should be independently capable of developing and implementing comparable services; moreover, we should be offering such services as a routine part of our practice. This situation is consistent with audiologists being uncertain how to use information derived from self-report measures. It also says a lot about our tendency to focus on hearing impairment rather than the person with hearing impairment; in short, our adherence to the biomedical model is directly responsible for unacceptable limitations in the scope of our clinical practice.

Although researchers from other professions have addressed important issues in relation to hearing impairment, a recurrent problem frequently limits the utility of their findings; specifically, degree of hearing impairment is often not taken into consideration. Hence, there are studies in which the findings are based on a nondifferentiated population of individuals who are categorized simply as "hard-of-hearing." The failure to distinguish between individuals with profound impairments versus those with usable residual hearing, or those with congenital versus acquired impairments essentially precludes meaningful findings. A surprising number of articles in which this problem occurs can be found in the nursing, vocational rehabilitation, and mental health literatures. The topics of these research endeavors, more often than not, are of relevance to audiology. The effects of hearing impairment on older couples, problems experienced by individuals with hearing impairment in nursing homes and assisted living facilities, and difficulties with job placements for those with hearing problems are among the issues being addressed by other professions. Every one of these issues touches on audiologists' scope of practice. Nevertheless, ongoing research in these areas is not benefiting from our expertise nor are we adequately addressing such issues ourselves. Recent statements in the nursing literature include, "Hearing impairment is a significant, often debilitating, problem for many older adults, but assessment and intervention by nurses can help," (Wallhagen, Pettengill, & Whiteside, 2006, p. 40) and " . . . Given the extensive nature of hearing impairment in elders, its impact on psychosocial well-being, and the potential for significant improvements in quality of life through the use of advanced hearing technology and assistive devices, nurses have the potential to play important roles in this unexplored area" (Wallhagen, 2002). A longitudinal investigation of the effects of hearing impairment on spouses was conducted in which hearing measures consisted of three questions pertaining to communication (1) in quiet, (2) on the telephone, and (3) in a noisy setting. Each had a response set ranging from 0 to 3. No audiometric data were obtained and no standardized self-report measures of hearing difficulty were employed (Wallhagen, Strawbridge, Shema, & Kaplan, 2004). Audiology's entrenchment in the biomedical model has narrowed our focus to the point that others are encroaching on our scope of practice by investigating issues we are not investigating and providing services we are not providing. Moreover, other professionals are obtaining funding to conduct research in areas in which audiologists are more qualified.

A traditional basic science model has dominated Ph.D. programs in audiology, a factor that is certainly implicated in audiology's move to the professional doctorate. The health care crisis and the unsettling lack of progress in addressing chronic illness and disease, however, are beginning to shift research priorities. Although the biomedical model is still pervasive, the health care crisis is resulting in critically needed change. The mandate to modify medical school curriculum is a bottom-up approach that will produce gradual but steady change. Health psychology and behavioral medicine are introducing innovative approaches to health care. The results of these approaches are mounting evidence of the invalid tenets underlying the biomedical model. At the same time, they are yielding evidence that the biopsychosocial model's underpinnings provide a sound and more realistic and productive means of understanding disease and illness, as well as impairment and disability. A similar infusion of social and behavioral sciences into audiology's curriculum is needed to enhance our understanding of the relationships and interactions among biopsychosocial variables that determine the individual's experience of hearing impairment.

A Biopsychosocial Approach to Audiologic Counseling

The times, they are a-changin. ♪
Robert Dylan (1963)

Our hard look at the world around us has forced us to acknowledge the inadequacies of the biomedical model and the limitations necessarily imposed on audiology by our adherence to it. We have also had the opportunity to recognize that the rest of health care has similarly been limited and that a logical and valid, albeit more complex approach, the biopsychosocial model, is increasingly being viewed as a viable and necessary alternative. In the face of a health care system in crisis and growing demands for change, it is evident that the old way of doing things does not suffice and will not survive. The biomedical model in audiology forces a band-aid solution, in the form of a hearing aid, on a problem that, more often than not, requires motivation, self-efficacy, complex psychosocial and behavioral adaptations, and a reintegration of self, not to mention the development of compensatory communication skills.

Audiologists provide services for one of the most common chronic conditions in our society. Audiology is a health care profession, but it is not a medical profession. It is a rehabilitative profession. To optimize our success as a profession, rehabilitation is an identity we must embrace fully. Diagnostic audiology is an essential component of audiologic rehabilitation, but it is just one component. It represents the "bio" portion of the biopsychosocial model. Adhering to a biopsychosocial model in audiology brings counseling to the forefront as the therapeutic context in which all services are provided, as the process guiding services, and as essential ingredients of the therapeutic process. The effectiveness of counseling throughout this three-tiered conceptualization ultimately determines the extent to which treatment outcome is successful.

The context of audiologic counseling is biopsychosocial, patient-centered, empathic, interactive, and facilitative. The therapeutic context guides the counseling process and the audiologist's role and responsibilities in it for each patient. As the ongoing process, counseling includes several key phases: establishing the practitioner/patient relationship, engaging the patient in the therapeutic process, creating opportunities and mechanisms to enhance and nurture patients' engagement and self-efficacy, and ensuring that counseling goals are met and maintained. Counseling activities can include ongoing exchanges between the clinician and the patient; dedicated sessions such as hearing aid orientations; cognitive, affective, and/or behavioral interventions targeted at relevant communication and adjustment issues; and family and group sessions. The characteristics of counseling as the therapeutic context of rehabilitative audiology extend to and infuse all aspects of the counseling process and counseling activities. This is easily achieved by ensuring that all aspects of intervention are patient-centered. Examining the biopsychosocial, patient-centered, empathic, interactive, and facilitative elements of audiologic counseling reveals a promising framework for rehabilitation planning, evaluation, and research as well as professional education.

Framework for a Biopsychosocial Approach to Audiologic Counseling

The IOM (2001) identified a continuous healing relationship as the most critical ingredient in improving the quality of patient care. It is in exactly this vein that patient-centered care is enhanced by relationship-centered care; the quality of the relationship ultimately determines treatment success (Gelso & Carter, 1994; Gelso & Hayes, 1998; Norcross, 2002; Norcross & Lambert, 2006; Rogers, 1957, 1958; Safran & Muran, 1998; Truax et al., 1966; Truax & Mitchell, 1971). Squire's (1990) model of an empathic practitioner-patient relationship illustrates how affective and cognitive components of empathy facilitate engagement of the patient in the management of his or her health condition resulting in adherence to a treatment regimen to achieve the desired health benefit. In Figure 9–3, Squire's model is shown adapted to illustrate such a process in audiologic care.

Briefly, in the model, the audiologist strives to understand, both cognitively and affectively, the patient's experience of hearing impairment as revealed in the patient's story. The practitioner must then articulate an empathic understanding of this experience to the patient. This understanding is based on (1) an accurate perspective of the patient's experience and (2) appropriate emotional reactivity. In doing so, the accuracy of the empathy conveys important information to the patient;

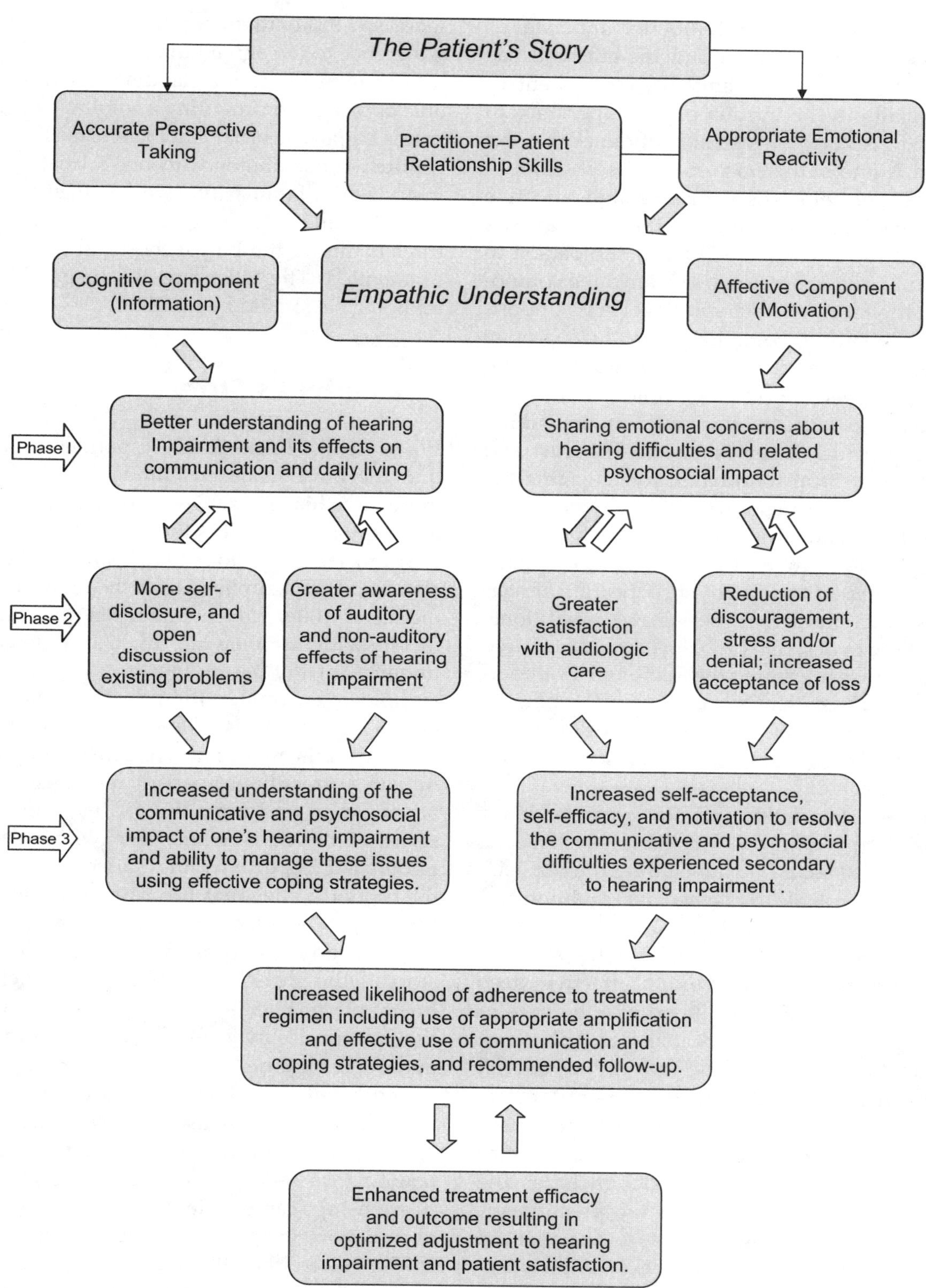

Figure 9–3. The role of empathic understanding in AR counseling based on Squier (1990) and Erdman (1993a).

it provides the patient with a better understanding of hearing impairment and the effects it has on communication. The affective component of empathy allows the burden of the experience to be shared instilling a sense of confidence that the problem is one with which it will be possible to cope. The audiologist's cognitive and affective communications (indicated by the solid arrows leading to the Phase 1 level) allow the person to know he/she is understood. The affective component of empathic understanding, which is supportive and reassuring, combined with the cognitive exchange, facilitates the development of a trusting relationship between the audiologist and the patient. Phase 1 of the empathic understanding model represents development of this trust and rapport, the critical foundation for engaging the patient in the treatment process.

The bidirectional arrows between Phase 1 and Phase 2 are indicative of a working, therapeutic alliance. Increased understanding of hearing impairment permits the patient to volunteer additional information, to describe problems more accurately, thereby further informing the audiologist's understanding of the patient's experience. The parallel affective-motivational process reduces the level of overall distress and enhances satisfaction with treatment thus far.

Successful cognitive and affective interactions during Phase 2 ultimately facilitate psychosocial and behavioral adjustment including the requisite knowledge and skills to manage the condition and the self-acceptance, self-efficacy and motivation to do so as indicated at the Phase 3 level. A successful Phase 3 in the cognitive and affective areas results in an increased likelihood of adherence to the agreed upon treatment regime. Adherence enhances treatment outcome in terms of overall adjustment, benefits derived, and patient satisfaction. These, in turn, solidify adherence (as indicated by the bidirectional arrows between adherence and outcome). Hence, the model includes the patient's story, development of the practitioner-patient relationship; engagement of the patient in the rehabilitative process; interaction of the working/therapeutic alliance; facilitation of the patient's management of hearing impairment through increased motivation, hope, and self-efficacy; and adherence to the agreed upon treatment regimen.

The empathic understanding model is a reasonable approach to providing audiologic counseling that is biopsychosocial, interactive, facilitative, and conducive to adherence to one's treatment regimen. Hence, familiarity with key elements of the empathic understanding model and their relation to elements of the biopsychosocial model is recommended. The following are areas with which audiologists should be familiar.

The Patient's Story

When George Engel (2005) responded to concerns that the biopsychosocial model was difficult to implement his primary response was, " . . . the key is the interview . . . it is the basic scientific tool of the clinician—the door that opens to everything else. Successful application of the biopsychosocial model is 100% dependent upon the clinician's facility with interviewing" (p. 378). When hearing impairment and the audiogram are the focus of an audiologic encounter, the patient's experience of hearing loss receives little to no attention. Unfortunately, this makes it virtually impossible to initiate a practitioner-patient relationship that is based on an understanding of the patient's concerns. Without this relationship, without a shared understanding of why the patient is presenting, the basis for engaging the patient in the rehabilitation process does not exist. Hence, our first responsibility is to hear each patient's story. Each story is the spark that activates biopsychosocial intervention. Eliciting that story is the clinician's first responsibility in each new encounter; ultimately, it may be the determining factor in the patient's outcome. Engel was fascinated by Margaret Mead's (1975) use of video-recordings to study human behavior as this supported his contention that behavior, feelings, transactions, and relationships can be scientifically studied through observation, introspection, and dialogue (Engel, 1977a, 1977b, 1987, 1997). He advocated allowing patients to talk about themselves, their families, and symptoms and observing their verbal and nonverbal communication. All of this he considered scientific data.

In contrast, what usually occurs during the audiology patient's first visit is an interview focused on the etiology and progression of the hearing impairment. Obviously, information regarding the onset of hearing impairment is vital in establishing a diagnosis. Additionally, the nature and cause of a patient's hearing impairment undoubtedly can play a part in how the loss is experienced. Nonetheless, questions that focus on auditory disorder and impairment are specific in nature and elicit responses that are similarly limited in scope. In fact, many answers are simply two or three word phrases or yes-no answers. They do not reveal the essence of the patient's experience.

The quotes included in Table 9–6 are "sound bites" from actual patient stories. Even these brief snippets are compelling, poignant, warm, funny, sad, and, at times, joyful. They are distinctly human elements that provide the critical, initial link between the audiologist and the patient. Listening to patients' stories, clinicians come to share their patients' experience of hearing loss in ways simply not possible through an audiogram, case history, or even self-report measures. The clinician who listens intently to the father as he laughingly describes his little girl grabbing his face to make sure he hears everything she has to say, cannot help but connect with him on a human level. In that connection, a patient recognizes that he is understood. The groundwork for empathy and rapport has been established.

Beginning clinicians often wonder how to elicit stories from patients that reveal such distinctively human elements. The fact is, every patient we see has a story. Moreover, the reason that patient is seeing you is to tell you that story. It is why an

Table 9–6. Excerpts From Patients' Stories

"My wife's small talk sometimes goes unanswered. I regret the difficulties she must endure. I know I must be a burden to her at times. It is more for her benefit than mine that I'm thinking about getting hearing aids."

"When someone has to repeat for me, I feel embarrassed and inadequate. I scold myself—you should be listening more closely, concentrating more! I get angry at myself. When I hear something incorrectly and respond inaccurately, then I am *really* embarrassed. I feel like my credibility is slipping away. In class, I try to cover up by saying, 'Speak up and talk clearly so the whole class can hear your question.' Inside though I don't think I'm really fooling anybody. Everyone must see through my sham. I feel so unsure of myself as a professional."

"I get annoyed when I don't hear someone and they yell loud enough for God and everyone to hear, 'What are you, deaf?' I tell them what they can do!"

"At parties, I have a terrible time. I move closer to the speaker and they back away. I ask them to speak up, but after a few words, their voices drop again. Not only am I a social loser, I'm a bore! When I'm in the backseat of our carpool, I have a terrible time understanding the conversation up front. So, I lean forward and ask them to speak louder. When they don't, which is most of the time, I sit back and drop out of the conversation. There I am again, the social outcast."

"My 5-year-old son has it figured out. He says, 'Daddy, come in here away from the TV so you can hear me. I got something to tell you!'"

"I work on a psychiatry ward and listen to patients 8 hrs. a day. Asking patients to repeat is not only frustrating for them and for me, it also alienates me from them. This is disastrous in a practitioner/patient relationship and causes extreme anxiety on my part."

continues

Table 9–6. *continued*

"My family has stopped trying to communicate with me anymore when we're watching TV in the evening. I feel like I am losing touch with my family."
"My husband's hearing loss has affected us all. We love him and want him back."
"At a crowded cocktail party, when I'm talking to women with high-pitched, or soft voices (small talk in which I may or may not be interested) I can't understand a thing they say. I get tired of faking it, kill my drink, and excuse myself to get a refill. It gets to the point where it's not worth the effort."
"A woman and I were talking soft and low like lovers do. I asked her to repeat something but she said, 'Never mind,' and the mood abruptly changed. It made me wonder how many 'yes's' I've missed."
"At a party where the music is already 3 times louder than I care for, three people are all trying to talk to me at once. I pick out the one who is talking the loudest and listen to him. Usually, I still can't understand what he's saying. So, if he smiles, I smile. If he frowns, I frown. When he is done talking I end up walking away wondering what the devil he was trying to tell me."
"I never purposely try to ignore anyone, but often it probably seems that way. Some may see me as unapproachable or think I'm rude."
"I don't think I will ever accept my hearing loss. I'll always believe this is just temporary."
"I cannot tell you what a difference my husband's hearing aids have made in our life. He wasn't listening to me. I was sure he didn't care enough to listen anymore. He just ignored me. I was so afraid there was someone else."
"I get very unhappy with myself when I don't hear something someone in my family tries to tell me. It's important to them. It must give them the impression I don't care which isn't true. If I ask someone to repeat what they said, they're put off. I know I've hurt my children's feelings. I have some fence-mending to do."
"My four-year-old daughter makes sure I hear her. She stands right in front of me or climbs on my lap. Sometimes she even grabs my face and looks straight at me! How can I miss what she has to say?"
"At work I attend and/or conduct meetings, participate in several counseling sessions, and communicate on the phone or in person all day. At the end of the day, I'm drained from the mental strain of concentrating and trying to compensate. After wearing a hearing aid for only 2 days, I can already see a marked difference in how I feel by 5 o'clock. I regret that I didn't pursue correcting my hearing loss earlier in my career." A month later she added, "I can stay up an hour to an hour and a half later than I did before. It's great getting to watch the late news with my husband."
"My teenage daughter gets away with murder. She'll tell my wife that she asked me if she could do something or have something and I said ok. When I say, 'You never asked me that!' She responds with, 'I did so! You said it was ok! It's not my fault if you didn't really hear what I said!'"
"I've been accused of being off in my own little world."
"I tried to go to college but the ambient noise in a classroom (papers rustling, background chatter, etc.) made listening to the professor difficult to impossible and not only made me anxious but also made him angry because he had to keep repeating. I stopped taking classes to remedy this particular situation."
"Telephone use at work is critical for task accomplishment. If I can't get this part down I may as well fold up my tent and say sayonara."

appointment was made. Open-ended statements such as "What brings you here today?" or "Tell me about the hearing problems you have been having," are appropriate ways to encourage patients to tell you about their experiences. Nonverbal factors are also important. As Perls (1969, 1973) succinctly and repeatedly pointed out, "the body does not lie." Ideally, you are in a private area, seated face-to-face, maintaining eye contact, and listening while your demeanor communicates your genuine interest in what a patient is telling you. You are not walking toward the test booth with the patient following you, or thumbing through a chart without looking at the patient. The challenge is not so much how to get them to reveal, as it is how to stay out of their way so they can. After asking that initial question, simply allow them to answer. They may not respond immediately. Giving someone room to answer, is actually giving them time to answer. It is always tempting to ask another question if the patient does not respond immediately. Allow patients time to gather their thoughts and to formulate an answer. To refrain from interrupting the patient's thoughts, mentally count to 10, slowly. Literally, do so. If necessary, count to 10 again. It is exceedingly rare for a patient not to respond within that amount of time. On the rare occasion that occurs, rephrase your question and again, wait. Allow the patient to see that you are genuinely interested in what he or she has been experiencing and that your question is a sincere and important one.

The goal is to understand the patient's story —to appreciate that story and come to a shared understanding of what the experience of hearing loss means to the individual. The intent of audiologic counseling is to bring about change in aspects of the patient's story that pertain to the difficulties and distress experienced in relation to hearing impairment. Our role is a facilitative one; we engage patients in the treatment process and we enable patients to make decisions that are both meaningful and acceptable to them. The narrative story is an increasingly common way of facilitating understanding. It is focal in personal construct theory (DasGupta & Charon, 2004; Kelly, 1963; Mahoney, 1991, 2003; Neimeyer & Raskin, 2000; Shapiro & Ross, 2002) which mirrors many facets of the biopsychosocial approach. In personal construct theory, patients are viewed as idiosyncratic; each person experiences his or her own world in a unique way. The clinician recognizes and appreciates the patient's uniqueness and establishes a shared understanding of his or her experience. In constructivist psychology, the clinician acknowledges patients' capacity for change and facilitates their efforts to change. This is a valuable area for audiologists to explore.

Counselor Characteristics

Listening is the application of the mind to sounds which the ear . . . may or may not hear.

Percy C. Buck (1944)

Effective counseling involves broad-based professional knowledge and skills combined with a set of personal aptitudes and characteristics. Typically, the knowledge and skills are acquired through academic programs and clinical training, whereas the personal aptitudes and characteristics often appear to be extensions of one's personality. Although many of the behaviors associated with these aptitudes and personality characteristics can be learned and honed, audiologists' counseling skills are rarely the focus of academic or clinical training or evaluation. Work by English and colleagues (2007) is a notable exception.

Counselor characteristics are an essential part of the therapeutic alliance, part of which is an interpersonal relationship and another part the task or work related component. The latter involves the critical functions of engagement in goal and treatment planning. Carl Rogers posited that empathy, congruence, positive regard and "unconditionality" are the necessary and sufficient conditions to effect therapeutic change. Moreover, he claimed that non-trained persons who demonstrate an interest in others and a desire to help, and who present with these necessary and sufficient conditions, can be as effective as trained counselors in the helping process. Since that time, others (Brammer & MacDonald, 2002; Corey & Corey, 2006; Egan, 2006) have stressed the veracity of Rogers' observation. Support for the idea that these factors are perhaps the most salient variables in treatment outcome has also been widespread (Blatt, Sanislow, Zuroff, & Pilkonis,1996; Castongay, Constantino, & Grosse Holtforth, 2006; Elvins & Green, 2008; Fierman, 1997; Truax et al., 1966; Truax & Mitchell, 1971). In Table 9–7, characteristics of effective counselors are categorized in terms of traits related primarily to personality, character strengths, and the core professional characteristics. Chief among these, of course is empathy. Throughout his career, Rogers maintained that empathy, unconditional positive regard, and congruence enable patients to be more positive, realistic, self-directed, and open in their experiencing. Rogers (1951) defined empathy as:

> *. . . the counselor's ability to assume, in so far as he is able, the internal frame of reference of the client, to perceive the world as the client sees it, to perceive the client himself as he is seen by himself, to lay aside all perceptions from the external frame of reference while doing so, and to communicate something of this empathic understanding to the client.* (p. 29)

Empathy is a prerequisite for the development of rapport, that is, an alliance based on trust and cooperation and on a shared understanding of the patient's perspective. As in the model discussed earlier, it is generally concurred that empathy has an emotive (affective) component and an intellectual (cognitive) component. Others expound further. Norfolk, Birdi, and Walsh (2007), for example, stress that an element of motivation, possibly fueled by openness and curiosity, must exist for empathy to occur. The motivation essentially consists of wanting to understand the patient. Another key element of their vision of empathy is the *ability* to understand another's experience and perspective. Listening is a critical skill required to achieve such understanding.

Stepien and Baernstein (2006) summarized a number of studies to develop strategies to teach empathy. The AAMC's stated goal of preparing physicians who are compassionate and empathetic coupled with evidence that empathy actually declines during professional training (Bellini & Shea, 2005; Chen, Lew, Hershman, & Orlander, 2007), highlights the need to focus on empathy throughout training. A literature review was conducted and identified 13 studies that described and evaluated educational interventions intended to increase student empathy. Although limitations including a lack of conceptual clarity, small sample size, brief and heterogeneous interventions, and shortcomings of assessment tools that plagued the studies, overall, the findings were encouraging. Brief, targeted interventions (e.g., theatrical

Table 9–7. Characteristics of Effective Counselors

Personality	Character Strengths	Professional
Patient	Self-awareness	Empathy
Warm personality	Cultural awareness	Warmth and caring
Good listener	Ability to analyze own feelings	Openness
Perceptive and sensitive	Ability to serve as a model	Positive regard and respect
Likes people	Altruism	Concreteness and specificity
Nonthreatening demeanor	Strong sense of ethics	Communication competence
Sense of humor	Responsible	Intentionality
Desire to help		
Positive attitude		
Problem-solver		

performances, literature courses, reflective writing, and experiential learning, i.e. admitting students to hospital with fake diagnoses) were among the strategies employed.

Pinkerton (2008) added to the list of important counselor characteristics in a wonderfully thought-provoking article entitled, *"I Apologize for Being Late": The Courteous Psychotherapist.* He emphasizes that above and beyond the obvious importance of responding courteously to the patients we serve, such behavior has positive effects on the therapeutic relationship. Inadvertent rudeness can have deleterious effects as in the case of the therapist who dozed off during a patient's session. It is sufficient to say, the patient became irate and left, never to return. Pinkerton also discusses the possibility that patients may feel insignificant or diminished by a practitioner's chronic tardiness. Taking telephone calls, checking the time, and mispronouncing patients' names are other potential pitfalls that clients should guard against. Novice and long-time clinicians can both benefit by reminding themselves periodically of the points Pinkerton raises.

It would be ideal if all clinicians were able to demonstrate the necessary characteristics and skills at all times with all patients. Needless to say, for the vast majority of us, it remains an ideal. Our professional responsibility, however, is to strive to achieve that ideal. Increasing emphasis is being placed on "self-monitoring" or "mindful practice" as a means of enhancing the likelihood that we convey empathy, warmth, and genuineness; that we eliminate bias and narrow thinking in our clinical judgments; and that we demonstrate attentiveness to our patients and to our clinical decision-making. Epstein (1999, 2003a, 2003b) stresses the need for self-awareness in practice and describes four key elements of mindful practice: attentive observation of oneself, the patient, and the problem; critical curiosity, "beginner's mind," and presence. The self-monitoring that Epstein advocates facilitates clear thinking, multitasking, and personal growth. Based on Eastern philosophies, those who practice yoga or who are familiar with ancient Buddhist thought will recognize the principles inherent in mindfulness. Remaining mindful in our interactions with our patients enables us to convey empathy, instill trust, and cultivate active patients who engage in the rehabilitative process.

Engaging Patients in the Rehabilitative Process

Clinicians are responsible for providing patients with the knowledge, self-efficacy, hope, and motivation to manage chronic health problems. Activating patients, making them partners in the management of their conditions, develops from a working alliance that is built on trust. Motivational interviewing (Miller & Rollnick, 2002) includes concepts from social psychology, attribution theory, cognitive dissonance, self-efficacy, and empathy (Britt, Hudson, & Blampied, 2004). Unlike Rogers' client-centered approach to counseling, however, motivational interviewing is a more directive approach that focuses on removing barriers to change. Wagner and McMahon (2004) point out the similarities between motivational interviewing and rehabilitation counseling citing the common emphasis on self-determination. The goal of motivational interviewing is to promote choice and responsibility in implementing change. Four guidelines in motivational interviewing include: (1) express empathy, (2) "roll" with resistance even when the patient is defensive and argumentative, (3) explore discrepancies between present behavior and behavioral goals, and (4) support self-efficacy.

Theories of hope (Snyder, 1989, 1994) and optimism (Scheier & Carver, 1985, 1987, 1992) have received attention in the audiology literature. Snyder, Lehman, Kluck, and Monsson (2006) have presented hope theory as a framework for understanding rehabilitation goals and designing effective interventions. This, of course, suggests that hope may have a role in audiologic rehabilitation. Kent and La Grow (2007) have conducted an investigation of the role of hope in the relationship between individual and disability characteristics and adjustment to hearing impairment. Their findings indicate that hope can be regarded as a principal component in the promotion of adjustment to hearing loss. Optimism has similarly been shown to have a role in adjustment to hearing impairment (Andersson, 1996; Andersson, Melin, Lindberg, & Scott, 1995). There are also similarities between the constructs of hope and optimism and that of self-efficacy.

Bandura's principle of self-efficacy (1977, 1982, 1997) has also been addressed in the audiological literature (Smith & West, 2006). Self-efficacy plays a major role in behavior change inasmuch as it represents one's perception of the ability to accomplish a specific task or behavior. In learning new behaviors, a sense of mastery is required that is achieved through practice. In audiologic counseling this may focus on adjusting to a new hearing aid, developing new communication skills, or becoming more assertive in difficult communication situations. Unlike self-efficacy, which is situation and goal specific, hope represents a generalized approach to goal attainment. Snyder and colleagues' (2006) discussion of the similarities and dissimilarities among these constructs and their relevance in rehabilitation should be required reading for anyone in the rehabilitation professions.

Successful rehabilitation results in patients capable of managing their disabilities effectively. Zubialde, Eubank, and Fink (2007) stress the need for a person- and relationship-centered approach to patient care that engages patients in ongoing learning, growth, and management of their health. Self-management programs have been developed in health education programs to address the management of chronic health conditions (Holman & Lorig, 2000, 2004; Lorig & Holman, 2003). The programs promote the development of six skills: problem-solving, decision-making, resource utilization, the formation of a practitioner-patient relationship, action planning, and self-tailoring. These skills are applied to three primary self-management tasks: medical management, role management, and emotional management. For individuals with chronic illness or disability, self-management, (i.e., management of the condition and the effects it has on daily living) becomes a lifelong responsibility. Stanford University's Patient Education Research Center has developed self-management programs for patients with arthritis, HIV-AIDS, back pain, as well as a program for individuals with varied chronic diseases, the Chronic Disease Self-Management Program (CDSMP), which has been replicated with diverse populations and outside the United States. Programs for other health issues have been developed based on comparable premises and the principles are highly relevant for inclusion in AR programs.

Holman and Lorig (2004) stress that although the health care system has failed to address adequately the current crisis and the unmet needs of those with chronic disease and disability, there are ways in which this can be done. Self-management education is one option. One strength inherent in the programs is their group approach that has long been advocated in AR. A second option involves group visits; groups of patients periodically meet with their practitioner. Comparable to group hearing aid orientations or hearing aid follow-up visits, this concept can be extended to address a range of issues including communication difficulties. The third option includes remote management. The Internet is permitting contact between practitioners and patients without involving appointment time and travel. Telephone follow-up procedures are also being implemented.

Summary

Modern health care is the product of the biomedical model. The result is a health care system that is designed for acute care rather than chronic illness and disability. Audiology's adherence to the biomedical model is evident in the emphasis placed on diagnosis of hearing impairment rather than on rehabilitation for the individual with hearing impairment. The biopsychosocial model espouses a patient-centered approach in which the subjective experience of illness and disability is the focus.

By shifting our focus to the patient and the experience of hearing impairment in a biopsychosocial approach, counseling is brought to the forefront of audiologic intervention. The patient's experience guides all aspects of intervention. Audiologists are the professionals who best understand the problems experienced by those who have hearing impairment and our counseling is necessary to enable them to resolve the communication difficulties and adjustment problems they and members of their families face because of hearing impairment.

As in other health care professions, audiology must be proactive and creative in developing ways to meet the needs of our patients. The increasing numbers of people who could benefit from audiologic services warrant a reappraisal of our service delivery to ensure that adherence to treatment recommendations, patient satisfaction and treatment success are maximized. Increased awareness and emphasis on the following areas is needed in our clinical training, practice, and research:

1. the critical nature of the client-clinician relationship
2. importance of clinician characteristics and counseling skills
3. supervision and evaluation of client-clinician interactions throughout graduate training
4. relevance of psychology and rehabilitation counseling perspectives
5. psychosocial adjustment issues including stigma, denial, loss and grieving, and the impact of hearing impairment on affective well-being
6. evaluation of the impact of hearing impairment on daily living and quality of life
7. approaches to individual, group, marital, and family counseling
8. limitations of the biomedical model on the scope of our clinical practice.

By addressing these areas, audiologic counseling will emerge as the foundation upon which all of our services are offered within a biopsychosocial context.

References

Abrams, H., Chisolm, T. H., & McArdle, R. (2002). A cost-utility analysis of group adult audiologic rehabilitation: Are the benefits worth the cost? *Journal of Rehabilitation Research and Development, 39*, 549–558.

American Academy of Audiology. (2004). *Audiology: Scope of practice.* McLean, VA: Author.

American Psychiatric Association. (2000). *Diagnostic and Statistical Manual of Mental Disorders DSM-IV-TR* (4th ed.). Arlington, VA: Author.

American Speech-Language-Hearing Association. (2001). *Knowledge and skills required for the practice of audiologic/aural Rehabilitation* [Knowledge and Skills]. Available from www.asha.org/policy

American Speech-Language-Hearing Association. (2004). *Scope of practice in audiology* [Scope of practice]. Available from www.asha.org/policy

American-Speech-Language-Hearing Association. (2006). *Preferred practice patterns for the profession of audiology* [Preferred practice patterns]. Available from ww.asha.org/policy1

American Speech-Language-Hearing Association. (2008). *Guidelines for audiologists providing informational and adjustment counseling to families of infants and young children with hearing loss birth to 5 years of age* [Guidelines]. Available from www.asha.org/policy

Anderson, D., & Noble, W. (2005). Couples' attributions about behaviours modulated by hearing impairment: Links with relationship satisfaction. *International Journal of Audiology, 44*(4), 197–205.

Anderson, G., & Horvath, J. (2004 May-June). The growing burden of chronic disease in America. *Public Health Reports, 11*, 263–270.

Andersson, G. (1996). The role of optimism in patients with tinnitus and in patients with hearing impairment. *Psychology and Health, 11*(5), 697–707.

Andersson, G., Melin, L., Lindberg, P., & Scott, B. (1995). Dispositional optimism, dysphoria, health, and coping with hearing impairment in elderly adults. *Audiology, 34*, 76–84.

Bandura, A. (1977). Self-efficacy: Toward a unifying theory of behavioral change. *Psychological Review, 84*, 191–215.

Bandura, A. (1978). The self-system in reciprocal determinism. *American Psychologist, 33*, 344–358.

Bandura, A. (1982). Self-efficacy mechanism in human agency. *American Psychologist, 37*,122–147.

Bandura A. (1997). *Self-efficacy: The exercise of control.* New York: Freeman.

Bandura, A. (2004). Health promotion by social cognitive means. *Health Education & Behavior, 31*(2), 143–164.

Beckman, H. B., & Frankel, R. M. (1984). The effect of physician behavior on the collection of data. *Annals of Internal Medicine, 101*, 692–696.

Bellini, L. M., & Shea, J. A. (2005). Mood change and empathy decline persist during three years of internal medicine training. *Academic Medicine, 80*, 164–167.

Bervan, N. L., Thomas, K. R., & Chan, F. (2004). An introduction to counseling for rehabilitation health professionals. In F. Chan, N. L. Berven, & K. R. Thomas (Eds.), *Counseling theories and techniques for rehabilitation health professionals* (pp. 3–16). New York: Springer.

Beynon, G. J., Thornton, F. L., & Poole, C. (1997). A randomized, controlled trial of the efficacy of a communication course for first time hearing aid users. *British Journal of Audiology, 31*(5), 345–352.

Biderman, A., Yeheskel, A., & Herman, J. (2005). The biopsychosocial model—have we made any progress since 1977? *Families, Systems, & Health, 23*(4), 379–386.

Blatt, S. J., Sanislow, C. A. III, Zuroff, D. C., & Pilkonis, P. A. (1996). Characteristics of effective therapists: Further analyses of data from the National Institute of Mental Health Treatment of Depression Collaborative Research Program. *Journal of Consulting and Clinical Psychology, 64*(6), 1276–1284.

Bodenheimer, T., Wagner, E., & Grumbach, K. (2002). Improving primary care for patients with chronic illness. *Journal of the American Medical Association, 288*, 1909–1914.

Borrell-Carrió, F., Suchman, A., L., & Epstein, R. M. (2004). The biopsychosocial model 25 years later: Principles, practice, and scientific inquiry. *Annals of Family Medicine, 2*(6), 576–582.

Brainerd, S. H., & Frankel, B. G. (1985). The relationship between audiometric and self-report measures of hearing handicap. *Ear and Hearing, 6*, 89–92.

Brammer, L. M., & MacDonald, G. (2002). *The helping relationship: Process and skills* (8th ed.). Needham Heights, MA: Allyn & Bacon.

Brennan, M., & Bally, S. J. (2007). Psychosocial adaptations to dual sensory loss in middle and late adulthood. *Trends in Amplification, 11*(4), 281–300.

Britt, E., Hudson, S. M., & Blampied, N. M. (2004). Motivational interviewing in health settings: A review. *Patient Education and Counseling, 53*(2), 147–155.

Buck, P. C. (1944). *Psychology for musicians*. London: Oxford University Press.

Carr, J. E., Emory, E. K., Errichetti, A., Johnson, S. B., & Reyes, E. (2007). Integrating behavioral and social sciences in the medical school curriculum: Opportunities and challenges for psychology. *Journal of Clinical Psychology in Medical Settings, 14*, 33–39.

Castonguay, L. G., Constantino, M. J., & Grosse, M. H. (2006). The working alliance: Where are we and where should we go? *Psychotherapy: Theory, Research, Practice, Training, 43*(3), 271–279.

Chan, F., Berven, N. L., & Thomas, K. R. (2004). *Counseling theories and techniques for rehabilitation health professionals*. New York: Springer.

Chen, D., Lew, R., Hershman, W., & Orlaner, J. (2007). A cross-sectional measurement of medical school empathy. *Journal of General Internal Medicine, 22*(10), 1434–1438.

Chisolm, T. H., Abrams, H. B., & McArdle, R. (2004). Short- and long-term outcomes of adult audiological rehabilitation. *Ear and Hearing, 25*, 464–477.

Christensen, A. J. (2004). *Patient adherence to medical treatment regimens: Bridging the gap between behavioral science and biomedicine*. New Haven, CT: Yale University Press.

Corey, G. (2008). *Theory and practice of counseling and psychotherapy* (8th ed.). Pacific Grove, CA: Brooks/Cole.

Corey, M. S., & Corey, G. (2006). *Becoming a helper* (5th ed.). Pacific Grove, CA: Brooks/Cole.

Crandell, C. C. (1997). An update on counseling instruction within audiology programs. *Journal of the Academy of Rehabilitative Audiology, 15*, 77–86.

Crandell, C. C., & Weiner, A. (2002). Counseling in competencies in audiologists: Efficacy of a distance-learning course. *Hearing Journal, 55*(9), 42–47.

Crombez, G., Vlaeyen, J. W., Heuts, P. H., & Lysens, R. (1999). Pain-related fear is more disabling than pain itself: Evidence on the role of pain-related fear in chronic back pain disability. *Pain, 80*, 329–339.

Cubbage, M. E., & Thomas, K. R. (1989). Freud and disability. *Rehabilitation Psychology, 34*, 161–173.

Cuff, P. A., & Vanselow, N. A. (2004). *Improving medical education: Enhancing the behavioral and social science content of medical school curricula*. Washington, DC: National Academies Press.

Culpepper, B., Mendel, L. L., & McCarthy, P. A. (1994). Counseling experience and training offered by ESB-accredited programs. *Asha, 36*, 55–58.

Danermark, B. D. (1998). Hearing impairment, emotions, and audiological rehabilitation: A sociological perspective. *Scandinavian Audiology, 27*(Suppl. 49), 125–131.

DasGupta, S., & Charon, R. (2004). Personal illness narratives: Using reflective writing to teach empathy. *Academic Medicine, 79*, 351–356.

Dell Orto, A. E., & Power, P. W. (2007). *The psychological and social impact of illness and disability* (5th ed.). New York: Springer.

Demorest, M. E., & Erdman, S. A. (1986). Scale composition and item analysis of the Communication Profile for the Hearing Impaired. *Journal of Speech and Hearing Research, 29*(4), 515–535.

Demorest, M. E., & Erdman, S. A. (1987). Development of the Communication Profile for the Hearing Impaired. *Journal of Speech and Hearing Disorders, 52*(2), 129–143.

Dobie, S. (2007). Reflections on a well-traveled path: Self-awareness, mindful practice, and relationship-centered care as foundations for medical education. *Academic Medicine, 82*(4), 422–426.

Dunstan, D. A., & Covic, T. (2006). Compensable work disability management: A literature review of biopsychosocial perspectives. *Australian Occupational Therapy Journal, 53*, 67–77.

Dylan, R. (1963). The times, they are a changin'. On *"The times, they are a changing"* (1964). New York: Columbia.

Earp, J. A., French, E. A., & Gilkey, M. B. (2007). *Patient advocacy for health care quality: Strategies for achieving patient centered care.* Sudbury, MA: Jones and Bartlett.

Egan, G. (2006). *The skilled helper: A problem management and opportunity development approach to helping* (8th ed.). Belmont, CA: Wadsworth.

Elvins, R., & Green, J. (2008). The conceptualization and measurement of the therapeutic alliance: An empirical review. *Clinical Psychology Review, 28*, 1167–1187.

Engel, G. L. (1977a). The need for a new medical model: A challenge for biomedicine. *Science, 196*, 129–136.

Engel, G. L. (1977b). The care of the patient: Art or science? *Johns Hopkins Medical Journal, 140*, 222–232.

Engel, G. L. (1980). The clinical application of the biopsychosocial model. *American Journal of Psychiatry, 137*(5), 535–544.

Engel, G. L. (1987). Physician-scientists and scientific physicians. Resolving the humanism-science dichotomy. *American Journal of Medicine, 82*, 107–111.

Engel, G. L. (1996). Biomedical to biopsychosocial: II. A personal odyssey. *Families, Systems, & Health, 14*, 434–449.

Engel, G. L. (1997). From biomedical to biopsychosocial. Being scientific in the human domain. *Psychosomatics, 38*, 521–528.

Engel, G. L. (2005). A response from George Engel to Joseph Herman—May 5, 1989. *Families, Systems, & Health, 23*(4), 377–378.

English, K., Naeve-Velguth, S., Rall, E., Uyehara-Isono, J., & Pittman, A. (2007). Development of an instrument to evaluate audiologic counseling skills. *Journal of the American Academy of Audiology, 18*, 675–687.

Epstein, R. M. (1999). Mindful practice. *Journal of the American Medical Association, 282*(9), 833–839.

Epstein, R. M. (2003a). Mindful practice in action (I): Technical competence, evidence-based medicine, and relationship centered care. *Families, Systems, & Health, 21*(1), 1–9.

Epstein, R. M. (2003b). Mindful practice in action (II): Cultivating habits of mind. *Families, Systems, & Health, 21*(1), 11–17.

Erdman, S. A. (1993a). Counseling the hearing-impaired adult. In J. G. Alpiner & P. A. McCarthy (Eds.), *Rehabilitative audiology: Children and adults* (2nd ed., pp. 374–413). Baltimore: Williams & Wilkins.

Erdman, S. A. (1993b). Self-assessment in audiology: The clinical rationale. *Seminars in Hearing, 14*, 303–313.

Erdman, S. A. (1994). Self-assessment: From research focus to research tool. In J-P. Gagné & N. Tye-Murray (Eds.), *Research in audiological rehabilitation: Current trends and future directions, Journal of the Academy of Rehabilitative Audiology, 27*(Monogr. Suppl.), 67–90.

Erdman, S. A. (1995, June). *Insights from the results of the CPHI-Spousal Form.* In R. Hétu (Chair), *The spouse in audiological rehabilitation: Their role and their needs.* Roundtable Discussion at the Academy of Rehabilitative Audiology Summer Institute, Howey-in-the-Hills, FL.

Erdman, S. A. (2000). Counseling adults with hearing impairment. In J. G. Alpiner & P. A. McCarthy (Eds.), *Rehabilitative audiology: Children and adults* (3rd ed., pp. 435–470). Baltimore: Lippincott Williams & Wilkins.

Erdman, S. A. (2001, June). *Hearing impairment and depression: Facts vs. fiction.* Presented at the Academy of Rehabilitative Audiology Summer Institute, Vancouver, British Columbia, Canada.

Erdman, S. A. (2006). Clinical interpretation of the CPHI. *Perspectives on Aural Rehabilitation and Its Instrumentation, 13,* 3–11. Available at http://div7 perspectives.asha.org/cgi/reprint/13/1/3-2.1KB-Perspectives

Erdman, S.A. (June, 2007). *Hearing loss and depression.* Invited presentation at the Hearing Loss Association of America Convention, Oklahoma City, OK.

Erdman, S. A., & Demorest, M. E. (1987). Post-treatment evaluations using the CPHI. *Asha, 29*(10), 77.

Erdman, S. A., & Demorest, M. E. (1996, June). *Psychological and marital correlates of adjustment to hearing impairment.* Paper presented at the Academy of Rehabilitative Audiology Summer Institute, Snowbird, UT.

Erdman, S. A., & Demorest, M. E. (1998a). Adjustment to hearing impairment I: Description of a heterogeneous clinical population. *Journal of Speech, Language, and Hearing Research, 41,* 107–122.

Erdman, S. A., & Demorest, M. E. (1998b). Adjustment to hearing impairment II: Audiological and demographic correlates. *Journal of Speech, Language, and Hearing Research, 41,* 123–136.

Erdman, S. A., Wark, D. J., & Montano, J. J. (1994). Implications of service delivery models in audiology. *Journal of the Academy of Rehabilitative Audiology, 27,* 45–60.

Falvo, D. R. (2004). *Effective patient education: A guide to increased compliance* (3rd ed.). Sudbury, MA: Jones and Bartlett.

Falvo, D. R. (2005). *Medical and psychosocial aspects of chronic illness and disability* (3rd ed.). Sudbury, MA: Jones and Bartlett.

Fava, G. A., & Sonino, N. (2008). The biopsychosocial model thirty years later. *Psychotherapy and Psychosomatics, 77,* 1–2.

Fierman, L. B. (1997). *The therapist is the therapy: Effective psychotherapy* (Vol. 2.). Northvale, NJ: Jason Aronson.

Frankel, R. M., Quill, T. E., & McDaniel, S. H. (Eds). (2003). *The biopsychosocial approach: Past, present, future.* Rochester, NY: University of Rochester Press.

Gaeth, J. H. (1979). A history of aural rehabilitation. In M. A. Henoch (Ed.), *Aural rehabilitation for the elderly* (pp. 1–21). New York: Grune & Stratton.

Gagné, J.-P., Southall, K., & Jennings, M. B. (2009). The psychological effects of social stigma: Applications to people with an acquired hearing loss. In J. J. Montano & J. B. Spitzer (Eds.), *Adult audiologic rehabilitation: Advanced practices* (pp. 63–92). San Diego, CA: Plural.

Gatchel, R. J., & Okifuji, A. (2006). Evidence-based scientific data documenting the treatment- and cost-effectiveness of comprehensive pain programs for chronic pain management. *Journal of Pain, 7,* 779–793.

Gatchel, R. J., Peng, Y. B., Fuchs, P. N., Peters, M. L., & Turk, D. C. (2007. The biopsychosocial approach to chronic pain: Scientific advances and future directions. *Psychological Bulletin, 133*(4), 581–624.

Gelso, C. J., & Carter, J. A. (1994). Components of the psychotherapy relationship: Their interaction and unfolding during treatment. *Journal of Counseling Psychology, 41*(3), 296–306.

Gelso, C. J., & Hayes, J. A. (1998). *The psychotherapy relationship: Theory, research, and practice.* New York: Wiley.

Getty, L., & Hétu, R. (1991). Development of a rehabilitation program for people affected with occupational hearing loss 2. Results from group intervention with 48 workers and their spouses. *Audiology, 30,* 317–329.

Goubert, L., Crombez, G., & Van Damme, S. (2004). The role of neuroticism, pain catastrophizing and pain related fear in vigilance to pain: A structural equations approach. *Pain, 107,* 234–241.

Greenberg, L. (2008). Emotion and cognition in psychotherapy: The transforming power of affect. *Canadian Psychology, 49*(1), 149–159.

Hallam, R., Ashton, P., Sherbourne, K., & Gailey, L. (2006). Acquired profound hearing loss: Mental health and other characteristics of a large sample. *International Journal of Audiology, 45*(12), 715–723.

Hallberg, L. R.-M., & Carlsson, S. G. (1991). Hearing impairment, coping and perceived hearing handicap in middle-aged subjects with acquired hearing loss. *British Journal of Audiology, 25*, 323–330.

Hallberg, L. R.-M., Hallberg, U., & Kramer, S. E. (2008). Self-reported hearing difficulties, communication strategies and psychological general well-being (quality of life) in patients with acquired hearing impairment. *Disability and Rehabilitation, 30*(3), 203–212.

Hallberg, L., Ringdahl, A., Holmes, A., & Carver, C. (2005, December). Psychological general well-being (quality of life) in patients with cochlear implants: Importance of social environment and age. *International Journal of Audiology, 44*(12), 706–711.

Hardick, E. J., & Gans, R. E. (1982). An approach to rehabilitation with amplification. *Ear and Hearing, 3*(3), 178–182.

Hawes, N. A., & Niswander, P. S. (1985). Comparison of the Revised Hearing Performance Inventory with audiometric measures. *Ear and Hearing, 6*(2), 93–97.

Hawkins, D. B. (2005). Effectiveness of counseling-based aural rehabilitation programs: A systematic review of the evidence. *Journal of the American Academy of Audiology, 16*, 485–493.

Heaton, E. M. (1992). The numerous facets of quality care. *Journal of Speech-Language-Pathology and Audiology, 16*, 263–272.

Helvik, A-S., Jacobsen, G., & Hallberg, L. R-M. (2006). Psychological well-being of adults with acquired hearing impairment. *Disability and Rehabilitation, 28*(9), 535–545.

Herman, J. (1989/2005). The need for a transitional model: A challenge for biopsychosocial medicine? *Families, Systems, & Health, 23*(4), 372–376. [Previously published in *Families, Systems Medicine, 7*(1), (1989)].

Hétu, R. (1996). The stigma attached to hearing impairment. *Scandinavian Audiology, 25(*Suppl. 43), 12–24.

Hétu, R., & Getty, L. (1991). Development of a program for people affected with occupational hearing loss. I. A new paradigm. *Audiology, 30*, 305–316.

Hétu, R., & Getty, L. (1993). Overcoming difficulties experienced in the workplace by employees with occupational hearing loss. *Volta Review, 95*, 391–402.

Hétu, R., Getty, L., Beaudry, J., & Philibert, L. (1994). Attitudes towards co-workers affected by occupational hearing loss I: Questionnaire development and inquiry. *British Journal of Audiology, 28*, 299–311.

Hétu, R., Getty, L., & Waridel, S. (1994). Attitudes towards co-workers affected by occupational hearing loss II: Focus groups interviews. *British Journal of Audiology, 28*, 313–325.

Hétu, R., Lalonde, M., & Getty, L. (1987), Psychosocial disadvantages associated with occupational hearing loss as experienced in the family. *Audiology, 26*, 141–152.

Hétu, R., Riverin, L., Getty, L., Lalande, N. M., & St-Cyr, C. (1990). The reluctance to acknowledge hearing difficulties among hearing-impaired workers. *British Journal of Audiology, 24*, 265–276.

Hétu, R., Riverin, L., Lalande, N. Getty, L., & St-Cyr, C. (1988). Qualitative analysis of the handicap associated with occupational hearing loss. *British Journal of Audiology, 22*, 251–264.

Hewa, S., & Hetherington, R. W. (1995). Specialists without spirit: Limitations of the mechanistic biomedical model. *Theoretical Medicine, 16*, 129–139.

Hideki, H., Kyoko, N., & Eiji, Y. (2004). Psychosomatic status affects the relationship between subjective hearing difficulties and the results of audiometry. *Journal of Clinical Epidemiology, 57*(4), 381–385.

High, W. S., Fairbanks, G., & Glorig, A. (1964), Scale for self-assessment of hearing handicap. *Journal of Speech and Hearing Disorders, 29*, 251–230.

Holman, H. R. (1976). The "excellence" deception in medicine. *Hospital Practice, 11*(4), 11, 18, 21.

Holman, H. R., & Lorig, K.R. (2000). Patients as partners in managing chronic disease. *British Medical Journal, 320*, 526–527.

Holman, H. R., & Lorig, K. R. (2004). Patient self-management: A key to effectiveness and efficiency in care of chronic disease. *Public Health Reports, 119*(3), 239–243.

Hunt, M. A., Birmingham, T. B., Skarakis-Doyle, E., & Vandervoort, A. A. (2008). Towards a biopsychosocial framework of osteoarthritis of the knee. *Disability and Rehabilitation, 30*(1), 54–61.

Institute of Medicine (2000). Hurtado, M. P., Swift, E. K., & Corrigan, J. M. (Eds.). Committee on the National Quality Report on Health Care Delivery, Board on Health Care Services, *Envisioning the National Health Care Quality Report* (p. 224). Washington, DC: National Academy Press.

Institute of Medicine. (2001). *Crossing the quality chasm: A new health system for the 21st century*. Washington, DC: National Academy Press.

Jones, E., (1951). The madonna's conception through the ear. In *Essays in applied psychoanalysis* (Vol. II). London: Hogarth.

Kelly, G. A. (1963). *Theory of personality: The psychology of personal constructs*. New York: Norton.

Kent, B., & La Grow, S. (2007). The role of hope in adjustment to acquired hearing loss. *International Journal of Audiology, 46*, 328–340.

Kielinen, L. L., & Nerbonne, M. A. (1990). Further investigation of the relationship between hearing handicap and audiometric measures of hearing impairment. *Journal of the Academy of Rehabilitative Audiology, 23*, 89–94.

Knapp, P. H. (1953). The ear, listening and hearing. *Journal of the American Psychoanalysis Association, 1*(4), 672–689.

Kramer, S. E., Kapteyn, T., Festen, J. M., & Tobi, H. (1996). The relationships between self-reported hearing disability and measures of auditory disability. *Audiology, 35*, 277–287.

Kricos, P. B., Erdman, S., Bratt, G. W., & Williams, D. W. (2007). Psychosocial correlates of hearing aid adjustment. *Journal of the American Academy of Audiology, 18*, 304–322.

Lee, D. J., & Gomez-Marin, O. (1997). Major depressive disorder, depressive symptoms, and bilateral hearing loss in Hispanic adults. *Journal of Affective Disorders, 44*(2–3), 189–195.

Livneh, H., & Antonak, R. F. (1997). *Psychosocial adaptation to chronic illness and disability*. Gaithersburg, MD: Aspen.

Livneh, H., & Siller, J. (2004). Psychodynamic therapy. In F. Chan, N. L. Berven, & K. R. Thomas (Eds.), *Counseling theories and techniques for rehabilitation health professionals*, (pp. 20–52). New York: Springer.

Lorig, K. (2000). *Patient education: A practical approach*. Thousand Oaks, CA: Sage.

Lorig, K. R., & Holman, H. R. (2003). Self-management education: History, definition, outcomes, and mechanisms. *Annals of Behavioral Medicine, 26*(1), 1–7.

Mahapatra, S. B. (1974). Deafness and mental health: Psychiatric and psychosomatic illness in the deaf. *Acta Psychiatrica Scandinavica, 50*, 596–611.

Mahoney, M. J. (1991). *Human change processes: The scientific foundations of psychotherapy*. New York: Basic Books.

Mahoney, M. J. (2003). *Constructive psychotherapy: A practical guide*. New York: Guilford Press.

Mahoney, M. J. (2005). Suffering, philosophy, and psychotherapy. *Journal of Psychotherapy Integration, 15*(3) 337–352.

Marcus-Bernstein, C. (1986). Audiologic and nonaudiologic correlates of hearing handicap in black elderly. *Journal of Speech and Hearing Research, 29*, 301–312.

Martz, E., & Livneh, H. (2007). *Coping with chronic illness and disability: Theoretical, empirical, and clinical aspects*. New York: Springer.

McCarthy, P. A., & Alpiner, J. G., (1983). An assessment scale of hearing handicap for use in family counseling. *Journal of the Academy of Rehabilitative Audiology, 16*, 256–270.

McCarthy, P. A., Culpepper, N.B., & Lucks, L. (1986). Variability in counseling experiences and training among ESB-accredited programs. *Asha, 28*(9), 49–52.

McCartney, J., Maurer, I., & Sorenson, F. (1976). A comparison of the Hearing Handicap Scale and the Hearing Measurement Scale with standard audiometric measures on the geriatric population. *Journal of Auditory Research, 16*, 51–58.

Mead, M. (1975). Towards a human science. *Science, 191*, 903–909.

Meadow-Orlans, K. P. (1985). Social and psychological effects of hearing loss in adulthood: A literature review. In H. Orlans (Ed.), *Adjustment to adult hearing loss* (pp. 35–57). San Diego, CA: College-Hill Press.

Miller, W. R., & Rollnick, S. (2002). *Motivational interviewing: Preparing people for change* (2nd ed.). New York: Guilford Press.

Morrissett, L. E. (1957). The aural-rehabilitation program for the deafened and hard of hearing. In J. B. Coates (Ed.), *Surgery in World War II: Ophthalmology and otolaryngology*. Washington, DC: Office of the Surgeon General, Department of the Army.

National Council on the Aging. (1999). *The consequences of untreated hearing loss in older people.* Washington, DC: Author.

Neimeyer, R. A., & Raskin, J. D. (2000). *Constructions of disorder: Meaning-making frameworks for psychotherapy*. Washington, DC: American Psychological Association.

Newman, C. W., & Weinstein, B. E. (1986). Judgments of perceived hearing handicap by hearing-impaired elderly men and their spouses. *Journal of the Academy of Rehabilitative Audiology, 19,* 109–115.

Newman, C. W., Weinstein, B. E., Jacobson, G. P., & Hug, G. A. (1990). The Hearing Handicap Inventory for Adults: Psychometric adequacy and audiometric correlates. *Ear and Hearing, 11,* 430–433.

Norcross, J. C. (2002). Empirically supported therapy relationship. In J. C. Norcross (Ed.), *Psychotherapy relationships that work: Therapist contributions and responsiveness of patients* (pp. 3–16). New York: Oxford University Press.

Norcross, J. C., & Goldfried, M. R. (Eds). (2005). *Handbook of psychotherapy integration*. New York: Oxford University Press.

Norcross, J. C., & Lambert, M. J. (2006). The therapy relationship. In J. R. Norcross, L. E. Beutler, & R. F. Levant (Eds.), *Evidence-based practices in mental health: Debate and dialogue on fundamental questions* (pp. 208–218). Washington, DC: American Psychological Association.

Norfolk, T., Birdi, K., & Walsh, D. (2007). The role of empathy in establishing rapport in the consultation: A new model. *Medical Education, 41,* 690–697.

Northern, J. L., Ciliax, D. R., Roth, D. E., & Johnson, R. J. (1969). Military patient attitudes toward aural rehabilitation. *Asha, 11*(9), 391–395.

Nuovo, J. (Ed.). (2006). *Chronic disease management*. New York: Springer.

O'Donahue, W. T., & Levensky, E. R. (2006). *Promoting treatment adherence: A practical handbook for health care providers*. Thousand Oaks, CA: Sage.

Parker, R. M., Szymanski, E. M., & Patterson, J. B. (2004) *Rehabilitation counseling: Basics and beyond.* Austin, TX: Pro-Ed.

Perls, F. S. (1969). *Gestalt therapy verbatim.* Lafayette, CA: Real People Press.

Perls, F. S. (1973). *The gestalt approach and eye witness to psychotherapy.* Palo Alto, CA: Science and Behavior Books.

Peters, M. L., Vlaeyen, J. W., & Weber, W. E. (2005). The joint contribution of physical pathology, pain-related fear and catastrophizing to chronic back pain disability. *Pain, 113,* 45–50.

Pinkerton, R. (2008). "I apologize for being late": the courteous psychotherapist. *Psychotherapy Theory, Research, Practice, Training 45*(2), 273–277.

Pope, K. S., & Vasquez, M. J. T. (2007). *Ethics in psychotherapy and counseling: A practical guide* (3rd ed.). San Francisco: Jossey-Bass.

Rogers, C. R. (1942). *Counseling and psychotherapy: Newer concepts in practice.* Boston: Houghton Mifflin.

Rogers, C. R. (1951). *Client-centered therapy.* Boston: Houghton Mifflin.

Rogers, C. R. (1957). The necessary and sufficient conditions of therapeutic personality change. *Journal of Consulting Psychology, 21,* 95–103.

Rogers, C. (1958, September). The characteristics of a helping relationship. *Personnel and Guidance Journal, 37,* 6–16.

Rooney, J. P., & Perrin, D. (2008). *America's health care crisis solved: Money-saving solutions, coverage for everyone.* Hoboken, NJ: Wiley.

Rousey, C. L. (1971). Psychological reactions to hearing loss. *Journal of Speech and Hearing Disorders, 37*(30), 382–389.

Rowland, J. P., Dirks, D. D., Dubno, J. R., & Bell, T. S. (1985). Comparison of speech recognition-in-noise and subjective communication assessment. *Ear and Hearing, 6*(6), 291–296.

Safran, J. D., & Muran, J. C. (1998). The therapeutic alliance in brief psychotherapy: General principles. In J. D. Safran & J. C. Muran (Eds.), *The therapeutic alliance in brief psychotherapy* (pp. 217–229). Washington, DC: American Psychological Association.

Sarafino, E. P. (2005). *Health psychology: Biopsychosocial interactions*. New York: John Wiley.

Scarinci, N., Worrall, L., & Hickson, L. (2008, March). The effect of hearing impairment in older people on the spouse. *International Journal of Audiology, 47*(3), 141–151.

Scheier, M. F., & Carver, C. S. (1985). Optimism, coping, and health: Assessment and implications of generalized outcome expectancies. *Health Psychology, 4*, 219–247.

Scheier, M. F., & Carver, C. S. (1987). Dispositional optimism and physical well-being: The influence of generalized outcome expectancies on health. *Journal of Personality, 55*, 169–210.

Scheier, M. F., & Carver, C. S. (1992). Effects of optimism on psychological and physical well-being: Theoretical overview and empirical update. *Cognitive Therapy and Research, 16*, 210–228.

Scherer, M. J., & Frisina, D. R. (1998). Characteristics associated with marginal hearing loss and subjective well-being among a sample of older adults. *Journal of Rehabilitation Research and Development, 35*(4), 420–426.

Schow, R. L., & Nerbonne, M. A. (1980). Hearing Handicap and Denver Scales: Applications, categories, interpretation. *Journal of the Academy of Rehabilitative Audiology, 13*, 66–77.

Seaburn, D. B. (2005). Is going "too far" far enough? *Families, Systems, & Health, 23*(4), 396–399.

Shapiro, J., & Ross, V. (2002). Applications of narrative theory and therapy to the practice of family medicine. *Family Medicine, 34*, 96–100.

Sharf, R. S. (2007). *Theories of psychotherapy and counseling: Concepts and cases* (4th ed.). Pacific Grove, CA: Brooks/Cole.

Sharp, T. (2007, May/June). Kooser helps others accept, understand hearing loss. *RSC NewsNet, 23*(3), 2–4.

Shontz, F. C. (1977). Six principles relating disability and psychological adjustment. *Rehabilitation Psychology, 24*(4). 207–210.

Smith, G. C., & Strain, J. J. (2002).George Engel's contribution to clinical psychiatry. *Australian and New Zealand Journal of Psychiatry, 36*, 458–466.

Smith, S. L., & West, R. L. (2006). The application of self-efficacy principles to audiologic rehabilitation: a tutorial. *American Journal of Audiology, 15*, 46–56.

Snyder, C. R. (1989). Reality negotiation: From excuses to hope and beyond. *Journal of Social and Clinical Psychology, 8*, 130–157.

Snyder, C. R. (1994). *The psychology of hope: You can get there from here.* New York: Free Press.

Snyder, C. R., Lehman, K. A., Kluck, B., & Monsson, Y. (2006). Hope for rehabilitation and vice versa. *Rehabilitation Psychology, 51*(2), 89–112.

Speaks, C. S., Jerger, J., & Trammell, J. (1970). Measurement of hearing handicap. *Journal of Speech and Hearing Research, 13*(4), 768–776.

Squier, R. W. (1990). A model of empathic understanding and adherence to treatment regimens in practitioner-patient relationships. *Social Science and Medicine, 30*(3), 325–339.

Stepien, K. A., & Baernstein, A. (2006). Educating for empathy: A review. *Journal of General Internal Medicine, 21*, 524–530.

Stewart, M., Belle-Brown, J., Weston, W. W., & McWhinney, I. R. (2003). *Patient-centered medicine: Transforming the clinical method.* New York: Radcliffe Medical Press.

Stewart, M., Brown, J. B., Donner, A., McWhinney, I. R., Oates, J., Weston, W. W., et al. (2000). The impact of patient-centered care on outcomes. *Journal of Family Practice, 49*(9), 796–804.

Stewart, M., Brown, J., & Weston, W. (1989). Patient-centered interviewing: Five provocative questions. *Canadian Family Physician, 35*, 159–161.

Stika, C. J. (1997, May/June). Mental health services for persons with hearing loss: The Rehabilitation Research and Training Center survey. *Hearing Loss*, pp. 20–25.

Swan, I. R. C., & Gatehouse, S. (1990). Factors influencing consultation for management of hearing disability. *British Journal of Audiology, 24*, 155–160.

Tambs, K. (2004). Moderate effects of hearing loss on mental health and subjective well-being: Results from the Nord-Trøndelag hearing loss study. *Psychosomatic Medicine, 66*, 776–782.

Thomas, A. J. (1984). *Acquired hearing loss: Psychological and psychosocial implications.* London: Academic Press.

Truax, C. B., & Mitchell, K. M. (1971). Research on certain therapist skills in relation to process and outcome. In A. E. Bergin & S. L. Garfield (Eds.), *Handbook of psychotherapy and behavior change: An empirical analysis.* New York: John Wiley.

Truax, C. B., Wargo, D. G., Frank J. D., Imber, S. D., Battle, C. C., Hoehn-Saric, R., et al. (1966). Therapist empathy, genuineness, and warmth and patient therapeutic outcome. *Journal of Consulting Psychology, 30*, 395–401.

Truchon, M., & Fillion, L. (2000). Biopsychosocial determinants of chronic disability and low-back pain: a review. *Journal of Occupational Rehabilitation, 10*(2), 117–140.

Truex, E. H. (1957). Follow-up study of deafened and hard of hearing patients. In J. B. Coates, Jr. (Ed.), *Surgery in World War II; Ophthalmology and otolaryngology* (pp. 573–579). Washington, DC: Office of the Surgeon General, Department of the Army.

Turk, D. C., & Okifuji, A. (2002). Psychological factors in chronic pain: Evolution and revolution. *Journal of Consulting and Clinical Psychology, 70*(3), 678–690.

van den Brink, R. H. S., Wit, H. P., Kempen, G. I. J. M., & van Heuvelen, M. J. G. (1996). Attitude and help-seeking for hearing impairment. *British Journal of Audiology, 30*, 313–324.

Vlaeyen, J. W. S., Crombez, G., & Goubert, L. (2007). The psychology of chronic pain and its management. *Physical Therapy Reviews, 12*, 179–188.

Vlaeyen, J. W., & Morley, S. (2005). Cognitive-behavioral treatments for chronic pain: What works for whom? *Clinical Journal of Pain, 21*, 1–8.

Vuorialho, A., Karinen, P., & Sorri, M. (2006). Counselling of hearing aid users is highly cost-effective. *European Archives of Otorhinolaryngology, 263*(11), 988–995.

Wagner, C. C., & McMahon, B. T. (2004). Motivational interviewing and rehabilitation counseling practice. *Rehabilitation Counseling Bulletin, 47*(30), 152–161.

Wallhagen, M. I. (2002). Hearing impairment. *Annual Review of Nursing Research, 20*, 341–368.

Wallhagen, M. I., Pettengill, E., & Whiteside, M. (2006). Sensory impairments in older adults Part I: Hearing loss. *American Journal of Nursing, 106*, 40–48.

Wallhagen, M. I., Strawbridge, W. J., Shema, S. J., & Kaplan, G. A. (2004). Impact of self-assessed hearing loss on a spouse: A longitudinal analysis of couples. *Journal of Gerontology: Social Sciences, 59B*(3), S190–S196.

Wampold, B. E. (2001). *The great psychotherapy debate: Models, methods, and findings*. Mahwah, NJ: Erlbaum.

Wampold, B. E., Ahn, H., & Coleman, H. L. K. (2001). Medical model as metaphor: Old habits die hard. *Journal of Counseling Psychology 48*(3), 268–273.

Wampold, B. E., & Brown, G. S. (2005). Estimating variability in outcomes attributable to therapists: A naturalistic study of outcomes in managed care. *Journal of Consulting and Clinical Psychology, 73*(5), 914–923.

Wear, D. (1998). On white coats and professional development: The formal and the hidden curricula. *Annals of Internal Medicine, 12*, 734–737.

Weinstein, B. E., & Ventry, I. M. (1983a). Audiologic correlates of hearing handicap in the elderly. *Journal of Speech and Hearing Research, 26*, 148–151.

Weinstein, B. E., & Ventry, I. M. (1983b). Audiometric correlates of the Hearing Handicap Inventory for the Elderly. *Journal of Speech and Hearing Disorders, 48*, 379–384.

Welfel, E. R., & Patterson, L. E. (2004). *The counseling process: A multitheoretical integrative approach* (6th ed.). Belmont, CA: Brooks/Cole.

Wylde, M. A. (1987). Psychological and counseling aspects of the adult remediation process. In J. G. Alpiner & P. A. McCarthy (Eds.), *Rehabilitative audiology: Children and adults*. Baltimore: Williams & Wilkins.

Yueh, B., Collins, M., & Souza, P. (2007, March). *Effects of depression on self-report hearing outcomes*. Paper presented at the meeting of the American Auditory Society, Phoenix, AZ.

Zubialde, J. P., Eubank, D., & Fink, L. D. (2007). Cultivating engaged patients: A lesson from adult learning. *Families, Systems, & Health, 25*(4), 355–366.

10

Conversation Repair Strategies in Audiologic Rehabilitation

Christopher Lind

Introduction

Conversational difficulties have been identified as the major activity limitation amongst adults who have acquired hearing impairments, leading to participation restrictions in many aspects of everyday social interaction (Erber, 2002; Stephens, Giannopolous, & Kerr, 2001). In response, therapy in audiologic rehabilitation has followed three general lines of activity, namely, sensory-perceptual, linguistic, and psychosocial approaches. Using the World Health Organization ICF classification (World Health Organization, 2001), these interventions have been directed at individuals' impairment, activity limitation and participation restriction, respectively. In each therapy model, clinicians rely on clinical assessment and self-report to judge the effectiveness of their intervention.

It is the thesis of this chapter that communication difficulties arising from acquired hearing impairment manifest in everyday conversations and, as such, assessment and intervention in the context of everyday interaction most directly address these communication difficulties. However, still little is known of the particulars of these problems in conversation, and how they might be remediated.

This chapter outlines a conversationally oriented assessment and intervention model which focuses on the interactional and sequential aspects of conversation behaviors as they may be influenced by one participant's acquired hearing impairment. Specifically, this program focuses on bringing patterns of conversational repair under conversation partners' control in order to minimize the effects of conversation breakdown or miscommunication on conversational flow. This clinical work is not new, yet there has been little concerted effort to bring under one theoretical approach the research findings that allow the development of this clinical activity.

Insights into conversation behavior and the influences of hearing impairment on its conduct have been provided by studies using several different research methods. Studies using speech perception tasks to investigate the effectiveness of repair strategies have tended to use information transfer to explain conversation repair (Gagné, Stelmacovich, & Yovetich, 1991; Gagné & Wylie, 1989; Marzolf, Stewart, Nerbonne, & Lehman, 1998; Tye-Murray, 1991; Tye-Murray, Purdy, Woodworth, & Tyler, 1990). These studies have shown that repetition is the most commonly requested repair. This is perhaps not surprising in tasks requiring repetition of the stimulus in the absence of a requirement to comprehend it. Discourse studies, including storytelling (Chelst, Tait, & Gallagher, 1990), simulated conversation breakdowns (Wilson, Hickson, & Worrall, 1998), and continuous discourse tracking (Lunato & Weisenberger, 1994) have used more interactive speech reception paradigms to analyze sequential aspects of repair behavior. However, in doing so, the researchers have labeled and categorized the turns comprising these sequences without reference to each other or to the turn in which the breakdown occurred, limiting the ability to mirror the sequential nature of conversational talk.

Studies using free and unstructured conversation as the research paradigm (Caissie, Dawe, Donovan, Brooks, & MacDonald, 1998; Caissie & Rockwell, 1993; Johnson & Pichora-Fuller, 1994; Pichora-Fuller, Johnson, & Roodenburg, 1998; Tye-Murray & Witt, 1997; Tye-Murray, Witt, Schum, 1995) have analyzed turns comprising repair in sequence, making commentary on the relation between the content of the turn initiating the repair and the content of the turn undertaking the repair. These studies have also indicated that repetition-type repairs commonly follow general repair initiators (i.e., those in which no information is given about the location or the content of the breakdown, such as "What?," or "Pardon?"). Repair initiators containing information that identifies the content of the miscommunication are likely to be followed either by repairs of repetition or by repairs in which additional information is provided, presumably in an attempt to clarify the miscommunicated portion of talk. These studies have provided important insights into sequential patterns of conversation repair.

A View of Conversation, Its Structure and Analysis

Everyday conversation is a complex interactive task, yet adults are able to traverse its complexities with family, friends, and strangers alike, and all with seemingly little effort. We manage to talk about topics we know very well and about which we know little. We take our turns at talk easily, and we swap readily from the role of speaker to the role of listener. In doing so, we speak one at the time with surprisingly little overlap. Yet, adults are by and large naive communicators. That is, we successfully communicate with each other every day, yet, we have little or no *overt* understanding of the rules or regularities by which conversation is successfully conducted.

So how do adults structure talk so successfully? According to sociologists, the key to successful communication is the maintenance of *intersubjectivity* (Verhagen, 2005). Intersubjectivity is the theoretical concept that underpins our shared views of the world and the mutual understanding that allows coordinated, concerted effort between individuals toward social goals. The sociolinguists who developed the Conversation Analysis (henceforth, CA) approach apply this concept to everyday conversation by suggesting it is the basis for establishing and extending mutually shared views, opinions, understanding, and knowledge through communication (Sacks, Schegloff, & Jefferson, 1974; Schegloff, 1991, 1996a, 1996b, 2007; Schegloff, Jefferson, & Sacks, 1977). In everyday talk, this theoretical construct of intersubjectivity is established and maintained by several important conversational actions.

The first of these is *recipient design*. Every time we take a turn at talk we design that turn with our current audience in mind (Hutchby & Wooffitt, 1998). That is, we take into account the knowledge, beliefs and ideas that we expect or believe our conversation partner or partners have brought to the interaction. The uttering of turns with one's communication partner(s) in mind, and the constant renewing and extending of context, allows participants to establish and maintain a mutual or shared understanding of the meaning of a conversation. This mutual understanding is maintained at a level sufficient for the purpose of the current talk whether that talk is for a job interview, a shopping transaction, or a chat over the back fence. That is, speakers establish and maintain *sufficient ongoing mutual understanding* (Foppa, 1995) as the criterion for the successful undertaking and continuation of a conversation.

If a talker's task is to establish and maintain sufficient mutual ongoing understanding, that is, if we are to agree with our conversation partners that the turns we take in a conversation are (perceived as) sequentially meaningful, how might we achieve this? Listeners do not make it overt that they have understood the content, meaning and/or the intent of their partner's previous turn at the beginning of every subsequent turn at talk. Rather, conversation partners simply present what they consider to be a logical and meaningful turn in the context of the prior turn(s) in the conversation. This is referred to as *sequential implicature*; that each turn in a conversation can only be understood in the context of what has been communicated before (Clayman & Maynard, 1995; Schegloff, 2007). Clark and colleagues (Clark & Schaefer, 1987, 1989; Clark & Wilkes-Gibbs, 1986) suggest that the *presentation* of conversationally relevant new information in each turn implies *acceptance* of the previous turn(s). That is, acceptance of a conversational turn is taken to have occurred if *both speakers* perceive it to be a logical and conversationally appropriate consequence of the previous turn. Some important consequences arise from this perspective. First, acceptance is not equated with agreement. One may disagree, even violently, with a view expressed in another's spoken turn, yet, accept the turn they disagree with as a conversationally appropriate act. In this context, acceptance reflects the conduct of successful sequential conversational behavior. Second, as acceptance is most commonly implicit, it is seldom directly apparent to the person speaking that they have been understood. Rather, it can only be inferred from the sequential meaning implied by the turn that follows.

To take this point further, third party observation of the flow of conversation provides particular hurdles for researcher and clinician alike. As no direct insight can be gleaned of the meaning of a particular turn especially in the face of referential or pragmatic ambiguities, proponents of CA use the *next turn proof procedure*. The meaning applied to a particular conversational turn can only be understood in the context *of the turn that follows*. This highlights that clinicians and researchers, as third party observers, must be careful to rely on the interpretation given to a particular turn by the participants in the conversation. This third party observer problem is made more complex in the study of repair as breakdowns are only observable by reference to the initiation of the repair that follows later in the same turn, or in subsequent turns. That is, a stretch of talk that results in a breakdown or miscommunication is likely in many cases not to be recognized as such by a third party until the talk that follows indicates that a miscommunication has occurred.

Third, acceptance of a spoken turn may be compromised by its phonetic, phonological, lexico-grammatical, morphologic, semantic, and/or pragmatic inarticulateness. Everyday talk is full of speech substitutions or omissions, word repetition, ellipses, false starts, nonword verbalizations, and grammatical, semantic, and pragmatic ambiguities. Talk cannot be easily divided up into clear grammatical units of syntactic and lexico-semantic meaning in the same way that written text may be analyzed. As a consequence, the CA theorists proposed conversational turns may be composed of *turn constructional units* (TCUs) which cover turns as simple as a vocalization such as "Hmm?," and at the same time full, complex grammatical phrases and clauses (Ford & Thompson, 1996).

Each TCU is followed by a brief pause labeled a *transition relevant place* (TRP) at which turn-taking is negotiated. By far, the most common event at a TRP has the current speaker continue their turn talking. Alternatively, the current speaker may relinquish his or her turn at talk, or the listener may vie to take up the role of speaker (Sacks, Schegloff, & Jefferson, 1974; Schegloff, 1996b). Thus, conversation turns may be seen to be composed of TCUs, followed by TRPs in sequence; and at certain of these TRPs, participants swap roles as speaker and listener. Ford and Thompson (1996) suggest that several factors mark a TCU, and that TCUs marking an upcoming change of speaker (i.e., turn-taking at a TRP) may be differentiated from those in which the current speaker intends to continue by their grammatical structure, suprasegmental patterns (particularly slowing and lengthening of TCU-final sounds), as well as their use of turn markers such as tag questions. Indeed the authors suggest that it is the combination of these factors that allows the split second timing that marks conversational turn taking.

It is common to suggest that in conversation, individuals swap easily and readily from speaker to listener and that these roles are defined by the act of speaking and listening respectively. This implies turn-taking is both consensual and inviolate, yet neither of these attributes is exhibited in conversation. The speaker's role is not only to talk but to listen and often the listener's role is not only to listen but to talk. Indeed this occurs when individuals vie for the role of speaker via simultaneous talk. As a more common example, *backchanelling* is the interactional label given to talk uttered by the person in the role of listener during another's turn at talk. It is the act of talking while maintaining the role as listener, while not jostling for a change of turn during another's talk (Jefferson, 1984). Talk labeled as backchanelling is seen often to be uttered by the person in the role of the listener by way of encouragement to the speaker to continue, to mark the listener's understanding, surprise or sympathy for example with talk currently under way (Mulac, Erlandson, Farrer, Hallett, Molloy, & Prescott, 1998).

Together, the constructs outlined briefly in this section provide a useful vocabulary by which clinicians and researchers might understand the structure and sequence of conversation. CA has proven to be a useful model by which to shape our understanding of the contextual nature of conversation. CA is by no means the only model of conversational behavior that might be used for these purposes (see Eggins and Slade [1997] for a summary of most current theories). However, its benefit is in its focus on the sequentiality or flow of conversation and, by extension, the manner by which interlocutors deal with instances at which this flow is disrupted. It is these instances to which we now turn our attention.

Repair Sequences in Everyday Conversation

As mentioned above, the CA criterion for successful conduct of a conversation is the establishment and maintenance of intersubjectivity through sufficient mutual ongoing understanding between participants. How sufficient ongoing mutual undestanding manifests is difficult to quantify or qualify, yet its centrality to conversational success is marked by the fact that repair sequences are initiated at any point in a conversation at which this criterion is violated. At these points in conversation, one or other of the participants makes overt that a miscommunication has occurred, and overwhelmingly, the flow of the conversation ceases almost immediately, a repair is initiated, the breakdown is resolved (i.e., such that the criterion of sufficient ongoing mutual understanding is re-established sufficient for the conduct of the conversation at hand), and the conversation recommenced. To this end, conversation repair is an exceptionally powerful activity in which instances of miscommunication are addressed in the immediate vicinity of their occurrence, not at some distant point in the conversation.

The repair sequences presented in this chapter have all been extracted from audio- and video-recorded free and unstructured conversations involving adults who have acquired hearing impairments and their normally hearing conversation partners (Lind, Hickson, & Erber, 2004, 2006). In each case, participants were left to converse in a quiet, well lit clinic room. No instructions were given prior to the conversation recordings other than that the topic of the conversation was of no importance to the research. A small collection of topic cards was supplied to stimulate new topics at times when participants fell quiet. All conversations were transcribed orthographically and the resulting text and recordings were scoured for instances of repair. Repairs were identified as sequences of talk in which conversation turn taking momentarily ceased while one participant undertook a stretch of talk that identified a (possible) miscommunication had occurred.

Schegloff and colleagues identified seven distinct sequences of conversation repair (Schegloff et al., 1977; Schegloff, 1992) (Table 10–1).

Table 10–1. Descriptions and Examples of Seven Repair Sequence Types (after Schegloff et al, 1977; Schegloff, 1992)

Repair type	Description	Example
Within-turn repairs		
Self-initiated self-repair	Speaker A utters the trouble source ("mos-"), the repair initiator (1.0 sec pause) and repair ("sometimes") all within a single turn constructional unit	B um (2.8) are you still using your computers Darren? A yeah mos- (1.0) sometimes 'coz I'm not at uni this year= B =no↓
Self-initiated self-repair at transition relevant place	Speaker A utters the trouble source ("writing a resume up") and then utters the repair (". . . writing a letter . . . ") in a subsequent turn constructional unit	A yeah (0.6) [that's] what I've been doing for jobs B [w-] B have you? A writing a resume up [writing] a letter then sending it away B [oh] B oh that's a good idea
Across-turn repairs		
Third turn self-initiated self-repair	Speaker A utters the trouble source ("and we got twelve pound here") in one turn and then utters the repair initiator ("no") and repair (. . . that was here when I got to Australia") following an intervening turn by Speaker B that *does not* identify the need for repair	A . . . and I'd only been earning four pound in- four pound ten A in England B twelve pound A and we got twelve [pound here B [well that's pretty good A no that was **here** when I got to Australia B yeah:↓ A yeah
Other-initiated self-repair	Speaker A utters a turn containing the trouble source (lines 1 to 3) which is followed by the Speaker B uttering the repair initiator ("pardon") and Speaker A addressing the miscommunication with the repair (" . . . wouldn't think they'd be shoplifting . . . ").	A . . . I think the main one was they picked up four girls A who were shoplifting you wouldn't think they'd be (0.5) A shoplifting in a place like Minlaton would you B pardon A wouldn't think they'd be **shoplifting** in a place like Minlaton B oh↓ there is is there↑

continues

Table 10–1. *continued*

Repair type	Description	Example
Other-initiated other repair	Speaker A utters a turn containing the trouble source (" . . . for Easter . . .) which is followed by the Speaker B uttering the repair initiator ("yeah, oh . . .) as well as the repair turn (" . . . not Easter").	A oh that's wonderful ((A.Insp.)) an- and you're going **away** A on: (0.9) for Easter and some of the first part of the holidays B yeah- [oh] **not** Easter A oh no you've gotta come [home at Easter] that's right yes A **oh**: well it'll be nice to have a few days away (.) **fishing**
Self-initiated other repair	Speaker A utters the trouble source as well as the repair initiator (. . . its seven isn't it") and Speaker B utters the repair in the following turn ("yes").	A its:: seven isn't it B yes: A er [seven pm I think hm] B [yeah they go on at seven] hm they go on at seven= A yeah= B =so that's alright you know
Third-position repair	Speaker A utters the trouble source (" . . . what about Andrew's lot") in one turn and then utters the repair initiator and repair turns (Andrew's is, what about his kids") following an intervening turn by Speaker B ("he's next week") that does identify the need for repair	B when's Cara's birthday A oh not until: Christmas time next year B yes (0.5) and Jessie↑ A u::m: October B October (.) what about Andrew's lot A he's next week B Andrew's is (.) [what] about his (0.3) kids A [yes] A they're all finished (.) January February March (.) one each

Note: Transcription conventions are presented in Appendix 10–A.

For the purposes of this chapter, these seven sequences of repair divide themselves into two broad categories. In the first category, the breakdown and all subsequent repair activity occurs within a single turn at talk. These *within-turn* repair sequences are commonly marked as those in which the speaker pauses and re-phrases, reframes, or otherwise addresses a portion of his or her own talk which he or she believes to have resulted in the conversation breakdown. These within-turn repair sequences are not the focus of this chapter. However, Skelt (2006) provides a detailed insight into the way these repairs reflect conversation partners' sensitivity towards another's hearing impairment. The second category comprises five conversational repair sequences of quite different sequential structure, all of which involve both speakers in the negotiation of the repair. Labeled *across-turn* sequences, it is these negotiated repairs that are the focus of the assessment and therapy model addressed in this chapter.

It should be noted that there is no one-to-one relationship between the sequential structure of the repair and the nature of the miscommunication that causes it. This notwithstanding, our research has indicated that two of these across-turn repair sequences are the most likely to arise as a result of one participant having an acquired hearing impairment, and we will return to this later in the chapter (Lind, Hickson, & Erber, 2004, 2006). Dialogue 10–1 exemplifies a common type of across-turn repair sequence. (*Note:* Transcription conventions are presented in Appendix 10–A).

Repair sequences all comprise four constituent actions, demonstrated in Dialogue 10–1:

- The trouble source (TS) is the portion of talk which has been miscommunicated. It may be as brief as a word or a long and complex as an entire turn.
- The second element of the repair sequence is the repair initiator (RI). The repair initiator is the talk uttered by one or other participant that identifies the need to address a miscommunication that has arisen in the immediately prior talk.
- The third element of the repair sequence is the repair (R) itself. This is the turn at talk in which one or other speaker addresses the trouble source.
- The final element of the repair sequence is the repair confirmation (RC). The repair confirmation is the brief portion of talk by which the listener marks their revised understanding of the miscommunicated talk.

In this sequence, the FCP asks a question about Frank Ifield (a popular Australian country singer of the early 1960s) in line 1. Following a brief pause in line 2, the HI participant simply asks "Pardon?" This is the repair initiator marking some portion of the previous turn as the trouble

Dialogue 10–1. Sample of an across-turn repair sequence

Line	Participant	Repair Activity	Text
1	FCP[1]	TS	Frank Ifield doesn't do them any more does he
2			(0.4)
3	**HI**[2]	RI	pardon?
4	FCP	R	Frank Ifield doesn't do them any more
5	**HI**	RC	I don't know **where** he is what happened (1.0) have you
6	**HI**	RC	read anything about him

[1]Frequent communication partner
[2]Hearing-impaired adult

source. In response to which the FCP replies with the repair turn by repeating his line 1 utterance without the final tag question. In turn, the HI participant marks her understanding of the repair in lines 5 and 6 by uttering a sequentially implicated turn (i.e., a turn that can be readily interpreted in the context of the previous turns) in which she responds to the question asked by the FCP. This four turn sequence marks the repair behavior most commonly undertaken in conversations involving adults who have acquired hearing impairments (Lind et al., 2004).

Repair is a complex and intricate interactive process, and one in which we have only indirect evidence for individuals' understanding of others' spoken turns. We cannot apply traditional clinical and research methods of accuracy and/or speed of identification or discrimination in the analysis of conversational behavior. The next section contains a brief summary of relevant research findings in the area of conversation repair and acquired hearing impairment. In the subsequent sections, we discuss the clinical sampling of conversation repair behavior, and some of the current rehabilitation techniques that may directly address conversation repair as a rehabilitation goal.

Common Patterns of Repair

As discussed earlier, Schegloff et al. (1977) who introduced the CA analysis of repair behavior identified seven sequential patterns of repair. Two of these seven sequences have been shown to be influenced by the presence of one participant's acquired hearing impairment (Lind et al., 2004). These two particular sequential forms of repair, labeled by Schegloff et al. (1977) and Schegloff (1992) as other-initiated self-repair (OISR) and third position repair (3PR) are the focus of the remainder of the chapter.

The Other-Initiated Self-Repair Sequence

The OISR sequence may be recognized as the stereotypical repair sequence instigated to address a miscommunication uttered by one's conversation partner. The sequence is labeled as an "other-initiated self-repair" (or OISR) sequence as the person uttering the problematic talk (i.e., the *self*) undertakes the repair after the conversation partner (i.e., the *other*) requests or initiates the repair. The dialogue extracts below taken from Lind (2006) highlight the key elements of the OISR sequence.

In Dialogue extracts 10–2 and 10–3, the same sequence of turns arises as presented in extract Dialogue 10–1 above. Both Dialogues 10–2 and 10–3 exemplify the interruption of a speaking turn; the trouble source (line 1 in each case) in the middle of a TCU (i.e., mid-grammatical unit of talk) with a repair initiator in lines 3 and 2, respectively. In Dialogue 10–2 the repair initiator is a simple "Hm?" in response to which the FCP repeats the inter-

Dialogue 10–2. OISR sequence "Devil on his shoulder"

Line	Participant	Repair Activity	Text
1	FCP	TS	he might have a little devil on his shoulder saying
2			(0.2)
3	**HI**	RI	hm?
4			(0.3)
5	FCP	R	he might have a little devil on his shoulder saying go on
6	FCP	R	do it [do it]
7	**HI**	(RC)	[((laugh))]

Dialogue 10–3. OISR sequence "Holiday plans"

Line	Participant	Repair Activity	Text
1	FCP	TS	y'know they might say they can't see us in [all]
2	**HI**	RI	[sorry] they might?
3	FCP	R	**say** that they can't see us in all of (0.6) June↑
4			(2.3)
5	**HI**	RC	ye:s but the problem **then** is if it can't be (1.0) the end of June
6	**HI**		what happens in (1.2) the four weeks **prece:ding**

rupted turn word for word, completing the previously interrupted portion of talk. The laugh in line 7 may be taken as a response to the understanding of the utterance in lines 5 and 6 previously miscommunicated in line 1. In Dialogue 10–3 the HI participant uses a more specific repair initiator (line 2) by apologizing ("sorry") and then identifying a portion of the previous turn with a questioning inflection. In response the FCP repeats the trouble source turn in line 1 from the point following the words uttered by the HI participant in line 3. Again, the response in lines 5 and 6 may be taken as a repair confirmation marking understanding of the previous utterance miscommunicated in line 1.

OISR sequences are characterized by the uttering of a trouble source (TS) in which a portion of talk is miscommunicated, followed by a repair initiator (RI) indicating a miscommunication has occurred. The request for repair is followed by a repair turn (R). In both Dialogues 10–2 and 10–3 the repair is uttered in the form of a repetition of the TS. The final element of the sequence is the repair confirmation (RC) in which the individual requesting the repair makes it apparent that the repair sequence has been completed, either by acknowledging the repair or by uttering a sequentially appropriate turn following the repair.

These seemingly straightforward sequences demonstrate several important issues in repair behavior:

- From the turn containing the trouble source in each sequence, it is not possible in either case or indeed in the vast majority of instances of OISR sequences to identify where or how a stretch of talk resulted in a trouble source and as such, no allocation of "blame" or responsibility for the breakdown can be made. The concept of error by speaker or listener is thus replaced with the concept of miscommunication for which the responsibility is shared.
- The stretch of talk that is the focus of the repair may not always be identifiable prior to the repair being initiated. Nor is it always apparent why a particular portion of talk has given rise to a turn implying the need to repair.
- Repair initiators tend to follow two forms. The first is the general repair initiator (as in Dialogue 10–1 above) in which no direction is given about the exact location or type of miscommunication that has arisen. This has been labeled an *open class* repair initiator (Drew, 1997). The second is the specific repair initiator (Dialogue 10–2) in which either the location and/or the type of trouble source is indicated in the content of the repair initiator.
- Repetition of some or all of the turn containing the TS is the most common response to general repair initiators. Variations in syntactic and phonetic characteristics may be noted between

the TS and its repetition in the repair turn, the repetition is seldom an exact repetition in either its grammatical or its suprasegmental presentation (Curl, 2002, 2004). Repairs uttered in response to specific repair initiators either take the form of repetitions or the provision of additional information (Lind, 2006).

- Repair confirmations take two forms. They are either overt comments of a change of state of understanding (e.g., "Oh!") (Schiffrin, 1987) or they are assumed in the re-uptake of the topic at hand.
- It cannot always be inferred what type of miscommunication resulted in the initiation of the repair sequence. It should not be assumed that all repairs arise from mishearings or that they are the sole preserve of the hearing-impaired participants in the conversation.

The Third Position Repair (3PR) Sequence

The 3PR sequence has also been implicated in the effects of acquired hearing impairment on conversation repair (Lind et al., 2006). Lind (2006) reported that this sequence occurs less commonly in free conversation amongst familiar conversation partners than does the OISR sequence. However it has much greater impact potentially on conversational fluency than does the OISR sequence. In the 3PR sequence, a breakdown is only recognized to have occurred when a subsequent turn is noted to be "sequentially non-implicated" (Schegloff, 1992); that is, when one participant's turn is not able to be understood by the other in the context of his or her own prior turn. In this case, the responsibility falls to the one participant to identify the repair initiator, to clarify what has been misunderstood and then to undertake the repair to clarify the original utterance. Two examples of 3PR sequences appear in Dialogues 10–4 and 10–5.

These 3PR sequences highlight two important points:

- The turn that first identifies the need for repair is not the repair initiator, rather it is the sequentially non-implicated prior turn (lines 4 and 3, respectively, in the dialogue extracts) in which the loss of sufficient mutual ongoing understanding is lost (albeit temporarily).
- The responsibility falls to the person uttering the trouble source to also take on the burden of both the repair initiation and repair. That is, there is no recognition by the speaker of the sequentially non-implicated turn that a miscommunication has occurred. As such this sequence type places greater emphasis on the monitoring of the conversation by the speaker of the trouble source.

Dialogue 10–4. 3PR sequence "Automatic teller"

Line	Participant	Repair Activity	Text
1	FCP	TS	yeah did you w- did you see where the other machine's
2	FCP	TS	gone?
3			(0.3)
4	**HI**	turn	it's **gone**
5	FCP	RI/R	yeah but (0.3) on the board it had (0.8) had in pen that it
6			had gone somewhere else down the road
7	**HI**	RC	oh::

Dialogue 10–5. 3PR sequence "Fishing"

Line	Participant	Repair Activity	Text
1	**HI**	TS	it was a nice catch you got last week
2			(0.9)
3	FCP	turn	yeah (1.7) there weren't [that many
4	**HI**	RI/R	[nice a nice **s:ize**
5	FCP	RC	they're a good size weren't they (0.6) what size were they↑
6			(0.7)
7	**HI**		oh over forty centimeters not bad for whiting
8	FCP		ah very good

In Dialogue 10–4 the turn uttered in lines 1 and 2 is recognized as having been miscommunicated by the sequentially nonimplicated turn that follows in line 4. That is, the line 4 turn does not directly address the line 1 comment concerning the whereabouts of the ATM that had moved, instead it comments that it HAS moved. In response the FCP utters "Yeah, but . . . " as the repair initiator and then undertakes the repair by qualifying the trouble source with additional information about the moved ATM. The repair confirmation is a simple "oh?" Similarly, in Dialogue 10–5, the line 1 turn is responded to in line 3 with a turn that seems to the reader to be a reasonable response but which the HI individual marks in line 4 by correcting the implication drawn by the FCP that there had been lots of fish caught with the comment that she was referring to the size not the number of the fish they caught. The conversation follows on from this point as it is made clear that both participants have re-established mutual ongoing understanding. In both these examples the central issue of the 3PR sequence is the uttering of a sequentially nonimplicated turn as a marker of miscommunication by one participant. This is followed by a turn containing both a repair initiator and a repair undertaken by the participant. In these cases it is the person recognizing the miscommunication and then having to undertake both the initiator and the repair who carries the major onus of this repair sequence.

In the following sections a number of sequential aspects of these repair sequences are discussed with particular reference to the impact of hearing impairment on the occurrence of these sequences outlined above. Finally, this view of repair is applied to audiologic rehabilitation (AR) assessment and intervention techniques in order to suggest how they might incorporate attention on lessening the effects of miscommunications and the time spent in repair on everyday conversations.

Conversation Repair and Adult Acquired Hearing Impairment

In the context of this chapter, the questions arise, how postlingual hearing loss influences conversational repair behavior and what type(s) of repair arise most commonly in interaction involving adults with acquired hearing impairment? The following section outlines some recent research by the author and others to address these questions. The key sequential issue is the way that the repair initiator addresses the trouble source and, in turn, how this influences the content of the repair and ultimately the resolution of the miscommunication. Analysis of repair initiators indicated six different repair initiator types, when categorized by grammatical structure and the relationship to the prior turn (Lind, 2006). These are summarized below.

- **General inquiry.** These repair initiators ask a general question of the speaker, but do not identify any portion of talk in the prior turn to inform the speaker of the nature of the trouble source (see also Dialogue 10–2, above). In Dialogue 10–6 below, the general inquiry appears in line 3 as a simple "hm?" This turn provides no guidance to the communication partner of the exact content of the trouble source, simply that there has been a miscommunication and as such is labeled as a "general repair initiator."
- **Metacommentary.** These repair initiators direct the speaker to the reason for or locus of the trouble source, but do not identify directly or indirectly the content of the trouble source. In Dialogue 10–7, the repair initiator (line 4) contains both an apology (a general RI) and a commentary about the HI participant's reception of the previous turn (" . . . I'm not . . . following."), also a general RI. Metacommentaries comment on transmission of another's speech rather than on the content of the turn. In this case the FCP responds with a long and grammatically complex turn in lines 5 to 7, possibly as a consequence of the absence of direction in the initiator about the exact content of the TS.
- **Partial repetition.** These repair initiators comprise brief sequences (commonly three or four words in length), which are

Dialogue 10–6. OISR sequence with general inquiry as repair initiator

Line	Participant	Repair Activity	Text
1	FCP	TS	how would that do for a birthday present
2			(0.5)
3	**HI**	RI	hm::?
4	FCP	R	how would it do for a birthday present?
5			(0.8)
6	**HI**	RC	yeah you could do that ((whispered laugh))

Dialogue 10–7. Metacommentary as repair initiator

Line	Participant	Repair Activity	Text
1	FCP	TS	we always used to camp in the winter (1.0) so (0.7) camping
2	FCP	TS	in the winter in Victoria is (0.7) is no different
3			(1.7)
4	**HI**	RI	sorry I'm not (0.7) not following
5	FCP	R	I mean if you're going to end up south (1.0) sooner (1.6)
6	FCP	R	that's no different to short holidays we used to have we
7	FCP	R	always used to go **away** in the winter time=
8	**HI**	RC	=yeah

exact (or nearly exact) repetitions of a portion of talk in the immediately prior turn. In response to the partial repetition repair initiator, the speaker of the trouble source on almost all occasions repeats a portion of their previous turn, commencing with the content of the partial repetition and continuing to the end of that TCU or to the next. In Dialogue 10–8, the initiator in line 3 addresses the content of the line 1 trouble source by uttering a portion of that turn with an upward inflection. In response the FCP repeats the word immediately following from line 1, the revised understanding of which is then clearly identified in line 5.

- **Specific *Wh* question.** These repair initiators repeat a portion of the content of the prior spoken turn and either precede or follow this with a *Wh* question. In Dialogue 10–9, the HI participant asks a direct *Wh* question ("What am I gonna do?") identifying the content of the trouble source and resulting in the FCP repeating the part of her turn commencing with the portion of the turn that answers the question asked in the initiator. Note that this initiator also interrupts the turn containing the trouble source mid-TCU which may help mark the portion of the turn to be addressed in the repair.
- **Candidate interpretation.** These repair sequences involve a repair initiator in which a portion of the TS is repeated with an upward inflection. In response the

Dialogue 10–8. Partial repetition as repair initiator

Line	Participant	Repair Activity	Text
1	FCP	TS	. . . they're (0.3) they (0.3) they're in Tuscany at
2	FCP	TS	the moment
3	**HI**	RI	they're in?
4	FCP	R	Tuscany
5	**HI**	RC	*oh are they* ((whispered)) [I] didn't know
6	FCP		[yeah]

Dialogue 10–9. Specific Wh question as repair initiator

Line	Participant	Repair Activity	Text
1	FCP	TS	. . . **if you're going to have** some of this (1.2) u:m asthma
2	FCP	TS	induced (0.8) **heat** induced [asthma]
3	**HI**	RI	[w: what] am I gonna do↑
4			(0.9)
5	FCP	R	if you're going to have some more (0.9) **heat** induced
6	FCP	R	asthma (0.9) /jə/ know the concept of getting away from
7	FCP	R	the cold might be one thing . . .

speaker of the trouble source commonly confirms the content of the repair initiator or provides the correct text of the trouble source. In Dialogue 10–10, the repair initiator contains a candidate portion of the previous turn ("trade in?") with a questioning inflection. The repair turn provides an alternative ("training . . . ") for the content of the RI followed by a definition of the term (" . . . they have to learn things").

- **Multiple-choice question.** In these repair sequences the person uttering the repair initiator commonly provides two alternative choices of interpretation of the trouble source. In response to this the speaker of the trouble source either confirms one of the choices or offers a third alternative. In Dialogue 10–11, a long passage uttered by the FCP in lines 1 to 8 is interrupted in line 10 by an initiator in the form of a multiple choice question concerning the identity of the main character in the preceding turns. In response to this, a repair is undertaken to clarify the identity in line 12. The revised understanding is, in turn, confirmed by the turn in line 14.

Although these sequences have been presented to demonstrate the various categories of repair initiators, it is important to pay attention to the sequentiality of the initiator/repair turns. For this purpose, repair initiators labeled general inquiry and metacommentary have been grouped together under the heading of general repair initiators. The remaining four types have been classified as specific repair initiators. It is the overwhelming, but not only, occurrence that general initiators are followed by repairs of repetition. However, Dialogue 10–7 is an example of a general initiator followed by a repair in which additional information is provided rather than simply repeating the trouble source. Although specific initiators are also often followed by repairs of repetition, there are substantial numbers which are followed by repairs in which information is provided in addition to the content of the trouble source. In Dialogue 10–10, the repair turn (line 5) combines repetition with additional information in the form of a definition of the trouble source.

Schegloff and colleagues (1977) suggested that there was a hierarchy of strength of understanding implied by the content of the repair initiator. As a general rule, specific repair initiators were seen to be more direct than general repair initiators as they contained content of the turn containing the trouble source. Among the specific repair initiators certain were seen to be more powerful markers of the listener's understanding of the trouble source than others. Those repair initiators reporting a candidate interpretation of the trouble source and those reporting a portion of talk leading up to the trouble source (and thus directly locating the trouble source) were considered to be the "strongest" repair initiators. Those asking a specific *Wh* question (e.g., "Where?," "When?," or "Who?") were considered to be less overt and

Dialogue 10–10. Candidate interpretation as repair initiator

Line	Participant	Repair Activity	Text
1	FCP	TS	I mean they'll obviously be involved for the Olympics but I
2	FCP	TS	don't know how much (1.1) how much **training** time there
3	FCP	TS	might be
4	**HI**	RI	**trade in:?**
5	FCP	R	training they might have to **learn** things
6	**HI**	RI	*oh right* ((whispered))

Dialogue 10–11. Multiple choice question as repair initiator

Line	Participant	Repair Activity	Text
1	FCP	TS	yeah Ron did say to me last night he said (0.8) when they
2	FCP		(0.7) when Ron when Bob come up and asked me would I be
3	FCP		secretary (1.1) and (2.1) he said you don't have to answer me
4	FCP		now (0.5) have a think about it (0.5) and after he'd (0.7) Bob
5	FCP		had gone back up to the table (1.0) he said uh he said
6	FCP		((unintell)) of these small towns are (0.6) one or two people
7	FCP		(0.5) get looked to (0.5) to do all the work (1.9) but I didn't
8	FCP		answer him
9			(1.2)
10	**HI**	RI	this is eh- eh- Bluey saying this or Bob?
11			(0.8)
12	FCP	R	this is Ron
13			(0.5)
14	**HI**	RC	oh Ron↓

thus 'weaker' repair initiators (Schegloff et al., 1977, p. 267).

Despite the compelling nature of this argument, our research found no difference in the length or complexity of OISR sequences when categorized by repair initiator type in free conversation between familiar adults in quiet environments, with conversation as the focal activity (Lind et al., 2004). This is not to suggest that under conditions less conducive than those in our research, there won't be an advantage in the use of specific repair initiators over general repair initiators. However, this has not been demonstrated to this point. There was also no difference in length of repair sequence noted when repairs were allocated by hearing status of the speaker uttering the repair initiator. Repair sequences initiated by adults with acquired hearing losses did not take more turns to resolve than those initiated under the same circumstances by their familiar communication partners (Lind, 2006). These results were surprising as it had been expected that both the HI listeners' hearing acuity and the use of general repair initiators might conspire against a successful completion of a miscommunicated sequence of talk.

In one particular dyad, it was apparent that another force was in play in directing the speaker of the trouble source to its content, despite the use of a general repair initiator (Lind et al., 2006). On several occasions in their conversation, the hearing impaired partner, interrupted (or perhaps more appropriately *interjected*) his partner's talk mid-TCU using a general repair initiator. In response to this, the conversation partner would on every occasion repeat the final or penultimate TCU prior to the interruption. Having done so, in each case the conversation partner's repeated segment of talk was accepted as an appropriate and adequate repair by the hearing impaired adult as he would either confirm understanding of the repaired content or continuing with the conversation. In Dialogue 10–12, the repair initiator ("No, sorry") in line 4 interrupts the previous turn mid-TCU. Despite the general nature of the initiator and the length of the previous turn, both of which militate against the accurate identification of the

Dialogue 10–12. Interjection using a general repair initiator mid-TCU

Line	Participant	Repair Activity	Text
1	FCP	TS	well we used to camp in Victoria previously when it was (1.3) wet
2	FCP	TS	and cold didn't we (0.7) I mean we (0.7) always used to do most
3	FCP	TS	of our **winter** camping (0.7) when we **lived**
4	**HI**	RI	no [sorry]
5	FCP	R	[w-] when we **lived** over there
6	**HI**	RC	yeah

trouble source, the FCP has no hesitation in repeating the last portion only of her previous turn as the candidate repair. This is accepted by the HI participant in line 6, indicating that the repair was indeed successfully identified, the only marker of that portion of text being its proximity to the interruption with the repair initiator.

This finding, limited as it is to the conversation between these two participants, indicates that interjection may indeed be a useful tool in identifying trouble sources of such a complexity that the speaker of the repair initiator has not been able to incorporate any content into the repair initiator. This result also highlights the salience of the TCU as a functional unit of conversation. As in every case, it was either the interrupted TCU alone or with the TCU immediately preceding it that was offered up as the repair. More recent work has indicated that interjection of repair initiators may be limited to interaction between familiar communication partners (Lind & West, in preparation). When OISR sequences are analyzed in conversations between adults with acquired hearing impairment and *unfamiliar* communication partners, there were fewer instances of OISR sequences and importantly, no instances of interjection were noted.

That there were fewer instances of repair possibly reflects changes in the dynamics of politeness between familiar and unfamiliar conversations (Brown & Levinson, 1987; Lind & West, in preparation; Skelt, 2006). Despite a substantially reduced number of OISR sequences in the unfamiliar conversations, there remained a substantial and statistically significant asymmetry in the initiation of these sequences when allocated by hearing status of the individual initiating the repair. It may be speculated that the social tension associated with identifying miscommunications arising in the talk of someone with whom one is unfamiliar, may be greater than in the same situation arising with a familiar communication partner. As such, the potential for the unfamiliar communication partner to *lose face* (Brown & Levinson, 1987) is increased and, thus, the repair is not initiated. The absence of interjection suggests that it may be a characteristic of familiar conversations rather than of conversations in general. It may also reflect differences in perceived politeness as interruptions may be taken as a *face-threatening acts*, and thus less likely to occur in unfamiliar conversations.

The second finding of interest concerns the relationship between topic changes and instances of OISR sequences (Caissie, 2002; Lind, Mann, Coonan, Kane, Miller, & West, in preparation). Topic change was noted to occur in several different forms. Following the analysis of Crow (1983), topic change was identified by its degree, that is, whether it was full or partial topic change and how the topic change related to previous topics in the conversation. Two important points arose from this analysis. Although it may be assumed that abrupt and unexpected topic changes were more likely to result in repairs being initiated, almost all instances of repair occurring in the turn immediately following a topic change did so following a partial rather than a full topic shift. Second, it was no more likely that OISR sequences would follow a topic change than not. OISR sequences seemed to arise in response to misperceived words or phrases whether they were embedded in a topic change or not.

Reliability and Validity in Sampling Conversation Behavior

A further question arises whether repair behavior identified in the clinical setting is a reliable and valid reflection of repair behavior in everyday conversation. Reliability measures were undertaken by comparing the number of sequences of each type (e.g., OISR, 3PR) across each of four 20-minute conversational recordings for four different conversation pairs (Lind, Hickson, & Erber, in preparation). The four 20-minute samples of conversation did not reliably sample across turn repair behavior, but when samples were combined into two 40-minute samples a substantial increase in reliability was noted. This finding remains to be verified by more detailed analysis of the repair behaviors in each of the recording samples. At this point, these results provide initial evidence that sampling techniques for free and unstructured conversation between familiar communication partners in the clinic setting provide reliable insights into patterns of across turn repair behavior.

Sample validity was also assessed by comparing quantitative and qualitative aspects of repair behavior of familiar conversation dyads in their home environments with recordings undertaken in the clinic setting (Lind, Hickson, & Erber, in preparation). Quantitative analysis indicated that the proportion of OISR sequences initiated by the hearing impaired adults and by their normally hearing communication partners did not vary between the clinic and home settings. It was noted also that the same set of repair initiators were used in both settings, and that sequences most commonly resolved in the minimum number of (i.e. three or four) turns. Although clinic recordings were undertaken with conversation as the focal activity, in the home recordings it was apparent that conversation was often undertaken in conjunction with other activities. In some cases conversation was conducted, while both participants undertook separate activities. As such, the lack of mutual focus on the topic associated with one participant's activity may have led to the need to gain attention, or indeed to gain focus on a particular item of context. Despite this important difference, sampling of OISR sequences in the clinic and home demonstrated substantial similarities.

Rehabilitation Techniques in Addressing Patterns of Repair

The CA approach presented in this chapter has demonstrated that each turn in a repair sequence (and indeed in any conversational sequence) can only be considered in the context of the preceding and subsequent turns. To this point the chapter has outlined the behaviors that may potentially influence the sequencing of conversation and conversation repair involving adults with acquired hearing impairment. This section outlines how clinicians might best address repair behaviors in the clinic setting in order to reduce their effect on conversational fluency.

The first question arises as to what format the conversational task might take for assessment and intervention purposes? Free conversation remains the most realistic and thus the most readily generalizable task in the clinic setting. However, for those clients whose difficulties are sufficiently severe to prevent them from participating in conversation, other methods are available to allow the gathering of information about patterns of repair behavior. More structured tasks may be the appropriate clinical tools in these situations.

Clinical conversation sampling implies analysis of repair sequences in real time. Analyses conducted in the studies reported throughout this chapter have been based on both audiotape and fully transcribed conversations of free and unstructured conversation samples. The experienced clinician may be able to identify the OISR and the 3PR sequences and identify the key issues of their sequential structure as they occur or from transcribed material. As an alternative, Pedley et al. (2005) published a simple checklist of repair initiator and repair behaviors in a tabulated form in which the key issues of the repair sequence might be checked off as repairs occur. The checklist divides the analysis of repair behavior into requests for repair (i.e., repair initiators) and repairs. The requests for repair are further divided into general and specific requests, including elliptical and full requests. Repairs are divided into repetitions, rephrasings (commonly simplifications) and reframings (including changes in syntactic structure and semantic cues). The list allows clinicians easier access to on-line analysis of repair behavior and provides useful summary data for assessment and intervention.

An Adaptive Speech Reception Assessment Task

Erber (1996, 2002) introduced the sentence-based speech perception task Sent-Ident as an *adaptive* assessment method. The task requires a substantially more active role to be played by the presenter of the speech material than in traditional speech reception tasks. Although it uses a standard stimulus repetition paradigm, it allows multiple presentations of each stimulus. Furthermore, each presentation of the stimulus is altered as a consequence of the accuracy of the HI adult's performance in response to the prior presentation. In its original form Sent-Ident is conducted in such a manner that any incomplete or inaccurate repetition of the stimulus item leads the presenter to re-present the item with additional visual and/or auditory cues. An individual's performance is scored by the number of times the stimulus is uttered in order for them to reach 100% accurate repetition. It also identifies the auditory-visual conditions under which accurate reception is most likely to occur. However, as noted above, all conversational turns are best understood in the context in which they occur. As such, a modified Sent-Ident procedure may be employed in which the HI recipient is given the opportunity to direct the speaker of the stimulus material to the manner in which it might be best re-presented, rather than relying on a predetermined hierarchy of repair strategies.

In this modified version of the test, the stimulus sentence is read aloud and the client either repeats accurately or initiates a repair. The sender's task is then to incorporate the requested changes into the repeated version of the stimulus utterance. In many ways this modified method mimics some of the essential issues in conversation repair but at a sentence rather than at a textual level. The outcome of the assessment changes from a judgment of which repair strategy works most efficiently to a judgment of which repair initiator/repair sequence works best for the individual.

Continuous Discourse Tracking as Intervention for Repair

Should the clinician feel that conversation sampling is not able to be conducted without placing the client with hearing impairment and/or his or her communication partner under strain or threat of failure, the most conversation-like clinical activity in the AR armamentarium for many years has been continuous discourse tracking (or *tracking*) (deFilippo & Scott, 1978). In its original format, tracking was designed as a measure of information transfer and as a result, is commonly assessed by the number of words repeated accurately by the receiver in a specified period of time (commonly 5 or 10 minutes). Researchers and clinicians alike have been aware for many years of the drawbacks associated with comparing word per minute scores in tracking across texts or sessions. So many potential contaminating influences prevent an accurate assessment of the speed of information processing (LeRoux & Turton, 1990). A second, more conversationally oriented, use of tracking focuses not on the speed of information transfer but on the instances in which the transfer of information is disrupted or breaks down. Each instance in which repair is undertaken is analyzed in order to provide insights into the way participants address conversation breakdown and repair. To this end, many of the "contaminating" variables are rendered inconsequential as transfer of text becomes a means to an end (i.e., practicing repair behaviors) rather than an end in itself.

In the standard form of tracking there are three possible outcomes following the reading of a brief passage of text by the *sender*. In the first instance, the *receiver*, whose task it is to repeat the text back as accurately as possible, does so with 100% accuracy. In response, the sender moves on to the next phrase or clause and no repair is required. In the second instance, the receiver recognizes that they have not fully received the sequence of talk uttered by the sender, and as such the receiver instigates a repair. This pattern of response mirrors exactly the OISR sequences outlined earlier. In the context of tracking, we might refer to this as a *receiver-initiated repair*. In the third instance, the sender reads a portion of text, and the receiver faithfully attempts to repeat that portion of text with 100% accuracy. Following the repetition the sender recognizes that the portion of text has not been accurately repeated, and the sender instigates the repair, the receiver having not recognized that their repetition was not an accurate representation of the passage. This repair sequence follows the 3PR sequences outlined earlier and in the context of tracking might be referred to as a *sender-initiated repair*. Each instance of repair may be analysed for its structure, content, and number of turns taken to reach resolution.

Tracking holds a special place among intervention tools in AR as it mimics aspects of conversation by allowing turn-taking and the development of conversational topics through themes, characters, plots and storylines of the text being transmitted. Its limitations lie in the inability of the recipient to direct the conversation, other than to repeat what they have heard. The key difference between the repairs arising in the context of tracking and their occurrence in a free and unstructured conversation is that all repairs in tracking represent mishearings as tracking requires repetition without any level of contextual or pragmatic understanding. In free conversation, OISR and 3PR sequences may arise as a result of the mishearings, misunderstanding of content and context or of pragmatic intent. This difference highlights the use of tracking for the purpose of addressing surface structure mishearings in a structured clinical task and in a carefully structured clinical setting.

It remains for the clinician to identify the repair turns and to make decisions about which behaviors are adaptive in overcoming mishearings. At the simplest level, sequences which take more than the minimum number turns to resolve are likely to be the first targets for intervention. The clinician might ask what characteristics arose in the repair initiator, and in the repair turn itself and whether they were useful in assisting participants to resolve the breakdown. In summary, issues in assessment and intervention may include:

- Use specific repair initiators wherever possible, and among these repairs those that identify the text of the trouble source or the text immediately preceding it have been suggested to be the most effective initiators.
- General repair initiators are not a lesser option. They are often used strategically to mark a depth of miscommunication that prevents the formulation of a specific initiator.
- Interjection may indeed be a useful repair initiation strategy, especially in conjunction with general repair initiators, although its effectiveness may be limited to conversations between familiar conversation partners.
- Abrupt topic changes do not result in repair more often than turns spoken mid-topic (see also Caissie, 2002). Rather, it seems that more local contextual (e.g., sentence, clausal, phrasal, and lexico-grammatical) forces are at work in miscommunications.
- 40 minute samples of free and unstructured conversation undertaken in a quiet environment by familiar communication partners contain examples of across turn-repair behaviors that are both reliable and valid representations of the number and sequencing of similar repairs uttered in the home environment.
- Repair sequences may vary in conversations with familiar and unfamiliar conversation partners. Furthermore, clients should undertake

this intervention with more than one individual as communication partner, and that the communication partners participating in the exercise should cover a range of familiarity with the hearing impaired individual.

- Intervention might usefully target repair sequences taking more than the minimum number of turns to resolve (commonly, three or four turns).

Ultimately, the aim of AR programs is the generalization of skills learned in the clinic to an individual's everyday communication in order to lessen the effects of their hearing impairment. The selection of appropriate techniques remains largely a matter of speculation and clinical experience rather than evidence. The very great drawback of many of the current audiologic rehabilitation techniques is that there is little or no evidence of generalization from clinical assessment and intervention to everyday talk. Tracking is no exception, and the technique described here remains to be investigated for its efficiency and effectiveness. Any rehabilitation technique must be embedded in a thoughtful progression of clinical activities aimed toward educating both the hearing-impaired adult and his or her chosen communication partners in the technique as a form of practice for the resolution of conversation difficulties outside clinical time and activity.

Conclusion

Conversation repair remains one of the key aspects of communication difficulty arising subsequent to an acquired hearing impairment. Yet, clinicians share little or no common vocabulary in discussing the content, sequence or structure of repair behavior. The therapy technique outlined in this chapter reflects the CA model of repair behavior and its use as an intervention technique relies on an understanding of the nature of conversation and conversation repair. Clinical experience indicates that this technique provides individualized intervention that can be readily and easily adapted by the client into his or her everyday conversational activity.

As clinicians and researchers, we remain at the early stages of understanding of repair behavior. This chapter has aimed to redesign one or two simple assessment and intervention techniques focused on conversation-level work. Their great benefits lie in the relatively brief periods of intervention required to instigate these techniques by contrast with more traditional synthetic and analytic speech perception rehabilitation paradigms. As pressure increases to provide efficient and effective intervention in the face of extremely limited private and or public funds for rehabilitation, the imperative is to provide techniques that are as immediately generalizable to everyday life as possible. The simple ideal behind the work presented in this chapter is the focus on clinical tasks which will allow clients and their communication partners to rapidly and easily apply principles and skills learned in the clinic to everyday conversation.

Further Reading

Interested readers are directed toward research into the effects of adult acquired hearing impairment on conversation activity by Nancy Tye-Murray (Tye-Murray, 1991, 2004; Tye-Murray, Purdy, Woodworth, & Tyler, 1990; Tye-Murray, Witt, & Schum, 1995; Tye-Murray & Witt, 1997), Rachel Caissie (Caissie, 2002; Caissie & Rockwell, 1993; Caissie, Dawe, Donovan, Brooks, & MacDonald, 1998), and Kathy Pichora-Fuller (Pichora-Fuller, Johnson, & Roodenburg, 1998), and their colleagues. Clinically oriented texts by Tye-Murray (2004), Erber (1996, 2002), Erber and Lind (1994), Kaplan, Bally, and Garrettson (1998), Pedley, Giles, and Hogan (2005), and Pedly, Lind and Hunt (2006) may also prove useful. Those wishing to read further may look to the literature in child language development (Brinton, Fujiki, Loeb, & Winkler, 1986) adult second language learning (Bremer, Roberts, Vasseur, Simonot, & Broeder 1988; van Lier, 1988; Zuengler, 1991), as well as aphasia and other adult neurogenic communication disorders (Ferguson, 1994; Goodwin, 2003; Perkins, 1995; Perkins, Crisp, & Walshaw, 1999) for similar analyses of conversation repair. For more general texts on conversation, conversation repair and in particular the Conversation Analytic approach readers are directed to Eggins and Slade (1997), Hutchby and Woffitt (1998), Schegloff (2007), and Schiffrin, (1994).

References

Atkinson, J. M., & Heritage, J. (Eds.). (1984). *Structures of social action: Studies in conversation analysis*. Cambridge: Cambridge University Press.

Bremer, K., Roberts, C., Vasseur, M.-T., Simonot, M., & Broeder, P. (1988). *Achieving understanding: Discourse in intercultural encounters*. London: Longman.

Brinton, B., Fujiki, M., Loeb, D. F., & Winkler, E. (1986). Development of conversational repair strategies in response to requests for clarification. *Journal of Speech and Hearing Research*, *29*, 75–81.

Brown, P., & Levinson, S. (1987). *Politeness: Some universals of language use*. Cambridge: Cambridge University Press.

Caissie, R (2002). Conversational topic shifting and its effect on communication breakdowns for individuals with hearing loss. *Volta Review*, *102*(2), 45–56.

Caissie, R., Dawe, A. L., Donovan, C., Brooks, H., & MacDonald, S. M. (1998). Conversational performance of adults with a hearing loss. *Journal of the Academy of Rehabilitative Audiology*, *31*, 45–67.

Caissie, R., & Rockwell, E. (1993). A videotape analysis procedure for assessing conversational fluency in hearing-impaired adults. *Ear and Hearing*, *14*, 202–209.

Chelst, T. S., Tait, C. A., & Gallagher, T. M. (1990). Linguistic strategies used by normally hearing caregivers in conversations with elderly hearing-impaired spouses. In D. E. Biegel & A. Blum (Eds.), *Aging and caregiving: Theory, research and policy* (pp. 204–218). Newberry Park, CA: Sage.

Clark, H. H., & Schaefer, E. F. (1987). Collaborating on contributions to conversation. *Language and Cognitive Processes*, *2*, 19–41.

Clark, H. H., & Schaefer, E. F. (1989). Contributing to discourse. *Cognitive Science*, *13*, 259–294.

Clark, H. H., & Wilkes-Gibbs, D. (1986). Referring as a collaborative process. *Cognition*, *22*, 1–39.

Clayman, S. E., & Maynard, E. W. (1995). Ethnomethodology and conversation analysis. In P. ten Have & G. Psathas (Eds.), *Situated order: Studies in the social organization of talk and embodied activities* (pp. 1–30). Washington DC: University Press of America.

Crow, B. (1983). Topic shifts in couples' conversations. In R. T. Craig & K. Tracy (Eds.), *Conversational coherence: Form, structure and strategy* (pp. 136–156). Beverley Hills, CA: Sage.

Curl, T. S. (2002). *The phonetics of sequence organization: An investigation of lexical repetition in other-initiated repair sequences in American English*. Unpublished Ph.D. thesis. University of Colorado. Retrieved 10 January, 2008 from http://www-users.york.ac.uk/~tsc3/diss.pdf

Curl, T. S. (2004). "Repetition" repairs: The relationship of phonetic structure and sequence organization. In E. Couper-Kuhlen & C. E. Ford, (Eds.), *Sound patterns in interaction* (pp. 273–298). Amsterdam: John Benjamin.

de Filippo, C. L., & Scott, B. L. (1978). A method for training and evaluating the reception of ongoing speech. *Journal of the Acoustical Society of America*, *63*, 1186–1192.

Drew, P. (1997). "Open" class repair initiators in response to sequential sources of troubles in conversation. *Journal of Pragmatics*, *28*, 69–101.

Eggins, S., & Slade, D. (1997). *Analysing casual conversation*. London: Cassell.

Erber, N. P. (1996). *Communication therapy for adults with sensory loss* (2nd ed.). Clifton Hill, Australia: Clavis.

Erber, N. P. (2002). *Hearing vision communication and older people*. Melbourne: Clavis.

Erber, N. P., & Lind, C. (1994). Communication therapy: Theory and practice. In J.-P. Gagné & N. Tye-Murray (Eds.), *Research in audiological rehabilitation: Current trends and future directions. Journal of the Academy of Rehabilitative Audiology*, *27 (monograph supplement)*, pp. 267–287.

Ferguson, A. (1994). The influence of aphasia, familiarity and activity on conversational repair. *Aphasiology*, *8*(2), 143–157.

Foppa, K. (1995). On mutual understanding and agreement in dialogues. In I. Markovà, C. Graumann & K. Foppa (Eds.), *Mutualities in dialogue* (pp. 149–175). Cambridge: Cambridge University Press.

Ford, C., & Thompson, S. (1996). Interactional units in conversation: Syntactic, intonational and pragmatic resources for the management of turns. In E. Ochs, E. A. Schegloff, & S. Thompson (Eds.), *Interaction and grammar* (pp. 134–184). Cambridge: Cambridge University Press.

Gagné, J.-P., Stelmacovich, P., & Yovetich, W. (1991). Reactions to requests for clarification used by hearing-impaired individuals. *Volta Review, 93*, 129–143.

Gagné, J.-P., & Wylie, K. A. (1989). Relative effectiveness of three repair strategies on the visual-identification of misperceived words. *Ear and Hearing, 10*, 368–374.

Goodwin, C. (Ed.). (2003). *Conversation and brain damage*. New York: Oxford University Press.

Hutchby, I., & Wooffitt, R. (1998). *Conversation analysis: Principles, practices and applications*. Cambridge: Polity Press.

Jefferson, G. (1984). Notes on a systematic deployment of the acknowledgement tokens "yeah" and "Mm hm." *Papers in Linguistics, 17*, 197–216.

Johnson, C. E., & Pichora-Fuller, M. K. (1994). How communication goals may alter handicap. *Journal of Speech-Language Pathology and Audiology, 18*, 235–242.

Kaplan, H., Bally, S. J., & Garretson, C. (1985). *Speechreading: A way to improve understanding*. Washington DC: Gallaudet University.

Le Roux, L., & Turton, R. W. (1990). Methodological considerations in employing the continuous discourse tracking procedure with hearing-impaired adults. *South African Journal of Communication Disorders, 37*, 51–57.

Lind, C. (2006). *Conversation repair and adult acquired hearing impairment*. Unpublished Ph.D. thesis. University of Queensland.

Lind, C., Hickson, L., & Erber, N. P. (2004). Conversation repair and acquired hearing impairment: A preliminary quantitative clinical study. *Australian and New Zealand Journal of Audiology 26*, 40–52.

Lind, C., Hickson, L., & Erber, N. P. (2006). Conversation repair and adult cochlear implantation: A qualitative case study. *Cochlear Implants International, 7*, 33–48.

Lind, C., Hickson, L., & Erber, N. P. (manuscript in preparation). *Conversation repair and acquired hearing impairment: Reliability and validity of clinical sampling*.

Lind, C., Mann, G., Coonan, E., Kane, M., Miller, S., & West, T. (manuscript in preparation). *Conversation repair and acquired hearing impairment: Effects of topic change on frequency and resolution of repair.*

Lind, C., & West, T. (manuscript in preparation). *Conversation repair and adult-acquired hearing impairment: Influences of conversation partner familiarity.*

Lunato, K. E., & Weisenberger, J. M. (1994). Comparative effectiveness of correction strategies in Connected Discourse Tracking. *Ear and Hearing, 15*, 362–370.

Marzolf, C. A., Stewart, M., Nerbonne, M. A., & Lehman, M. E. (1998). Effects of two repair strategies on speechreading of words and sentences. *Journal of the American Academy of Audiology, 9*, 243–248.

Mulac, A., Erlandson, K. T., Farrer, W. J., Hallett, J. S., Molloy, J. L., & Prescott, M. E. (1998). "Uh-huh. What's that all about?" Differing interpretations of conversational backchannels and questions as sources of miscommunication across gender boundaries. *Communication Research, 25*, 641–668.

Pedley, K., Giles., E., & Hogan, A. (2005). *Adult cochlear implant rehabilitation*. London: Whurr.

Pedley, K., Lind, C., & Hunt, P. (2006). *Adult aural rehabilitation: A guide for CI professionals*. Sydney: Cochlear.

Perkins, L. (1995). Applying conversation analysis to aphasia: Clinical implications and analytic issues. *European Journal of Disorders of Communication, 30*, 372–383.

Perkins, L., Crisp, J., & Walshaw, D. (1999). Exploring conversation analysis as an assessment tool for aphasia: The issue of reliability. *Aphasiology, 13*(4/5), 259–281.

Pichora-Fuller, M. K., Johnson, C. E., & Roodenburg, K. E. J. (1998). The discrepancy between hearing impairment and handicap in the elderly: Balancing transaction and interaction in conversation. *Journal of Applied Communication Research, 26*(1), 99–119.

Sacks, H., Schegloff, E. A., & Jefferson, G. (1974). A simplest systematics for the organization of turn-taking in conversation. *Language, 50*, 696–735.

Schegloff, E. A. (1991). Reflections on talk and social structure. In D. Boden & D. Zimmerman (Eds.), *Talk and social structure* (pp. 44–70). Cambridge: Polity Press.

Schegloff, E. A. (1992). Repair after next turn: The last structurally provided defence of intersubjectivity in conversation. *American Journal of Sociology, 97*, 1295–1345.

Schegloff, E. A. (1996a). Confirming allusions: Toward an empirical account of action. *American Journal of Sociology, 102*, 161–216.

Schegloff, E. A. (1996b). Turn organization: One intersection of grammar and interaction. In E. Ochs, E. A. Schegloff, & S. Thompson (Eds.), *Interaction and grammar* (pp. 52–133). Cambridge: Cambridge University Press.

Schegloff, E. A. (2007). *Sequence organization in interaction: A primer in Conversation Analysis*. Cambridge: Cambridge University Press.

Schegloff, E. A., Jefferson, G., & Sacks, H. (1977). The preference for self-correction in the organization of repair for conversation. *Language, 53*, 361–382.

Schegloff, E. A., & Sacks, H. (1973). Opening up closings. *Semiotica, 8*, 289–327.

Schiffrin, D. (1987). *Discourse markers*. Cambridge: Cambridge University Press.

Schiffrin, D. (1994). *Approaches to discourse*. Oxford: Blackwell.

Skelt, L. (2006). *Prevention and repair of problems in talk with adults with acquired hearing impairment*. Unpublished Ph.D. thesis. Australian National University.

Stephens, D., Giannopolous, I., & Kerr, P. (2001). Determination and classification of the problems experienced by hearing-impaired elderly people. *Audiology, 40*, 294–300.

Tye-Murray, N. (1991). Repair strategy usage by hearing-impaired adults and changes following communication therapy. *Journal of Speech and Hearing Research, 34*, 921–928.

Tye-Murray, N. (2004). *Foundations of aural rehabilitation: Children, adults, and their family members* (2nd ed.). San Diego, CA: Singular.

Tye-Murray, N., Purdy, S. C., Woodworth, G. G., & Tyler, R. S. (1990). Effects of repair strategies on visual identification of sentences. *Journal of Speech and Hearing Disorders, 55*, 621–627.

Tye-Murray, N., & Witt, S. (1997). Communication strategies training. *Seminars in Hearing, 18*, 153–165.

Tye-Murray, N., Witt, S., & Schum, L. (1995). Effects of talker familiarity on communication breakdown in conversation with adult cochlear-implant users. *Ear and Hearing, 16*, 459–469.

van Lier, L. (1988). *The classroom and the learning language learner; Ethnography and second-language classroom research*. London: Longman.

Verhagen, A. (2005). *Constructions of intersubjectivity. Discourse, syntax, and cognition*. Oxford: Oxford University Press.

World Health Organization. (2001). *International Classification Of Functioning, Disability and Health*. Geneva, Switzerland: Author.

Wilson, J., Hickson, L., & Worrall, L. (1998). Use of communication strategies by adults with hearing impairment. *Asia Pacific Journal of Speech, Language and Hearing, 3*, 29–41.

Zuengler, J. (1991). Accommodation in native-nonnative interactions: Going beyond the "what" to the "why" in second-language research. In H. Giles, N. Coupland, & J. Coupland (Eds.), *Contexts of accommodation: Developments in applied sociolinguistics* (pp. 223–244). Cambridge: Cambridge University Press.

Appendix 10–A
Transcription Conventions and Notations

Note: Superscripts following symbol descriptions refer to the texts (cited below) from which these notations have been taken, as in some cases the definitions provided below have been copied directly from the original sources.

1. Words and word units

coz — **Nonstandard pronunciation** indicates word or word unit pronounced in non-standard form (e.g., shortened, lengthened, or mispronounced) for which orthography adequately represents individual production or token

/ksz/ — **Phonetic transcription** presented between "/ /," indicates word or word unit that cannot be adequately represented by standard or nonstandard orthography. Summer Institute of Linguistics (2001) IPA (Sophia 93 font) phonetic symbols used.

2. Transcriber's commentary

( )
( )/( ) — **Empty parentheses**[1,2,3] indicate talk in doubt or too obscure to transcribe, symbols (letters, phonetic symbols) inside such parentheses indicate the transcriber's best estimate of what was said. Sometimes multiple possibilities may be identified, appearing either side of a "/"

((points)) — **Double parentheses**[1,2] indicate transcriber's comments, not transcriptions, and may include:

- vocalizations and nonspeech sounds that cannot be spelled recognizably (e.g., ((cough)), ((snort)), ((sniff)), or ((laugh))—abbreviated nonspeech vocalizations (e.g., ((TC))—throat clearing, ((tc))—tongue click, and ((A.Insp.))—audible inspiration),
- other environmental details of the conversational scene (e.g., ((telephone rings))), or
- other characterizations of talk (e.g., ((falsetto)), or ((whispered)), ((laughing)))—where the characteristic of talk is superimposed across a series of words, the words are italicized (e.g., *that's funny* ((laughing)))

3. Overlapping and contiguous talk

[— **Left-side brackets**[1,2] indicate where overlapping talk begins

] — **Right-side brackets**[1,2] indicate where overlapping talk ends, or marks alignment within a continuing stream of overlapping talk

[[— **Double left-side brackets**[2] indicate the overlap of entire utterances

= — **Equals sign**[1,2] indicates a "latched" relationship, or contiguous talk, no silence between items (usually at the end of one line and the start of another) especially when contiguous or overlapping talk has occurred, they are placed at the end of one utterance and the beginning of the contiguous utterance

4. Pausing

(0.8) **Numbers in parentheses**[1,2] indicate periods of silence, in seconds and tenths of seconds. Pauses greater than 0.2 seconds occurring between turns by different speakers have been given "unattributable" status and are noted on a separate line without a speaker label

(.) **Dot in parentheses**[1] indicate a pause equal to or less than two-tenths of a second

5. Segmental timing

::: **Colon or colons**[1,2] indicate lengthening of a sound that just precedes them, the amount of lengthening is proportional to the number of colons

becau- **Hyphen/dash**[1,2] indicates an abrupt cutoff or self-interruption of the sound in progress indicated by the preceding letter(s) or phoneme(s).

6. Stress

he says **Bolding**[2,3] indicate increased stress or emphasis. May occur across one or two letters/phonemes for all or part of word token (e.g., em**ployee**)

he says (underlined) **Bolding with underlining**[3] Indicate additional or further increased stress (e.g., em**ploy**ee, with "ploy" underlined)

7. Intonation

↓ **Downward arrow**[2] indicates a stopping fall in tone, not necessarily at the end of a sentence

↑ **Upward arrow**[2] indicates a rising inflection , not necessarily a question

? **Question mark** Questioning inflection

↕ **Upward/downward arrow**[2] indicates an animated tone not necessarily an exclamation

8. Textual ellipsis

. . . . **Widely spaced row of dots**[2] indicate "horizontal ellipses" (A & H, 1984) in which intervening portions of an utterance are omitted as unnecessary or irrelevant

.
.
. **Vertically placed dots**[2] indicate "vertical ellipses" (A & H, 1984) in which intervening turns are omitted as unnecessary or irrelevant

---

References cited by superscript
[1]Schegloff (1996b)
[2]Atkinson and Heritage (1984, pp. ix–xvi)
[3]Schegloff and Sacks (1973)

11

Visual Speech Perception in Spoken Language Understanding

Charissa R. Lansing

Introduction

In producing spoken language, a talker creates patterns of kinematic patterns that may be externally observable in the opening and closing gestures of the lips, displacements of the jaw, and dynamic deformations of the skin within different face regions. These motions are inherent in the production of the segmental and prosodic elements that constitute spoken language. Motions in the eye regions of the talker, such as deformations of the eyebrows, eye-widening, and shifts in gaze may also be used to assist the perceiver in language understanding. In addition, speech-related head and body movements, supplemented with manual gestures, may help to convey prosodic, linguistic information. These sets of complex, and highly redundant streams of acoustic and optical stimuli in spoken language production, elicit behavioral and physiologic responses by the human perceiver who attempts to extract meaningful information and integrate it efficiently to achieve language understanding. The discussion of visual speech perception that follows embraces the premise that the cross-modal stimulation from optical and acoustic events contribute to multisensory enhancement in speech perception. The conceptual framework is described that human perceivers utilize a body of cognitive/linguistic knowledge and visual processes to facilitate spoken language understanding.

In the literature on audiologic rehabilitation (AR), the terms lipreading or speechreading are applied to visual speech perception, a form of information processing. Some authors interchange these terms, but others limit the term "lipreading" to visual speech perception without sound, specifically. For the purposes of this chapter, the term speechreading will be used to refer to " . . . a process of perceiving spoken language using vision as the sole source of sensory evidence . . . " (Boothroyd,

1988, p. 77). Facial motion in speech production is thought to augment or replace degraded auditory information (Erber, 1969). Several investigators have demonstrated that speech understanding is improved under conditions in which perceivers have access to audible information supplemented with the visible information conveyed by movements of the talker's lips and other facial regions in speech production, compared to that achieved with audible information alone (for a review, see Summerfield, 1979). Human perception of a talking person, however, is tied to the synchrony between audible and visible aspects of the talker's speech, and accuracy in identification may be reduced when this synchrony is disrupted (Dodd, 1977; Grant, van Wassenhove, & Poeppel, 2004).

Contribution of Visual Information in Spoken Language Understanding

In everyday communication situations in which humans typically observe one another, the perception of spoken language consists of concurrent and multiple sensations in auditory and visual sensory modalities. Instead of perceiving a separate stream of audible vocalizations, related in time and space to a sequence of visible face and body movements, humans perceive a person talking, a unified cross-modal object or event.

The term "visual hearing," introduced by Cotton (1935), is applied to the unconscious use of vision in everyday communication situations. Cotton demonstrated the contribution of vision in understanding spoken language for sentences partially masked by the presence of a loud buzzing noise which reduced its quality and introduced ambiguity into the speech signal. When participants were permitted to see the talker's face movements simultaneously, concurrent with speech production, sentence understanding improved compared to that for listening alone. Similarly, Sumby and Pollack (1954) have demonstrated that word understanding in noise may be enhanced when the talker can be seen. Their data have been interpreted to illustrate that access to a talker's face movements may be functionally equivalent to improving the signal-to-noise ratio. These findings have been supported more recently by Grant and Seitz (2000) who have demonstrated that access to a talker's congruent speech movements improves accurate detection of sentences partially masked by white noise compared to that for the degraded auditory signal alone. Methodologies that degrade the quality of the audible signal reduce vision to a supportive role; however, there is a growing body of empirical evidence to demonstrate that vision penetrates speech communication. This is true, not only when perceivers see the talker's speech movements for speech that is difficult to hear and ambiguous, but also for speech that is easy to hear and understand. In a series of experiments, Reisberg, McLean, and Goldfield (1987) required perceivers to rapidly repeat back messages in a foreign language, produced with an unfamiliar accent, or consisting of syntactically and semantically complex narratives. They demonstrated that performance was improved if the perceivers both saw and heard the talker, compared to only hearing the talker. More recent findings by Arnold and Hill (2001) and Massaro, Cohen, Gesi, Heredia, and Tsuzaki (1993) support the conclusion that auditory, as well as visual, sensory stimulation can influence the identification of speech segments. These findings further support the contention that visual information not only supplements but complements auditory information (Summerfield, 1987).

Visual information also contributes to verbal and nonverbal forms of learned and innate social behaviors in humans and other animals (Argyle & Cooke, 1976). Evidence from studies that measure eye gaze in auditory-visual tasks of speech understanding demonstrates that perceivers attend to mouth movements as well as movements in the upper face regions (e.g., the eyes) of a talker (Lansing & McConkie, 2003). Watching the talker's face not only improves the accuracy with which perceivers understand segmental aspects of spoken language, but it influences understanding of human communication at many levels. Visual information serves to regulate interactions in conversation, for example, talkers may use eye contact, shifts in gaze, or facial expressions to signal the end of an utterance or a new conversational turn (Argyle & Cook, 1976). The talker's face also conveys valuable information about prosody as it relates to: emotions, intent (asking a question, making a statement, etc.), force (timid, bland, excited, expressive, cynical, etc.), emphasis, and phrasing. To interpret spoken language, perceivers must recognize not only what is said, but also how it is said. A simple optical image, such as the display of a static facial expression, has been shown to impact judgments of the emotion in a heard voice (Vroomen, Driver, & DeGelder, 2001). Depending on the talker's emotional attitude and willingness to share information about his or her emotional state, changes in acoustic cues, such as intonation (voice pitch register), or optical cues, such as facial expressions, may influence interpretation and response in speechreading (Johansson, 1997; Lidestam, 2002).

Results from psychophysical experiments in visual speech perception demonstrate the usefulness of observable kinematic patterns produced by talkers to convey segmental and prosodic information for speech understanding. Although expert speechreaders report that movements in a talker's cheeks may aid speechreading, it is critical to understand the stimulus-response characteristics for visual processing in language understanding. For example, facial motion may be characterized in spatial and temporal domains as a unified percept (Gestalt) or in terms of parallel and/or simultaneous dynamic motions for facial features across multiple locations. In speech production, quantifiable motion produced by kinematic activity and observable in the regions of the talker's jaw, cheeks, and mouth is closely related to the temporal and acoustic characteristics of speech (Yehia, Rubin, & Vatikiotis-Bateson, 1998). In addition, there are extensive correlations among motions at different facial regions (Vatikiotis-Bateson, Eigsti, Yano, & Munhall, 1998).

Several researchers have attempted to identify critical face motion in visual perception of spoken language. Greenberg and Bode (1968) compared the visual perception in word recognition under two viewing conditions: full-face versus lips-only (in which the lips, jaw, and upper larynx region of the talker were visible). The latter condition was achieved by mounting an opaque mask over the video display of a television monitor to obscure the talker's nose and upper face regions. Their data supported the usefulness of the entire face for accurate consonant recognition in words. Other researchers report results that demonstrate observable speech gestures from the lips and mouth region of a talker are sufficient for accurate word recognition and access to observable motion in other face regions does not increase perception significantly (Ijsseldijk, 1992; Marassa & Lansing, 1995). Some individuals have been shown to discriminate among a small set of syllable segments without directly gazing at the phonetic gestures produced by the mouth of the talker (Massaro, 1998). Although masking of the talker's mouth limits speech perception, perceivers have been shown to identify 70% of visually distinct categories of consonants (visemes) in /a/ and /aw/ vowel contexts with the mouth masked (Preminger, Lin, Payen, & Levitt, 1998). In addition to facial motion, perceivers have been shown to be sensitive to speech-related head movements of the talker that may facilitate language processing (Munhall, Jones, Callan, Kuratate, & Vatikiotis-Bateson, 2004).This diverse set of findings supports the hypothesis that facial motion at the mouth and in other face regions, as well as head movement, provide useful cues about speech production, linguistic segments, and language.

Monitoring Visual Processes

Perceivers use vision to acquire information about visual objects and events in the world and to monitor anticipated or actual objects/events. To obtain maximal visual resolution perceivers produce abrupt, high velocity rotations of their eyes (saccades) to direct the highly specialized, densely packed, cone receptor cells that lie within the fovea, a small region on the retina, toward an event, object, or region of interest (for a review, see Hallett, 1986).

Eye monitoring techniques have been used to study a variety of information processing tasks, such as reading, face recognition, and scene analyses (for a review, see Rayner, 1998). Data from eye monitoring may also be useful in understanding the role of visual processes in speechreading (Lansing & McConkie, 1994). Information, acquired in real time, about the perceiver's dynamics of eye gaze (e.g., frequency, location, and duration) may further our understanding of the eye-mind connection, that is, how the brain controls the eyes to select, extract, and process visual information in spoken language understanding. Although foveal fixation is related to concurrent cognitive and attentional processing, it is possible for a perceiver to direct gaze toward one region of interest but attend to a different one (Posner, 1980). Therefore, the validity of the eye-mind connection requires appropriate experimental controls.

The basic methodological approach to interpreting eye monitoring data is to define the spatial and temporal characteristics of the speech-reading stimulus and to study these in relation to the record of eye movement data in a task that requires spoken language processing, indexed by some quantifiable performance measure (e.g., for a review, see Lansing, 2004). For example, Lansing and McConkie (2003) displayed video clips on a computer monitor of everyday sentences (presented with and without sound) spoken by a talker using natural facial expression. Perceivers with some speechreading proficiency were instructed to recall each sentence and then to say it aloud, immediately after each clip. Eye movements (saccadic activity) of the perceivers were monitored as each clip was displayed to obtain a detailed record of the sequence and duration for eye gazes directed to different parts of the video display. The eye movement records were then time-linked to the frames of the video clips and mapped onto corresponding regions of interest on the face of the talker.

Results reported by Lansing and McConkie (1994) documented that perceivers shift their eye gaze from the mouth to the cheeks, chin, or jaw of the talker to understand spoken language without sound, in tasks that require understanding of phonetic information. A working hypothesis, the Gaze Direction Assumption, suggested by Lansing and McConkie (1999), is that perceivers have a strong tendency to direct their gaze (i.e., make direct foveal fixations) toward the talker's face regions from which visual information is being sought to carry out a particular speech perception task. For intonation judgments, perceivers spent more time and directed more gazes toward a talker's upper face regions (that displayed eyebrow movement and eye-widening) than for word recognition; and, results from a second experiment demonstrated that, when facial motion in the upper face was restricted, accuracy in intonation judgments was reduced significantly (Lansing & McConkie, 1999).

Vatikiotis-Bateson et al. (1998) reported that perceivers with normal hearing directed gaze primarily toward the eyes of the talker when given the opportunity to watch and listen to a talker producing long monologues against a background of noise, and that salient observable speech gestures did not appear to draw the perceiver's gaze toward the mouth of the talker. However, Lansing and McConkie (2003) reported that perceivers primarily shift their gaze toward the talker's mouth dynamically during periods of speech production, especially for difficult sentence identification tasks in which a verbatim word correct score is the goal and no access to audible speech is provided. Although present research suggests that information about detailed phonetic information is available at the mouth of the talker, in some instances, speechreading was successful with gaze directed at the eyes of the talker. This suggests that relevant facial motion for speech understanding may also be acquired peripherally. Therefore it is important to understand if perceivers typically direct their gaze toward the mouth of the talker during speech periods because this is the primary source of information, or if they are monitoring the full complexity of the visual stimulus configuration of the face. Further research questions should focus on understanding how attention is deployed in the speechreading process because the eye movement data do not reveal how broadly attention may be distributed or if covert shifts in attention are occurring in acquiring information for speech understanding.

Multisensory Enhancement

Given cross-modal input, the brain will characteristically integrate or bind cues across modalities. In the case of speech perception, this integration may heighten a perceiver's sensitivity to the stimulus as a whole and increase the speed of interpreting the stimulus. A growing body of research has developed models for behavioral processes and neural mechanisms consistent with physiological evidence to support the grouping of cues within visual and auditory modalities, the convergence of cross-modal cues, and neural substrates dedicated to multisensory integration. The brain's fundamental ability to perform this integration is consistent with the general theory of perception proposed by Gibson (1966), and the ecologically driven manner in which communication is conveyed in the direct realism approach to modeling speech perception (Fowler, 1986, 1996). The recovery of communicative intent from the visible and audible cues of speech gestures and facial expressions has implications for models of auditory-visual spoken language recognition and human perception and performance.

Perceptual models of multisensory enhancement may be useful in conceptualizing processes in spoken language understanding by a person with a hearing loss. It has been argued that the ability to fuse streams of information across different modalities is fundamental to the percept of similarity (Marks, 1978). This similarity, which Gibson (1966) refers to as intermodal invariance, and Lewkowicz (1994) terms intersensory equivalence, is one way in which multimodal information may enhance perception. Stimulation in different modalities with modality-specific attributes may also result in perceptual associative processes (e.g., hearing a child laugh, seeing her smiling mouth and crinkled appearance of the outer corners of her eyes are associated to signify the emotional state of happiness). Another effect is that of enhancing comprehension for cues in one modality by providing concurrent access to cues in another modality (e.g., accurate identification of audible place-of-articulation cues, such as voice-onset-time for "ba" versus "ga," in noise is enhanced when supplemented by visible cues of the observable phonetic gestures). In contrast, Lewkowicz (2000) reports that cues in one modality may dominate and reduce the sensitivity or responsiveness to cues from another modality (e.g., the visual modality dominates when seeing a talker produce the phonetic gesture for the syllable "va" accompanied by the vocalization for "ba," maintaining the percept in the visual modality of "va").

In adults with normal hearing, physiologic evidence from event-related potential (ERP) studies supports facilitation/inhibition effects in multimodal integration that occur by around 100 ms, corresponding to the N1/P2 event-related-potential (ERP), for identification of auditory-visual speech stimuli presented in quiet. Data reported by Besle, Fort, Delpuech, and Giard (2004) for audiovisual speech identification in quiet demonstrated suppressed neural activity of N1 generators which they suggest marks neural facilitation for bimodal stimulation. Similarly, Giard and Peronnet (1999) observed a similar effect for object recognition. More recently, van Wassenhove, Grant, and Poeppel (2005) reported decreased latencies (i.e., temporal facilitation) for auditory-visual speech compared to auditory-only speech recognition. These sets of data provide evidence to support the existence of underlying neural mechanisms in perceptual enhancement and may be useful in quantifying how quickly visual sensory stimulation penetrates acoustic information in speech perception. Less is known, however, about the time course of multimodal integrative processes and their neural underpinnings.

McGurk and Ventriloquism Effects

Two well-known phenomena demonstrate our proclivity for intersensory/perceptual unity: the McGurk effect (McGurk & MacDonald, 1976), and the ventriloquism effect (Jack & Thurlow, 1973). To demonstrate the McGurk effect, stimuli are created to show full-motion video of a talker producing a visible syllable, such as "ba," presented with a different audible syllable simultaneously, such as, "ga." Given this specific combination, most perceivers will report hearing "da." Depending on the particular syllables selected, the visual modality may dominate the percept or be partly influenced. This effect has been demonstrated with young infants (Rosenblum, Schmuckler, & Johnson, 1997), across a variety of languages (e.g., Massaro, Cohen, Gesi, Heredia, & Tsuzaki, 1993), and for pairings of visible and auditory components for speakers of different genders (Green, Kuhl, Meltzoff, & Stevens, 1991). The McGurk effect is more robust with some consonants than others (McGurk & MacDonald, 1976) and less sensitive to vowels than consonants (Summerfield & McGrath, 1984). Rosenblum and Saldaña (1996) observed the effect in perceivers who observed highly reduced faces, represented by points-of-light displays and often were not aware that they were looking at faces. It is also evident when perceivers touch, rather than see the face (Fowler & Dekle, 1991). Similarly, noncongruent, simultaneous visible and haptic sensations influence modality dominance in the perception of a variety of physical attributes, such as shape (Miller, 1972), texture (Lederman, Thorne, & Jones, 1986), depth (Singer & Day, 1969), and orientation (Over, 1966).

The ventriloquism effect (Jack & Thurlow, 1973) is illustrated by our adaptation to the discordance between concurrent visual and auditory modal stimulation (Radeau & Bertelson, 1977, 1978). In this illustration, the perceiver hears the voice of the ventriloquist and concurrently observes the opening and closing gestures of the puppet's mouth. Although the acoustic signals do not emanate from the puppet's mouth (and typically contain consonant substitutions due to the ventriloquist's closed-mouth postures), they are perceived as being closer to the puppet than they actually are. Consequently, the spatially discrepant stimulations in the auditory and visual sensory modalities are fused to perceive a talking puppet. A similar phenomenon occurs while watching movie scenes on a television equipped with a single, stationary loudspeaker. Although the sound emanates from a single loudspeaker, perceivers associate particular voices with particular characters as they are depicted in different locations within the scene (Stein & Stanford, 2008). The ventriloquism effect demonstrates spatial biases that can also be demonstrated with non-speech audiovisual stimuli such as sounds bursts paired with point flashes of light, as well as with other modality pairs such as audition by touch and touch by vision (De Gelder & Bertleson, 2003).

Although the McGurk and ventriloquism effect may be demonstrated in the laboratory and provide insights into multimodal integration and perception, De Gelder and Bertleson (2003) question their ecologic validity. Their concern is that these effects may not be genuine, automatic perceptual processes. Instead, they may be associated with strategies adopted by perceivers to meet the demands of experimental tasks. Additional information regarding the underlying neural basis of multimodal integration and perception is needed to enhance our understanding of these processes.

Impact of Hearing Loss

Although our perceptual systems have a proclivity for intersensory equivalence, this may not be desirable in complex auditory scenes, in which sensations in auditory modalities are degraded. This may be due to competition from stationary and nonstationary sound sources, such as background noises and other people talking, as well as alterations of sound transmission due to reflective properties of room surfaces, contributing to perceptual errors in understanding audible signals. Consequently, to achieve spoken language understanding under adverse listening situations human perceivers may need to depend on sensations in the visual modality to a greater extent than those in the auditory modality. One explanation for enhanced performance by the addition of visual cues is that some speech sounds are vulnerable to distortion in background noise, but their kinematic patterns (observable in speech production) are robust, for example, distinctions among sounds that differ in their place-of-articulation, such as /p/ versus /t/ (Summerfield, 1987). Enhancement from access to the talker's speech movements under audiovisual conditions may be directly related to the perceiver's ability to extract information in the auditory and the visual sensory modalities. Degraded information extraction due to the constraints of hearing loss, especially when exacerbated by adverse listening conditions, may require the perceiver to depend primarily on sensations in the visual modality to enhance, or perhaps to achieve, spoken language understanding.

Grant, Walden, and Seitz (1998) have proposed a model to help explain problems in understanding audiovisual speech, dependent on processes that involve: extracting information for auditory and visual modalities across various levels of linguistic complexity; recognition of prosodic, semantic, and syntactic constraints; processing speed for auditory, visual, and auditory-visual sensory modalities; and the integration of auditory and visual cues. These researchers suggest that difficulties in any one of these processes may affect speech understanding under audiovisual conditions. One theoretical controversy focuses on conclusions about individual differences in the ability to integrate acoustic and optical cues for speech understanding (Grant, 2002). Grant and Seitz (1998) argue that perceivers differ in the efficiency with which they integrate cross-modal information with support from results of stepwise multiple regression analyses; however, Massaro and Cohen (2000) suggest that when these same data are submitted to their fuzzy logic model of speech perception (FLMP), a probabilistic goodness of fit model, the results do not support the hypothesis of individual differences in integration efficiency. One challenge in understanding differences in extracting information and its integration is that there are no established methods for assessing integration efficiency (Grant, 2002). Nevertheless, there is a substantial body of evidence to demonstrate that vision penetrates speech perception and contributes synergistically to enhance speech understanding compared to that achieved with hearing alone.

Limitations of Visual Information in Spoken Language Understanding

The task of the speech-reader is to detect, select, and interpret meaningful cognitive/linguistic optical cues from the complex movements produced by the talker's facial expressions, speech gestures, and possibly head and body motions that are congruent with the acoustic stream of spoken language. When fused, these cross-modal cues may enhance spoken language understanding. A complex of multidimensional factors, however, constrains the visual perception of spoken language. Three primary factors include: (a) stimulus characteristics, (b) talker-specific characteristics, and (c) the proficiency of the perceiver. The perceptual weighting of these factors and the differences among their potential synergistic effects in cross-modal stimulation are not well understood, but may account for the large variance associated with performance outcomes in speech understanding observed across perceivers.

Stimulus Characteristics

In spoken conversational English, much speech information is indistinguishable through vision alone (e.g., distinctions between voiced vs. voiceless sounds, Lisker & Abramson, 1964). This is because many sounds are hidden in the mouth, produced with indistinguishable speech gestures or closely related places of articulation, or produced with variation in their production that is influenced by neighboring sounds (coarticulation). Some speech gestures are more visible than others. For example, salient place-of-articulation cues (Binnie, Montgomery, & Jackson, 1974) and extended-rounded and vertical lip-separation cues (Montgomery & Jackson, 1983) contribute to the visibility of linguistic segments. Fisher (1968) coined the term "viseme," a possible analogy to the term "phoneme" applied to acoustic units of speech, to describe categories of vowels and consonants that are indistinguishable from one another. Although English contains approximately 40 phonemes, several phonemes may constitute a viseme. The number of visemes that a perceiver identifies, and the specific speech gestures for sounds that constitute a viseme cluster, may differ as a function of the talker (Kricos & Lesner, 1982). This variability may contribute to the observation that some talkers are easier to speechread than others. Under ideal speechreading conditions, in which the talker adopts a clear speaking style, many more visemes clusters may be distinguished than under usual daily conditions in which the talker adopts a conversational speaking style (for a review, see Jeffers & Barley, 1971). Independent of the number of viseme categories recognized by a perceiver, estimates by Berger (1972) indicate that approximately 50% of words in conversational English may be easily confused with one another based on visual information alone due to ambiguous or limited observable characteristics (e.g., consider the homophemes produced in the following phrases which are very difficult to distinguish through the visual sensory modality alone: "I love you . . . island view . . . olive, too").

Linguistic Constraints

In addition to sensory constraints (the visibility of sound movement patterns), linguistic factors influence speechreading performance. It is well known that spoken language contains a variety of linguistic constraints at the pragmatic, topical, semantic, syntactic, lexical, and phonological levels. The body of cognitive/linguistic knowledge that a perceiver brings to the speechreading task about these constraints, as well as variations in their redundancy may affect speechreading performance (Boothroyd, 1988; Summerfield, 1983). Facial expressions or gestures, common to a spoken language or culture, may also have a functional role in social communication unique to a language/cultural group (for example, Greeks may use an upward nod of their heads to signal disagreement and a downward nod to signal agreement which may be confusing to tourists from the United States or northern Europe who typically nod their heads up and down to signal agreement; for a review see Kirch, 1979). Additional linguistic rules of a particular language, for example, may constrain specific combinations or sequences of sounds in the lexicon of that language. Knowledge about these patterns may assist the speechreader in identifying a lexical unit when data about that unit are either incomplete or inaccessible due to signal distortion or other ambiguity. For more complex linguistic units, such as connected discourse, knowledge about the predictability of semantic or syntactic constraints may be useful in resolving ambiguities. Strategies to manipulate the level of redundancy or the complexity of linguistic segments are also utilized to change the difficulty of training/practice activities or in the assessment of speechreading proficiency. A richer linguistic context appears to facilitate sentence and word understanding (Auer & Bernstein, 1997; Lidestam & Besko, 2006). For example, it may be more difficult for a perceiver to recognize a string of unrelated lexical items than it would be to recognize these same items if organized to form a grammatically correct sentence. Speechreading has also been shown to improve when relevant contextual cues are provided to the perceiver, e.g., use of question-answer formats (Erber, 1992); contextual topical/situational cues (Gagné, Tugby, & Michaud, 1991; Garstecki & O'Neill, 1980). Lyxell and Rönnberg (1991) suggest that less skilled speechreaders may rely on available contextual information in word discrimination tasks to a greater extent than skilled speechreaders who rely primarily on differences in visible phonetic cues. Lansing and Helgeson (1995) report that spoken word recognition for pairs of unrelated words may be facilitated by sensory factors, such as word/viseme visibility, however it may be facilitated by linguistic factors, such as prime-association, in related semantic contexts.

Environmental Considerations

Lighting conditions, the viewing distance between the perceiver and talker and the angle of view are factors that may influence speechreading performance because they may impact the quality of an optical signal, however only a few controlled studies have been conducted to quantify their effects (for reviews, see O'Neill & Oyer, 1981; Sanders, 1993). In clinical practice several practical suggestions to facilitate speechreading performance are followed, based on findings reported by Erber (1974) for children. For example, the perceiver and talker may be made aware of the need for appropriate lighting conditions and to arrange for high contrast between the intensity of light on the face of the talker against low background light intensity levels. More recently, similar considerations regarding contrast in luminance at the talker's face have been addressed for the use of an audiovisual FM-system (Gagné, Laplante-Lévesque, Labelle, Doucet, & Potvin, 2006). Another consideration for the perceiver is that of moving from one area to another in which there is either a large increase or decrease in light intensity and may require a short time interval for some visual adaptation to occur, following which the level of lighting does not appear to be a critical factor given that there is enough light to see the talker's face. According to a review by Sanders (1993), the optimal separation between the perceiver and talker for efficient speechreading is approximately 5-feet; however, there is little difference in the variability of the viewing angle over a range of 0 to 35 degrees. The visual acuity of the perceiver plays a role at distances of 22 feet or more, and requires a minimum visual acuity of 20/30 for the better eye (Johnson & Snell, 1986). The synergistic characteristics of background noise or the competition of other people talking coupled with reverberation undoubtedly will degrade the quality of the acoustic signal. This will further affect speechreading performance, requiring the perceiver to rely on visual cues to a greater extent than auditory cues and may result in a superadditive effect for vision in multisensory enhancement.

Talker-Specific Characteristics and Variability in Speaking Style

Numerous reports on talker variability appear in the literature in auditory language processing (e.g., for a review, see Johnson & Mullennix, 1997). One source of variability in auditory speech perception occurs for iterations produced by the same talker and is associated with a magnitude of 10% for test-retest reliability in speech intelligibility (Brandy, 1996). Talker-specific characteristics, such as physical details about a talker's face and observable patterns of articulation, have also been shown to affect memory for spoken words (Sheffert & Fowler, 1995). There are some suggestions that the appearance of facial features (e.g., prominence of lip vermilion, lip thickness, facial hair) may influence the visibility of a talker (Berger, 1972). Additional sources of variance within and across talkers include differences in regional accents or social variations that affect speech sound production and coaraticulation, as well as differences in anatomical structures and kinematics in the speech mechanism. These factors may contribute to the significant variance in visual category classification of visemes that may differ as a function of the talker (Kricos & Lesner, 1982). Consequently, some talkers are easier to speechread than others, possibly because they are able to convey subtle phonemic information (Bernstein, Demorest, Coulter, & O'Connell, 1991; Kricos & Lesner, 1982). There is also some evidence that female talkers may produce more visible speech gestures than males, but this gender difference may not generalize to audiovisual speechreading conditions (Daly, Bench, & Chappell, 1996).

It is well known that differences in speaking style are a source of significant variation within a talker. Several investigators have used paradigms to elicit different speaking styles to address questions related to intra- and intertalker variance as a function of speaking style and modality with implications for AR. Picheny, Durlach, and Braida (1985, 1986, 1989) described a variety of linguistic and acoustic differences between clear versus conversational speech within and across talkers. "Clear speech" has widespread clinical relevance in AR; however, there is disagreement in the literature on how best to elicit a clear-speech speaking style. Hardison (2005) suggested that instructions to elicit clear speech speaking styles in research paradigms to study speech intelligibility for syllable-length units as a function of presentation modality (auditory, visual, and auditory-visual), may result in a dichotomy that reflects hyperarticulated (clear) versus hypoarticulated (conversational) speech. For example, Helfer (1997) instructed the talker to produce her speech as if communicating under adverse listening conditions with someone who has a hearing loss and to enunciate clearly and avoid slurring of words to define clear speech operationally, but provided no instructions to elicit conversation speech. Gagné, Rochette, and Charest (2002) elicited multiple iterations for "clear" versus "normal" speaking styles by instructing their talkers, who had no specific training in clear speech production, to speak clearly as if talking to a person who had difficulty understanding versus to speak normally as if talking to a familiar person. Talkers may differ in the specific behaviors they identify with clear or conversational speech and differ in their proficiency in executing these behaviors. These factors may contribute to the variability in the optical and acoustic parameters of speech production within and across talkers and impact perception. Two general findings emerge: one is that clear and conversation speech are two different speaking styles; the other is that the use of clear speech generally improves speech understanding for the perceiver compared to conversational speech. The variation in intelligibility within and across talkers for these two speaking styles as a function of modality, however, is not well understood (Gagné et al., 2002).

Overall, the literature on talker-specific characteristics suggests several sources of variability that may influence performance with a single talker over time or across different talkers. Similarly the literature suggests various sources of talker variation for the audibility and the visibility of speech. It is plausible that a talker's intelligibility in one sensory modality may not generalize to another, and that variance may also be observed for multisensory enhancement effects.

Proficiency of the Perceiver

Proficiency in visual perception of spoken language varies over a wide range of performance. Nevertheless, there are individuals who are expert speechreaders, demonstrating exceptional accuracy for visual phonetic perception and achieving scores in excess of 80% accuracy on spoken words in unrelated sentences without sound (Andersson & Lidestam, 2005; Bernstein, Demorest, & Tucker, 1998, 2000; Lyxell, 1994).

It is not clear why some individuals are better at selecting, extracting, and using visual information for language understanding than others or what factors may enhance the synthesis of information from cross-modal stimulation with cognitive/linguistic knowledge in language understanding. Numerous investigators have attempted to relate speechreading proficiency to other sensory, perceptual, and cognitive abilities (for a review, see Dodd & Campbell, 1987). Summerfield (1991) concluded that, in individuals with normal intellectual and language ability performance on intelligence and verbal reasoning tasks, these factors were not related to speechreading proficiency. Findings from a cross-sectional study of speechreading in adults suggest that females are better speechreaders than males (Dancer, Krain, Thompson, Davis, & Glenn, 1994), however this is not supported for results for young and old adults (Sommers, Tye-Murray, & Spehar, 2005) or in groups of young adults with early-onset hearing loss and normal hearing (Auer & Bernstein, 2007).

Initial results reported by Shepard, DeLavergne, Fruck, and Clobridge (1977) suggested that neurophysiologic responsiveness, as measured by visual evoked responses, may account for some of the variance in speechreading proficiency, however conflicting results reported by Samar and Sims (1984) have challenged this conclusion. There is also some conflicting evidence about the impact of aging in adults on their performance for visual speech perception tasks and for cross-modal enhancement. It is plausible that a complex of sensory, perceptual, and cognitive factors (e.g., changes in visual acuity and contrast sensitivity, processing of visual temporal information, working memory) may affect performance on tests of spoken language understanding in the older adult, further complicated by acquired hearing loss. Findings reported by Sommers, Tye-Murray, and Spehar (2005) indicate that groups of young adults achiever higher scores on tests of visual speech perception than those by old adults. Recent findings for speechreading performance for groups of old adults with acquired hearing loss, however, indicate that their performance on vision-only and auditory-visual speech perception task is similar to that of old adults without hearing loss (Cienkowski & Carney, 2002; Tye-Murray, Sommers, & Spehar, 2007).

Findings from a normative study reported by Bernstein, Demorest, and Tucker (2000) provide consistent evidence for superior visual speech perception skills across various linguistic segments for a large group of adults in their sample with early onset deafness and whose native language was English, compared to those demonstrated by all of the other adults in their sample with normal hearing. Recent findings for adults with early-onset of severe-to-profound hearing loss (Auer & Bernstein, 2007; Bernstein et al., 2000; Bernstein, Auer, & Tucker, 2001) have challenged prior conclusions reported in the literature that argued against superior speechreading skills for adults with early onset deafness.

Perhaps one salient characteristic of proficient speechreaders is that they make better use of the talker's observable speech gestures (Summerfield, 1987, 1991). A review of the literature reported by Gailey (1987) concluded that accuracy for visual perception of syllables and isolated words is associated with accuracy for spoken language understanding without sound. Additional support for this conclusion is reported by Bernstein et al. (2000). Recent findings reported by Lidestam and Beskow (2006) also support the hypothesis that proficiency on the part of the perceiver in distinguishing among the least visually distinct phonemes facilitates greater accuracy in word identification. Ideally, research findings to help explain variance for proficiency in visual speech perception may be applied to the clinical practice of AR for purposes of assessment and intervention. Given an understanding of those factors that contribute to enhanced proficiency, it may be feasible to structure intervention strategies to ameliorate difficulties in speech understanding for individuals with hearing loss.

Speechreading Assessment and Training/Practice Approaches

At the present time, there is insufficient evidence to conclude that visual speech perception for spoken language is innately "hard-wired" or that long-term training/practice is of limited value (for a review, see Arnold, 1997). Scientific understanding of perceptual learning and performance and cross-modal enhancement must be developed synergistically by clinicians and researchers to guide the development of evidence-based effective and efficient strategies in AR.

Background

Historically, speechreading (lipreading) was practiced in Europe until the 1890s, as a method to teach primarily speech production to young children with hearing loss. The approach was unisensory, relying on visual sensory stimulation only. Students focused on postures and movements of the speech articulators (lips, tongue, teeth, and jaw positions) to produce and recognize observable phonetic units at the syllable, word, and sentence levels. Early attempts at speechreading (lipreading) in America identified with analytic (bottom-up analysis of phonetic units) or synthetic (Gestalt, top-down analysis of message intent) philosophies of instruction. O'Neill and Oyer (1981) provide a review of the major distinctive methods of training that were adopted in America and their characteristics: (a) Bruhn (which focused on syllable drill and encouraged careful observation of lip gestures); (b) Nitchie (which later combined synthetic, message driven elements, with analytic phonetic unit recognition); (c) Kinzie (which merged Bruhn's phonetic unit classification with components of Nichie's psychological constructs); (d) Jena (which linked visual cues to kinematic patterns of speech production); and (e) film technique approaches (e.g., Mason's Visual Hearing, Markovin and Moore's Contextual System Approach).

Performance Evaluation

At the present time, no set of reliable and valid speechreading assessment tools has been universally accepted, but a variety of informal and formal measures, originally developed to evaluate auditory speech perception, have been used clinically with adults to screen speechreading proficiency and estimate post-training gains for the recognition of syllables, words, sentences, and paragraphs (For a review, see Gagné & Jennings, 2000; Hipskind, 2007). Recordings for some of these test materials are available in an audiovisual format and allow computations of speechreading enhancement: a simple percent correct difference score for accuracy achieved under vision-only (V) conditions compared to that for auditory-visual (AV) conditions (i.e., AV – V); and, a normalized ratio score that attempts to compensate for individual differences in visual perception (i.e., AV – V/100 – V). In addition, they may be used to evaluate performance in the auditory modality alone to allow for other computations of multisensory enhancement and guide AR intervention. Some examples of these tests include: The Iowa Phoneme and Sentence Test (Tyler, Preece, & Tye-Murray, 1986) and the CUNY Sentence Test (Boothroyd, Hanin, & Hnath-Chisholm, 1985) originally used for CASPER (computer assisted speechreading perception evaluation and training) as described by Boothroyd (1987) and currently marketed with updated software. In many clinical settings however, speechreading assessments are delivered with live-voice by the clinician. Due to variability between talkers and within a single talker, performance scores on live administration tests must be interpreted with caution.

Assessment tools are needed for which normative data are available, including test-retest reliability. Ideally, tools that are validated with functional performance under environmental conditions representative of daily communication situations should be designed. Another challenge is that a large set of stimuli are needed to track performance overtime and reduce the possibility that perceivers recall stimuli from previous test sessions, which is also a challenge in evaluating auditory speech perception. Given a very large *corpora* of stimuli representative of speech events in daily communication, it is plausible that choosing a large set of new items at random for each test condition may be one solution. Another remedy is to use different lists, balanced for linguistic segments and constraints, but this is further complicated by the issue of list-equivalency, especially for comparisons across modalities (in that speech segments differ in visible or auditory characteristics) or with different speech-to-noise ratios and/or types of noise.

Normative data sets and experimental paradigms reported in the recent research literature may guide the development of new clinical assessment tools. For example, it may be helpful to explain an individual's score on a speechreading test in the context of normative data that have been reported for a large sample of adults with normal hearing and for those with early-onset hearing loss across various levels of linguistic complexity (Bernstein, Demorest, & Tucker, 2000). Another useful set of data are sample distributions for proportions of words-correct on speechreading screening tests (high-quality recordings of 30-CID sentences for two talkers; Bernstein & Eberhardt, 1986) reported by Auer and Bernstein (2007). In addition, new phoneme-correct scoring techniques for sentence-level materials, derived from phoneme confusion data for nonsense-syllables, should provide more sensitive measures than key-word or word-correct scores, detecting enhanced perception at a phonemic level (Bernstein, Auer, & Tucker, 2001). Other recent developments are tools to assess identification of speech segments at various levels of linguistic complexity for a variety of talkers that employ a multiple-choice response format, minimizing the effects of spoken or written language proficiency (e.g., the Test of Adult Speechreading [TAS] developed by Ellis, MacSweeney, & Campbell, 2001). For the assessment of multisensory enhancement, examples of approaches to control for audibility using adaptive multi-talker babble noise backgrounds with old adults (e.g., Tye-Murray, Sommers, and Spehar, 2007) may guide clinical diagnosis and intervention approaches.

Present Day Approaches to Intervention for the Perceiver and the Talker

Present day approaches in intervention may include speechreading practice, when indicated, as one component of a comprehensive program of AR. Instead of a unisensory, vision-only approach, training is in the context of multisensory inputs for information extracted from auditory and visual sensations that is integrated into a unified percept. To optimize success in information extraction as well as functional hearing performance, personal amplification, assisitive listening systems and/or other sensory-prosthetic devices are appropriately fit, adjusted, and validated using best practice guidelines to maximize the use of residual hearing. Typically, practice in visual perception would be provided with access to auditory cues. Some orientation to distinctions among visual categories of phonetic units may be provided, but today's speechreading approaches are highly holistic.

In addition to Multimodal Speech Perception, Gagné (1994) highlighted trends that include Conversational Contexts: focused on employing question-answer formats (e.g., Erber, 1996), training in communication repair strategies and effective communication behaviors (e.g., Tye-Murray, 1994), as well as training for talkers to improve communication interactions (e.g., Erber, 1996; Schum, 1997; Schow, 2001); and Computer-Based Activities: focused on interactive learning algorithms and high-quality, full-motion video displays (e.g., Korpra, Korpra, Abrahamson, & Dunlop, 1986; Pichora-Fuller & Benguerel, 1991). Self-instructional videotapes, such as *I See What You Are Saying* (available from the League for the Hard of Hearing in New York) and speechreading tapes from the National Technical Institute for the Deaf, provide home-based practice. In addition, two commercially-available, interactive speechreading home-based training programs, recently reviewed by Ross (2005) are: *Seeing and Hearing Speech* (available from Sensimeterics) which features several talkers and six noise types, practice and test conditions; and *Conversation Made Easy* (available from the Central Institute for the Deaf) which features three training modules for adults and teenagers that are organized around a multiple choice response format and practice applying communication repair strategies. Both programs allow perceivers to: choose presentation modalities (visual, auditory, or auditory-visual); control loudness levels, and practice with syllable, phrase, and sentence length utterances.

Some clinicians have also incorporated the procedure first described by de Filippo and Scott (1978), *Continuous Discourse Tracking* (*CDT*) or some modification for training/practice to combine analytic and synthetic speechreading skills, practice with communication strategies, and for assessment purposes with adults. Typically, this procedure uses scripted material, such as a narrative or other discourse. It is structured so that one person takes the role of "sender" and delivers chunks of continuous discourse, such as phrases or clauses. A second person takes the role of "receiver" and must attempt to provide an accurate verbatim repetition of each chunk. If an error is made, the sender may use a specified strategy to assist the receiver in accurate identification. Some examples of the strategies include: simple repetition of full phrases or words, repetition with hyperarticulation, changes in rate and intonation, use of paraphrase, and oral spelling. Depending on the type of practice or purpose of the activity, the material may be presented under vision only, auditory only or auditory-visual conditions. Performance on CDT is quantified by the rate at which accurate verbatim word identification is achieved over a unit of time (typically reported as a word-per-minute score). Suggestions to use this procedure to encourage communication partners to discover effective expressive speech production and receptive communication repair strategies or to gain practice in requesting such strategies also appear in the literature (e.g., Erber, 1996). Results employing CDT as an assessment tool are reported in the research literature; however, there are many sources of variability that must be systematically controlled for purposes of replication or to provide reliable and valid comparisons as a function of presentation modality over time, or for individual or groups of participants (for a review, see Spens, 1995).

There also has been continued interest in approaches designed to modify the behaviors of talkers, family members and significant others, who want to facilitate success in communication interactions (and speechreading performance) for persons with hearing loss. These methods include raising awareness of physical and cognitive/linguistic communication constraints, encouraging proactive behaviors to avoid communication breakdowns, and modifying speech and voice behaviors to enhance speech understanding. A set of suggestions with the acronym SPEECH (Schow, 2001) outlines some possible strategies. For example, talkers are encouraged to strive for "clear speech," which Schow (2001) operationally defines as delivering speech at a moderate rate, with pauses between phrases and sentences, characteristic of the temporal patterns described by Picheny et al. (1985, 1986, 1989). Recommendations for communication partners to develop and use clear speech speaking styles to enhance speech understanding are a central component of many AR programs (Erber, 1996, Gagné & Jennnings, 2000; Schum, 1997; Tye-Murray & Schum, 1994).

Training Efficacy Needs

As reported in the literature, post-treatment gains from repeated speechreading training/practice are modest (Bernstein, Auer, & Tucker, 2001), with group average gains estimated in the range of approximately 15% improvement. Little is know about the efficacy of different approaches; however, some individuals do demonstrate clinically significant enhancements in speechreading. Following short-term training/practice, perceivers may distinguish among categories of visible phonetic gestures based on distinct differences in their place-of-speech-articulation (Walden, Prosek, Montgomery, Scherr, & Jones, 1977). Although it is not clear what factors contribute directly for gains in performance, the outcomes reported by Walden et al. (1977) may provide evidence that perception has been modified, that is, perceptual learning. Findings from other studies are more variable and suggest gains may be related to nonsensory factors, such as familiarity with the test procedure, test materials, talker, or improved attention and viewing strategies. For example, Massaro, Cohen, and Gesi (1993) demonstrated that experience with repeated testing was as beneficial as short-term training/practice. It is plausible, however, that remembering sentences presented initially under auditory-visual conditions may have resulted in improved scores (Bernstein et al., 2001). Long-term training/practice may provide perceivers with opportunities to learn to distinguish among a talker's specific patterns of observable phonetic patterns (Bernstein et al., 1991). Such learning may also require some normalization process to learn to categorize similar phonetic gestures produced with small kinematic variance inherent across iterations of an utterance or across different talkers.

The recent research literature represents improvements in treatment efficacy studies that may produce results to guide evidence-based practice in AR. Examples include: data analyses based on a large number of participants, the use of separate stimuli for training/practice versus assessment, and experimental designs that require homogeneous groupings of participants to investigate variables under experimental control. For replication purposes, it is critical to include details about the training methodology and stimuli. Performance data on unisensory and cross-modal tasks are needed to understand processes of information extraction and cross-modal integrative functions. Less is known about the effects of long-term training/practice and evidence for attaining asymptotic performance levels, or for the generalization of gains demonstrated in training sessions to daily communication situations. Experimental designs that control for individual participant factors such as motivation, self-efficacy, and test-taking behaviors are needed. In addition, designs that separate training/practice activities from the personal attention inherent in clinician-guided training/practice activities present new challenges.

New Developments in Visual Speech Perception: Research and Technology

In recent years, there has been increased interest in studying cross-modal human communication for gaining basic knowledge about how speech is perceived by the brain and the contribution of neural processes to human perception and behavior. Advances in brain imaging technologies have been a useful tool to test hypotheses about the neural correlates in human performance. In addition, a number of research groups worldwide have applied new knowledge in multisensory phenomena to guide the development of 3D avatars/electronic speaking faces (computer models of talking heads or synthetic talkers) that generate speech-related acoustic and optical information with applications for intelligent human computer interactions. Databases of human speech production and perception are needed to enhance this technology further. It has the potential to be a powerful tool for scientists and clinicians to test new hypotheses about perceptual processes and to guide the development of new approaches to assessment and intervention in spoken language understanding.

Neural Bases of Visual Contribution to Spoken Language Understanding

Although current scientific understanding into multisensory phenomena is at an intermediate stage, this area of research has experienced an explosive growth (Stein & Standford, 2008). New findings from brain imaging studies have expanded our understanding of multimodal processes in spoken language perception. Hemodynamic measures such as functional magnetic resonance imaging (fMRI) and MRI generate a loud noise, but they deliver good spatial resolution and may provide valuable insights into the neural underpinnings for the multimodal perception of spoken language. The findings demonstrate that a wide network of brain regions in the temporal, frontal, and parietal lobes are involved. Results reported by Calvert et al. (1997) indicate bilateral activation of the auditory cortex for visual perception (silent speechreading) by individuals without hearing loss. Some investigators have demonstrated that visual sensory stimulation influences processing in the auditory cortex directly, potentially via direct interconnections between visual and auditory cortical regions (MacSweeny et al., 2000; Molholm & Foxe, 2005; Pekkola et al., 2005). In contrast, results from perceivers with congenital-onset profound bilateral deafness (who must rely on visual sensory stimulation for spoken language understanding) do not indicate strong left temporal activation (MacSweeny et al., 2002).

Evidence of individual differences is also emerging. More recent findings reported for adults with normal hearing by Hall, Fussell, and Summerfield (2005) suggest that group average activation patterns do not always access acoustic-based representations in the auditory cortex. These findings provide evidence that supports the existence of individual differences in activation patterns (Ludman et al., 2000). Hall et al., (2005) argue that variance in efficiency of one or more component perceptual and cognitive processes may provide insights into individual differences.

Scientific knowledge about the contribution of specific brain regions to the rapid integration of information synthesis from cross-modal stimulation is also needed. Results from measures that have a high degree of temporal and spectral resolution, such as event-related optical signals (EROS) may prove useful in localizing the rapid time course of neural effects involved in the sequencing of auditory and/or visual information extraction and the integration of this information. (For a review, see Gratton & Fabiani, 2001.)

Neural Development and Plasticity

New theoretical models of neural development and physiologic changes in the central nervous system associated with plasticity for sensory stimulation across the life span are grounded in emerging evidence on the processing of auditory, visual and multisensory integration. Immature cortical structures and/or connections are linked with auditory deprivation that occurs early in human development, during an optimal period of learning (Ponton & Eggermont, 2001; Sharma, Dorman, & Spahr, 2002). Furthermore, because visual sensory stimulation penetrates speech perception since infancy, intersensory audiovisual capacities are affected and may have consequences for spoken language understanding and may potentially have an impact on other cognitive processes, such as attention, and memory. It is plausible that modified, reduced, or limited experience with auditory sensory stimuli during early brain development in people with hearing loss may be accentuated by compensatory plasticity in the cortex and associated with differences in visual processes in spoken language understanding (Bavelier & Neville, 2002; Bavelier et al., 2001). Results from longitudinal studies with children using cochlear implants demonstrate that children rely on either the auditory or visual cues in audiovisual speech tasks, depending on the age at which they are provided with access to auditory stimulation (Bergeson, Pisoni, & Davis, 2003). These findings have potential applications for AR following a period of auditory sensory deprivation or new sensory stimulation via hearing aids or cochlear implants (Trembly & Kraus, 2002). Rouger et al. (2007) present evidence that cochlear implant users with excellent speechreading proficiency compared to persons without hearing loss, maintain their speechreading skill several years after implantation and may also be better at integrating auditory and visual information. Rouger et al. (2007) purport that highly specialized visual systems in their participants may have been mediated by a reorganization of the cortical network involved in speech understanding. These researchers suggest that visually oriented rehabilitation strategies should be considered in rehabilitation strategies.

Use of Synthetic Talkers: Avatars

Embodied Conversational Agents or avatars, have the potential to enhance functional communication understanding by providing realistic, synchronized visual cues that convey observable speech gestures and emotional facial expressions to enhance the understanding of the content and intent of a message (Adjoudani & Benoît, 1996). Customized avatars, as personal clones or virtual actors, may also serve as assistive communication devices that enable individuals with hearing and speech/voice problems to participate in spoken communication interactions using spoken language (for a review, see Massaro, 2004). The work thus far has documented the benefit of visual face information in comprehending the spoken message under adverse listening conditions, and has provided some information about the nature of the cues involved, and of the facial regions from which different aspects of the communicated information are perceived (e.g., Martin et al., 2007). Examples of applications to language learning with "Baldy," a talking head, developed by Massaro and Cohen (1990), include: literacy, speech production training, vocabulary acquisition, and second language acquisition in the research lab. Data for audiovisual speech perception in noise, reported by Lidestam and Beskow (2006) for a natural human and synthetic talker that produced neutral, positive, and negative emotional expressions, revealed good accuracy for word and sentence identification; performance, however, was better with the natural talker than with the synthetic talker. Their analysis of within cluster (viseme) response rates revealed that perceivers did not make as many distinctions among the less visible speech sound gestures (e.g., among /d, s, h/) produced by the synthetic talker than for those by the natural talker.

Progress in the development of synthetic talkers is encouraging and holds great promise as a powerful tool to learn about human perception. The present day systems require further enhancement to capture naturalistic speech gestures integrated with facial expressions (Martin et al., 2007). Current systems are typically animated and synchronized with natural speech observed in video recordings (e.g., Theobald, Bangham, Mathews, & Cowley, 2004). The facial deformation modeling and synthesis algorithms are not based on empirical data or three-dimensional kinematic measures of real facial motion in speech combined with facial expression. In addition, they do not incorporate natural changes in the texture and geometry of the human face, or natural movements of the head and eyes of the talker. Emotional expression during speech is conveyed with changes in action units related to the activity of muscle groups to achieve primarily changes in the eye regions (e.g., eyebrow movement, eye-widening, gaze-shifts). Cues for emotional expression at the mouth (e.g., smile, frown) are not simultaneously displayed during speech activity. In these models, facial expressions are treated as an independent source of information from speech acts, rather than integrated to constrain the range of movement observable for naturalistic speech articulation production, similar to the avatar described by Lidestam and Beskow (2006). As Gagné et al. (2002) suggest, it would be ideal to develop synthetic faces that combine empirical kinematic and acoustic measures with perceptual data in an integrated framework. New advances in kinematic modeling (e.g., Lucerno et al., 2005) and 3D measurement and analysis-by-synthesis techniques (e.g., Odisio, Bailly, & Elisei, 2004) have the potential to yield significant data for understanding speechreading enhancement. Highly sophisticated avatars of the future may be developed to capture optimal cues for speech perception, producing naturalistic speech and emotional expressions in an unconstrained way and adapting to imitate different talkers in real time. It is plausible that avatars could be developed that would outperform natural talkers and exceed expectations for visual processes in spoken language understanding.

Conclusions

Vision penetrates the perception of spoken language. It is useful for persons with hearing loss and for persons with normal hearing who must communicate in noisy, cluttered, reverberant environments. Vision facilitates perception of complex spoken language, new vocabulary, or the learning of foreign language, albeit audible and clearly articulated! Visual cues related to speech are available on the face of the talker, but the stimulus of the talking face is highly complex and displays dynamic spatial and temporal variability. Human visual processes are utilized to integrate information extracted from the talker's face with that from the talker's voice and interpreted in the context of cognitive/linguistic knowledge to enhance perception of a unified event in spoken language.

Limitations on vision for spoken language understanding are due to a reduced set of speech gestures that may be categorized into representations of linguistic segments on the basis of observable, visible differences in movement patterns. Large sources of variability related to linguistic constraints, dynamic phonetic environments, different speaking styles, and talker-specific characteristics challenge speech understanding. Proficiency in visual speech understanding is due to a multifaceted combination of factors; however, it may be related to cortical development and plasticity, enhanced for individuals with early onset deafness and associated with the ability to make subtle perceptual distinctions among less visible speech gestures.

Proficiency in visual speech understanding may not be innate. Instead, perceptual learning activities, practice, and the use of clear speaking styles by talkers may enhance speech understanding. Training/practice in visual speech perception is only one component of a comprehensive program of AR. Assessment tools are not universally accepted and such tools must be developed. Similarly, systematic treatment efficacy studies for present day approaches to training/practice must be pursued.

New scientific information is becoming accessible with the development of technical tools such as advanced brain imaging. This new knowledge will contribute to our understanding of the neural correlates and the time course of visual perception in unisensory and cross-modal integration, cortical development and neural plasticity. Furthermore, new findings have the potential to have an impact on AR and may guide the development of effective and efficient approaches to assessment and intervention for persons with hearing loss. Translational research efforts to develop synthetic faces from an integrated framework of acoustic, kinematic, and perceptual empirical data hold much promise as powerful tools to learn about visual speech perception in spoken language understanding and contribute to the development of new technologies for assessment and intervention in AR.

References

Adjoudani, A., & Benoit, C. (1996). On the integration of auditory and visual parameters in an HMM-based ASR. In D. G. Stork, & M. E. Hennecke (Eds.), *Speechreading by humans and machines: Mod-*

els, systems and applications. NATO ASI Series (pp. 315–322), Berlin, Germany: Springer.

Andersson, U., & Lidestam, B. (2005). Bottom-up driven speechreading in a speechreading expert: The case of AA (JK023). *Ear and Hearing, 26*, 214–224.

Argyle, M., & Cook, M. (1976). *Gaze and mutual gaze*. Cambridge: Cambridge University Press.

Arnold, P. (1997). The structure and optimization of speechreading. *Journal of Deaf Studies and Education*, 2(4) 199–211.

Arnold, P., & Hill, F. (2001). Bisensory augmentation: A speechreading advantage when speech is clearly audible and intact. *British Journal of Psychology, 92*, 339–355.

Auer, E. T., Jr., & Bernstein, L. E. (1997). Speechreading and the structure of the lexicon: Computationally modeling the effects of reduced phonetic distinctiveness on lexical uniqueness. *Journal of the Acoustical Society of America, 102*, 3704–3710.

Auer, E. T., Jr., & Bernstein, L. E. (2007). Enhanced visual speech perception in individuals with early-onset hearing impairment. *Journal of Speech, Language, and Hearing Research, 50*, 1157–1165.

Bavelier, D., Brozinsky, C., Tomann, A., Mitchell, T., Neville, H., & Liu, G. (2001). Impact of early deafness and early exposure to sign language on the cerebral organization for motion processing. *Journal of Neuroscience, 21*(22), 8931–8942.

Bavelier, D., & Neville, H. J. (2002). Cross-modal plasticity: Where and how? *Nature Reviews Neuroscience, 3*, 443–452.

Berger, K. (1972). Visemes and homophenous words. *Teacher of the Deaf, 70*, 396–399.

Bergeson, T. R., Pisoni, D. B., & Davis, R. A. O. (2003). A longitudinal study of audiovisual speech perception by children with hearing loss who have cochlear implants. *Volta Review, 103*(4) (Monograph), 347–370.

Bernstein, L. E., Auer, E. T., Jr., & Tucker, P. E. (2001). Enhanced speechreading in deaf adults: Can short-term training/practice close the gap for hearing adults? *Journal of Speech, Language, and Hearing Research, 44*, 5–18.

Bernstein, L. E., Demorest, M. E., Coulter, D. C., & O'Connel, M. P. (1991). Lipreading sentences with vibrotactile vocoders. Performance of normal-hearing and hearing impaired subjects. *Journal of the Acoustical Society of America, 95*, 3617–3622.

Bernstein, L. E., Demorest, M. E., & Tucker, P. E. (1998). What makes a good speechreader? First you have to find one. In R. Campbell, B. Dodd, & D. Burnham (Eds.), *Hearing by eye II: The psychology of speechreading and auditory-visual speech* (pp. 211–228). East Sussex, UK: Psychology Press.

Bernstein, L. E., Demorest, M. E., & Tucker, P. E. (2000). Speech perception without hearing. *Perception and Psychophysics, 62*, 233–252.

Bernstein, L. E., & Eberhardt, S. P. (1986). *Johns Hopkins lipreading corpus I–II: Disc I* [Laser video disk]. Baltimore: Johns Hopkins University.

Besle, J., Fort, A., Delpuech, C., & Giard, M. H. (2004). Bimodal speech: Early suppressive visual effects in human auditory cortex. *European Journal of Neuroscience, 20*, 2225–2234.

Binnie, C. A., Montgomery, A. A., & Jackson, P. L (1974). Auditory and visual contributions to the perception of consonants. *Journal of Speech and Hearing Research, 17*, 619–630.

Boothroyd, A. (1987). CASPER: A computer system for speech-perception testing and training. *Proceedings of the 10th Annual Conference of the Rehabilitative Society of North America*, 428–430.

Boothroyd, A. (1988). Linguistic factors in speechreading. *Volta Review, 90*(5), 77–88.

Boothroyd, A., Hanin, L., & Hnath-Chisholm, T. (1985). *The CUNY Sentence Test*. New York: City University of New York.

Brandy, W. T. (1966). Reliability of voice tests of speech discrimination. *Journal of Speech and Hearing Research, 9*, 461–465.

Calvert, G., Bullmore, E., Brammer, M., Campbell, R., Woodruff, P., McGuire, P., et al. (1997). Activation of auditory cortex during silent speechreading. *Science, 276*, 593–596.

Cienkowski, K. M., & Carney, A. E. (2002). Auditory-visual speech perception and aging. *Ear and Hearing, 23*, 439–449.

Cotton, J. C. (1935). Normal "visual hearing." *Science, 82*, 592–593.

Daly, N., Bench, J., & Chappell, H. (1996).Gender differences in speechreadability. *Journal of the Academy of Rehabilitative Audiology, 29*, 27–40.

Dancer, J., Krain, M., Thompson, C., Davis, P., & Glenn, J. (1994). A cross-sectional investigation of speechreading in adults: Effects of gender, practice, and education. *Volta Review, 96*, 31–40.

de Filippo, C. L., & Scott, B. L. (1978). A method for training and evaluating the reception of ongoing speech. *Journal of the Acoustical Society of America, 63*, 1186–1192.

De Gelder, B., & Bertelson, P. (2003). Multisensory integration, perception and ecological validity. *Trends in Cognitive Science, 7*(10), 460–467.

Dodd, B. (1977). The role of vision in the perception of speech. *Perception*, 6(1), 31–40.

Dodd, B., & Campbell, R. (1987). *Hearing by eye: The psychology of lip-reading*. London: Erlbaum.

Ellis, T., MacSweeney, M., Dodd, B., & Campbell, R. (2001). TAS: A new test of adult speechreading—deaf people really can be better speechreaders. *Proceedings of the International Conference on Auditory-Visual Speech Processing* (AVSP-2001), pp. 13–17.

Erber, N. P. (1969). Interaction of audition and vision in the recognition of oral speech. *Journal of Speech and Hearing* Research, *12*(2), 423–425.

Erber, N. P. (1974). Effects of angle, distance and illumination on visual speech perception by profoundly deaf children. *Journal of Speech and Hearing Research, 17*, 99–112.

Erber, N. (1992). Effects of a question-answer format on visual perception of sentences. *Journal of the Academy of Rehabilitative Audiology, 25*, 113–122.

Erber, N. P. (1996). *Communication therapy for adults with sensory loss* (2nd ed.). Melbourne, Australia: Clavis.

Fisher, C. G. (1968). Confusions among visually perceived consonants. *Journal of Speech and Hearing Research, 12*, 796–804.

Fowler, C. A. (1986). An event approach to the study of speech perception from a direct-realist perspective. *Journal of Phonetics, 14*, 3–28.

Fowler, C. A. (1996). Listeners do hear sounds, not tongues. *Journal of the Acoustical Society of America, 99*, 1730–1741.

Fowler, C. A., & Dekle, D. J. (1991). Listening with eye and hand: Cross-modal contributions to speech perception. *Journal of Experimental Psychology: Human Perception and Performance, 17*, 816–828.

Gagné, J.-P. (1994). Visual and audiovisual speech perception training: Basic and applied research needs. In J.-P. Gagné & N. Tye-Murray (Eds.), *Research in audiolgocial rehabilitation: Current trends and future directions* [Monograph supplement]. *Journal of the Academy of Rehabilitative Audiology*, pp. 133–160.

Gagné, J.-P., & Jennings, M. B. (2000). Audiologic rehabilitation: Intervention services for adults with an acquired hearing loss. In M. Valente, A. Hosford-Dunn, & R. J. Roeser (Eds.), *Audiologic treatment* (pp. 547–579). New York: Thieme Medical.

Gagné, J.-P., Laplante-Lévesque, A., Labelle, M., Doucet, K., & Patvin, M.-C. (2006). Evaluation of an audiovisual-FM system: Investigating the interaction between illumination level and a talker's skin color on speech-reading performance. *Journal of Speech, Language, and Hearing Research, 49*, 628–635.

Gagné, J.-P., Rochete, A.-J., & Chares, M. (2002). Auditory, visual and audiovisual clear speech. *Speech Communication, 37*, 213–230.

Gagné, J.-P., Tugby, K. G., & Michaud, J. (1991). Development of a speechreading test on the utilization of contextual cues (STUCC): Preliminary findings with normal hearing subjects. *Journal of the Academy of Rehabilitative Audiology, 24*, 157–170.

Gailey, L. (1987). Psychological parameters of lip reading skill. In B. Dodd & R. Campbell (Eds.), *Hearing by eye: The psychology lip-reading* (pp. 115–142). London: Erlbaum.

Garstecki, D. C., & O'Neill, J. J. (1980). Situational cue and strategy influence on speechreading. *Scandinavian Audiology, 9*, 147–151.

Giard, M. H., & Peronnet, F. (1999). Auditory-visual integration during multimodal object recognition in humans: A behavioral and electrophysiological study. *Journal of Cognitive Neuroscience, 11*(5), 473–490.

Gibson, J. J. (1966). *The senses considered as perceptual systems*. Boston: Houghton-Mifflin.

Grant, K. W. (2002). Measures of auditory-visual integration for speech understanding: A theoretical perspective (L). *Journal of the Acoustical Society of America, 112*(1), 30–33.

Grant, K. W., & Seitz, P. F. (1998). Measures of auditory-visual integration in nonsense syllables and sentences. *Journal of the Acoustical Society of America, 104*, 2438–2450.

Grant, K. W., & Seitz, P. F. (2000) The use of visible speech cues for improving auditory detection of spoken sentences. *Journal of the Acoustical Society of America, 108*(3), 1197–1208.

Grant, K. W., van Wassenhove, V., & Poeppel, D. (2004). Detection of auditory (cross-spectral) and auditory-visual (cross-modal) synchrony. *Speech Communication, 44*, 43–45.

Grant, K. W., Walden, B. E., & Seitz, P. F. (1998). Auditory-visual speech recognition by hearing-impaired subjects: Consonant recognition, sentence recognition, and auditory-visual integration. *Journal of the Acoustical Society of America, 103*, 2677–2690.

Gratton, G., & Fabiani, M. (2001). Shedding light on brain function in the event-related optical signal. *Trends in Cognitive Science, 5*(8), 357–363.

Green, K. P., Kuhl, P. K., Meltzoff, A. N, & Stevens, E. B. (1991). Integrating speech information across talkers, gender, and sensory modality: Female faces and male voices in the McGurk effect. *Perception and Pshychophysics, 50*(6), 524–536.

Greenberg, H. J., & Bode, D. L. (1968). Visual discrimination of consonants. *Journal of Speech and Hearing Research, 11*, 466–471.

Hall, D. A., Fussell, C., & Summerfield, A. Q. (2005). Reading fluent speech from talking faces: Typical brain networks and individual differences. *Journal of Cognitive Neuroscience, 17*, 939–953.

Hallett, P. E. (1986). Eye movements. In K. R. Boff, L. Kaufman, & J. P. Thomas (Eds.), *Handbook of perception and human performance I: Sensory processes and perception* (Chapter 10, pp. 1–102). New York: Wiley.

Hardison, D. M. (2005). Variability in bimodal spoken language processing by native and nonnative speakers of English: A closer look at effects of speech style. *Speech Communication, 46*, 73–93.

Helfer, K. S. (1997). Auditory and auditory-visual perception of clear and conversational speech. *Journal of Speech and Hearing Research, 40*, 432–443.

Hipskind, N. M. (2007) Visual stimuli in communication. In Schow, R. L., & Nerbone, M. A. (Eds.), *Introduction to audiologic rehabilitation* (pp. 151–196). Boston: Allyn and Bacon.

Ijsseldijk, F. J. (1992). Speechreading performance under different conditions of video image, repetition, and speech rate. *Journal of Speech and Hearing Research, 35*, 466–477.

Jack, C. E., & Thurlow, W. R. (1973). Effects of degree of visual association and angle of displacement on the "ventriloquism" effect. *Perceptual and Motor Skills, 37*, 967–979.

Jeffers, J., & Barley, M. (1971). *Speechreading (lipreading)*. Springfield, IL: Thomas.

Johansson, K. (1997). The role of facial approach signals in speechreading. *Scandinavian Journal of Psychology, 38*(4), 335–341.

Johnson, D., & Snell, K. B. (1986). Effects of distance visual acuity problems on the speechreading performance of hearing-impaired adults. *Journal of the Academy of Rehabilitative Audiology, 19*, 42–55.

Johnson, K., & Mullennix, J. W. (Eds.). (1997). *Talker variability in speech processing*. San Diego, CA: Academic Press.

Kirch, M. S. (1979). Non-verbal communication across cultures. *Modern Language Journal, 63*(8), 416–423.

Kopra, L., Kopra, M., Abrahamson, J., & Dunlop, R. (1986). Development of sentences graded in difficulty for lipreading practice. *Journal of the Academy of Rehabilitative Audiology, 19*, 71–86.

Kricos, P. B., & Lesner, S. A. (1982). Differences in visual intelligibility across talkers. *Volta Review, 84*, 219–225.

Lansing, C. R. (2004). Speechreading training and visual tracking. In R. M. Kent (Ed.), *The MIT encyclopedia of communication disorders* (pp. 543–547). Cambridge, MA: MIT Press.

Lansing, C. R., & Helgeson, C. L. (1995). Priming the visual recognition of spoken words. *Journal of Speech and Hearing Research, 38*, 1377–1386.

Lansing, C. R., & McConkie, G. W. (1994). A new method for speechreading research: Tracking observers' eye movements. *Journal of the Academy of Rehabilitative Audiology, 27*, 25–43.

Lansing, C. R., & McConkie, G. W. (1999). Attention to facial regions in segmental and prosodic visual speech perception tasks. *Journal of Speech, Language, and Hearing Research, 42*, 1–14.

Lansing, C. R., & McConkie, G.W. (2003). Word identification and eye fixation locations in visual and visual-plus-auditory presentations of spoken sentences. *Perception and Psychophysics, 65*(4), 536–552.

Lederman, S. J., Thorne, G., & Jones, B. (1986). Perception of texture by vision and touch: Multidimensionality and intersensory integration. *Journal of Experimental Psychology: Human Perception and Performance, 12*, 169–180.

Lewkowicz, D. J. (1994). Development of intersensory perception in human infants. In D. J. Lewkowicz & R. Lickliter (Eds.), *The development of intersensory perception: Comparative perspectives* (pp. 165–203). Hillsdale, NJ: Lawrence Erlbaum Associates.

Lewkowicz, D. J. (2000). The development of intersensory temporal perception: An epigenetic systems/limitations view. *Psychological Bulletin, 126*(2), 281–308.

Lidestam, B. (2002). Effects of displayed emotion on attitude and impression formation in visual speechreading. *Scandinavian Journal of Psychology, 43*(3), 261–268.

Lidestam, B., & Beskow, J. (2006). Visual phonemic ambiguity and speechreading. *Journal of Speech, Language, and Hearing Research, 49*, 835–847.

Lisker, L., & Abramson, A. S. (1964). Crosslanguage study of voicing in initial stops. *Journal of the Acoustical Society of America, 35*(11),1889–1890.

Lucero, J. C., Maciel, S. T. R., Johns, D. A., & Munhall, K. G. (2005). Empirical modeling of human face kinematics during speech motion clustering. *Journal of the Acoustical Society of America, 118*(1), 405–409.

Ludman, C. N., Summerfield, A. Q., Hall, D., Elliott, M., Foster, J., Hykin, J. L., et al. (2000). Lip-reading ability and patterns of cortical activation studied using fMRI. *British Journal of Audiology, 34*, 225–230.

Lyxell, B. (1994). Skilled speechreading: A single case study. *Scandinavian Journal of Psychology, 35*, 212–219.

Lyxell, B., & Rönnberg, J. (1991). Visual speech processing: Word-decoding and word-discrimination related to sentence-based speechreading and hearing-impairment. *Scandinavian Journal of Psychology, 32*, 9–17.

MacSweeney, M., Amaro, E., Calvert, G. A., Campbell, R., David, A. S., McGuire, P., et al. (2000). Silent speechreading in the absence of scanner noise: An event-related fMRI study. *NeuroReport, 11*, 1729–1733.

MacSweeney, M., Calvert, G. A., Campbell, R., McGuire, P. K., David, A. S., Williams, S. C. et al. (2002). Speechreading circuits in people born deaf. *Neuropsychologia, 40*, 801–807.

Marassa, L. K., & Lansing, C. R. (1995). Visual word recognition in two facial motion conditions: Full-face versus lips-plus-mandible. *Journal of Speech and Hearing Research, 38*, 1387–1394.

Marks, L. (1978). *The unity of the senses*. New York: Academic Press.

Martin, J.-C., d'Alessandro, C., Jacquemin, C., Katz, B., Max, A., Pointal, L., et al. (2007). 3D audiovisual rendering and real-time interactive control of expressivity in a talking head. In J. G. Carbonell & J. Siekmann (Eds.), *Intelligent Virtual Agents. Proceedings IVA 2007* (pp. 29–36). Berlin, Germany: Springer LNCS.

Massaro, D. W. (1998). *Perceiving talking faces: From speech perception to a behavioral principle*. Cambridge, MA: MIT Press, Bradford Books.

Massaro, D. W. (2004). From multisensory integration to talking heads and language learning. In G. Calvert, C. Spence, & B. E. Stein (Eds.), *Handbook of multisensory processes* (pp. 153–176). Cambridge, MA: M.I.T. Press.

Massaro, D. M., & Cohen, M. M. (1990). Perception of synthesized audible and visible speech. *Psychological Science, 1*, 1–9.

Massaro, D. W., & Cohen, M. M. (2000). Tests of auditory visual integration efficiency within the framework of the fuzzy logic model of perception. *Journal of the Acoustical Society of America, 108*, 784–789.

Massaro, D. W., Cohen, M. M., & Gesi, A. T. (1993). Longterm training, transfer, and retention in learning to lipread. *Perception and Psychophysics, 53*, 549–562.

Massaro, D. W., Cohen, M. M., Gesi, A., Heredia, R., & Tsuzaki, M. (1993). Bimodal speech perception: An examination across languages. *Journal of Phonetics, 21*, 445–478.

McGurk, H., & MacDonald, J. (1976). Hearing lips and seeing voices. *Nature, 264*, 746–748.

Miller, E. A. (1972). Interaction of vision and touch in conflict and nonconflict form perception tasks. *Journal of Experimental Psychology, 96*, 114–123.

Molholm, S., & Foxe, J. J. (2005). Look "hear," primary auditory cortex is active during lipreading. *Neuroreport, 16*, 123–124.

Montgomery, A. A., & Jackson, P. L. (1983). Physical characteristics of the lips underlying vowel lipreading performance. *Journal of the Acoustical Society of America, 73*(6), 2134–2144.

Munhall, K. G., Jones, J. A., Callan, D. E., Kuratate, T., & Vatikiotis-Bateson, E. (2004). Visual prosody and speech intelligibility: Head movement improves audiovisual speech perception. *Psychological Science, 15*(4), 133–137.

O'Neill, J. J., & Oyer, H. J. (1981). *Visual communication for the hard of hearing* (2nd ed.) Englewood Cliffs, NJ: Prentice-Hall.

Odisio, M., Bailly, G., & Elisei, F. (2004). Tracking talking faces with shape and appearance models. *Speech Communication, 44*, 63–82.

Over, R. (1966). An experimentally induced conflict between vision and proprioception. *British Journal of Psychology, 57*, 335–341.

Pekkola, J., Ojanen, V., Autti, T., Jaaskelainen, I. P., Mottonen, R., Tarkianen, A., et al. (2005). Primary auditory cortex activation by visual speech: An fMRI study at 3 T. *NeuroReport, 16*, 125–128.

Picheny, M. A., Durlach, N. I., & Braida, K. D. (1985). Speaking clearly for the hard of hearing I: Intelligibility differences between clear and conversational speech. *Journal of Speech and Hearing Research, 28*, 96–103.

Picheny, M. A., Durlach, N. I., & Braida, K. D. (1986). Speaking clearly for the hard of hearing II: Acoustic characteristics of clear and conversational speech. *Journal of Speech and Hearing Research, 29*, 434–446.

Picheny, M. A., Durlach, N. I., & Braida, K. D. (1989). Speaking clearly for the hard of hearing III: An attempt to determine the contribution of speaking rate to differences in intelligibility between clear and conversational speech. *Journal of Speech and Hearing Research, 32*, 600–603.

Pichora-Fuller, M. K., & Benguerel, A.-P. (1991). The design of CAST (computer-aided speechreading training). *Journal of Speech and Hearing Research, 34*, 202–212.

Ponton, C. W., & Eggermont, J. J. (2001). Of kittens and kids: Altered cortical maturation following profound deafness and cochlear implant use. *Audiology and Neuro-Otology, 6*, 363–380.

Posner, M. I. (1980). Orienting of attention. *Quarterly Journal of Experimental Psychology, 32*, 3–25.

Preminger, J. E., Lin, H.-B., Payen, M., & Levitt, H. (1998). Selective masking in speechreading. *Journal of Speech, Language, and Hearing Research, 41*, 564–575.

Radeau, M., & Bertelson, P. (1977). Adaptation to auditory-visual discordance and ventriloquism in semirealistic situation. *Perception and Psychophysics, 22*(2), 137–146.

Radeau, M., & Bertelson, P. (1978). Cognitive factors and adaptation to auditory-visual discordance. *Perception and Psychophysics, 23*(4), 341–343.

Rayner, K. (1998). Eye movements in reading and information processing: 20 years of research. *Psychological Bulletin, 124*, 372–422.

Reisberg, D., McLean, J., & Goldfield, A. (1987). Easy to hear but hard to understand: A speechreading advantage with intact auditory stimuli. In B. Dodd & R. Campbell (Eds.), *Hearing by eye: The psychology of lip-reading* (pp. 97–113). London: Erlbaum.

Rosenblum, L. D., & Saldaña, H. M. (1996). An audiovisual test of kinematic primitives for visual speech perception. *Journal of Experimental Psychology: Human Perception and Performance, 22*(2), 318–331.

Rosenblum, L. D., Schmuckler, M. A., & Johnson, J. A. (1997). The McGurk effect in infants. *Perception and Psychophysics, 59*(3), 347–357.

Ross, M. (2005 November/December). Home-based auditory and speechreading training. *Hearing Loss, 26*, 30–34.

Rouger, J., Lagleyre, S., Fraysse, B., Deneve, S., Deguine, O., & Barone, P. (2007). Evidence that cochlear-implanted deaf patients are better multisensory integraters. *Proceedings of the National Academy of Sciences (PNAS), 104*(17), 7295–7300.

Samar, V. J., & Sims, D. G. (1984). Visual evoked response components related to speechreading and spatial skills in hearing and hearing impaired adults. *Journal of Speech and Hearing Research, 27*, 23–26.

Sanders, D. A. (1993). *Aural rehabilitation* (3rd ed.) Englewood Cliffs, NJ: Prentice-Hall.

Schow, R. L. (2001). A standardized AR battery for dispensers. *Hearing Journal, 54*(8), 10–12.

Schum, D. J. (1997). Beyond hearing aids: The Clear Speech training technique. *Hearing Journal, 50*(10), 36–40.

Sharma, A., Dorman, M. F., & Spahr, A. J. (2002). A sensitive period for the development of the central auditory system in children with cochlear implants: Implications for age of implantation. *Ear and Hearing, 23*(6), 532–539.

Sheffert, S. M., & Fowler, C. A. (1995). The effects of voice and visible speaker change on memory for spoken words. *Journal of Memory and Language, 34*, 665–685.

Shepard, D. C., DeLavergne, R. W., Fruek, F. X., & Clobridge, C. (1977). Visual-neural correlate of speechreading ability in normal-hearing adults. *Journal of Speech and Hearing Research, 25,* 521–527.

Singer, G., & Day, R. H. (1969). Visual capture of haptically judged depth. *Perception and Psychophsyics, 5,* 315–316.

Sommers, M. S., Tye-Murray, N., & Spehar, B. (2005). Auditory-visual speech perception and auditory-visual enhancement in normal-hearing younger and older adults. *Ear and Hearing, 26,* 263–275.

Spens, K. E. (1995). Evaluation of speech tracking results: Some numerical considerations and examples. In G. Plant, & K. E. Spens (Eds.), *Profound deafness and speech communication* (pp. 417–437). London: Whurr.

Stein, B. E., & Stanford, T. R. (2008). Multisensory integration: current issues from the perspective of the single neuron. *Nature Reviews Neuroscience, 9,* 255–266.

Sumby, W. H., & Pollack, I. (1954). Visual contribution to speech intelligibility in noise. *Journal of the Acoustical Society of America, 26*(2), 212–215.

Summerfield, A. Q. (1979). Use of visual information in phonetic perception. *Phoneticia, 36,* 314–331.

Summerfield, A. Q. (1991). Visual perception of phonetic gestures. In I. G. Mattingly & M. Studdert-Kennedy (Eds.), *Modularity and the motor theory of speech perception* (pp. 117–137). Hillsdale, NJ: Erlbaum.

Summerfield, Q. (1983). Audio-visual speech perception, lipreading, and artificial stimulation. In M. Lutman & M. Haggard (Eds.), *Hearing science and hearing disorders* (pp. 131–182). New York: Academic Press.

Summerfield, Q. (1987). Some preliminaries to a comprehensive account of audio-visual speech perception. In B. Dodd & R. Campbell (Eds.), *Hearing by eye: The psychology of lipreading* (pp. 3–51). Hillsdale, NJ: Erlbaum.

Summerfield, Q., & McGrath, M. (1984). Detection and resolution of audiovisual incompatibility in the perception of vowels. *Quarterly Journal of Experimental Psychology, 36A,* 51–74.

Theobald, B. J., Bangham, J. A., Mathews, I. A., & Cawley, G. C., (2004). Near videorealistic synthetic talking faces: Implementation and evaluation. *Speech Communication, 44,* 127–140.

Trembly, K. L., & Kraus, H. (2002). Auditory training induces assymetrical changes in cortical neural activity. *Journal of Speech, Language, and Hearing Research, 45*(3), 564–572.

Tye-Murray, N. (1994). Communication breakdowns in conversations: Adult-initiated repair strategies. In N. Tye-Murray (Ed.), *Let's converse! A how-to guide to develop and expand the conversational skills of children and teenagers who are hearing impaired* (pp. 85–121). Washington, DC: Alexander Graham Bell Association for the Deaf.

Tye-Murray, N., & Schum, L. (1994). Conversational training for frequent communication partners. In J.-P. Gagné & N. Tye-Murray (Eds.), *Research in audiological rehabilitation: Current trends and future directions* [Monograph supplement]. *Journal of the Academy of Rehabilitative Audiology*, pp. 209–222.

Tye-Murray, N., Sommer, M. S., & Spehar, B. (2007). Audiovisual integration and lipreading abilities of older adults with normal an impaired hearing. *Ear and Hearing, 28,* 656–668.

Tyler, R., Preece, J., & Tye-Murray, N. (1986). *The Iowa Phoneme and Sentence Tests*. Iowa City, IA: University of Iowa Hospitals and Clinics.

van Wassenhove, V., Grant, K. W., & Poeppel, D. (2005). Visual speech speeds up the neural processing of auditory speech. *Proceedings of the National Academy of Science (PNAS), 102*(4), 1181–1186.

Vatikiotis-Bateson, E., Eigsti, I-M., Yano, S., & Munhall, K. G. (1998). Eye-movement of perceivers during audiovisual speech perception. *Perception and Psychophysics, 60*(6), 926–940.

Vroomen, J., Driver, J. , & De Gelder, B. (2001). Is cross-modal integration of emotional expressions independent of attentional resources? *Cognitive, Affective, and Behavioral Neuroscience 1*(4), 382–387.

Walden, B. E., Prosek, R. A., Montgomery, A. A., Scherr, C. K., & Jones, C. J. (1977). Effects of training on the visual recognition of consonants. *Journal of Speech and Hearing Research, 20,* 130–145.

Yehia, H., Rubin, P., & Vatikiotis-Bateson, E. (1998). Quantitative association of vocal-tract and facial behavior. *Speech Communication, 26*(1), 23–43.

12

Auditory Training

Robert W. Sweetow
Jennifer Henderson Sabes

Introduction

The objective of audiologic rehabilitation (AR) is to enhance the ability to communicate for individuals with hearing impairment. Several elements lead to communication (Kiessling et al., 2003). The most basic components are *hearing*, "a passive function providing access to the auditory world via the perception of sound" and *listening*, the "process of hearing with intention and attention." Listening is an active process requiring effort that is then followed by *comprehending*, "the reception of information, meaning, and intent." Comprehending is unidirectional, that is, altering the speaker's characteristics does not necessarily alter the listener's comprehension. The final element is *communicating*, " . . . the bi-directional transfer of information, meaning, and intent." The listener can impact communication by altering the speaker's and the environment's characteristics. In this chapter, we scrutinize Auditory Training (AT), one of the key components of AR that can potentially impact the processes of listening, comprehending and receptive communication. We consider the following questions in detail:

- What is auditory training?
- What limitations are imposed by impaired sound processing and why is AT important?
- What considerations are necessary in designing and incorporating AT into an AR program?
- Does AT work?
- Why isn't AT used more frequently?
- What has been the impact of technologic advances on auditory training?
- What AT programs are available, and what are the similarities and differences in these methods?
- What are the roles of the Audiologist and Speech-Language Pathologist in AT?

What Is Auditory Training?

Auditory training is a process designed to enhance the ability to interpret auditory experiences by maximally utilizing residual hearing. Training can be analytic, synthetic, or a combination of the two approaches. Analytic training uses exercises with small segments of the speech signal such as phonemes or syllables. Analytic training employs bottom-up tactics. This implies that perception (hearing) influences cognition (communication). Synthetic training refers to training based on recognition of the overall meaning of discourse. It does not require awareness, identification or comprehension of every single small segment of the speech signal. Instead, it focuses on communication strategies and top-down processing. This is based on the concept that cognition influences perception. The reality is two-fold; that is, perception influences cognition and cognition influences perception. Therefore, as discussed below, many AT programs utilize both types of training.

AT can be performed in either an individual or group format. A major limitation of group therapy is the lack of individualized attention to patients, many of whom present unique problems and a wide range of abilities. Thus, the question of individual AR and AT becomes relevant. The advantages of individual AR include personal treatment plans along with training at an optimal pace for the patient. However, it can be expensive from both a time and cost perspective. Although a substantial body of literature exists supporting the positive impact from group informational AR, there are fewer reports available regarding the efficacy of individual auditory training. These studies are discussed in greater detail below.

What Limitations Are Imposed by Impaired Sound Processing and Why Is AT Important?

Sensorineural hearing loss not only affects the ability to detect sounds, but also the capacity to process them. Damage to outer hair cells raises thresholds and broadens peripheral spectral and temporal filters (Florentine & Buus, 1984; Moore & Glasberg, 1986). As a result, speech perception may be impaired even when the speech signal is audible. Most hearing-impaired individuals and hearing aid users' brains receive incoming acoustic signals that are, to some degree, different, and presumably inferior, to that which the individual with normal hearing receives. As a result, the hearing aid user generally receives a fragmented or partially degraded signal, either because of extrinsic sources such as noise interference or limited bandwidth, or from underlying intrinsic limitations such as inaudibility, cochlear distortion, and impaired frequency and temporal resolution. Hearing aids can provide audibility, but may not rectify impaired frequency and temporal resolution. In fact, wearable amplification can easily improve speech reception thresholds, but frequently does not adequately solve problems with suprathreshold processing and, in fact, may exacerbate them, particularly in difficult listening situations. Hearing aid and other sensory technology are constantly improving. However, in contrast to the rapid advances in amplification in the last decades, satisfaction with hearing aids is only recently starting to change for the better (Kochkin, 2007). This disparity is likely due to the components of optimal auditory processing that modern hearing aids cannot improve, such as restoring resolution caused by a damaged cochlea, replicating the ability of the auditory system to parse the auditory scene, improving ingrained maladaptive listening and communication strategies, reversing plastic or degenerative changes in the central auditory system, or correcting for declines in cognitive function.

Listeners with hearing loss may develop compensatory tactics that may be maladaptive to optimal listening. There is a fundamental difference between hearing and listening. A person can have normal hearing, but may still be a poor listener. On the other hand, a person with hearing impairment may be an excellent listener. Hearing requires audibility; but to be a good listener, the listener must integrate a number of skills including attending, understanding, and remembering. Patients presenting similar audiometric profiles often obtain very different benefits from amplification. Various factors may account for this observation. One factor relates to an individual's assimilation of acoustic, linguistic, and environmental cues. To optimize integration, a person must call upon many skills and processes, including cognition, auditory memory, auditory closure, auditory learning, application of metalinguistics, usage of pragmatics, semantics, grammatical shape, localization, visual cues, repair tactics, and effective interactive communication strategies (Hickson & Worrall, 2003; Keissling et al., 2003; Pichora-Fuller, 2003). Further hindering many individuals with hearing impairment is the fact that certain cognitive skills (such as speed of processing and auditory working memory) that are important for comprehending speech in adverse acoustic environments tend to diminish with age (Pichora-Fuller & Singh, 2006, Wingfield & Tun, 2007). van Hooren, et al. (2005) concluded hearing aids alone cannot improve central cognitive processes.

Cognitive function typically is an area not addressed in AR programs, even though the average new hearing aid user is roughly 70 years old (Kochkin, 2007). Studies have shown that older listeners require a greater signal-to-noise ratio to perform as well as younger listeners with similar thresholds (Dubno et al., 1984; Gordon-Salant & Fitzgibbons, 1995; Pichora-Fuller et al., 1995). Although declines in areas of cognitive processing speed and working memory are observed in this population, recent studies have shown that rehabilitative training can improve these skills (Ball et al., 2002; Mahncke et al. 2006).

Threshold elevation can account for nearly all of the changes in speech perception with age, in quiet or in less demanding listening environments (Humes, 1996), but most of the problems associated with hearing impairment relate to attempts to communicate in more adverse listening conditions. Older normal hearing subjects perform approximately the same as young hearing-impaired subjects in noisy and difficult listening situations (Gordon-Salant & Fitzgibbons, 1999). Pichora-Fuller et al. (2006) has raised the possibility that the need for greater signal-to-noise ratio (SNR) places a greater strain on the already restricted cognitive resources of the elderly patient, thus creating more effortful listening.

Adjunctive therapies are used for many sensory and motor disorders. When a person injures an arm or leg, for example, professionals and patients recognize the importance of physical therapy to strengthen adjacent muscles (the physiologic adaptation) and instruction to optimize function (behavioral modification). Therapy also is commonly recommended for patients displaying central auditory processing disorders. It has been shown that peripheral hearing disorders lead to central auditory changes (Irvine et al., 2001; Kim et al., 2004). It is possible that the mere introduction of amplification will not produce optimal readaptation of the auditory system and most advantageous auditory skills unless augmented by training.

What Considerations Are Necessary in Designing and Incorporating AT into an AR Program?

A number of factors must be considered in establishing an AT program. They include the type of training (analytic versus synthetic), the difficulty level and progression of the training, the type of stimuli to be employed, the aspects of processing to be targeted, the time frame, and the impact of the training (particularly the likelihood of generalization and the duration of the benefits).

Type of Training

Analytic training typically utilizes phonemes or small elements of speech, in addition to non-speech sounds. Analytic training is influenced predominantly by peripheral perception, and as such, can be considered bottom-up processing. Synthetic training focuses on the ability to utilize all auditory and linguistic skills to interpret the speech message. Synthetic training programs teach skills for the listener to use optimally various communication strategies, including attention, use of contextual cues, repair strategies, knowledge about linguistics and communication, and the redundancies therein, to communicate effectively. This type of training is considered to be influenced by top-down processing and generally utilizes longer speech stimuli, such as words, sentences, or conversational discourse. Analytic and synthetic training, while quite different, may be most effective when combined with a comprehensive auditory training program. Synthetic training, much more so than analytic training, can be employed in group settings.

Progression of Analytic Training

There are four main levels of skills that can be trained progressing from basic to complex.

1. Sound awareness: (the recognition that an acoustic event has occurred).
2. Discrimination: (the recognition that one sound is different from another).
3. Sound identification: (the ability to correctly label or identify an acoustic event).
4. Comprehension: (understanding the meaning or implication of the acoustic event).

Note that this continuum of skills can be compared to the elements of communication that were described previously.

Training typically progresses from easy to difficult so that the trainee can experience early success. For example, training with a closed stimulus set is easier than with an open set. Dissimilar words are easier to discriminate than similar words. Stimuli containing high contextual cues are easier than those with low contextual cues. Structured content is easier than spontaneous content. High SNRs are easier than low SNRs. This is especially important to recognize for AT with older patients, because, even in the absence of hearing loss, older subjects require higher SNRs than young listeners (Schneider, Daneman & Murphy, 2005).

Carhart (1960) described a systematic analytic auditory training program, beginning with awareness of sound, progressing sequentially to gross sound discrimination using non-speech stimuli, to discrimination of dissimilar speech sounds, and finally to discrimination of highly similar speech sounds. For example, training can commence with discrimination between broadly different acoustic stimuli (like the vowels in the words /mat/ and /moot/); then slowly the sound discrimination task gradually becomes increasingly difficult (e.g., discriminating between /beet/ and /bit/, or /deed/ and /beed/bead). Similarly, consonant training can start by training discrimination of voiced (/b,d,g,v,z,m,n,l,w,j, and r/) versus unvoiced (/p,t,k,t,f,ʃ,h,s/) phonemes. This can be followed by training in discrimination of manner of articulation, for example, utilizing stop consonants (p,t, k,b,d,g) versus fricatives, or affricatives (f,v,h,s,ʃ,z). After that, training can use nasal consonants such as n and m, versus glides or liquids such as w,j,r, and l. Then one can progress to training for place of articulation discrimination with bilabial consonants like /m/, labiodentals like /v/, linguadentals like /θ/ as in thumb), alveolars /d/, palatals /ʃ/, and velar /g/ consonants (as these are the toughest for people with high-frequency hearing loss).

Carhart's early contributions to systematic organization were subsequently embraced by audiologists such as Norman Erber, who continued to refine and promulgate this auditory training protocol (Erber, 1996). Erber played a major role in designing and propagating a comprehensive (analytic and synthetic) communication therapy program for adults with hearing loss, including practical, hierarchical auditory training activities.

Types of Stimuli

When speech stimuli such as those utilized in the Carhart program are employed, it is likely that generalization from training could be enhanced by using multiple talkers (e.g. males versus female versus child). Although many analytic training programs use speech stimuli, analytic training may include exercises with nonspeech sounds. For example, Moore and Amitay (2006) described a frequency training task, in which subjects determined whether tones are higher or lower in pitch. The determination of which stimuli should be used was based on the specific processing skills targeted during the training. Among the auditory skills that can be targeted by AT are pitch, loudness, and duration discrimination; temporal integration and resolution, temporal masking; temporal ordering; binaural interaction using intensity and time differences; and binaural separation using selective attention. Similar to the use of speech sounds for analytic training, a number of factors must be considered in both the frequency and time domain when training with non-speech stimuli. Among these stimuli factors are the rise-fall times, inter-stimulus intervals, presentation levels, and mode of delivery, that is, whether the stimuli are monotic, diotic, or dichotic. Synthetic training programs include sentence identification, as well as strategies and information for better speech understanding and communication.

Note that whereas training typically progresses from easy to difficult, or utilizes randomly presented stimuli, adaptive training can also be employed. Tye-Murray (1998) suggests the difficulty of the task should be set so that the patient does not achieve more than 80% or less than 50% success so that the task can remain challenging without creating fatigue or frustration.

Length of Time Required and Training Schedule

Establishing the minimal time frame required for lasting learning and generalization is important in order to create AT programs that will be recommended by professionals and completed by hearing impaired individuals. Learning may be categorized into procedural and perceptual learning. Procedural learning refers to improvements that are a result of learning how to perform the exercise. It occurs rapidly but does not necessarily generalize to real world performance on tasks that contain different stimuli. Perceptual learning refers to the integration of skills learned in the training that may be, but are not always, consistently generalized and/or long-lasting. Obviously, the objective of AT is perceptual learning. The exact time frame required to produce maximal perceptual learning is undoubtedly a function of multiple factors. Ideally, training should be able to be completed in as short a time frame as possible while still yielding the desired outcome. Merzenich et al. (1996) suggest that the optimal conditions for perceptual learning to occur include successive sessions with intense practice and conditions that motivate the subjects. Most studies reporting successful training of speech perception have included numerous training sessions conducted over a short period of time (Bernstein et al., 2001; Logan et al., 1993; Massaro et al., 1993; Stecker et al., 2006; Sweetow & Henderson Sabes, 2006; Walden et al., 1981; Walden, Prosek, Montgomery, Scherr, & Jones, 1977). Walden et al. (1981) demonstrated that adults with sensorineural hearing loss who wear hearing aids could be trained to improve their recognition of syllables (analytic training) after a short-term analytic individual training program (7 hours over a 10-day period), with most of the improvement in speech perception completed after 5 hours of training. Stecker et al. (2006) found continued improvement on Nonsense Syllable Test (NST) syllables throughout an 8 week period, with most of the improvement occurring in the first 2 weeks. Nogaki et al. (2007) found that similar improvements were seen in subjects trained once a week, three times a week or five times a week, providing the amount of overall training time was similar. Even initial, rapid learning, can be surprisingly long-lasting. Hawkey et al. (2004) reported that training for just a few minutes on a phoneme discrimination task can result in improved performance a week after the training.

Data from experiments reported by Moore and Amitay (2006) showed that learning can occur for certain tasks with passive, as opposed to active, listening. This may be an important consideration for future program design that could improve patient participation and compliance. It is also possible that analytic training, although it is focused on bottom-up sensory processing, may improve other detection and discrimination skills beyond those that are directly trained (Moore & Amitay, 2006, Fu & Galvin, 2008). Moreover, most training drills target multiple auditory processing skills. Sweetow and Henderson Sabes (2006) have outlined a number of principles and assumptions that should be considered in creating individualized audiologic rehabilitation auditory training programs. For example, they indicated that training should be interactive. Training should be practical and easily accessible. Therapy conducted at home has the advantages of being more cost-effective than repeated clinic visits with a professional and can allow the patient to practice in a nonthreatening atmosphere. It also allows for training to proceed at the patient's optimal pace. Training should be difficult enough to maintain the patient's interest and attention while being easy enough so that it minimizes fatigue and frustration. To effectively accomplish this, training should be adaptive so that exercises are conducted near the patient's performance threshold. As studies (to be discussed shortly) have demonstrated benefits from either analytic (bottom-up) or synthetic (top-down) training, it may be useful to integrate listening training with presentation of communication strategies. Elderly patients, those comprising the bulk of individuals wearing hearing aids, have additional cognitive and central auditory deficits to consider when implementing a rehabilitation protocol. Performance must be measurable and patients should be given feedback regarding their progress or lack of progress. Feedback should be provided on a trial-by-trial basis, as well as at the conclusion of each training session.

Does AT work?

Sweetow and Palmer (2005) conducted a systematic evidenced-based review of the AT literature. They identified 213 articles for review, eliminated 171 based on abstracts, and conducted a final review of 42 manuscripts. Of these, 6 met the rigid inclusion criteria for evidenced-based papers. These papers, although producing evidence supporting efficacy, did not produce unanimous or indisputable conclusions regarding the efficiency of individual auditory training. However, certain trends were supported. These trends suggest that synthetic training might be capable of teaching individuals with hearing-impairment to utilize more effectively active listening strategies that can translate into improved psychosocial function (Sweetow & Palmer, 2005). Some studies further supported the finding that speech recognition skills, particularly in noise, can be improved by synthetic or combined training Greater uncertainty remains regarding the contribution of analytic training alone. For example, Walden et al. (1981) showed that analytic auditory and lipreading training (e.g., training perception and discrimination of individual consonants) were useful in improving speech recognition in noise for younger adults. However, improvements were less with older adults and the efficacy of analytic speech perception training for this group was questioned. Rubinstein and Boothroyd (1987) found modest improvements in speech recognition in 20 older adults using either purely synthetic or combined analytic and synthetic approaches. Kricos and Holmes (1996) studied the efficacy of AR for older adults, using 78 adults with hearing loss. Analytic training did not help the older adults improve their speech perception or reduce their perceived problems associated with hearing loss. The use of an active listening approach, however, was proven to be effective for improving audiovisual speech recognition in noise. These findings are particularly important because many older adults with hearing impairment report their greatest difficulties in understanding speech when background noise is present. In addition to improved speech recognition, Kricos and Holmes' active listening group showed significant improvement in several aspects of psychosocial functioning, as measured by the Communication Profile for the Hearing Impaired (CPHI) (Demorest & Erdman, 1987). Specifically, the active listening group demonstrated improved verbal and nonverbal strategies, as well as increased ability to modify the behavior of others to improve their potential for successful communication. Improvements in the CPHI subscales (attitudes of others, acceptance of loss, withdrawal, and problem awareness) were noted for research participants in the active listening group whose pretraining scores suggested greater difficulties. Thus, these results offer evidence that when older adults exhibit personal adjustment problems such as withdrawal as a result of their hearing difficulties, they may benefit from learning coping strategies to help deal with communication breakdowns.

Recent discoveries in the field of neuroscience suggest that auditory skills might be enhanced with training that exploits neural plasticity and reorganization (Draganski & May, 2008; Polley et al., 2006; Zhou & Merzenich, 2007). However, questions persist regarding how to identify individuals who might benefit from training, how to determine the most efficient parameters of training, and how to measure progress. In addition, advances in electrophysiology and neural imaging, have demonstrated that these training procedures can actually produce measurable changes in cortical neural activity (Song et al., 2008; Tremblay & Kraus, 2002).

Why Isn't AT Used More Frequently?

Only the most skeptical audiologist would deny the likelihood that additional therapy beyond the use of wearable amplification can potentially benefit patients. Unfortunately, most audiologists do not offer or prescribe many of the additional therapies introduced in this book that comprise the broad scope of AR, and most patients do not ask for, or even wish to participate in, additional rehabilitation. There are many possible reasons for this reluctance. From the patients' perspective, many believe that they have spent enough money on products and professional services. Thus, they acquire the common, but unrealistic, expectation that the responsibility for success should rest solely with the hearing aids and the expertise of the audiologist. This is a primary reason why expectations (which tend to be based on the product and thus carry no responsibility for active participation on the part of the patient) should be replaced by goals (which have a rehabilitative foundation, and which require the active participation of the patient). From the audiologists' perception, some believe there is a perceived lack of evidence-based data, as illustrated by Ross (1997). This belief may be due to outcome measures typically concentrating on auditory training and speechreading, and not routinely considering the emotional and psychological byproducts. Furthermore, clinicians may have the unsubstantiated view that modern technology is sufficient to negate the need for additional auditory training. Moreover, and perhaps most importantly, some audiologists may believe that additional auditory training for the patient will require additional responsibilities and valuable, and frequently unavailable, professional time, for which they will not likely be reimbursed. Results of a survey of audiologists conducted by Schow et al. (1993) showed a major decline in the provision by audiologists of formal training in speechreading and auditory training. From 1980 to 1990, for example, the percentage of audiologists reporting the provision of auditory training to their patients dropped from 31% to 16%. Even viable alternatives, such as group AR, tend to be underutilized by professionals.

What Has Been the Impact of Technologic Advances on Auditory Training?

As described by Sweetow and Palmer (2005), auditory training can result in improvements in communication strategies. Such training on a one-to-one basis can be both time- and cost-intensive, however. Fortunately, there are alternatives available in our high-tech world via computerized auditory training. Computerized training has been shown to be effective in sensory training for visual disorders (Ciuffreda, 2002), as well as for cognitive disorders such as aging-associated memory deficits and early-stage Alzheimer's (Gunther et al., 2003). Also, well-established rules of perceptual learning can be easily implemented in a computerized protocol. For example, it is essential that the patients being trained maintain a high level of interest. Visual graphics and dynamic interaction between the patient and the computer program help maintain attention. In addition, the task must be difficult enough to present a challenge, but not so hard as to create frustration. One can accomplish this by adapting the difficulty level of the training to the individual subject. This model has long been a tenet of learning theory (Wolfle, 1951) and been proven effective in driving neural plasticity in animal models (Linkenhoker & Knudsen, 2002). As computerized training can be performed off-site, it can proceed in a comfortable environment and at a pace based on the individual patient's progress. By carefully defining the patient's communication profile, one can further devise deficit-specific training to fit that person's needs. Moreover, progress can be measured remotely.

A completely different approach to AT enhancement has been examined by Tobey and colleagues (2005). They investigated the potential benefit of pharmacologically enhanced (using d-amphetamine) AR therapy as a means of increasing speech-tracking skills in adult cochlear implant users. Following therapy, they measured regional cerebral blood flow (rCBF) in cochlear implant patients using Single Photon Emission Tomography (SPECT). Results showed that individuals with minimal open-set speech perception scores demonstrated unilateral cortical activation of the hemisphere contralateral to the implanted ear. Speech-tracking scores for the placebo and treatment groups were similar prior to intervention. In the placebo group, speech-tracking performance increased by 13.5% for visual plus auditory and auditory-only presentations as a function of aural therapy alone. The subjects in the d-amphetamine facilitated program yielded small increases in visual plus auditory tracking scores (2%) but showed a 43% increase for auditory-only speech tracking. Preliminary conclusions were that cortical imaging reveals important aspects of responsiveness in cochlear implant users and that pharmacologically enhanced AT subjects show increased neuroplastic changes. The optimal dosage and frequency of d-amphetamine remains to be determined, as does the ideal type and duration of AR intervention combined with a pharmacologic approach.

What AT Programs Are Available, and What Are the Similarities and Differences in These Methods?

A number of synthetic, analytic, and combined approaches have been developed. Examples of synthetic and combined programs include speech tracking procedures (DeFilippo & Scott, 1978; Owens & Raggio, 1987), the Active Communication Education program (Hickson et al., 2007), and the Learning to Hear Again program, (Wayner & Abrahamson, 1996). AR programs and many curricula have been suggested in the literature (Erber, 1982, 1996; Spitzer et al., 1993; Tye-Murray, 1997). Many clinicians have developed their own individualized AT activities including missing word (fill-in-the-blank), direction following, and topic or category determination from phrases and sentences.

The proliferation of home computers also has encouraged the development of individualized computer-based AT programs that allow for at-home training as a complement to group AR, or as a stand-alone training program. The most cost-effective and likely to be viable of these programs are delivered by a user-friendly computer program, are automated and adaptive, usually track some aspect of the patient's skill level or threshold, and retain the listener's responses and scores for easy access for the clinician. The exercises contained within these programs may include any or all of the following: auditory training (AT), AT combined with speechreading, behavioral and lifestyle changes, information and instruction regarding communication repair strategies, and cognitive training. All of these approaches are designed to maximize everyday performance and quality of life of the hearing-impaired individual. Although some of these programs have been designed specifically for cochlear implant recipients, all are intended to exploit the flexibility and plasticity of the central nervous system.

A number of efforts to produce computerized speechreading and assertive listening training programs have been discussed and proposed (Pichora-Fuller & Bengeural, 1991; Sims et al., 1979; Tye-Murray et al., 1988). Applications for speech perception training also have been developed, such as, Computer-Assisted Speech Perception Evaluation and Training (CASPER) (Boothroyd, 1987), and Computer-Assisted Tracking Simulation (CATS) (Dempsey et al., 1992). Although these programs relieve the audiologist from having to prepare and administer auditory training sessions, there has been limited interest in their use in most audiology clinics and these training programs have had limited impact for most clinicians. More recently, software-based programs have become easier to use, more adaptive and more engaging. Among these are Sound and Beyond™ (Cochlear Corporation of America, Englewood, CO) and Hearing Your Life™ (Advanced Bionics Corporation, Valencia, CA) programs based on the Computer-Assisted Speech Training (CAST) program and primarily used by cochlear implant recipients; Seeing and Hearing Speech (Boothroyd, 2003, Sensimetrics, Somerville MA), a program designed for both auditory and visual speech perception training; Conversation Made Easy (Tye-Murray, 2002), a program offering structured auditory and visual speech perception training, as well as exercises in conversational strategies on CD-ROM; SPATS (Speech Perception Assessment and Training System) (Miller et al., 2007), an adaptive program that trains phoneme, syllable, word, and sentence recognition; and Listening and Communication Enhancement (LACE™ from Neurotone, Redwood City, CA) a software-based program that may also be used with a DVD player that includes auditory training, as well as cognitive exercises that focus on aspects like auditory memory and cognitive processing speed (Sweetow & Henderson Sabes, 2006).

Examples of Auditory Training Programs

It is beyond the scope of this chapter to discuss all available programs in detail, but for the purpose of illustrating some of the deliberation that goes into designing computerized AT, four programs with different approaches and objectives will be summarized.

Computer-Assisted Speech-Perception Testing and Training at the Sentence Level (CasperSent)

CasperSent is an expansion of the original CASPER program (Boothroyd, 1987). The software, which is also available on DVD, was created with the Gallaudet Rehabilitation Engineering Research Center. The program trains and assesses auditory, visual, and auditory-visual speech understanding. The stimuli consist of 60 sets of CUNY sentences with 12 topics and 3 sentence types (statements, questions, and commands) that are presented in one of three conditions: lipreading only, hearing only, or a combination of the two. The sentence length ranges from 3 to 14 words. When self-training, the patient hears and/or sees (in the case of visual training) a spoken sentence, repeats as much of the sentence as possible, views the text, clicks on the words correctly identified, hears and/or sees the sentence again, and then continues on to the next sentence. The software can be adapted to remove all feedback to the patient. The training may be completed independently, or with the aid of a scorer. Scores are based on sets of 12 sentences, and are saved for analysis at a later time. A newer version of this software includes low-pass speech as a demonstration mode for significant others.

Computer-Assisted Tracking Simulation (CATS)

Dempsey et al. (1992) reported on an updated approach to the Continuous Discourse Tracking (speech tracking) method originally developed at CID by de Filippo and Scott (1978). This AT software program is based on the Kungliga-Tekniska-Högskolan (KTH) speech-tracking protocol developed at the Royal Institute of Technology in Sweden and refined by Gnosspelius and Spens (1992). Like most of the computerized programs, it is designed both to train and assess the skills of the patient and is adaptive to the patient's needs and abilities. Unlike other programs, however, it is designed to be used face-to-face, so this computer AT program is *not* home-based and requires a clinician for administration. The advantages of this tracking approach are that it can cover a wide range of communication skills and can be employed with all communication modes (i.e., auditory, visual, auditory/visual).

The protocol is as follows: a display shows text that is read by the clinician (talker) to the patient (listener) using a conversational manner of speech. The listener then repeats as much of the text as possible. If the listener is incorrect, the talker enters the information into the computer, and repeats the utterance or the incorrect portion of it, (and may provide correction strategies) until the utterance is correctly repeated in its entirety. Up to two repetitions are provided to the listener. If the word is still not correctly identified, the incorrect word is shown as text on the listener's computer screen. The results of each session are saved and training information is saved for later analysis. The patient's scores are based on the speed of tracking (words per minute). The CATS tracking protocol has new rules the patient must follow, in order to provide consistency in the tracking program, a drawback to previous programs (Tye-Murray & Tyler, 1988). For example, there are a set number of available correction strategies, and the difficulty of the material is controlled. The goal of the CATS program is to reduce the variability of previous tracking programs while preserving the interactive qualities of communication. CATS also may be adapted for self-training applications using prerecorded materials.

Computer-Assisted Speech Training (CAST)

CAST software was developed at the House Ear Institute (Fu & Galvin, 2008). CAST is a home-based computer-assisted speech training program used by CI recipients. The program monitors progress and saves data for analysis by the clinician. Versions of CAST have been produced commercially by CI companies: Sound and Beyond™ for Cochlear Corporation, and Hearing Your Life™ for Advanced Bionics. CAST provides auditory training that is specific to the needs of CI users, but could be used by others with significant hearing loss. It is primarily an analytic approach, focusing on the acoustic contrasts and signals that are especially problematic for the CI user, as opposed to more synthetic exercises. Training materials include pure tones, environmental sounds, monosyllabic words, consonant stimuli (VC, VCV, and CV), familiar words, and sentences, melodic sequences and melodies. CAST uses more than 1,000 monosyllabic and nonsense words spoken by multiple talkers. The program is adaptive, in that the level of difficulty is automatically adjusted according to individual patient performance by increasing the number of response choices and/or reducing the acoustic differences between response choices. During training, both auditory and visual feedback is provided. At the end of each testing and training session, the program offers training recommendations. For example, CAST may suggest that the user move to an easier or more difficult training level, based on performance. Additional training materials and/or training modules can be added. CAST also can incorporate noise or competing speech to simulate a difficult listening environment.

Several studies have been conducted using AT with variations of the CAST program for recognition of phonemes, melodic sequences, and Chinese tones (Galvin et al. 2007; Nogaki, 2007). The data from these studies indicate improved performance in the targeted listening task. Improvement sometimes generalized to tasks that were not explicitly trained, such as improved sentence recognition after training with phonetic contrasts, or improved familiar melody identification after training with simple melodic sequences (Fu & Galvin, 2007). Nearly all of the subjects had at least one year of experience with their CI device prior to training, indicating that training could be used to improve speech performance at early as well as later stages of the implantation rehabilitative process. Although other studies have shown preservation of skills gained during auditory training (Stecker et al., 2006; Sweetow & Henderson Sabes, 2006), these authors report that performance on measured tasks may revert to baseline levels as soon as 1 to 2 months post-training. The current CAST program task and training protocol has been modified from those used in previous studies and the CAST recommendations for training protocols are more flexible.

Listening and Communication Enhancement (LACE™)

Listening and Communication Enhancement (LACE™) (Sweetow & Henderson Sabes, 2006) is an interactive computer software program designed to be used in the patient's home, but is now also available in a clinic version for an in-office training lab as well as a DVD version. LACE™ is designed for use by the adult hearing-impaired listener. The main objectives of LACE™ are to build skills and confidence by providing AT exercises and communication strategies with the goal of enhancing listening and communication skills. The program was designed to provide exercises in the types of situations most difficult for hearing-impaired listeners and to address cognitive changes characteristic of the aging process that may interfere with effective communication. LACE™ utilizes an adaptive training algorithm so that the training difficulty level occurs near the individual's skill threshold and proceeds at the patient's optimal pace. The training combines listening training (analytic) with repair strategies (synthetic), and gives the patient feedback regarding performance. LACE™ provides a variety of tasks that are divided into three main categories (degraded speech, cognitive skills, and communication strategies).

Degraded Speech. The degraded speech exercises represent some of the situations in which the individual with hearing loss has difficulty functioning. The components include Speech-in-Noise (speaker with multitalker babble background), Rapid Speech (time-compressed speech to challenge the temporal processing of the auditory system and make demands on cognitive speed of processing), and Competing Speaker (speaker with a single talker background as masking). The sentence-length stimuli are organized into topics (health issues, money matters, exercise, etc.) that are selected by the trainee at the beginning of each training session. This reinforces the importance of utilizing contextual cues by keeping the general topic in mind when listening. Stimuli are presented by male, female, and child talkers, in order to present acoustic variation and enhance generalization. The stimuli are varied in difficulty (signal-to-noise ratio or time-compression ratio), based on the patient's performance. The patient is asked to repeat as much of the stimuli as possible, and the difficulty of the stimuli is modified trial-by-trial, based on performance.

Cognitive Training. Because of cognitive changes and the effects they may have on listening (Pichora-Fuller, 2007), exercises based on improving speed of cognitive processing and auditory memory, two elements of listening that are particularly important in difficult listening environments, and are particularly affected in older listeners, are included in the LACE™ training.

Communication Strategies. Additionally, LACE™ provides over 150 communication strategies to enhance communication (managing acoustic environment, realistic expectations, hearing aid information, effective communication strategies, etc). These strategies are interspersed throughout the training and are accompanied by visual images.

Training is provided for 20 half-hour sessions, and is recommended to be completed over the course of approximately one month. Additional training time is available on demand. In addition to the immediate feedback given for each trial of each task, LACE™ creates a graph depicting previous and current performance at the end of each training session. Furthermore, the results of the training are tracked and may be electronically transmitted to a HIPAA compliant secure Web site accessible by the audiologist so that the patient's progress can be monitored.

In a multisite study of the effectiveness of a pilot version of LACE™ on 65 subjects, Sweetow and Henderson Sabes (2006) reported significant improvements, not only on the training tasks, but also on a variety of "off-task" standardized outcome measures including the Quick Sin (Killion et al., 2004; Etymotic Research, Inc., Elk Grove Village, IL), Hearing Handicap Scale for the Elderly (HHIE) (Ventry & Weinstein, 1982), and Communication Scale for Older Adults (CSOA) (Kaplan et al., 1997).

Differences and Similarities of Individual Aural Rehabilitation Programs

Although the programs outlined above were designed for different purposes and populations, they share many similarities. Some of the programs (LACE™ and CAST) incorporate adaptive difficulty levels. Some programs (CATS and CasperSent) include both auditory and visual training. The frequency and duration of training sessions differ. Some programs are designed for more bottom-up training using phonemes, syllables, and melodies (CAST), whereas others (LACE™) use a more combined bottom-up and top-down approach by including contextually related sentence length training materials, communication strategies, and cognitive exercises. Training stimuli also vary. LACE™ and CasperSent use topic-related sentences. CATS uses sentences or longer discourse. CAST includes environmental sounds, pure tones, nonsense syllables, words, sentences, and melodies. Some programs are specifically designed for training in noise or with other degraded signals (LACE™ and CAST), though all can be adapted so that noise is included. Some programs can be used both for training and testing, others just for training. All include the provision of feedback to patients, though at different intervals, and all allow for data retrieval and later analysis. Table 12–1 compares some of the program features for these and other available programs.

The Roles of the Audiologist and Speech-Language Pathologist in AT

As stated earlier, the adult with hearing loss must call upon many skills and processes to communicate effectively. These include hearing, cognition, auditory memory, auditory closure, auditory learning, metalinguistics, usage of pragmatics, semantics, grammatical shape, localization, visual cues, repair tactics, and effective interactive communication strategies (Keissling et al., 2003). In addition, many elderly individuals with hearing impairment have diminished cognitive skills. The study and treatment of these skills and processes fall within the purview of both audiologists and Speech-Language-Pathologists (SLPs). The decline in the practice and provision of comprehensive AR by audiologists has occurred, in part, because of the restricted definition of audiology as a diagnostic, rather than as both a diagnostic and therapeutic profession. Thus, reimbursement frequently is difficult to obtain for audiologists. SLPs do not have similar restrictions because it is considered a therapeutic profession. Therefore, it is important that SLPs continue to provide (and perhaps expand upon) these services. This is particularly significant when face-to-face individualized AT, as opposed to home-based programs, are necessary. (*Note:* For further discussion of reimbursement issues related to AR services, the reader is referred to Chapter 2 of this text.)

Conclusions and Final Remarks

Auditory training can be a great asset to adults with hearing impairment. It is an underutilized therapy for a number of reasons, some of which have been described in this chapter. In order for AT to regain its rightful place as an important component of AR, more data will be required to

Table 12–1. Components of the Four Training Programs Are Shown (Filled circles indicate that the training program includes this aspect of aural rehabilitation)

	Bottom-up AT	Top-down AT	Feed-back	Communication Strategies	Adaptive	Video	Data Retrieval	Remote Access
LACE™		●	●	●	●		●	●
CasperSent		●	●			●	●	
CATS		●	●	●		●	●	
CAST	●		●		●		●	
SPATS	●		●		●		●	
Seeing/Hearing Speech		●	●		●	●	●	
Conversation Made Easy	●	●	●			●		

convince audiologists of its efficacy. As with any training program, one can question whether positive outcomes are a result of completing specific training parameters or merely a function of patient practice. Regardless of the cause, if it benefits the patient, it should be promoted by professionals. Questions remain regarding the optimal training parameters and outcome measures. The combination of AT with other aspects of AR (amplification, assistive listening devices, speechreading, cognitive therapies, communication repair strategies, group meetings, etc.) must continue to be investigated. In addition to the need for additional behavioral data, electrophysiologic evidence of changes associated with enhanced performance may help convince professionals, patients, and perhaps third-party payers of the importance of AT.

It is our hope that in the near future, auditory training programs will be embraced with the same confidence and fervor as amplification and that all patients entering an audiologist's office will exit with a therapeutic plan that focuses on communication, not just hearing.

Disclosure. The authors have a financial interest in Neurotone, the company licensed by UCSF to produce LACE.

References

Ball, K., Berch D. B., Helmers, K. F., Jobe, J. B., Leveck, M. D., Marsiske, M., et al. (2002). Effects of cognitive training interventions with older adults: A randomized controlled trial. *Journal of the American Medical Association, 288*, 2271–2281.

Bernstein, L. E., Auer, E. T., & Tucker, P. E. (2001). Enhanced speechreading in deaf adults: Can short-term training/practice close the gap for hearing adults? *Journal of Speech, Language, and Hearing Research, 44*, 5–18.

Boothroyd A. (1987). CASPER, computer-assisted speech-perception evaluation and training. In *Proceedings of the 10th Annual Conference of the Rehabilitation Society of North America* (pp. 734–736). Washington DC: Association for Advancement of Rehabilitation Technology.

Boothroyd, A. (2003). Seeing and hearing speech: Lessons in lipreading and listening. *Ear and Hearing, 24*(1), 96.

Carhart, R. (1960). Auditory Training. In H. Davis & R. Silverman (Eds.), *Hearing and deafness* (2nd ed., pp. 346–359). New York: Holt Rinehart and Winston.

Ciuffreda, K. J. (2002). The scientific basis for and efficacy of optometric vision therapy in nonstrabismic accommodative and vergence disorders. *Optometry, 73*, 735–762.

Dempsey, J., Levitt, H., Josephson, J., & Porrazzo, J. (1992). Computer-assisted tracking simulation (CATS). *Journal of the Acoustical Society of America, 92*, 701–710.

de Filippo, C. L., & Scott, B. L. (1978). A method for training and evaluating the reception of ongoing speech. *Journal of the Acoustical Society of America, 63*(4), 1186–1192.

Demorest, M. E., & Erdman, S. A. (1987). Development of the communication profile for the hearing impaired. *Journal of Speech and Hearing Disorders, 52*, 129–143.

Draganski, B., & May, A. (2008). Training-induced structural changes in the adult human brain. *Behavioural Brain Research* (Feb 17, epub).

Dubno, J. R., Dirks, D. D., & Morgan, D. E. (1984). Effects of age and mild hearing loss on speech recognition in noise. *Journal of the Acoustical Society of America, 76*(1), 87–96.

Erber, N. P. (1982). *Auditory training*. Washington DC: Alexander Graham Bell Association for the Deaf.

Erber, N. P. (1996). *Communication therapy for hearing-impaired adults* (2nd ed.). Melbourne, Australia: Clavis.

Florentine, M., & Buus, S. (1984) Temporal gap detection in sensorineural and simulated hearing impairments. *Journal of Speech and Hearing Research, 27*, 449–455.

Fu, Q.-J., & Galvin, J. J. (2008). Maximizing cochlear implant patients' performance with advanced speech training procedures. *Hearing Research, 242*, 198–208.

Galvin, J. J., Fu, Q.-J., & Nogaki, G. (2007). Melodic contour identification in cochlear implants. *Ear and Hearing, 28*(3), 302–319.

Gordon-Salant, S., & Fitzgibbons, P. J. (1995). Comparing recognition of distorted speech using an equivalent signal-to-noise ratio index. *Journal of Speech and Hearing Research, 38*(3), 706–713.

Gordon-Salant, S., & Fitzgibbons, P. J. (1999). Profile of auditory temporal processing in older listeners. *Journal of Speech, Language, and Hearing Research, 42*, 300–311.

Gnosspelius, J., & Spens, K.-E. (1992). A computer-based speech tracking procedure. *Speech Transmissions Laboratory Quarterly Progress and Status Report, 1*, 131–137.

Gunther, V. K., Schafer, P., Holzner, B. J., & Kemmler, G. W. (2003). Long-term improvements in cognitive performance through computer-assisted cognitive training: A pilot study in a residential home for older people. *Aging Mental Health, 7*, 200–206.

Hawkey, D. J., Amitay, S., & Moore, D. R. (2004). Early and rapid perceptual learning. *Nature Neuroscience, 7*, 1055–1056.

Hickson, L., & Worrall, L. (2003) Beyond hearing aid fitting: Improving communication for older adults. *International Journal of Audiology, 42*(Suppl. 2), 2S84–2S91.

Hickson, L., Worrall, L., & Scarinci, N. (2007). A randomized controlled trial evaluating the active communication education program for older people with hearing impairment. *Ear and Hearing, 28*(2), 212–230.

Humes, L. E. (1996). Speech understanding in the elderly. *Journal of the American Academy of Audiology, 7*, 161–167.

Irvine, D. R., Rajan, R., & Brown, M. (2001). Injury- and use-related plasticity in adult auditory cortex. *Audiology and Neuro-otology, 6*, 192–195.

Kaplan, H., Bally, S., Brandt, F., Busacco, D., & Pray, J. (1997) Communication Scale for Older Adults (CSOA). *Journal of the American Academy of Audiology, 8*(3), 203–217.

Keissling, J., Pichora-Fuller, M. K., Gatehouse, S., Stephens, D., Arlinger, S., Chisholm, T., et al. (2003). Candidature for and delivery of audiological services: Special needs of older people. *International Journal of Audiology, 42*, S92–S101.

Killion, M. C., Niquette, P. A., Gudmundson, G. I., Revit, L. J., & Banerjee, S. (2004). Development of a quick speech-in-noise test for measuring signal-to-noise ratio loss in normal-hearing and hearing-impaired listeners. *Journal of the Acoustical Society of America, 116*(4 Pt. 1), 2395–2405.

Kim, J. J., Gross, J., Morest, D. K., & Potashner, S. J. (2004). Quantitative study of degeneration and new growth of axons and synaptic endings in the chinchilla cochlear nucleus after acoustic overstimulation. *Journal of Neuroscience Research, 15*, 829–842.

Kochkin, S. (2007). MarkeTrak VII: Obstacles to adult non-user adoption of hearing aids. *Hearing Journal, 60*, 27–43.

Kricos, P. B., & Holmes, A. E. (1996). Efficacy of audiologic rehabilitation for older adults. *Journal of the American Academy of Audiology, 7*, 219–229.

Linkenhoker, B. A., & Knudsen, E. I. (2002). Incremental training increases the plasticity of the auditory space map in adult barn owls. *Nature, 419*, 293–296.

Logan, J. S., Lively, S. E., & Pisoni, D. B. (1993). Training listeners to perceive novel phonetic categories: How do we know what is learned? *Journal of the Acoustical Society of America, 94*, 1148–1151.

Mahncke, H. W., Connor, B. B., Appelman, J., Ahsanuddin, O. N., Hardy, J. L., Wood, R. A., et al. (2006). Memory enhancement in healthy older adults using a brain plasticity-based training program: A randomized, controlled study. *Proceedings of the National Academy of Sciences of the United States of America, 103*, 12523–12528.

Massaro, D. W., Cohen, M. M., & Gesi, A. T. (1993). Long-term training, transfer, and retention in learning to lipread. *Perception and Psychophysics, 53*, 549–562.

Merzenich, M. M., Jenkins, W. M., Johnston, P., Schreiner, C., Miller, S. L., & Tallal, P. (1996). Temporal processing deficits of language-learning impaired children ameliorated by training. *Science, 271*, 77–81.

Miller, J. D., Watson, C. S., Kewley-Port, D., Sillings, R., Mills, W. B., & Burleson, D. F. (2007). SPATS: Speech perception assessment and training system. Abstract. *Journal of the Acoustical Society of America, 122*, 3063.

Moore, B. C., & Glasberg, B. R. (1986). Comparisons of frequency selectivity in simultaneous and forward masking for subjects with unilateral cochlear impairments. *Journal of the Acoustical Society of America, 80*, 93–107.

Moore, D. R., & Amitay, S. (2006). Auditory training: Rules and applications. *Seminars in Hearing, 28*, 99–109.

Neurotone. Redwood City, CA. Retrieved March 2007 from http://www.neurotone.com

Nogaki, G., Fu, Q. J., & Galvin, J. J., 3rd. (2007). Effect of training rate on recognition of spectrally shifted speech. *Ear and Hearing, 28*, 132–140.

Owens, E., & Raggio, M. (1987). The UCSF tracking procedure for evaluation and training of speech reception by hearing-impaired adults. *Journal of Speech and Hearing Disorders, 52*(2), 120–128.

Pichora-Fuller, M. K. (2003) Cognitive aging and auditory information processing. *International Journal of Audiology, 42*(Suppl. 2), S26–S32.

Pichora-Fuller, M. K. (2007). Rehabilitative audiology: Using the brain to reconnect listeners with impaired ears to their acoustic ecologies. *Journal of the American Academy of Audiology, 18*, 536–583.

Pichora-Fuller, M. K., & Benquerel, A. P. (1991). The design of CAST (Computer-aided speechreading training). *Journal of Speech and Hearing Research, 34*, 202–212.

Pichora-Fuller, M. K., Schneider, B. A., & Daneman, M. (1995). How young and old adults listen to and remember speech in noise. *Journal of the Acoustical Society of America, 97*(1), 593–608.

Pichora-Fuller, M. K., & Singh, G. (2006). Effects of age on auditory and cognitive processing: Implications for hearing aid fitting and audiologic rehabilitation. *Trends in Amplification, 10*, 29–59.

Polley, D. B., Steinberg, E. E., & Merzenich, M. M. (2006). Perceptual learning directs auditory cortical map reorganization through top-down influences. *Journal of Neuroscience, 26*(18), 4970–4982.

Ross, M. (1997). A retrospective look at the future of aural rehabilitation. *Journal of the Academy of Rehabilitative Audiology, 30*, 11–28.

Rubinstein, A., & Boothroyd, A. (1987). Effect of two approaches to auditory training on speech recognition by hearing-impaired adults. *Journal of Speech and Hearing Research, 30*, 153–160.

Schneider, B. A., Daneman, M., & Murphy, D. R. (2005). Speech comprehension difficulties in older adults: Cognitive slowing or age-related changes in hearing? *Psychology and Aging, 20*, 261–271.

Schow, R., Balsara, N., Smedley, T., & Whitcomb, C. (1993). Aural rehabilitation by ASHA audiologists: 1980–1990. *American Journal of Audiology, 2*, 28–37.

Sensimetrics. Somerville, MA. Seeing and hearing speech. Retrieved March 2007 from: http://www.seeingspeech.com/

Sims, D. G., Feldt, J., von Dowaliby, F., Hutchinson, K., & Myers, T. (1979). A pilot experiment in computer-assisted speechreading instruction utilizing the Data Analysis Video Interactive Device (DAVID). *American Annals of the Deaf, 124*, 618–623.

Song, J. H., Skoe, E., Wong, P. C., & Kraus, N. (2008). Plasticity in the adult human auditory brainstem following short-term linguistic training. *Journal of Cognitive Neuroscience, 20*(10), 1892–1902.

Spitzer, J. B., Leder, S. B., & Giolas, T. G. (1993). *Rehabilitation of late-deafened adults: Modular program manual.* St Louis, MO: Mosby.

Stecker, G. C., Bowman, G. A., Yund, E. W., Herron, T. J., Roup, C. M., & Woods, D. L. (2006) Perceptual training improves syllable identification in new and experienced hearing aid users. *Journal of Rehabilitation Research and Development, 43*, 537–552.

Sweetow, R. W., & Henderson Sabes, J. (2006). The need for and development of an adaptive Listening and Communication Enhancement (LACE) Program. *Journal of the American Academy of Audiology, 17*, 538–558.

Sweetow, R. W., & Palmer, C. V. (2005). Efficacy of individual auditory training in adults: A systematic review of the evidence. *Journal of the American Academy of Audiology, 16*(7), 494–504.

Tobey, E. A., Devous, M. D., Buckley, K., Overson, G., Harris, T., Ringe, W., et al. (2005). Pharmacological enhancement of aural habilitation in adult cochlear implant users. *Ear and Hearing, 26* (Suppl. 4), 45S–56S.

Tremblay, K. L., & Kraus, N. (2002). Auditory training induces asymmetrical changes in cortical neural activity. *Journal of Speech, Language, and Hearing Research, 45*(3), 564–572.

Tye-Murray, N. (1997). *Communication training for older teenagers and adults: Listening speechreading and using conversational strategies.* Austin TX: Pro-Ed.

Tye-Murray, N. (1998). *Auditory training: In foundations in aural rehabilitation* (pp. 159–192). San Diego, CA: Singular.

Tye-Murray, N. (2002). *Conversation made easy: Speechreading and conversation strategies training for people with hearing loss.* Retrieved March 2007 from: http://www.cid.wustl.edu/deaf%20home/PUBLICATIONS/books.htm

Tye-Murray, N, & Tyler, R. S. (1988). A critique of continuous discourse tracking as a test procedure.

Journal of Speech and Hearing Disorders, 53(3), 226–231.

Tye-Murray, N., Tyler, R. S., Bong, B., & Nares, T. (1988). Computerized laser videodisc programs for training speech reading and assertive communication behaviors. *Journal of the Academy of Rehabilitative Audiology, 21*, 143–152.

van Hooren, S. A., Anteunis, L. J., Valentijn, S. A., Bosma, H., Ponds, R. W., Jolles, J., et al. (2005). Does cognitive function in older adults with hearing impairment improve by hearing aid use? *International Journal of Audiology, 44*, 265–271.

Ventry, I. M., & Weinstein, B. E. (1982). The hearing handicap inventory for the elderly: A new tool. *Ear and Hearing, 3*(3), 128–134.

Walden, B. E., Erdman, S. A., Montgomery, A. A., Schwartz, D. M., & Prosek, R. A. (1981). Some effects of training on speech recognition by hearing-impaired adults. *Journal of Speech and Hearing Research, 24*, 207–216.

Walden, B. E., Prosek, R. A., Montgomery, A. A., Scherr, C. K., & Jones, C. J. (1977). Effects of training on the visual recognition of consonants. *Journal of Speech and Hearing Research, 20*, 130–145.

Wayner, D. S., & Abrahamson, J. E. (1996). *Learning to hear again: An audiologic rehabilitation curriculum guide.* Austin, TX: Hear Again.

Wingfield, A., & Tun, P. A. (2007). Cognitive supports and cognitive constraints on comprehension of spoken language. *Journal of the American Academy of Audiology 18*, 548–558.

Wolfle, D. (1951) Training. In S. S. Stevens (Ed.), *Handbook of experimental psychology.* New York: John Wiley and Sons.

Zhou, X., & Merzenich, M. M. (2007). Intensive training in adults refines A1 representations degraded in an early postnatal critical period. *Proceedings of the National Academy of Sciences of the United States of America, 104*, 15935–15940.

13

Group Therapy and Group Dynamics in Audiologic Rehabilitation

Scott J. Bally

We're all in this together . . . by ourselves
Lily Tomlin

Groups as a Context for Audiologic Rehabilitation

Definitions of aural or audiologic rehabilitation (AR) abound in the professional literature. Recent efforts to capture the essence of AR have been offered by Ross (1997) as "any device, procedure, information, interaction, or therapy which lessens the communicative and psychosocial consequences of hearing loss" whereas Boothroyd (2007) defines AR as "the reduction of hearing-loss-induced deficits of function, activity, participation, and quality of life through a combination of sensory management instruction, perceptual training and counseling (2007, p. 63). AR can only be loosely defined because the scope of practice is so broad. In practice, a review of AR program components varies widely and may include such skill areas as: speechreading/lipreading and auditory training or more global areas including the use of hearing assistive technology systems (HATS), development of communication strategies, assertiveness approaches and systematic problem solving, and adaptation to the psychosocial effects of hearing loss. AR in the context of culturally Deaf populations may include both receptive and expressive communication skills with less emphasis on psychosocial adjustment.

Group intervention is a methodology frequently employed by audiologists to help achieve AR goals and objectives. The dynamics that commonly occur within therapy groups, self-help groups, and mutual support groups may be facilitated by professionals to help group members adapt to the biopsychosocial effects of hearing loss. The primary difference between group and individual rehabilitation is that groups offer the opportunity for mutual support and facilitate empowerment through self- or intermember help. Groups tend to be "powerful rather than weak, active rather than passive, fluid rather than static and catalyzing rather than reifying" (Forsyth, 2006, p. 16). Lewin (1947) selected the term *dynamics* to emphasize the powerful impact of these complex social processes on members of a given group.

Using an ecological systems perspective, this chapter will consider the psychological factors and social contexts that affect successful adaptation to hearing loss. It will explore the interpersonal dynamics that occur in change-oriented groups and provide suggestions for utilizing those dynamics to help participants meet the challenges of hearing loss more successfully.

Defining Group Therapy

Group therapy may be defined as a treatment mechanism that involves a small group of members who are guided by a professional with expertise in the area of intervention. The objective of groups is to promote psychological and social growth and to ameliorate psychosocial problems through exploration of the cognitive, behavioral and affective interactions among members and within micro- and mesosocial contexts. These elements distinguish therapy groups from self-help and support groups. Whereas group therapy seeks to affect psychological change, self-help and support groups have the more limited goal of assisting members in coping with their immediate problems. Fuhriman and Burlingame (1994) stress the critical nature of the opportunity for interation among group members, citing studies that demonstrate that without that interactive dynamic the potential benefits of formulating a group are not realized.

Professionally Guided Therapeutic, Self-Help, and Support Groups

AR groups vary in their appellation, degree of professional involvement and inclusion of significant others. Each may influence the functioning of the group in different ways and to varying degrees.

An informal survey of the literature, including that which is cited in this chapter, reveals that the nomenclature for therapeutic groups varies widely, using such terms as therapy group, support group, mutual support or mutual aid group and self-help group. The terms are used inconsistently and, often, interchangeably. The degree to which these groups are professionally guided also varies widely and does not always appear to have a direct relationship to the group labels. By definition, mutual support groups focus on providing psychosocial and spiritual support, while self-help and mutual aid groups focus on change or adaptation to the common problems. Not only are these appellations inconsistent, but they are also somewhat misleading. There are, however, some fundamental consistencies in the nature of these groups. They are all groups of individuals who come together because of a "single life problem or condition shared by all its members" (Kurtz, 1997, p. 4). They are all supportive, educational, and change-oriented and established for the accomplishment of a specific purpose; information, resources, and life experiences are exchanged (Brabender, Fallon, & Smolar, 2004; Edgerton & Hunter, 1985; Hollister, Katz, & Bender, 1976; Kurtz, 1997). All have a "great potential to alleviate psychological suffering" (Brabender, Fallon, & Smolar, 2004, p. 15). "Self-help or mutual aid groups provide a mechanism whereby individuals in a collective setting with others who face similar life situations can assume responsibility for their own bodies, psyches, and behavior and can help others do the same" (Sidel & Sidel, 1976, p. 67). Virtually all AR groups fall somewhere along this continuum, depending on the extent to which psychosocial issues are actively addressed and the degree of latitude and self-direction allowed by the professional who conducts the group.

Regardless of intent, psychosocial changes do occur as the result of group participation. Commonly occurring group dynamics can facilitate such changes. A characteristic of successful therapy groups is that they formalize change efforts by establishing group goals and objectives. Achieving these ends may be more successful when professionals facilitate or enhance the group dynamics to render desired outcomes.

The inclusion of significant others who do not have the common problem, but share its effects, is inconsistent across groups. Pray (1996) notes that hearing loss is a shared problem and results in *parallel reactions* by both communication partners when communication breakdown occurs (i.e., anxiety, frustration, guilt, feelings of incompetence).

Attributes of Self-Help Groups

To understand better their nature, it may be helpful to examine the attributes of self-help groups. Katz and Bender (1976, pp. 9–11) enumerate such characteristics as:

- involving other persons,
- having patterned small group or face-to-face interactions, of spontaneous origin,
- being limited in duration,
- having a variety of functions and characteristics,
- having personal participation,
- fostering sympathetic and empathetic relationships,
- providing a point of connection and identification with others,
- engaging is some form of action, and
- moving from being powerless to being empowered.

It should be noted that these attributes are consistent within all rehabilitation group types.

In contrast, Riessman and Carroll (1995) enumerate principles that distinguish true self-help groups including:

- self-direction,
- reduced dependency on institutions, such as the medical community,
- freely donated services,
- a democratic philosophy,
- nonhierarchic structure,
- emphasis on experiential learning, and
- struggle against expertism, mystification, exclusivity, elitism, and professional privatization of knowledge.

Although these attributes are less often associated with AR groups, the characteristics and principles, especially experiential learning, may be helpful in addressing the systemic needs of persons with hearing loss.

Answering a Need

Sidel and Sidel (1976) identify factors in our society that led to the development of a self-help and mutual aid movement to meet human needs. The primary tenet is that human services are either unavailable or are not responsive to those in need of them. Other societal factors include:

- the rapidly expanding and pervasiveness of technology;
- the multiplicity, complexity, and size of institutions and communities that are more frequently characterized by depersonalization;
- the alienation of people from each other, their institutions and communities, as well as from themselves; and
- the professionalization of many areas that were previously addressed by individuals for themselves or for each other.

More specific to AR is that traditional medically based professional perspectives and treatment models for disability, and especially hearing loss, have not adequately addressed individual needs for psychosocial adjustment.

Therapy groups have the capacity to make significant contributions toward dealing with problems that, for varying reasons are not being addressed by traditional professional approaches or institutions in our society. At the same time, such groups provide individuals with the opportunity to help others; such roles are increasingly more difficult to find in our society as trained professionals have usurped many of these volunteer or self-help roles. Katz (1984) refers to them as "the grass roots answer to our hierarchical, professionalized society—to a society which attempts in so many ways to render impotent the individual, the family, the neighbor. These [self-help] groups . . . enhance the use of the community's natural care-giving resources of family, extended family, informal friendship and workplace networks, religious organizations and the like" (p. 234). As early as 1963 Clinard noted that "Not only are self-help groups providing desperately needed services, but they are returning to the individual a feeling of competence and self-respect and they are forging new links, new connections among people" (p. 647). Gartner and Riessman (1977) state that "In each case, the group helps to integrate the individual, to change his conception of himself, to make him feel again the solidarity of the group behind the individual, and to combat social stigma. These group processes, it is felt, replace the 'I' feelings with 'we' feelings, give the individual the feeling of being in a group and redefine certain norms of behavior" (p. 647). These processes are not exclusive to self-help groups and may be applied to professionally guided AR groups.

The mutual support aspect of effectively managed AR groups has the capacity to meet a number of basic human needs. Maslow's Theory of Human Motivation provides us with some insights as to the bases of human need (Maslow, 1943). Maslow's hierarchy suggests that the need for biological homeostasis places physiologic needs as the most fundamental to human existence. Other critical human needs include those for safety, love, and self-esteem. Each of these fundamental needs may be best achieved through some use of interpersonal communication (Maslow, 1991; Trotzer, 2006). Although writing and sign language are viable options, the standard for our society is through aural/oral communication. This has fundamental implications for persons with hearing loss, whose ability to communicate is impaired. An AR group may be instrumental in assisting its members to overcome the challenges of communication within the context of hearing loss. From a societal perspective, any communication is "an act that sustains the self and the others in their statuses as full members of the human social world" (Noble, 1983).

Limitations and Weaknesses of Groups

Group approaches are not without their detractors or valid criticisms. Those most frequently cited in the literature are:

- rehabilitation groups espouse middle class values, and/or are inaccessible or irrelevant for individuals from lower socioeconomic classes,
- self-paced or limited time groups often try to do too much or move too fast,
- AR groups tend to focus on technology use at the expense of psychosocial adaptation,
- therapy groups have a continuing conflict between fulfilling individual and group needs, and
- small groups may not exert enough power to facilitate change.

Such criticism must be considered in the greater context that includes the many benefits of groups, as described above. These arguments can easily be refuted, professional guidance being the key factor in doing so. Smaller self-guided groups *are* likely to do too much or move too fast. A professional understanding of the varied learning styles and rates of adaptation of different people may increase sensitivity to individuals and temper the rate of group movement. Providing these groups with guidelines from a professional could help them limit or pace themselves, balance technology with skill development, identify realistic change efforts and enhance the ability to generalize group to individual change efforts.

The Value Systems of Groups

In a small group, both individual and group needs are often synonymous. Small group formats allow for identification of shared problems and the development of rehabilitation objectives that are broad enough to address them, yet incorporate individual needs. Professionally-run groups are likely to focus on common objectives and needs of group members and guide the group to address individual challenges and, at the same time, generalize for all members. There is a trend toward more holistic treatment wherein psychosocial systems are addressed (Boothroyd, 2007; Kricos, 2000).

Stewart, Banks, Crossman, and Poel (1995) interviewed an equal number of health care professionals and group members representing a cross section of rehabilitation groups. They identified specific tensions and barriers which contraindicated group success. These included: negative attitudes, competition, ideological conflicts and role ambiguity. The researchers recommended some strategies to address these issues including:

- building communication,
- clarifying role and goal,
- building trust,
- establishing credibility, and
- educating the public.

There are also a variety of personal reasons why some individuals may not join groups. Many people do not believe they need help; those with hearing loss may be in denial. Some individuals may not view the group setting as a *fit* for them. Individuals with disabilities may have lower self-esteem and may, therefore, perceive that their social and verbal skills render them inadequate for group participation and worthy contribution. Hurvitz (1974), in examining the reasons why individuals drop out of rehabilitation or self-help groups, explains they are likely to have acceptance issues because of low self-esteem, citing real or assumed differences which cause rejection including such characteristics as social status, educational level, income, race, ethnic background, and religious affiliation. Others may opt out of therapy because of real or perceived problems in the group such as poor organization or management or destructive conflicts between participants. A small percentage may leave because they reject some group principle or practice such as transferring responsibility for change to themselves. Finally, some participants are simply unable or uncomfortable disclosing personal information within the group forum.

An understanding of the values of groups provides additional evidence as to why people join them and why persons with hearing loss may be likely to ascribe to such values. Self-help, self-sufficiency, and mutual aid have long been held as American values. Traditionally, those values have been experienced through group efforts. Democracy is founded on the basis of people gathering together for a common good (Swift, 1928). The self-help, mutual aid ethos is a reaffirmation of basic core traditions of community, neighborhood, spiritual values and self-reliance (Kurtz, 1997).

Demographics show that the typical therapy group member is middle class, well-educated, middle-aged, European-American and male (Lieberman & Snowden, 1994). Membership predominantly holds those characteristics and with it, certain Caucasian, middle class values. These include, but are not limited to, self-sufficiency, strong work ethic, reciprocal giving, democracy, self-determination, self-production, and self-worth. In holding such values, these groups are immediately less attractive to members of racial or ethnic minorities and other social/economic classes.

The Hearing Loss Association of America (HLAA), the largest consumer organization for hard of hearing individuals in this country, reflects similar demographics except that the number of women exceeds that of men and the average age is older (Kleinrock, 1998). These two factors, in combination, in part may reflect the fact that women live longer than men and that hearing loss is a characteristic of aging. These differences do not suggest a significantly different set of values than those embraced by most other self-help or rehabilitation groups.

Criteria for Group Formation

Although some variety of membership is desirable to maximize the effects of some group dynamics (e.g., universality, collective experience, bringing to the table), by and large, homogeneous groups are more likely to be effective (Pollin, 1995). Ideally, members' communication ability and the degree and nature of hearing loss should be similar. Children, adolescents, working age adults and the elderly should be grouped separately as their needs and interests are substantially different. There are also criteria for exclusion. Although the clinician must use her professional judgment in selecting group members, there are some conditions that contraindicate group membership. These may include persons who:

- are in a state of crisis
- experience anxiety attacks
- exhibit pathologic behaviors
- have poor impulse control
- are perpetually argumentative
- have drug or alcohol dependency
- use groups purely as a means of making social contacts (Yalom, 2005).

Group leaders have the primary responsibility of orienting members to prepare them for participation. This may include:

- explaining objectives and functioning
- describing membership
- contracting for regular attendance
- orienting to rules or norms for appropriate behavior
- raising expectations for helpfulness of the group process in achieving objectives
- identifying potential problems
- planning interventions (Corey, 2008; Posthuma, 1996; Yalom, 2005).

Older Adults in Groups

Older adults constitute the largest demographic of individuals with hearing loss (Ross, 1997). Group rehabilitation may be helpful in guiding older adults to more fulfilling life experiences (Kemp, 1990). It provides some of the same important benefits for older adults as it does for their younger counterparts. In fact, there is a greater similarity between benefits enjoyed by older adult and those of adolescents. Corey (2008) notes that both group types "often feel unproductive, unneeded and unwanted by society" (p. 7). The psychosocial characteristics of therapy groups speak to these issues and address such effects.

An important factor when considering group AR is *ageism*, including that which is self-generated and sustained. Many older adults accept the myths and stereotypes related to aging; this in turn becomes a self-fulfilling prophecy. For example, "All old people have hearing loss so I should just accept it" or "I'm too old to change." AR groups for older adults may address the reality of such issues through such techniques as cognitive restructuring. Counseling groups can do a lot to help older people challenge these myths and deal with the developmental tasks that they, like any other age group, must face in such a way that they can retain their integrity and self-respect, provide support that helps older individuals to break out of their social isolation, and encourage them to find new meaning and direction in their lives as opposed to merely existing (Corey, 2008).

Research by Bliwise and Lieberman (1984) strongly supports the effectiveness of self-help groups for older adults with health-related problems. Although no systematic changes in health status were noted in their study, a substantial number of psychosocial benefits were accrued. Characteristics of therapy groups identified in the related literature which were particularly supportive to participation by older adults included: reductions in psychological distance between the helper and helpee promoting rapport and identification, and leading to openness to change (Karlsruher, 1974), greater client control increasing feelings of self-determination and self-benefit

(Gartner & Riessman, 1977), the opportunity to help others (i.e., helper-therapy principle, Riessman, 1998), and increased self-esteem resulting from seeing oneself as a positive and contributing group member (Riessman, 1965; Skovholt, 1974).

Unfortunately, and although the reasons are not completely clear, elderly people are less likely than their younger counterparts to join organizations for the hard of hearing, especially if they lost their hearing in later life (Miller, 1975; Thomas & Gilhome-Herbst, 1980).

Vocational concerns should be considered when planning AR for older adults. Although more and more older adults remain in the workplace, this trend is reversing (U.S. Bureau of Labor statistics as reported by Gregory Mott, 1999) including for persons with hearing loss, who are more likely to retire earlier, or volunteer in workplace or community settings (Bally, Pray, & Battat, 1997). Even in volunteer roles, communication skills and strategies are essential to older adults coping with hearing loss. Battat (1994, 1995a, 1995b, 1995c, 1996) has authored a series of self-help articles for the *HLAA Journal* (now *Hearing Loss*) that address workplace issues and suggest methods of coping with the biopsychosocial effects of hearing loss in job settings. Psychosocial assets which may be fostered in the group context may include development of assertive behavior (Bally, 1996; Erdman, 1993; Rezen, 1992; Trychin, 1990a) problem-solving skills (Brabender, 2004; Perlman, 1986; Pope, 1997; Toseland & Rivas, 2004; Trychin 1988a, 1998c; Trychin & Bonvillian, 1990, 1991; Trychin & Wright, 1988), ability to disclose (Mechem, 1994; Ross, 1996b), career modification or goal setting (Bally, Pray, & Battat, 1997), stress management and relaxation techniques (Trychin,1985a, 1985b, 1986a, 1986b, 1986c, 1986d, 1986e, 1987d, 1987e, 1987f, 1987g), adjustment to the use of amplification (Beebe & Masterson, 1989; Binnie, 1977; Brooks, 1979; Franks & Beckman, 1985; Ross, 1991, 1992, 1993, 1995, 1996a; Trychin, 1990b) and empowerment (Bally, Pray, & Battat, 1997). All of these areas may be incorporated into AR group approaches as topics for discussion or problem solving or for developing coping and communication strategies germane to the workplace.

Implications of Values and Attitudes Toward Older Adults and Persons with Hearing Loss

The need for, and usefulness of, groups in which there is mutual support may be further justified because they address the ways in which Americans value, and the attitudes they have toward, persons with disabilities. People with disabilities, including hearing loss, have suffered a long history of discrimination in the United States based on a perceived limited value. Generations of Americans equated deafness with being dumb or incapable of learning, a fallacy yet to be invalidated by much of the population. Early treatment for congenitally deaf persons focused on institutionalization and underemployment in menial labor. Educational opportunities were limited or nonexistent. Although these conditions have improved significantly, the understanding and attitudes of the general public have not improved to the same extent. Misperceptions related to the abilities of persons with disabilities, and those with hearing loss in particular, are still held by many citizens of the United States. Professionals, such as teachers, speech-language pathologists and audiologists have traditionally affected paternal attitudes toward people with disabilities and have treated them accordingly. Professional attitudes are changing, but, as yet, are far from ideal (Bauman, 2008; Christiansen & Barnartt, 1995; Gitterman & Shulman, 2005; Kricos, 2000; Shapiro, 1993). (*Note:* For further information regarding stigma, the reader is referred to Chapter 4 of this text.)

An Ecological Perspective and Systems Theory

Systems theory provides a functional model that illuminates our understanding of individuals functioning within their social environments. This ecological perspective, in turn, provides us with insights as to how systemic changes affect the individuals and the social contexts within which they communicate. Although there is some variation in the definitions of social systems, they are generally broken down into micro, meso and macro categories. Santrock (2004) defines microsystems as those relationships with individuals who have the strongest personal bonds and with whom a person communicates most often. This will vary depending on the individual and might include such dyads as husband-wife, mother or father-child, individual-caregiver, business associates, or closest friends. They are largely influenced by the affective, behavioral, and cognitive changes that occur in both individuals and their relationships as a result of hearing loss. Meso systems are the groups within the environment in which the individual functions on a regular basis. These may include such entities as the extended family, the work place, church group, school class, or neighborhood. Macrosystems are the larger societal systems in which people live. These may include the community, school as a whole, company or business as a whole, congregation, or cultural community. American society as a whole constitutes the largest macrosystem. Each of these systems provides a context for communication. The individual exerts influence of these systems through communication and they, in turn exert influence on the individual. The impact of a communication disorder that affects communication bares influence on all the systems within which the individual sustaining such as loss functions. Figure 13–1 illustrates a nested systems-ecological model (Bally, 1999) that looks at an individual within the contexts of these three social systems and would help to consider how a hearing loss or other disability would impact the individual and the social relationships and how they, in turn, respond.

Groups and Microsystems: Interpersonal Communication

Our primary interpersonal contacts are with other individuals, especially those who are most significant in our lives and those with whom we communicate most often. Given that hearing loss impedes our communication, those relationships are likely to be the most significantly affected. Both the person with the hearing loss and the significant other will endure the related psychosocial effects of the loss. Therefore, it is reasonable to place the primary focus of rehabilitation efforts on the individuals who comprise these primary relationships. This may be achieved in three ways: (1) by including significant others in AR groups; (2) focusing on interpersonal skills and abilities; and (3) reinforcing and integrating emerging skills with experiential tasks to be completed outside of the therapy room. Communication ability may be improved through the effective use of hearing

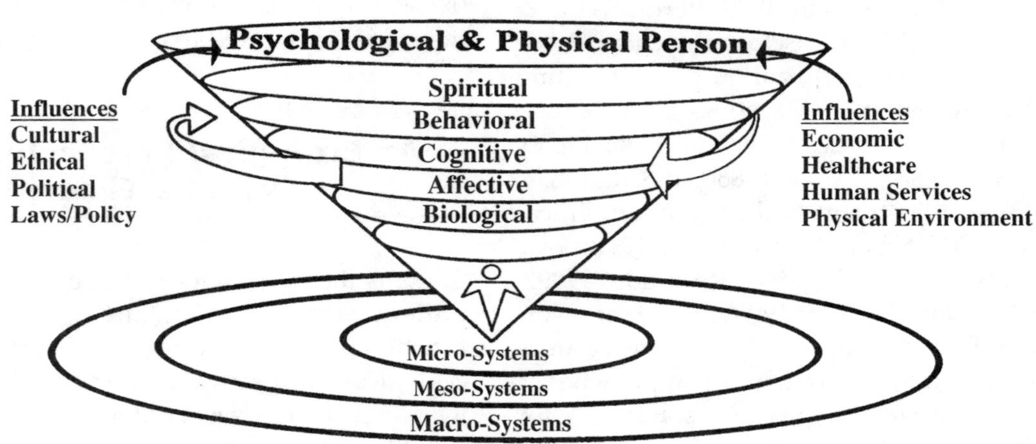

Figure 13–1. Nested systems—ecological model (Bally, 1999).

assistive technology systems (HATS) auditory and speechreading training, and the development of communication strategies. Such training may positively influence the biological, behavioral and social systems by easing interpersonal communication. In turn, this may influence the psychological systems by increasing the ability to meet life needs, empowering, and increasing self-esteem (Binnie, 1977).

"The greatest enemy of people with hearing impairments" asserts Lesner (1995) "is often the people they love the most, namely their significant others" (p. 204). Lesner describes a problematic lack of understanding of the challenges precipitated by hearing loss. She highlights the unrealistic expectations of significant others noting that they "expect that use of a hearing aid cures the hearing loss or that attendance at speechreading classes enables people with hearing impairments to speechread perfectly" (p. 204).

Research by Preminger (2003) identifies positive influences of significant others in AR groups including increased use of communication strategies and a significant reduction in overall hearing handicap across all areas assessed by the Communication Scale for Older Adults (CSOA) (Kaplan, Bally, Brandt, Busacco, & Pray, 1997) and the HHIE (Ventry & Weinstein, 1982) for both persons with hearing loss and their SOs.

Some of the more specific ways in which spouses and significant others who participate in AR groups benefit may include:

- understanding the impact of hearing loss on biopsychosocial systems of the person with hearing loss and the micro-, meso- and macrosystems of society,
- developing more realistic expectations about the abilities of the person with hearing loss and the technology that he uses,
- learning to actively participate in problem solving as related to hearing loss,
- developing a balance and sensitivity between efforts to be supportive and allowing for self-determination,
- learning to identify and use communication strategies that are supportive to the person with hearing loss, yet do not undermine their feelings of self-competence or self-esteem,
- practicing skills with significant others or as part of changing communication dyads within the group setting,
- learning to communicate more effectively in all communication contexts,
- helping to create or modify effective communication environments,
- learning to model effective communication behaviors for mutual friends and acquaintances and others with whom the couples might communicate together, and
- presenting themselves as the most logical practice partners for the person with hearing loss in the development of speechreading ability and communication strategies.

"Because communication between people with hearing impairments and significant others represents the most important communication dyad, both people need to be involved in the rehabilitative process" (Lesner, 1995, p. 205).

Training of communication partners can be a crucial element to successful communication for both the SO and the person with hearing loss. These internal microsystems may provide a model for external functioning. More recently, professionals have turned their attention to this practice and have developed materials for, and to use with, communication partners including: Bally and Hilley, 1996; Erber, 1996; Kaplan, Bally, and Garretson, 1987; Preminger, 2003; Trychin, 1990c; Tye-Murray and Schum, 1994; Tye-Murray, 1993, 1994, 1997, 2002; and Wayner and Abrahamson, 1996, 1998. As stated earlier, the small group provides a safe environment for exploring and addressing psychosocial issues that may not be generally understood, or may be uncomfortable.

Groups and Mesosystems

The rehabilitation group provides a systemic base parallel to that of other mesosystems. It provides a microcosm context that serves as a lab for the development of mesoskills with, or independent of, participation of significant others. AR groups are mesosystems and, as such, provide an effective context and laboratory for group interaction. From this model, and from the experiential knowledge of group members, the person with hearing loss may learn skills that may generalize and improve communication and psychosocial functioning in social or other group contexts such as the family, spiritual, workplace or social setting. As with the microcontext, members may learn to develop the communication skills and abilities including assertiveness needed to negotiate group contexts more effectively. These may include speechreading, auditory training, the use of communication strategies and the use of auxiliary devices and techniques such as group amplification systems or computer-assisted note taking (CAN). To foster these skills and abilities, group practice or role-play situations, when initiated, may include simulated family, work or social situations (Trychin, 1987a, 1987b, 1988a, 1988c, 1990b; Trychin & Bonvillian, 1990, 1991).

Family participation in self-help groups or specific group activities may be beneficial to individuals with hearing loss as well as to the family members (Preminger, 2003; Trychin, 1988b, 1990c, 1996, Trychin & Albright, 1996; Tye-Murray, 1998). Powell (1987) is emphatic that the family should be considered the "most fundamental support system" (p. 117) and therapy groups should not be viewed as competing with the family. The group as a model meso system should be regarded as "a specialized extrafamilial helping system that works best when they are articulated with the supportive features of the nuclear family and the extended family" (p. 117). Caplan (1976) wisely notes that "individuals who, for a variety of reasons, do not have a family of their own are often 'adopted' by a family to which they are not linked by blood or marriage" (p. 127) . . . such as a rehabilitation group.

Oyer and Oyer (1985) emphasize the importance of family in reducing the impact of hearing loss based on their understanding of multiple implications of hearing loss and their motivation to support the AR process of their family member. It is reasonable to assume that some judicious disclosure of this kind of information accompanied by concrete suggestions in vocational, spiritual and social settings could help open dialogues and result in adaptations and accommodations to create more accessible environments.

Focus areas for rehabilitation groups for addressing family issues may include an understanding of the nature of hearing loss, assertiveness training for family members, introduction of problem solving models and communication and coping strategies Cognitive restructuring may help address the emotional effects of hearing loss by introducing such concepts as parallel reactions (Pray, 1996), the psychosocial effects of hearing loss and the development of adaptive communication skills (Bally & Hilley, 1996; Erber, 1996; Hilley & Bally, 1996; Trychin, 1990c; Tye-Murray, 1993, 1994, 1997, 2002; Tye-Murray & Schum, 1994).

Therapy Groups and Macrosystems

Implicit in every self-help group . . . including those focused on individual adaptation, is the criticism of lacks or failures of the larger society

(Katz & Bender, 1976, p. 23)

Macrosystems include such entities as community, company or religious denomination or society as a whole and their respective sub cultures. These systems have significant influences on individuals with hearing loss as well as on micro- and mesosystems and how they respond to individuals with hearing loss. An important benefit of rehabilitation groups is that they have the capacity to identify macro and meso resources for their members. Larger consumer groups have demonstrated the ability to counter the negative effects of some external macro level influences that may impact on the lives of older adults with hearing loss. Macro-influences include ethics, politics, policy and legislation, economics, health care and human services, as well as physical environments. It is not unreasonable for therapy groups to empower members by providing the resources and problem-solving structures needed to facilitate social changes in each of these areas.

Cultural considerations are of utmost concern to the professional in participant selection and group functioning. Cultural differences have the capacity to impede group functioning, if ignored. Culturally diverse AR group mesosystems may provide a model for external functioning for members. When various cultures are represented in a group, the professional may identify potential features related to a given cultural group and consider how they might influence group functioning. DeLucia-Waack and Donigian (2004) suggest that individuals from some cultural groups or backgrounds may be reluctant to become active participants or share personal information in a group situation. They explain that many cultures prohibit the sharing of personal information that might bring shame on the individual or the family. Bloch (1983) provides an assessment structure that may be used to consider biological, cognitive, spiritual, behavioral, and psychological characteristics of cultures that can be considered in clinical settings. The extent to which a person from another culture or subculture has been assimilated or acculturated should also be weighed in order for the group leader to help participants be culturally sensitive and avoid pitfalls. Such characteristics as eye contact, communication affect, spiritual beliefs, and family and cultural roles have the potential to affect the therapy process. Group leaders may establish guidelines and safeguards relative to cultural differences. Skilled group leaders will highlight and frame differences in ways that will increase or enhance understanding and develop cultural sensitivity.

Important macroresources may be considered in AR groups to determine benefits that might be useful in meeting the challenges of hearing loss. These include:

- health care services and research programs related to hearing loss such as counseling, medical intervention, and speech language pathology,
- community accommodations including existing and potential or needed communication access in public places such as government buildings, places or worship, theaters, public transportation, and so forth,
- public laws which mandate accommodations for individuals with disabilities such as the Telecommunications Accessibility Act of 1988 (P. L. 100-542) and The Americans with Disabilities Act of 1990 (P. L. 101-336),
- approaches and strategies for advocating for accommodations in communities and public places under the laws listed above including affiliation with consumer organizations (e.g., HLAA, Association for Late Deafened Adults, ALDA),
- protocols and procedures for advocating for communication accessibility in such venues as the workplace and in places of worship.

Sidel and Sidel (1976) urge groups to become advocates within their communities so they can receive benefit from available resources.

Economic considerations are paramount for older adults with hearing loss. Many are on fixed incomes and, given their propensity toward chronic age-related illnesses must prioritize spending. The cost of amplification is perceived as inordinately high and therefore may be considered as less a priority than other medical needs such as medications or basic living expenses. From the professional perspective, Abrams, Chisholm, and McArdle (2002) provide evidence from a cost-utility analysis of adult group AR and conclude that providing hearing aids with supportive AR is more cost effective and results in an improved quality of life when compared to providing hearing aids without AR.

Ethical influences include discrimination, unfair treatment, and withholding of civil rights of persons with disabilities. These may be addressed indirectly through legislation, civil action, economic influence, public education, and exerting change on cultural norms. Each of these is addressed within this section. Self-help and mutual support groups have the opportunity to influence values and ethics on local, regional, state, and national levels through these venues.

Consumer groups have also influenced *communication access* on local, state, and national levels. "Communication access is a summary term for accommodations that provide an environment where persons with hearing loss can communicate" (Battat, 1993, p. 11). The Americans with Disabilities Act (ADA) requires reasonable accommodations for persons with disabilities including those with hearing loss. However, although the ADA is law, there is no single enforcement agency to oversee compliance (Mechem, 1998). Local self-help groups report efforts to move community meeting halls, senior centers and movie theaters to compliance with the ADA by community-based efforts to enhance communication through use of group amplification systems, elimination of background noise such as Muzak and installation of acoustic barriers. The Architectural Barriers Act (P.L. 90-480) also requires user-friendly environments for persons with disabilities. Both laws were passed through cooperative efforts that included national, state, regional, and local self-help groups representing a cross-section of persons with physical disabilities.

Psychosocial Dynamics of Groups

The primary objective of all rehabilitation groups is to facilitate change. Riessman and Carroll (1995) assert that such changes may be achieved through the promotion of "latent inner strengths" (p. 3). Groups foster the creation of caring communities and provide educational information to help improve coping skills for individuals with hearing loss (Gartner & Riessman, 1984). AR groups seek to identify and maximize the abilities and capabilities of their participants. Table 13–1 describes psychosocial objectives for AR groups.

With respect to hearing loss, *change* means adaptation in order to maximize communication and ameliorate the negative psychosocial effects of the loss. There are three possible outcomes to AR: the individual may maintain his diminished level of functioning; he may approximate his former level of functioning; or, in some instances, he may attain a higher level of functioning than before

Table 13–1. Desired Psychosocial Objectives for AR Groups

- Develop more realistic expectations related to hearing loss & amplification
- Adopt a more positive and proactive mindset
- Recognize the commonality of members needs and problems and develop a sense of connectedness
- Realize that their feelings related to hearing loss are normal and valid
- Develop a comfortable relationship with amplification
- Broaden a repertoire and improve the use of communication strategies
- Improve attending strategies and speechreading skills
- Work toward a more appropriate degree of assertiveness
- Increase familiarity with resources for independent coping with hearing loss
- Improve social skills
- Develop improved problem-solving ability: be aware of one's choices and make choices wisely
- Make specific plans for behavioral change, and make an ongoing commitment to those changes.
- Increase self-acceptance, self-confidence, self-respect, self-esteem, and achieve a new view of oneself and others
- Reduce stress
- Utilize hearing conservation strategies
- Assume personal responsibility for managing hearing loss
- Increase self-monitoring and regulating speech
- Develop an understanding of the behavioral, affective, behavioral, cognitive, and social effects of hearing loss on self, family, etc.
- Develop the ability to explain communication needs to others
- Develop a support system outside the group
- Internalize the shared responsibilities of communicating with others
- Identify resources within their extended families, and communities

the loss. For example, a participant in a Gallaudet University AR program was a self-described "couch potato." He lamented that his hearing loss had beaten him and he had retreated from public life. Following a successful experience with AR and armed with better problem solving skills, improved communication strategies and a more proactive mindset as well as an educated, committed and supportive spouse, he returned to many of his pre-hearing loss activities. He then moved above and beyond, becoming an active member of his condominium association board, and his local HLAA chapter. In the next few years he rose to the Presidency of the chapter and was an active advocate for state disability rights. Although atypical, he was able to harness and direct his inner strengths. He credited his group AR experience with jump starting him toward actively addressing the effects of his hearing loss.

The literature in the allied health and counseling professions identifies a number of dynamic phenomena that characterize rehabilitation groups and may help members identify and meet their psychosocial needs. In view of the dynamic interrelationships between the affective, cognitive and behavioral processes reported, each phenomenon should be considered within the context of the AR group as well as the individual's external social systems. Vinogradov and Yalom (1989) describe the group experience as "a therapeutic cafeteria in that many different mechanisms of change are available and each individual patient *chooses* those particular factors best suited to his or her needs and problems" (p. 28).

Group process provides the participant with a wealth of opportunities for personal growth and development. It can help the individual achieve comfort with his identity as a person with a hearing loss. There are multiple layers that lead to the facilitation of change for group participants. Table 13–2, adapted from Forsyth (2006, p. 537), describes the dynamics that facilitate change in groups and the perceived meaning to the participants. For example, instilling hope serves to increase optimism of the participant. Curry, Snyder, Cook, Ruby, and Rehm (1997) reported that individuals with high hope are significantly more likely to meet their objectives than those who have lesser degrees of hope.

As one reads through the contents of Table 13–2, it becomes apparent that aspects of the dynamics of change interact and are not mutually exclusive. For example, microcosm effects reflect the feeling of being with members of a representative population while universality contributes to the feeling of a shared experience. The collective experience highlights the individual contributions made by members of the group, whereas modeling allows participants to learn from others (Goodman, Schlossberg, & Anderson, 2006). Pearson (1992) describes benefits of modeling saying "members can catch functional attitudes such as hope, perseverance, concern for others" as well as learning coping strategies like asking for help, owning failures, and substituting adaptive communication strategies for maladaptive ones.

Professional Roles

The therapist's role within groups as based on systems theory is to be a boundary manager. Corey (2008) describes the group leader as having the following responsibilities:

- defining and monitoring the process and specific tasks,
- developing ground rules and setting norms,
- teaching the basics of group process,
- selecting members,
- serving as a catalyst for change,
- modeling appropriate behaviors (communication strategies),
- guiding goal setting,
- establishing a safe environment,
- providing safeguards for disclosure,
- reinforcing new behaviors and skills,
- fostering responsibility to self and group to achieve goals,
- processing and interpreting information, and
- assessing group functioning and redirecting as needed to achieve group/member objectives.

Table 13–2. Dynamics That Facilitate Change in Groups

Dynamic	Definition	Meaning to participant
INSTILLED HOPE	Increased sense of optimism	"If others can change, so can I"
MEMBERSHIP	Sense of belonging	"I'm not in this alone"
MICROCOSM EFFECT	Representative population	"That's like my life"
GROUP CLIMATE/ AFFIRMATIVE AFFECT	Mutual support	"Everyone's behind me"
SAFE ENVIRONMENT	Nonjudgmental, accepting, supportive	"I can share my thoughts and feelings without risk"
MUTUAL DEMAND	Expectations of each other	"We all need to do our part; I don't want to let down the group"
COLLECTIVE EXPERIENCE	Everyone has difference experiences to share	Bring to the table
MODELING (COMMUNICATION) BEHAVIORS	Demonstration of communication strategies	"Look what he's doing; I should do that"
PROBLEM-SOLVING	A methodical means to solve problems	"What's the best way to handle this?"
COGNITIVE REFRAME & RESTRUCTURING	Eliminate self-defeating thinking	"That's another way to look at it"
ALTRUISM/THE HELPER PRINCIPLE	Increased sense of efficacy from helping others	"It feels good to help others"
UNIVERSALITY/SHARED EXPERIENCES	Recognition of shared problems/ experiences; decreased sense of uniqueness	"I'm not the only one"
STRENGTH IN NUMBERS	The group is more powerful than the individual	"Look what we can accomplish together"
SENSE OF HUMOR	Find the humor in the situation, not the person.	"It does have its humorous side . . . "

Source: Adapted from Forsyth, 2006; Gazda, Gintner, & Horne 2001.

The group process may be facilitated through the use of reaction skills such as active listening, restatement, reflection, clarifying, summarizing, tracking, scanning, and reframing; and interactions skills including interpreting, linking, blocking, supporting, limiting, protecting and consensus taking, action skills such as questioning, probing, tone setting, confronting, personal disclosure, and modeling (Corey, 2008; Posthuma, 1996; Shipley, 2006; Trotzer, 2006). Each of these clinical techniques may be used to facilitate group dynamics and move groups and group members toward their objectives. When planning group AR programs, desired psychosocial outcomes will vary, depending on time, membership and members' personal needs. Appendix 13–A identifies means of facilitating helpful group dynamics in AR.

Information counseling is an especially significant part of the facilitator's responsibility. Practicing clinical professionals are familiar with clients' lack of information or misinformation garnered from hearsay and inaccurate or poorly understood published materials. The sources of misinformation are numerous (web sites, misleading advertisements, poorly written articles, etc.).

A facilitator's first order of business after convening a group is to educate members as to the rules, structures and policies which will enable maximum benefits for those who participate. Beyond that, AR group facilitators will provide information to the group, clarify information that is errant and provide more beneficial perspectives on the information with which they are working.

Assigning homework is used to foster the connection between the therapy context and life contexts in which learned skills will be put to use. Noting that homework is a means of intensifying short-term therapy experiences, Brabender (2004) and Spitz (1997) cite key elements essential for the success of homework assignments:

- careful planning of the homework assignment so that the group members knows what specifically is to be done,
- anticipation of obstacles to performing the assignment, and
- opportunity for the member to report back to the group on successes and failures in relation to its execution.

Changing Professional Attitudes and Perspectives

Rehabilitation groups related to medically based problems such as hearing loss must not only deal with the participants and their specific problems, but may also take on as their responsibility the humanizing of profession and its professionals. Participants in the "Hearing Loss in Later Years" Elderhostel program at Gallaudet University reported both insensitivity and misinformation related to hearing health professionals. Not infrequently, they told of doctors who said that "nerve deafness" has no treatment. They described situations in which hearing aid dealers or dispensers offered little in the way of hearing aid orientation, and seldom referred to AR programs. Few were introduced to the benefits of telecoils. Many reported that, after the initial sale of a hearing aid, less welcoming attitudes were noted when further help or adjustments were requested. Self-help groups may encourage consumer advocacy by sharing such observations and, as a result, prompting members, their friends and families to patronize businesses and professionals who have more positive, enlightened and proactive attitudes and perspectives. (*Note*: For more information on the consumer perspective, the reader is referred to Chapter 16.)

Some Important Needs and Consideration

It is difficult to champion the cause of group AR given the scarcity of comprehensive group AR services and quality efficacy studies that evaluate their approaches (Hawkins, 2005). Kricos (2000) speaks of a transformation of AR in recent years, moving from a model focusing on amplification and communication ability to adjustment to hearing loss, problem solving, repair strategies, and on collaboration. Indeed, counseling based models are more visible, but the number of all such programs remains extremely limited. From a more optimistic perspective, the advent of the Au.D. has given training institutions the opportunity to broaden their curricula to include counseling courses. The logical next step might be to recruit students who have a strong interest in AR.

There is much work to be done to demonstrate the efficacy of AR groups. Numerous assessment tools have been utilized to evaluate the efficacy of groups and of AR groups (Hawkins, 2005). Because of the enormous variation in content included in AR group approaches and the shortcomings of efficacy research, few conclusions can be drawn that may be generalized. Collectively, we may conclude that the use of assistive technology combined with comprehensive aural rehabilitation is effective in helping individuals adapt to hearing loss. Beyond that we must examine the results of efficacy studies in the context of intervention content. By doing so, we may determine which facets of AR are most helpful to group members.

The literature and research of social work, psychology, nursing, and counseling offers great insights for us to consider. These professions have proven strategies and approaches that may be adapted for AR groups. A few of the more important needs include:

- review and analysis of the literature of the allied health professionals. There are (additional) studies and therapy models that may have profound implications for AR groups,
- measurement of the impact of group dynamics to determine which facilitate better outcomes; scale to assess the impact of these dynamics needs to be developed,
- determination of which efficacy measures provide the most valid data and assess programs accordingly,
- determination of which therapeutic methodologies provide the most practical and positive results for group participants, and
- incorporation of professional training for group counseling into the Au.D. professional curricula.

Overall, more studies using randomized controlled trial designs are needed. Results of such studies should be analyzed and the results used to facilitate better group approaches and hone the types of objectives that are most likely to result in better outcomes.

Conclusions

In this chapter, an ecological systems model has been used to illuminate the interactive nature of human psychosocial systems and how they are affected by an individual's hearing loss. Group participants may be evaluated using this model as a basis. The external macrofactors that may influence successful adaptation to hearing loss have been described. Professionals should work with their clients to address those factors and, to the extent possible, ameliorate the negative influences on therapy and adaptation while enhancing those that facilitate it.

Significant dynamics that occur or may be facilitated to occur in group contexts have been identified and described. Each has proven to be a positive influence in other therapeutic group contexts. There is reason enough to support professional efforts to employ those dynamics in AR groups to evaluate their influences. Efficacy measures that look at these dynamics need to be developed or adapted. Methodology for the effective delivery of services based on these dynamics needs to be assessed. Those dynamics that prove more effective in helping individuals adapt to hearing loss should provide a basis for improved counseling based AR group methodology and approaches.

References

Abrams, H., Chisholm, T., & McArdle, R. (2002). A cost-utility analysis of adult group aural rehabilitation: Are the benefits worth the cost? *Journal of Rehabilitation Research and Development, 39*(5), 549–558.

Americans with Disabilities Act of 1990 (Public Law 101-336), 42 USC §§ 12101 et seq.

Architectural Barriers Act of 1968 (P.L. 90-480), 42 U.S.C. §§ 4151 et seq.

Bally, S. J. (1996). Communication strategies. In M. J. Moseley & S. J. Bally (Eds.), *Communication therapy: An integrated approach to aural rehabilitation for deaf and hard of hearing adolescents and adults* (pp. 41–91). Washington, DC: Gallaudet University Press.

Bally, S. J. (1999). *A self-help aural rehabilitation model for older adults with hearing loss.* Doctoral dissertation, The Union Institute: Cincinnati, OH.

Bally, S. J., & Hilley, M. H. (1996). Repair strategies hierarchy for communication partners. In M. J. Moseley & S. J. Bally (Eds.), *Communication therapy: An integrated approach to aural rehabilitation for deaf and hard of hearing adolescents and adults* (pp. 84–85). Washington, DC: Gallaudet University Press.

Bally, S. J., Pray, J. L., & Battat, B. (1997, June 14). *Achieving success in the workplace.* Presentation at the 12th International Conference of Self-Help for Hard of Hearing, Phoenix, AZ.

Battat, B. (1993). Advocacy and access: You can't have one without the other. *SHHH Journal, 14*(1), 11–13.

Battat, B. (1994). Breaking barriers for employees with hearing impairment. *SHHH Journal, 15*(4), 28–29.

Battat, B. (1995a). Getting a job: Let's put you in the successful employment picture. *SHHH Journal, 16*(4), 26–30.

Battat, B. (1995b). Putting you in the employment picture: Getting the equipment and services you need. *SHHH Journal, 16*(5), 9–11.

Battat, B. (1995c). Putting you in the employment picture: Getting promoted. *SHHH Journal, 16*(6), 10–12.

Battat, B. (1996). Putting you in the employment picture: Getting along with your supervisors and co-workers. *SHHH Journal, 17*(1), 11–12, 14.

Bauman, H. L. (Ed.) (2008). *Open your eyes: Deaf studies talking*. Minneapolis, MN: University of Minnesota Press.

Beebe, S. A., & Masterson, J. T. (1989). *Communicating in small groups*. Glenview, IL: Harper Collins.

Binnie, C. A. (1977). Attitude changes following speechreading training. *Scandinavian Audiology, 6*(6), 13–19.

Bliwise, N. G., & Lieberman, M. (1984). From professional help to self-help: An evaluation of therapeutic groups for the elderly, In A. Gartner & F. Riessman (Eds.), *Self-help in the human services* (pp. 217–231). San Francisco: Jossey-Bass.

Bloch, L. (1983) Bloch's Ethic/Cultural Assessment Guide. In M. Orque, B. Bloch, & L. Monrroy (Eds.), *Ethnic nursing care: A multicultural approach* (pp. 63–69). St. Louis, MO: C. V. Mosby.

Bloch, S., Browning, S., & McGrath, G. (1983). Humor in group psychotherapy. *British Journal of Medical Psychology, 56*(1), 89–97.

Boothroyd, A. (2007). Adult aural rehabilitation: What is it and does it work? *Trends in Amplification, 11*, 63–71.

Brabender, V. (2004). *Essentials of group therapy*. Hoboken, NJ: John Wiley & Sons.

Brabender, V. A., Fallon, A. E., & Smolar, A. I. (2004). *Essentials of group therapy*. Hoboken, NJ: John Wiley & Sons.

Brooks, D. N. (1979). Counseling and its effect on hearing aid use. *Scandanavian Audiology, 8*(2), 101–107.

Caplan, G. (1976). Spontaneous or natural support systems. In A. H. Katz & E. I. Bender (Eds.), *The strength in us: Self-help groups in the modern world* (pp. 125–136). New York: New Viewpoints.

Christiansen, J.B., & Barnartt, S. N. (1995). *Deaf president now! The 1988 revolution at Gallaudet University*. Washington, DC: Gallaudet University Press.

Clinard, M. (1963). *Sociology of deviant behavior*. New York: Holt, Rinehart and Winston.

Corey, G. (2008). *Theory and practice of counseling and psychotherapy* (7th ed.) Pacific Grove, CA: Brooks/Cole.

Curry, L. A., Snyder, C. R., Cook, D. L., Ruby, B. C., & Rehm, M. (1997). The role of hope in academic and sport performance. *Journal of Personality and Social Psychology, 73*(6), 1257– 1267.

DeLucia-Waack, J. L., & Donigian, J. (2004). *The practice of multicultural group work*. Belmont, CA: Brooks/Cole.

Erber, N. P. (1996). *Communication partners* (2nd ed.). Abbotsford, Victoria, Australia: Clavis.

Erdman, S. A. (1993). Counseling hearing impaired adults. In J. G. Alpine & P. A. McCarthy (Eds.), *Rehabilitative audiology: Children and adults* (2nd ed., pp. 374–413). Baltimore: Williams & Wilkins.

Fehr, S. S. (2003). *Introduction to group therapy* (2nd ed.). New York: Haworth Press.

Forsyth, D. R. (2006). *Group dynamics* (4th ed.). Belmont, CA: Thomson Wadsworth.

Franks, J., & Beckmann, N. (1985). Rejection of hearing aids: Attitudes of a geriatric sample. *Ear and Hearing, 6*(3), 161–166.

Fuhriman A., & Burlingame, G. M. (1994). *Handbook of group psychotherapy: An empirical and clinical synthesis*. New York: John Wiley & Sons.

Gartner, A., & Riessman, F. (1977). *Self-help in the human services*. San Francisco: Jossey-Bass.

Gartner, A., & Riessman, F. (1984). *The self-help revolution* (Vol. 10). *Community Psychology Series*. New York: Human Sciences Press.

Gazda, G. M., Ginter, E. J., & Horne, A. M. (2001). *Group counseling and group psychotherapy: Theory and application*. Needham Heights, MA: Allyn & Bacon.

Gitterman, A., & Shulman, L. (2005). *Mutual aid groups, vulnerable and resilient populations, and the life cycle* (3rd ed.). New York: Columbia University Press.

Goodman, J., Schlossberg, N. K., & Anderson, M. L. (2006). *Counseling adults in transition* (3rd ed.). New York: Springer.

Hawkins, D. (2005). Effectiveness of counseling-based adult group aural rehabilitation programs: A systematic review of the evidence. *Journal of the American Academy of Audiology, 16*(7), 485–493.

Hilley, M. H., & Bally, S. J. (1996). Repair strategies hierarchy. In M. J. Moseley & S. J. Bally (Eds.), *Communication therapy: An integrated approach to aural rehabilitation for deaf and hard of hearing adolescents and adults* (pp. 62–67). Washington, DC: Gallaudet University Press.

Hollister, W. G., Edgerton, J. W., & Hunter, R. H. (1985). *Alternative services in mental health: Programs and processes.* Chapel Hill, NC: The University of North Carolina Press.

Hurvitz, N. (1974). Peer self-help psychotherapy groups: Psychotherapy without psychotherapists. In P. M. Roman & H. M. Trice (Eds.), *The sociology of psychotherapy* (pp. 84–138). New York: Aronson.

Kaplan, H., Bally, S., Brandt, F., Busacco, D., & Pray, J. (1997). Communication scale for older adults. *Journal of the American Academy of Audiology, 8*, 203–217.

Kaplan, H., Bally, S. J., & Garretson, C. (1987). *Speechreading: A way to improve understanding* (2nd ed.). Washington, DC. Gallaudet University Press.

Karlsruher, A. E. (1974). The nonprofessional as a psychotherapeutic agent: A review of empirical evidence pertaining to his effectiveness. *American Journal of Community Psychology, 2*(1), 61–77.

Katz, A. (1984). Self-help groups: An international perspective. In A. Gartner & F. Riessman (Eds.), *The self-help revolution* (pp. 233–242). New York: Human Science Press.

Katz, A. H., & Bender, E. I. (Eds.). (1976). *The strength in us: Self-help groups in the modern world*. New York: New Viewpoints.

Kemp, B. (1990). The psychosocial context of geriatric rehabilitation. In B. Kemp, K. Brummel-Smith, & J. W. Ramsdell (Eds.), *Geriatric rehabilitation* (pp. 41–56). Boston: College-Hill Press.

Kleinrock, J. (1998). Membership Director, Self-Help for Hard of Hearing People, Inc. Personal Interview July 26, 1998.

Kricos, P. (2000). Preface. *Seminars in Hearing, 21*(3), 203–204.

Kurtz, E. (1979). *Not God: The history of Alcoholics Anonymous*. Center City, MN: Hazelden.

Kurtz, L. F. (1997). *Self-help and support groups: A handbook for practitioners.* Thousand Oaks, CA: Sage.

Lesner, S. A. (1995). Group hearing care for older adults. In P. B. Kricos & S. A. Lesner (Eds.), *Hearing care for the older adult: Audiologic rehabilitation* (pp. 203–225). Boston: Butterworth-Heinemann.

Lewin, K. (1947). Frontiers in group dynamics. *Human Relations, 1*, 143–153.

Lieberman, M. A., & Snowden, L. R. (1994). Problems in assessing prevalence and membership characteristics of self-help group participants. In T. J. Powell (Ed.), *Understanding the self-help organization: Frameworks and findings* (pp. 32–49). Thousand Oaks, CA: Sage.

Maslow, A. (1943). *Motivation and personality*. New York: Harper and Row.

Maslow, A. H. (1991). A theory of human motivation. In J. M. Shafritz & J. S. Ott, *Classics of organization theory* (pp. 159–173). Pacific Grove, CA: Brooks/Cole.

Mechem, J. (1994). *In search of a hard of hearing identity: An ethnography of Self-help for Hard of Hearing People, Inc.* Olympia, WA: Ethnography and Culture Program, Evergreen State College.

Mechem, J. (1998). P.L. 504 Representative, U.S. Department of Education, Personal Interview, May 14, 1998.

Miller, L. V. (1975). The adult and the elderly: Health care and hearing loss. *Volta Review, 77*(1), 57–63.

Mott, G. (1999, July 20). Gone fishin.' *The Washington Post, Health, The Cutting Edge*, p. 4.

Noble, W. G. (1983). Hearing, hearing impairment, and the audible world: A theoretical essay. *Audiology, 22*, 325–338.

Oyer, O. J., & Oyer, E. J. (1985). Adjustment to adult hearing loss. In H. Orlans (Ed.), *Adjustment to adult hearing loss*. San Diego, CA: College-Hill Press.

Pearson, R. E. (1992). Group counseling: Self-enhancement. In D. Capuzzi & D. R. Gross (Eds.), *Introduction to group counseling*. Denver, CO: Love.

Perlman, H. H. (1986). The problem-solving model. In F. J. Turner (Ed.), *Social work treatment: Interlocking theoretical approaches* (pp. 245–266). New York: The Free Press.

Pollin, I. (1995). *Medical crisis counseling*. New York: Norton.

Pope, A. (1997). *Hear: Solutions, skills, and sources for people with hearing loss*. New York: DK.

Posthuma, B.W. (1996). *Small groups in counseling and therapy: Process and Leadership* (2nd ed.). Needham Heights, MA: Allyn & Bacon.

Powell, T. J. (1987). *Self-help organizations and professional practice*. Silver Spring, MD: NASW.

Pray, J. L. (1996). Psychosocial aspects of hearing loss. In M. J. Mosley & S. J. Bally (Eds.), *Communication therapy: An integrated approach to aural rehabilitation for deaf and hard of hearing adolescents and adults* (pp. 128–148). Washington, DC: Gallaudet University Press.

Preminger, J. (2003). Should significant others be encouraged to join adult Audiologic rehabilitation classes? *Journal of the American Academy of Audiology, 14*(10), 545–555.

Rezen, S. V. (1992). Can't hear? Try being assertive. *Hearing Rehabilitation Quarterly, 17*(1), 4–5, 14.

Riessman, F. (1998). Ten self-help principles [online]. Perspectives [1998, March 27] Retrieved 1/3/08.

Riessman F., & Carroll, D. (1995). *Redefining self-help: Policy and practice*. San Francisco: Jossey-Bass.

Ross, M. (1991). Helpful hints to the new hearing aid user. *Hearing Rehabilitation Quarterly, 16*(3), 4–7.

Ross, M. (1992). Why people won't wear hearing aids. *Hearing Rehabilitation Quarterly, 17*(2), 8–11.

Ross, M. (1993). Self-administered auditory training from a personal and professional perspective. *Hearing Rehabilitation Quarterly, 18*(3), 4–15.

Ross, M. (1995). Maximizing residual hearing: Basic principles. *Hearing Rehabilitation Quarterly, 20*(4), 4–13.

Ross, M. (1996a, June). A modest proposal: Group hearing instrument orientations. *Hearing Review, 3*, 8–11.

Ross, M. (1996b, August 6). *Personal and social identity of hard of hearing people*. Paper presented at the annual convention of the International Federation of the Hard of Hearing, The Hague, The Netherlands.

Ross, M. (1997). A retrospective look at the future of aural rehabilitation. *Journal of the Academy of Rehabilitative Audiology, 30*, 11–28.

Santrock, J. W. (2004). *Children* (9th ed.). Dubuque, IA: Wm C. Brown.

Shapiro, J. P. (1993). *No pity*. New York: Time Books.

Shipley, K. G. (2006). *Interviewing and counseling in communicative disorders* (3rd ed.). Austin, TX: Pro-Ed.

Sidel, V. W., & Sidel, R. (1976). Beyond coping. *Social Policy, 7*(2), 67–69.

Skovholt, T. M. (1974). The client as helper: A means to promote psychological growth. *Counseling Psychologist, 4*(3), 58–64.

Spitz, H. I. (1997). Brief group therapy. In S. Sauber (Ed.), *Managed mental health care: Major diagnostic and treatment approaches* (pp. 103–132). Philadelphia: Brunner/Mazel.

Stewart, M., Banks, S., Crossman, D., & Poel, D. (1995). Partnerships between health professionals and self-help groups: Meanings and mechanisms. In F. Lavoie, T. Borkman, & B. Gidron (Eds.), *Self-help and mutual aid groups: International and multicultural perspectives* (pp. 199–240). New York: Haworth.

Swift, L. B. (1928). *How we got our liberties*. Indianapolis, IN: Robbs-Merrill.

Telecommunications Accessibility Enhancement Act of 1988. (P.L. 100-542), 40 USC 762a-d.

Thomas, A., & Gilhome-Herbst, K. (1980). Social and psychological implications of acquired deafness. *British Journal of Audiology, 14*(3), 76–85.

Toseland, R. W., & Rivas, R. F. (2004). *An introduction to group work practice* (4th ed.) Boston: Allyn & Bacon.

Trotzer, J. P. (2006). *The counselor and the group*. New York: Routledge.

Trychin, S. (1985a). Stress management-I. *SHHH Journal, 6*(5), 9–11.

Trychin, S. (1985b). Stress management-II. *SHHH Journal, 6*(7), 9–12.

Trychin, S. (1986a). *Relaxation training for hard of hearing people* [Audiotapes]. Washington, DC: Gallaudet University.

Trychin, S. (1986b). *Relaxation training for hard of hearing people: Trainee's manual*. Washington, DC: Gallaudet University.

Trychin, S. (1986c). *Relaxation training for hard of hearing people* [Videotapes]. Washington, DC: Gallaudet University.

Trychin, S. (1986d). Stress management-III. *SHHH Journal, 7*(1), 8–9.

Trychin, S. (1986e). Stress management-IV. *SHHH Journal, 7*(2), 14–16.

Trychin, S. (1987a). *Communication rules for hard of hearing people*. Bethesda, MD: SHHH.

Trychin, S. (1987b). *Did I do that*? Bethesda, MD: SHHH.

Trychin, S. (1987c). *Relaxation training for hard of hearing people* [Videotapes]. Bethesda, MD: SHHH.

Trychin, S. (1987d). *Relaxation training for hard of hearing people: Trainee's manual*. Bethesda, MD: SHHH.

Trychin, S. (1987e). *Relaxation training for hard of hearing people: Practitioner's manual*. Bethesda, MD: SHHH.

Trychin, S. (1987f). *Stress management* (Information Series, #203). Bethesda, MD: SHHH.

Trychin, S. (1988a). *Is THAT what you think*? Bethesda, MD: SHHH.

Trychin, S. (1988b, Sept/Oct). Relationships: Managing the "huhs" and "whats"—and coping with your loved ones, *The Voice*, pp. 13–14.

Trychin, S. (1988c). *So THAT'S the problem*! Bethesda, MD: SHHH.

Trychin, S. (1990a). *Speak out: Tips on speaking in public for individuals with a hearing loss*. Washington, DC: Gallaudet University.

Trychin, S. (1990b). Why people don't acquire and/or use hearing aids from a psychologists point of view. *SHHH Journal, 11*(3), 13–16.

Trychin, S. (1990c). You . . . me . . . and hearing loss makes three. *SHHH Journal, 11*(1), 7–11.

Trychin , S. (1996, June 24). *Coping strategies for people who are hard of hearing and their families*. Presentation at Self-Help for Hard of Hearing People 11th International Convention, Orlando, FL.

Trychin, S., & Albright, J. (1996, June 24). *Coping with hearing loss from the perspective of hearing family members and friends*. Self-Help for Hard of Hearing People 11th International Convention, Orlando, FL.

Trychin, S., & Bonvillian, B. (1990). *Speak out: Tips for putting on skits relating to hearing loss*. Washington, DC: Gallaudet University.

Trychin, S., & Bonvillian, B. (1991). *Actions speak louder: Tips for putting on skits relating to hearing loss*. Washington, DC: Gallaudet University.

Trychin, S., & Wright, F. (1988). *Is THAT what you think*? Washington, DC: Gallaudet University.

Tye-Murray, N. (1993). *Communication training for hearing-impaired children and teenagers*. Austin, TX: Pro-Ed.

Tye-Murray, N. (1994). *Let's converse: A how-to guide to develop and expand conversational skills of children and teenagers who are hearing impaired*. Washington, DC: A.G. Bell.

Tye-Murray, N. (1997). *Communication training for older teenagers and adults: Listening, Speechreading and using conversational strategies*. Austin, TX: Pro-Ed.

Tye-Murray, N. (1998). *Foundations of aural rehabilitation: Children, adults and their family members*. San Diego, CA: Singular.

Tye-Murray, N. (2002). *Conversation made easy: Speechreading and conversation strategies for adults and teenagers with hearing loss*. St. Louis, MO: Central Institute for the Deaf.

Tye-Murray, N., & Schum, L. (1994). Conversation training for frequent communication partners. *Journal of the Academy of Rehabilitative Audiology, 27* (Monograph supplement), 209–236.

Ventry, I., & Weinstein, B. (1982) The Hearing Handicap Inventory for the Elderly: A new tool. *Ear and Hearing, 3*, 128–133.

Vinogradov, S., & Yalom, I. D. (1989). *Group psychotherapy*. Washington, DC: American Psychiatric Press.

Wayner, D. S., & Abrahamson, J. E. (1996). *Learning to hear again: An audiologic rehabilitation curriculum guide*. Austin, TX: Hear Again.

Wayner, D. S., & Abrahamson, J. E. (1998). *Learning to hear again with a cochlear implant: An audiologic rehabilitation curriculum guide*. Austin, TX: Hear Again.

Yalom, I.D. (2005). *Theory and practice of group psychotherapy* (4th ed.) New York: Basic Books.

Appendix 13–A
Means of Facilitating Group Dynamics in Group AR

Instills Hope	Recognize that joining the group is a positive first step toward achieving goals Create microgoals which are easier to achieve Encourage group members to share success stories, achievement of microgoals Reinforce decision to participate in group to achieve objectives Summarize accomplishments at termination of group; reinforce that this is the beginning of a process of change Create realistic microgoals and monitor progress; recognize progress Note that professionals have developed a significant number of therapy approaches and materials to help meet their goals
Membership	Establish a group identity Reinforce the universality of experience and challenges of the group Establish an intersupportive relationship between members Reflect on the power of the group after group activities
Microcosm Effect	Vary dyads in practice activities Encourage varying perspective for problem-solving
Group Climate/ Affirmative Affect	Recognize achievements of group members microgoals; acknowledge efforts to achieve goals
Safe Environment	Stress confidentiality Encourage self-disclosure; encourage reinforcement of both content and the fact of disclosure Create a positive reinforcement atmosphere Initiate turn-taking disclosure activities Invite members to try out strategies. "this is the environment in which to make mistakes and see what 'fits' for you" Encourage members to share their defeats as well as successes May allow for catharsis, emotional purging within limits
Mutual Demand	Encourage members to set goals for outside the therapy situation; report back to the group on success/failure; open for discussion/suggestions Hold members accountable when microgoals are not met when appropriate
Collective Experience, "Bringing to the Table"	Initiate activities where each group member is expected to disclose or to put forth a perspective or idea. Provide ample opportunities for brainstorming and group problem-solving Give homework for identifying resources Allow for advice; research and education

Communication Behaviors/ Modeling	Facilitators should model use of communication strategies Provide a communication model; identify source of communication breakdown (sender, receiver, environment, etc.) Reinforce use of communication strategies Establish a proactive problem-solving orientation in which participants perceive problems as inherent to daily life and are amenable to solution. Encourage members to air their problem situations in sessions; point out common themes and challenges or allow members to do so
Problem-Solving	Discourage a one problem-one solution model. Facets of multifaceted problems are easier to address and are generally more successful Introduce a structured problem-solving model. Provide case studies which parallel members issues; gradually use member's actual problems Encourage members to brainstorm multiple solutions to the same problem problems; have the person whose problem is being solved evaluate the viability of each solution (what works for one may not work for another) Consider the assertiveness factor of each proposed solution. Scenerio-based or scripted role-play may bring problem situations to life and allow for problem-solving activities Start with more concrete scenerios, such as hostile physical environments; move on to more complex or abstract situations (e.g., indifferent or uncooperative communicators)
Cognitive Reframing/ Restructuring	Allow for spontaneous interaction to introduce alternative perspectives Generate activities that will challenge invalid thinking and generalizations Solicit examples from group members' personal experiences that demonstrate the invalidity of invalid assumptions or conclusions Provide opportunities for members to modify their counterproductive assumptions
Altruism/Helper-Therapy Principal	Foster supportive interrelationships among members Help members transition from receiving help, to helping others
Universality/Shared Experience	Allow each member to tell his/her "story" early in the process Encourage members to share topic related experiences throughout the process Solicit experiences with both successful and unsuccessful strategy use
Strength in Numbers	Emphasize the collective contributions of the group Encourage group efforts or projects Discuss instances wherein groups were successful in achieving objectives related to policy, law, and public accommodation
Maintain a Sense of Humor	Encourage members to share humorous anecdotes related to communication breakdown Use cartoons to highlight situations/perceptions Encourage members to laugh at the folly of the human condition, put their challenges into perspective and occasionally laugh at themselves (and with each other)

14

Hearing Assistance Technology Systems as Part of a Comprehensive Audiologic Rehabilitation Program

Linda M. Thibodeau

Introduction

Hearing assistance technology systems (HATS) refers to the systems used by persons with hearing loss to facilitate reception and identification of speech and non-speech signals. This term, HATS, essentially encompasses all technology used by individuals with hearing impairment, including the personal hearing aid. Although personal hearing aids facilitate the reception of both speech and nonspeech signals, over the years, they have been considered the primary technology whereas HATS have been considered when communication difficulties still remain. The possible chain of events for someone with an acquired hearing loss as a result of aging is shown in Figure 14–1.

When communication difficulties begin because of hearing loss, often people just ask for repetition. As hearing loss progresses, this behavior may become so frequent that changes may occur at work and in one's social life. For example, one may not accept new responsibilities or withdraw from social activities. Eventually, after months and possibly years, the individual seeks amplification. Typically, they receive an audiologic evaluation and hearing aid fitting in two appointments. When the person returns for another hearing aid check near the end of the trial period and still reports difficulties, an audiologic rehabilitation (AR) program may be considered. During this program, they will also learn about many therapeutic communication techniques including environmental modifications, repair strategies, and other assistive

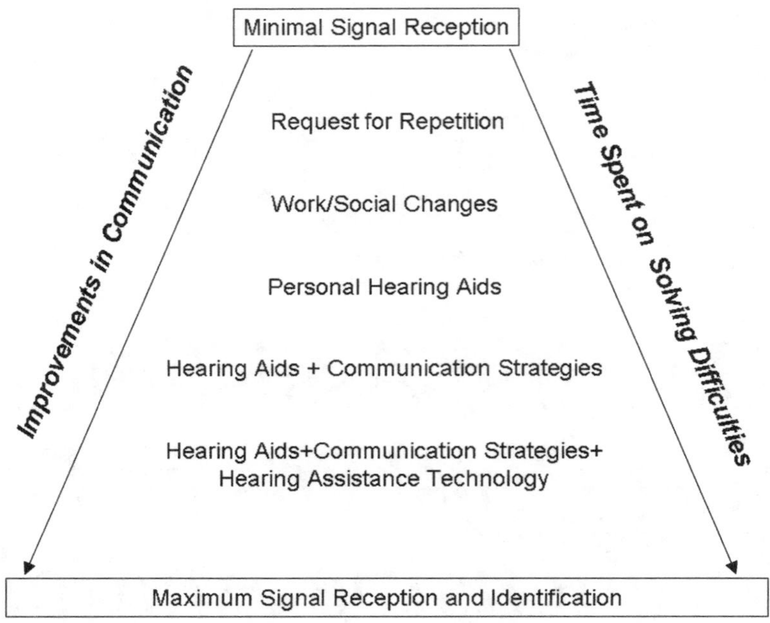

Figure 14–1. Lengthy process to optimal communication when solutions are presented sequentially.

technology. Finally, maximal communication may be obtained through a combination of the personal amplification, strategies, and HATS.

An alternative time sequence is shown in Figure 14–2 where the options of personal amplification, communication strategies, and HATS are presented as a combined program. This saves the consumer and audiologist considerable time and frustration, represented by the shorter time lines in the figure. The frustrations are not only experienced by the person with impaired hearing but also by his or her family. Many times, it is the family member who benefits as much or more from the addition of technology such as the use of a remote microphone. The focus in this discussion regarding HATS is to consider a broader approach to helping persons with hearing loss than simply providing a hearing aid to increase the intensity of the signal. Increasing intensity of the signal is a very small part of the vast resources that could dramatically improve one's communication.

Addressing the communication difficulties with only a hearing aid is like sending an elderly person home with only a cast on a broken leg. After experiencing frustration while moving around the house, she realizes many other accommodations could be offered including a wheelchair, bedside commode, shower chair, and so forth. It would certainly be most efficient for the person to have these items from the beginning rather than experience the frustration and then have to seek the additional support. Now it is possible that not everyone needs all the accommodations which is exactly why the trial period is necessary whether it is orthopedic supports or HATS.

Another consideration to support the broad notion of improving communication through a variety of means is the distinction between hearing assistance technology and assistive listening devices. The major distinction is between the words "hearing" and "listening." "Listening" requires an active process of attending to the auditory environment. HATS can provide signals while persons are sleeping to awaken them to danger. Therefore, "hearing" technology has become the preferred term rather than "listening" devices. Use of this word "hearing" is also a reminder that persons with hearing loss have needs even when not wearing

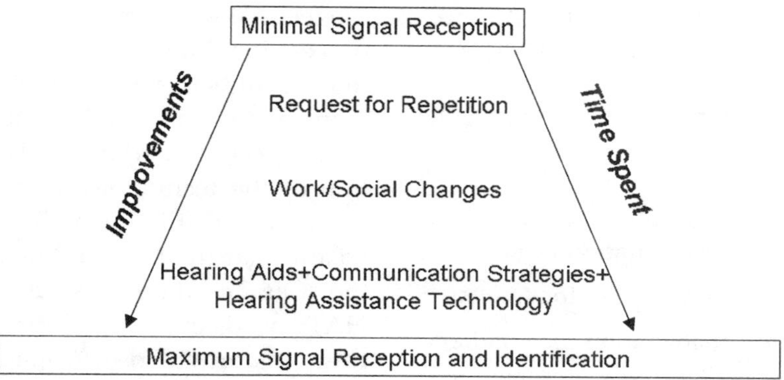

Figure 14–2. Efficient path to optimal communication when possible solutions are presented in the combined program.

personal hearing aids. For example, serving the total communication needs would include consideration of a flashing smoke alarm or vibrating alarm clock when these signals are not audible during sleep.

It is interesting to note some historical influences on the terminology. Twenty-five years ago, Vaughn et al. (1981) argued that the advent of smaller hearing aids resulted in certain communication limitations and that it was imperative that greater attention be focused on communication-centered environments and effective listener/talker devices. So, as the industry moved toward smaller hearing aids, the distinction between "hearing aids" and other devices such as "hearing assistance technology" developed. There evolved a focus on fitting hearing aids by the audiologist and assistive technology received less attention in clinical practice. The technology became so separate in fact, that in 1982, the notion of an Assistive Device Demonstration Center was recommended (Fellendorf, 1982). Nearly 15 years later, Sandridge and Lesner (1995) encouraged audiologists no longer to ask "whether or not" to provide ALDs, but rather, ask "how to" incorporate ALDs within one's service delivery. Wayner (2004) described the inclusion of assistive technology as part of the fitting process:

> It was an underlying belief that most persons with hearing loss could receive some benefit from amplification and that hearing aids were only one of a number of aids for successful rehabilitation and improved communication. (p. 43)

The inclusion of HATS was also supported by professional organizations. The "Preferred Practice Patterns (PPP) for the Profession of Audiology," as developed by the American Speech, Language, and Hearing Association (ASHA, 2006), reflect the collective judgments of practitioners and researchers in the field. In the current PPP, there are 27 audiologic practices. Specifically, practice 19.0 addresses Hearing Assistive Technology Systems. In addition, it is referenced in several other practice areas, as seen in Table 14–1.

Now, with technologic advances, there is a movement to include more options to interface the personal hearing aid with assistive technology. Hearing aids are capable of receiving signals from remote MP3 players, cell phones, and microphones. Therefore, the notion that the "assistive" devices are a separate category of devices that requires special mention in PPP may actually disappear. The fewer components to manage and to keep charged, the easier it will be to use HATS. For example, recent developments in FM systems are comprised of a multimicrophone FM transmitter(s) and a behind-the-ear hearing aid with integrated FM receiver. In addition to the noise reduction circuitry in the hearing aid, the multimicrophone transmitter will allow transmission of

Table 14–1. Audiology Preferred Practice Pattern Items That Reference Hearing Assistive Technology Systems (HATS)

Preferred Practice Pattern	Focus
14.0	Audiologic (Re)Habilitation Evaluation
15.0	Audiologic Rehabilitation for Adults
16.0	Audiologic Rehabilitation for Children
17.0	Hearing Aid Selection and Fitting
18.0	Product Repair and Modification
19.0	Hearing Assistive Technology Systems
20.0	Audiologic Management of the Cochlear Implant Patient

Source: ASHA, 2006.

the primary speaker with an improved signal-to-noise ratio compared to the signal arriving at the hearing aid microphone via the traditional airborne pathway. Studies have shown that use of multi-microphone arrays has resulted in significantly improved speech recognition and quality of life (Lewis et al., 2003, 2004). The FM transmitter may contain a Bluetooth receiver so that, when paired with a Bluetooth phone, the signal will be transmitted to the hearing aid and processed with optimal amplification. As more technology becomes integrated into the hearing aid, the programming options increase. For example, the FM receiver may be programmed for optimal transmission frequencies and FM advantage as described below in the verification process.

As technology increases, the integration of devices will also increase along with the demand for the audiologist's expertise, including interfacing HATS with bone-anchored hearing aids and with cochlear implants (Chisolm, McArdle, Abrams, & Noe, 2004; Schafer & Thibodeau, 2004). Today's consumers will likely bring more technologic experience than previous generations because of their increased use of devices such as cell phones with built-in cameras, electronic organizers with MP3 players, and multifunction printers that copy, scan, and fax. Regardless of the sophistication of the technology or programming options, the basic process for obtaining and successfully using HATS remains the same. Initially, there must be an assessment of the communication difficulties that will lead to recommendations. There must be verification of the technology to document appropriate settings and finally, validation must occur to ensure that the intended benefits are received by the user. To summarize the benefits meeting the HATS needs of an individual, a light-hearted illustration is provided in Appendix 14–A. Of course, the overall challenge is to integrate these steps into the routine clinical practice so that HATS are no longer considered an "option," much like checking one's blood pressure during a physical exam.

Needs Assessment

There is a variety of assessments that evaluate the communication difficulties facing a person with hearing loss. One common, efficient tool is the Client Oriented Scale of Improvement (COSI) (Dillon, James, & Ginis, 1997). This assessment is particularly useful because the individual provides the five most difficult communication situations, which are rated before and after amplification. Although this and other scales such as the Abbreviated Profile of Hearing Aid Benefit (APHAB) (Cox & Alexander, 1995) are very helpful in documenting the benefits of amplification, they only indirectly evaluate the need for HATS. There are no questions to prompt exploration of hearing alarms such as the smoke detector or alarm clock. In addition, traditional scales do not assess one's knowledge of laws that provide these accommodations in hotels while traveling. Therefore, a new tool was developed in a convenient format for the audiologist to use with every client to ensure a comprehensive assessment of communication needs. Tools are most useful if the name in some way implies their function. In this case, a novel acronym was chosen to convey the desire to improve communication across distances.

The new assessment is the TELEGRAM and it is designed to be completed following the routine audiologic evaluation (Thibodeau, 2004). As shown in Figure 14–3, the TELEGRAM is intended to be a convenient prompt for the areas that must be considered: Telephone, Employment, Legal issues, Entertainment, Group Communication, Recreation, Alarms, and Members of the family. Obtaining information regarding one's functioning in each of these areas will lead to recommendations for HATS or other rehabilitative strategies. The questions provided in Table 14–2 are based on critical areas recommended by Ross (2004) to be explored with every patient. Associated rating scales are suggested to quantify the difficulties. By providing a graphic form that is analogous to the audiogram, the audiologist should find it easy to document one's current functioning and determine areas of need.

Symbols are provided at the bottom with room for unique items for each client to be added. These can represent the patient's specific situations such as his/her recreational preferences. For example, the degree of difficulty with phone conversations can be recorded from 1 (no difficulty) to 5 (great difficulty) with an "L" for landline phones and a "C" for cell phones. Based on the difficulty, a recommendation may be made for intervention. At the next evaluation, the degree of difficulty may be compared to the initial levels to determine if improvement has occurred.

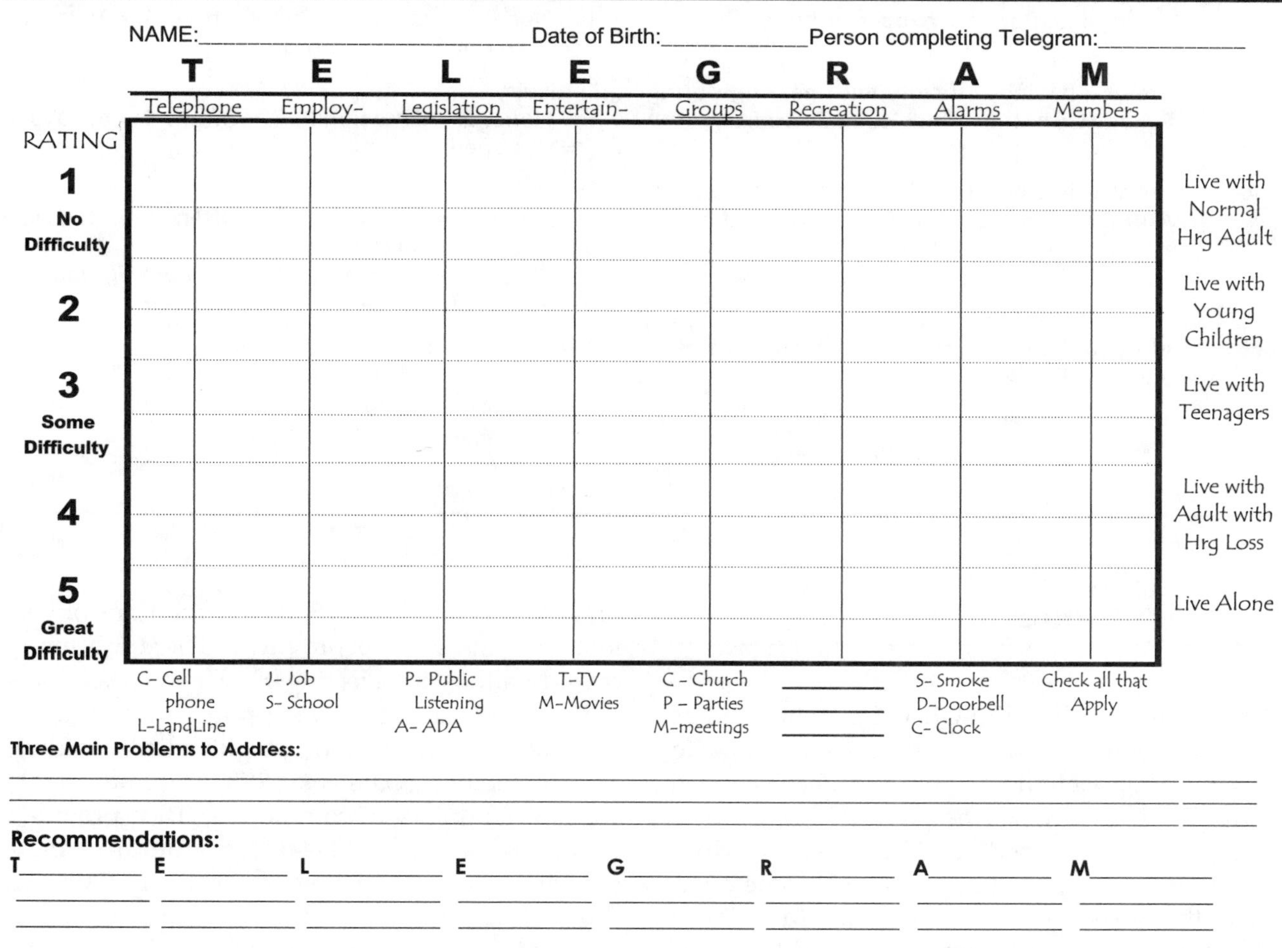

NAME:__________ Date of Birth:__________ Person completing Telegram:__________

RATING	T Telephone	E Employ-	L Legislation	E Entertain-	G Groups	R Recreation	A Alarms	M Members	
1 No Difficulty									Live with Normal Hrg Adult
2									Live with Young Children
3 Some Difficulty									Live with Teenagers
4									Live with Adult with Hrg Loss
5 Great Difficulty									Live Alone
	C- Cell phone L-LandLine	J- Job S- School	P- Public Listening A- ADA	T-TV M-Movies	C - Church P - Parties M-meetings	_____ _____ _____	S- Smoke D-Doorbell C- Clock	Check all that Apply	

Three Main Problems to Address:

____

____

____

Recommendations:

T_____ E_____ L_____ E_____ G_____ R_____ A_____ M_____

Figure 14–3. The TELEGRAM form that can be used as a prompt for gaining comprehensive information about difficulties and needs of adults with hearing loss.

Table 14–2. TELEGRAM Rating Scale Key

Topic	Question	Rating
T	Are you having difficulty with communication over the **telephone**?	Difficulty 1 = None, 2 = Occasional, 3 = Often, 4 = Always, 5 = Can't use the phone *Use "L" to designate Landline and "C" to designate Cell phone.*
E	Are you having any difficulty with communication in your **employment** or **educational** environment?	Difficulty 1 = None, 2 = Occasional, 3 = Often, 4 = Always, 5 = Stopped working
L	Do you know about **Legislation** that provides assistance for you to hear in public places or in hotels when you travel?	Knowledge 1 = Vast, 2 = Considerable, 3 = Some, 4 = Limited, 5 = None
E	Are you having difficulty with hearing during **Entertainment** activities that you enjoy such as television, movies, or concerts?	Difficulty 1 = None, 2 = Occasional, 3 = Often, 4 = Always, 5 = Stopped Going
G	Are you having difficulty with communication in **Group** settings?	Difficulty 1 = None, 2 = Occasional, 3 = Often, 4 = Always, 5 = Can't hear at all in groups
R	Are you having difficulty with hearing during **Recreational** activities such as sports, hunting, or sailing?	Difficulty 1 = None, 2 = Occasional, 3 = Often, 4 = Always, 5 = Stopped the activity
A	Are you having difficulty hearing **Alarms** or **Alerting** signals such as the smoke alarm, alarm clock, or the doorbell?	Difficulty 1 = None, 2 = Occasional, 3 = Often, 4 = Always, 5 = Can't hear alarm *Use "S" for Smoke Alarm, "D" for Doorbell, and "A" for Alarm Clock*
M	Are you communicating with **Members** of your family?	1 = Live with Normal Hrg Adult, 2 = Live with Young Children, 3 = Live withTeenagers, 4 = Live with Adult with Hrg Loss, 5 = Live Alone *Check all that apply*

Intervention

The answers on the TELEGRAM may be used as guides to determine appropriate technology. To review the possible items of benefit, each section of the TELEGRAM will be presented relative to the possible devices that might be used to reduce activity limitations. Although there is some overlap in the areas, use of the TELEGRAM helps to address all aspects of communication difficulties. While not within the scope of this chapter to review all possible HATS, the descriptions of various systems will be provided. There are many considerations in selecting HATS, such as: individual needs, age, family support, familiarization with technology, current amplification features, and preference (Garstecki, 1982; Holmes et al., 2000). A summary of common HATS is provided in Tables 14–3 and 14–4 for reception of non-speech and speech signals, respectively (Wayner, 2004). Resources to obtain HATS are provided in Table 14–5 so that current information may be obtained when working a particular individual's needs. Appendix 14–B also includes all the state contacts for programs for assistance for those with hearing loss.

Table 14–3. Hearing Assistance Technology Systems for Persons with Hearing Impairment-Nonspeech Enhancement Devices

NONSPEECH ENHANCEMENT DEVICES		
Visual	**Auditory**	**Tactile**
Call Alert	Ring Max	Shake Awake
Ring Indicator/Lamp	Fone Alert	Pillow Vibrator
Phone Flash/Strobe	Loud Ringer	Bed Vibrator
Baby Cry	Buzzer	Fan
Knock Light	Gong	Wrist Vibrator

Source: Adapted from Wayner (2004).

Table 14–4. Hearing Assistance Technology Systems for Persons with Hearing Impairment-Speech Enhancement Devices

SPEECH ENHANCEMENT DEVICES		
Telephone	**Television**	**Groups**
Portable Amplifier	Amplified Speaker	Infrared System
Handset Amplifier	Transistor Radio/ TV Band	Induction Loop
Telelink	Closed Caption	FM System
Telephone Typewriter (TTY)	Personal Listening Extension Cord	
Relay System	Pocketalker	
	Stereo Amplified Listener	
	Infrared Transmitter/Receiver	

Source: Adapted from Wayner (2004).

Table 14–5. Resources for Hearing Assistance Technology Systems

General Hearing Assistance Technology	www.assistedaudio.com www.oaktreeproducts.com www.dogsforthedeaf.org www.harc.com www.hitech.com www.sprintcaptel.com
Legislative and State Programs Regarding Accommodations for those with Impaired Hearing	http://www.fcc.gov/cgb/dro/ http://www.fcc.gov/cgb/consumerfacts/711.html http://www.tedpa.org/tedpainfo/stateprograms.html
FM Systems	www.phonak.com www.oticon.com www.avrsono.com http://www.comtek.com/assistive_listening/personal_fm_systems.html www.audioenhancement.com
Professional Organizations with information regarding HATS	www.hlaa.org www.asha.org www.audiology.org www.agbell.org www.audrehab.org

Telephone

Almost everyone needs to communicate by phone, particularly with the increasing popularity of mobile phones. Therefore, communication by phone is nearly as important as face-to-face conversations. It is important to distinguish problems with land-line phones versus cell phones because the solutions may vary depending on the features on the personal hearing aid. For example, difficulty with landline phones may be addressed by a phone amplifier or increasing the gain of the telecoil, whereas difficulties with cell phone communication may be addressed by setting up direct audio input or a Bluetooth connection.

For mild communication difficulties on the phone, a simple phone amplifier that fits over the handset may be sufficient. Others may need a phone that provides an amplified handset as shown in Figures 14–4 and 14–5. The features of the phone, such as cordless (Figure 14–4) or large numbers (Figure 14–5), will need to be considered relative to the patient's needs. If the phone communication is severely limited, a Telecommunication Device for the Deaf (TDD) may be considered where the communication occurs through typing messages on a keyboard and seeing responses on a small scrolling display. These are now widely available in public places and may provide a stress-free communication system when auditory solutions are not sufficient for clear reception. To communicate this way, both the caller and the receiver must have the TDD. When a person with a TDD wants to call someone without a TDD, a relay service may be used. The person with the TDD can call the relay service who will then call the other party without the TDD. The relay service will speak the typed message from the TDD to the person without the TDD. The service will also type messages back to the person with the TDD.

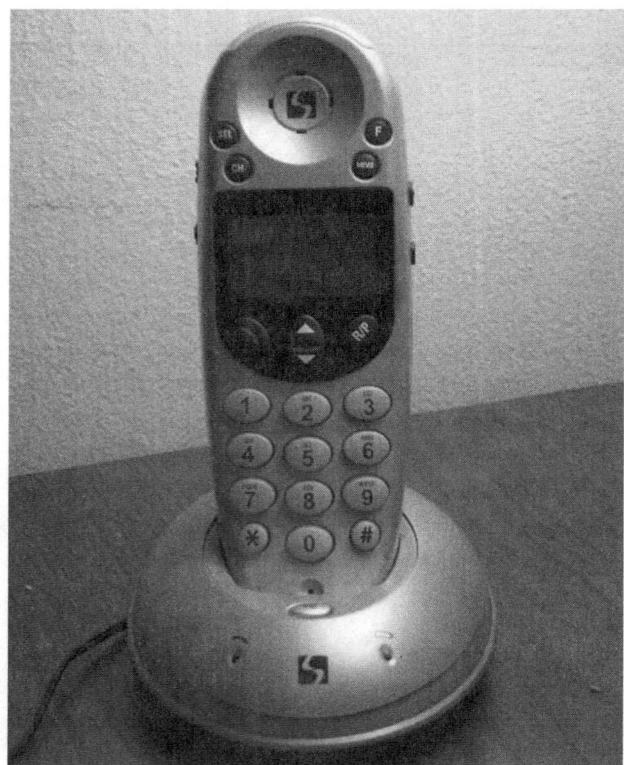

Figure 14–4. ClearSounds A50 Amplified Cordless Phone.

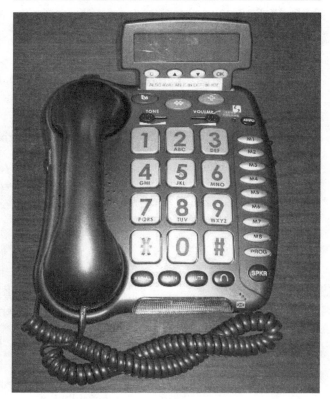

Figure 14–5. ClearSounds CSC50 Amplified Phone.

Another text-based solution is called Internet-Protocol Relay or IP where the person with hearing loss may communicate through an Internet site and does not need the TDD to enter the text. There are also captioned phones now that have visual displays where the speech is converted to text by an operator. The text scrolls across a small screen on the phone and the person with hearing impairment speaks naturally into the phone. A final text-based solution for phone communication is to use text messaging between cell phones, which is a common option on most cell phones. With this messaging, the information is typically typed in abbreviated format because of the limitations of the small keyboard and displays on cell phones. Further information regarding these options may be obtained through resources provided in Table 14–5.

The ability of the listener to hear the phone ring should also be considered. A common solution for the inaudibility of the typical high-pitched ring of a landline phone is to add an amplified ringer. An accommodation that does not involve HATS is to recommend the user purchase a cordless phone with a high volume ringer and with multiple receivers that can be placed in rooms of frequent use.

Employment

Communication difficulties at the workplace can be minimized in a variety of ways. This section is included to prompt discussion of challenges at work that can be addressed through specific programs on the personal hearing aids or perhaps through group amplification systems. In addition, there may be challenges on the phones at work that can be reduced through HATS. A referral to a state program that provides services to assist with employment may be necessary. Appendix 14–B includes contact information for all the state programs that provide services such as assistive technology, college tuition, and/or interview/resumé coaching to facilitate gaining employment.

HATS required in the workplace depend on the type of job requirements.. Through exploring the challenges the individual may have in the workplace, many possible solutions can be offered. In addition to phone solutions, communication issues may be addressed through the use of an FM system. Such a system includes a wireless microphone and a receiver that delivers the signal directly to the hearing aid or cochlear implant as shown in Figure 14–6. The advantage is significant improvement in speech recognition in noise as a direct result of microphone location (Lewis et al., 2003). Some microphones can be worn by the speaker, whereas others can be pointed directly at the speaker (held by the listener) for optimum reception. A particularly useful feature in small meetings is the use of a conference microphone that can be placed in a center location to pick up conversation ranging around the table.

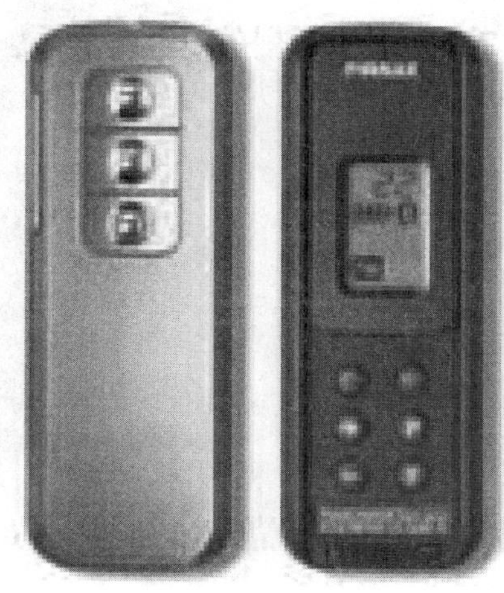

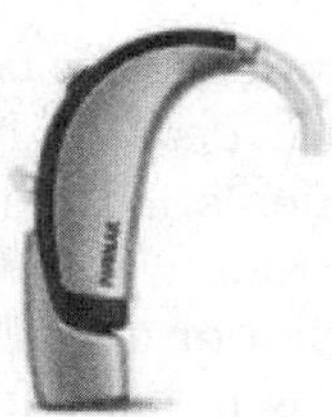

Figure 14–6. Front and back of an FM transmitter (*left*) and FM receiver attached to base of personal hearing aid (*right*). Photos courtesy of Phonak.

Legislation

As part of a comprehensive service to persons with hearing impairment, audiologists should determine if laws and state programs that provide assistive devices are known by the individual with hearing loss. Persons with hearing impairment can use this information to become advocates for their needs in employment, travel, or educational situations. Probably the most useful legislative action is the Americans with Disabilities Act (ADA). The ADA requires employers and/or businesses that provide services to the public to make accommodations for persons with disabilities such as hearing loss. This could include amplified telephones, infrared devices in theatres, vibrating alarm clocks in hotels, or an FM system with a conference microphone in staff meetings. (*Note:* Development of legislation providing for use of HATS is described in Chapter 15 in this text.)

Knowledge of legislation regarding phone communication is also important. The Telecommunications Relay Service (TRS), mentioned earlier, that allows persons with hearing or speech disabilities to place and receive telephone calls is available in all states for local and/or long distance calls. The Federal Communications Commission has adopted a convenient code, 711, for access to TRS regardless of the state. More information regarding 711 may be found in the Web sites provided in Table 14–5.

Many states have legislation that provides telephone assistance for persons with hearing loss. A list of state offices that provide services for persons with disabilities is in Appendix 14–B. For example, in Texas, the Division for Rehabilitation Services provides the Specialized Telecommunications Assistance Program (STAP) for people who are deaf or hard-of-hearing. Eligibility requirements for the program include proof of a Texas residency and an application signed by a physician or audiologist documenting that the person has impaired hearing. A STAP voucher is mailed to the recipient's home, which is brought to a certified vendor. At these sites, a variety of devices is offered, such as amplified telephones, signaling devices, and telephone listening systems.

Entertainment

Entertainment is often provided in group formats, such as theatrical productions or concerts, thus requiring the assistance of a large-area system. Three main systems may be used in large auditoriums, including, infrared, FM, and induction loop. The first two transmission methods involve receivers offered by the establishment at no cost to the person with hearing impairment. Whether the client watches television at home or attends concerts, the audiologist should determine the need and recommend possible solutions. An example of a personal infrared system is shown in Figure 14–7. Another solution for improved reception of the sound from the television is to purchase a TV-band radio that can be placed next to the chair of the

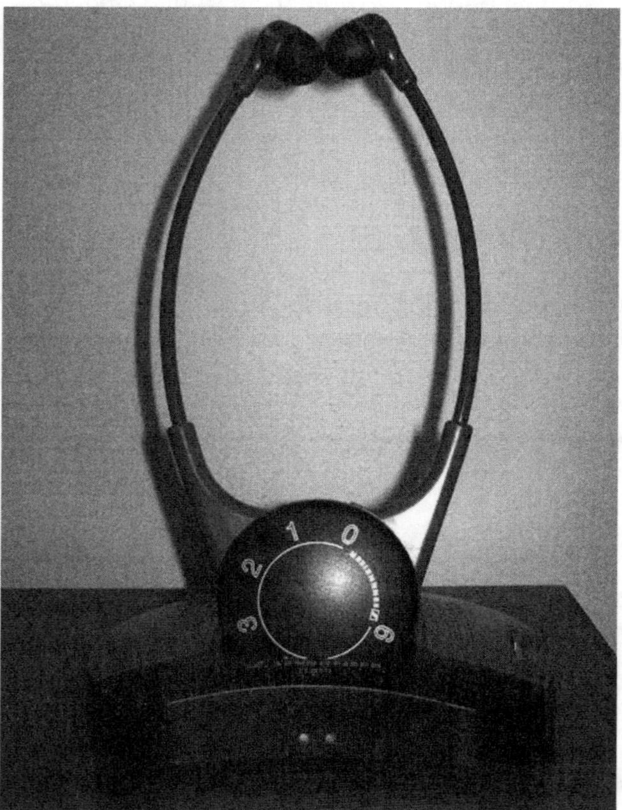

Figure 14–7. Sennheiser 810 Infrared TV Listening Headphones.

person with hearing loss. By having the radio speaker close to the listener, the signal-to-noise ratio is improved. In addition, personal earphones may be used with the radio to reduce unwanted ambient sound.

Groups

Communication in groups is often difficult because of distance from the speaker and noise and/or reverberation in the background. An FM system has been shown to reduce the deleterious effects of these factors and may be interfaced with the personal hearing aid in two primary ways. A small FM receiver may be attached to the hearing aid or implantable hearing device through a direct audio input connection. The receiver may be secured to the aid with an audio shoe or directly attached to the aid as shown in Figure 14–6. The FM signal may also be received via a neck loop attached to a body-worn FM receiver and the personal hearing aid set to t-coil. In group situations where there is one primary speaker, such as a lecture, the FM microphone can be worn by the presenter. For small group conversations the FM microphone may simply be pointed towards the speaker of interest. New developments in FM technology allow the use of multiple transmitters to one receiver. This will allow members of a group to use their own microphone and communicate directly with the person with hearing loss.

Recreation

Hobbies, of course, vary with personal preference and the dependence on hearing for full enjoyment should be considered. For example, if a retired couple enjoys traveling in a recreational vehicle across the country, communication may be limited because of road noise. An eight-hour trip could be significantly more enjoyable with a hard-wired amplifier with an extended microphone cord to be worn by the speaker. Some persons prefer to use the FM system described earlier for more freedom of movement. Providing a tour guide with an FM transmitter can significantly improve the quality of an organized vacation for a traveler with hearing loss. Assistive technology should always be explored for those with hobbies that involve noise such as woodworking or boating depending on their communication needs. For example, an amplified phone and intercom system may reduce frustrations for a wife trying to communicate with her husband who spends considerable time in a woodworking shop. Individuals may be wearing ear protection in these noisy environments which further necessitates assistive technology such as vibrating signals described in the next section.

Alarms

Hearing assistance technology is often a necessity to detect alarms, phone ringers, and warning signals in the environment. Most common alarm-type signals include doorbells, alarm clocks, and smoke alarms. There can be a single device used for all these alarms that convert the auditory signal into a tactile alert through a band worn on the wrist or into a code of all flashing lights. For example, a wristband with six lights may code the smoke alarm by all flashing, and code the doorbell and the phone by the first and second light, respectively.

Although not considered technology, the benefit of Hearing Dogs should not be overlooked when considering options for hearing alarms. Hearing Dogs are specially trained to help an individual hear the specific alarms in their environments. The dogs are selected from animal shelters and are trained over several months before being matched with an individual and receiving the more specific training for that person's environment. More information may be obtained from the resource provided in Table 14–5.

Members of Household

Members of the household certainly provide hearing assistance and should be considered when addressing the needs of the person with hearing impairment. If there is a spouse or life partner, he or she should be an integral part of the technology and communication strategy training. Small children or teenagers present a special set of challenges with high-pitched voice and rapid speech. HATS may be an integral solution for these challenges but simple communication rules, such as not talking until in the same room or facing the listener, will often be of great assistance. Solutions can also be creative, such as wearing a button or t-shirt with a printed reminder to "Thank you for facing me when you speak!"

Fitting and Verification

After determining the need for assistive technology, the particular device should be verified in some way. The techniques to do this vary with the device. Ideally, verification can include both electroacoustic and behavioral measures. Those that deliver the signal via the personal hearing aid, such as an FM system with a direct audio input FM receiver, can be evaluated using existing electroacoustic test equipment and couplers. When the coupling does not allow use of standard couplers for evaluation, behavioral evaluation should be performed.

There are two documents that relate to the verification of HATS. They are both in review at the time of this writing, but are expected to be adopted soon. The one that has been in progress the longest is the ANSI standard for *Specification of Hearing Assistance Devices/Systems* (ANSI, 2008). This standard will address the electroacoustic evaluation of technology that is packaged as a personal system (rather than large area group systems). Recommended electroacoustic measurements are similar to those for hearing aids in the ANSI S3.22 standard, but have specific requirements for placement of the transmitting microphone and the receiver. These procedures will allow for comparison to manufacturer specifications, as well as comparison across equipment models because prescribed input levels and equipment arrangements are used (Schafer, Thibodeau, Whalen, & Overson, 2007). Many devices can be evaluated with existing couplers used to test hearing aids whereas other devices, such as those with headphones, may not. The manufacturer will then report the coupling method used to obtain the electroacoustic results.

The second document is the *AAA Clinical Practice Guidelines: Remote Microphone Hearing Assistance Technologies* (AAA, 2008). This comprehensive guide focuses on hearing assistive technology for individuals from birth to 21 years. It is an expansion of the original guidelines developed by an ASHA (2002) Task Force which focused on real-ear, electroacoustic, and behavioral evaluation procedures. As technology has expanded, the need for a more comprehensive document emerged. The new AAA guidelines include information to consider in determining candidacy, device selection, fitting/evaluation, and staff in-service. A supplement is included with specific protocols for the evaluation of ear-level FM systems when used with children who wear hearing aids, cochlear implants, or who have normal hearing. Additional supplements will be forthcoming to address evaluation of soundfield and induction loop systems.

Although written for children, these fitting protocols are applicable to adult populations. When fitting FM Systems, it is important that electroacoustic verification be performed to measure that the FM signal is received at a level above the environmental signals processed through the hearing aid resulting in a favorable signal-to-noise ratio (S/N). This is determined by comparing the output of the hearing aid alone to that of the combined hearing aid and FM system when tested with a 65 dB SPL complex input. The two curves should be closely aligned. Then when the FM microphone receives the typical input of 80 dB SPL from the speaker, the optimal signal-to-noise ratio will be accomplished. If the two curves are not similar, then adjustments must be made in the FM receiver to compensate for the "offset." The AAA Task Force has proposed a taxonomy that includes the type of measure (electroacoustic), the system receiving the input (HA or FM), and the input level (65 dB SPL). For example, the first measurement is EHA65 which is an electroacoustic measure performed with the HA in the test box and a 65 dB SPL input.

The next measure is EFMHA65 which is performed with the FM microphone in the test box to receive the input and the HA outside the test box. In summary, the difference between the output curves for EHA65 and EFMHA65 should be close to zero.

Although the benefit of assistive technology is best measured in one's real life environment, the AAA Guidelines include procedures for behavioral verification of remote microphone technology. The listener with the technology is seated in the sound booth at zero degrees azimuth, while the examiner with the microphone is seated at the audiometer outside the booth. Using appropriate speech recognition materials, the first score is obtained via live-voice presentation in a 0 dB S/N. Following the proposed terminology, this condition is BHA50/50, which designates a behavioral evaluation with the hearing aid alone with speech and noise presented at 50 dB HL. The next condition is BFM/HA50/50, which is similar to the first measure except now the examiner has turned on the remote microphone. When BHA50/50 doesn't result in a score below 80%, the noise may be increased to create a poorer S/N so that the benefit from the assistive technology can reach significance. The 20% change in scores required for significant difference is based on a 25-word list. The average benefit for 10 adults when tested with this protocol with FM technology was 34% (Thibodeau, 2007).

Following verification, the individual and possibly a family member will need instruction on the care and use of the chosen technology. Although some HATS can be very simple to operate such as a vibrating alarm clock, others may involve multiple components such as an FM system that interfaces with one's personal hearing aids or implantable device. Not only is there technology added to the hearing aid, but there is a remote microphone, which may also have several features. In addition to the verbal instruction and practice at the AR appointment, written materials should be provided for review at home. Conveniently, one FM manufacturer provides instruction sheets via a "Configurator" on their Web page where the information can be customized for a user depending on the equipment they will be using.

Validation

Once HATS have been appropriately fit, the final step is validation. This is necessary to determine if the intended benefits are received by the individual. Although an FM system could be precisely fit and significant benefit shown in the FM fitting evaluation, if the individual forgets how to operate the device when she gets home and does not use the system, then the intended benefits are not realized. Therefore, the TELEGRAM or COSI should be administered three to six months following the fitting to determine if there is reduction in the degree of difficulty. In a study using the TELEGRAM, it was determined that all individuals showed improvement in six of the seven areas (Thibodeau, 2007). By reviewing the TELEGRAM at the annual audiologic evaluation, the benefit received through the technology that was recommended the previous year could be documented and new recommendations made if necessary.

Integrating into Clinical Practice

Prendergast and Kelley (2002) reported that more than 80% of audiologists were providing information regarding HATS to their patients. However, the extent to which patients were actually provided HATS or information to obtain devices is unknown. It may be difficult for the audiologists to maintain a stock of equipment in addition to keeping current versions of manufacturer software for fitting hearing aids. Lesner and Klinger (1995) provided several considerations for incorporating HATS into a clinical practice including room size, furnishings, environment, and organization of special equipment. There are, however, several alternatives to a dedicated hearing technology room. Some of these resources can be offered with minimal effort by providing a simple resource brochure of commonly used HATS for the telephone, television, and alarm clocks (cf. www.oaktreeproducts.com). These brochures can be customized with contact information and provided to each patient following the recommendations provided on the TELEGRAM.

It still may be challenging for audiologists to follow up with their patients regarding appropriate use and benefit from the system that has been dispensed. Fortunately, there are some resources to consider to assist with the initial exploration of devices as well as the follow-up. One such resource is the Hearing Loss Association of America (HLAA) National Center for Hearing Assistive Technology (NCHAT), which promotes the use of technology to maximize the residual hearing of people who are hard of hearing (www.hlaa.org). They offer intensive regional training sessions regarding HATS to selected HLAA members from specific states. More information can be obtained at www.hearingloss.org . Following training, the participants agree to provide outreach efforts at the local level about HATS. These trained persons may be actively using HATS and can be a significant asset to the professional who adopts this broad approach to addressing the needs of persons with hearing impairment (Wayner, 2004).

Another program that will train support personnel to specialize in assistive technology is the Peer Mentoring Certification Program offered at Gallaudet University as part of the Rehabilitation Engineering Research Center on Hearing Enhancement (RERC). Laypersons develop skills to support the use of hearing assistance technology and several other services through a 13-credit distance-learning program (Bally & Bakke, 2007).

In addition to incorporation of these HATS resources into clinical practice, the benefits of group sessions focused on HATS should be considered. Patients may increase their acceptance of HATS when sharing communication frustrations and HATS solutions in group discussions (Thibodeau & Cokely, 2003). Furthermore, clinical efficiency is increased when device explanation occurs in group formats. (Chisolm, McArdle, Abrams, & Noe, 2004). One recently evaluated format involves four, weekly, one-hour meetings focused on trials with wireless technology. The program is referred to as AALTA or Application of Advanced Listening Technology in Adults is offered with support from manufacturers of wireless technology so that individuals may have personal experiences which can then be shared in the weekly AALTA meetings (Thibodeau, 2007).

Summary

The needs of the adult with hearing loss extend into many aspects of life. The first solution that is considered is to provide amplification that can restore audibility of acoustic information. However, there are many instances in which noise, reverberation, and distance render the acoustic signal inaudible, regardless of the amplification technology. In addition, hearing aids are not worn all hours of the day, yet there are alarms that can convey life-saving information, such as a smoke detector, that need to be heard. Therefore, it is part of basic audiologic care to consider the assistive technology that a person may need in their everyday lives.

Despite the basic needs of persons with hearing loss, audiologists typically view assistive technology as accessories and consequently many needs are unmet. A routine tool is proposed as part of the basic audiological evaluation to prompt the audiologist to address these needs. The format of the TELEGRAM allows for a quick review of problems that can lead to recommendations for technology or acquiring knowledge (such as learning about legislative issues).

Once the needs are identified, the next challenge is for the audiologist to provide the technology or a system by which patients can get the technology. In addition to having a demonstration center within the audiology practice, there are trained laypersons with considerable experience that may be called on to meet with patients to review operation and troubleshooting of devices. After the appropriate technology is received, the audiologist's responsibility includes follow-up to ensure that it is being used properly and is effectively meeting patient needs. The progress can be noted on the TELEGRAM so that areas may be reassessed at subsequent evaluations. Hearing aids alone are sufficient for some persons with hearing loss, and many can benefit from assistive technology. Audiologists are best suited to see that the process of acquiring and fitting assistive technology occurs efficiently without weeks or months of frustration. With this comprehensive audiologic care, those with impaired hearing may reduce their communication challenges and continue to live enjoyable and productive lives.

References

American Academy of Audiology. (2008). Remote microphone hearing assistance technologies for children and youth birth–21 years. In review.

American National Standards Institute. (2008). ANSI S.3.47 Specification of Hearing Assistance Devices/ Systems. In review.

American Speech-Language-Hearing Association. (2002). Guidelines for fitting and monitoring FM systems. *ASHA Desk Reference.*

American Speech, Language, and Hearing Association. (2006). Preferred practice patterns for the profession of audiology. Available at www.asha .org/policy

Bally, S. J., & Bakke, M. H. (2007). A peer mentor training program for aural rehabilitation. *Trends in Amplification, 11*(2), 125–131.

Chisolm, T., McArdle, R., Abrams, H., & Noe, C. (2004). Goals and outcomes of FM use by adults. *Hearing Journal, 57*(11), 28–35.

Cox, R. M., & Alexander, G. C. (1995). The abbreviated profile of hearing aid benefit (APHAB). *Ear and Hearing, 16*, 176–186.

Dillon, H., James, A., & Ginis, J. (1997). Client-Oriented Scale of Improvement (COSI) and its relationship to several other measures of benefit and satisfaction provided by hearing aids. *Journal of the American Academy of Audiology, 8*, 27–43.

Fellendorf, G. W. (1982). A model demonstration of assistive devices for hearing-impaired people. *Journal of the Academy of Rehabilitative Audiology, 15*, 70–82.

Garstecki, D. C. (1988). Considerations in selecting assistive devices for hearing-impaired adults. *Journal of the Academy of Rehabilitative Audiology, 21*, 153–157.

Holmes, A. E., Saxon, J. P., & Kaplan, H. S. (2000). Assistive listening devices and systems: Amplification technology for consumers with hearing loss. *Journal of Rehabilitation, 66*(3), 56–59.

Lesner, S., & Klinger, M. (1995). Considerations in establishing an optimum assistive listening device center. *Journal of the Academy of Rehabilitative Audiology, 14*, 60–67.

Lewis, S., Crandell, C., Valente, M., & Enrietto Horn, J. (2004). Speech perception in noise: Directional microphones versus frequency modulation (FM) systems. *Journal of the American Academy of Audiology, 15*, 426–439.

Lewis, S., Crandell, C., Valente, M., Enrietto, J., Kreisman, N., Kreisman, B., et al. (2003). Study measures impact of hearing aids plus FM on the quality of life in older adults. *Hearing Journal, 56*, 30–33.

Prendergast, S. G., & Kelley, L. A. (2002). Aural rehab services: Survey reports who offers which ones and how often. *Hearing Journal, 55*, 30–35.

Ross, M. (2004). Hearing assistive technologies: Making a world of difference. *Hearing Journal, 57*(11), 12–17.

Sandridge, S., & Lesner, S. (1995). Practical considerations in providing assistive devices. *Journal of the Academy of Rehabilitative Audiology, 28*, 68–77.

Schafer, E., & Thibodeau, L. (2004). Speech recognition abilities of adults using cochlear implants with FM systems. *Journal of the American Academy of Audiology, 15*, 678–691.

Schafer, E., Thibodeau, L., Whalen, H., & Overson, G. (2007). Electroacoustic evaluation of frequency-modulated receivers interfaced with personal hearing aids. *Language, Speech, Hearing Services in Schools, 38*, 1–12.

Thibodeau, L. (2004). Maximizing communication via hearing assistance technology: Plotting beyond the audiogram! *Hearing Journal, 57*(11), 46–51.

Thibodeau, L. (2007) Application of advanced listening technology in adults, AALTA. *Proceedings of Hearing Care in Adults* (pp. 3–13). Chicago: Phonak.

Thibodeau, L., & Cokely, C. (2003). Maximizing auditory rehabilitation training for clients, students, and faculty through SIARC: Summer Intensive

Aural Rehabilitation Conference. *Journal of the Academy of Rehabilitative Audiology*, *36*, 67–82.

Vaughn, G. R., Lightfoot, R. K., & Arnold, L. C. (1981). Alternative listening devices and delivery systems for audiologic habilitation of hearing-impaired persons. *Journal of the Academy of Rehabilitative Audiology*, *14*, 62–77.

Wayner, D. (2004). Integrating ALDS into your daily dispensing practice. *Hearing Journal*, *57*(11), 43–45.

Appendix 14–A
Illustration of Benefits of HATS

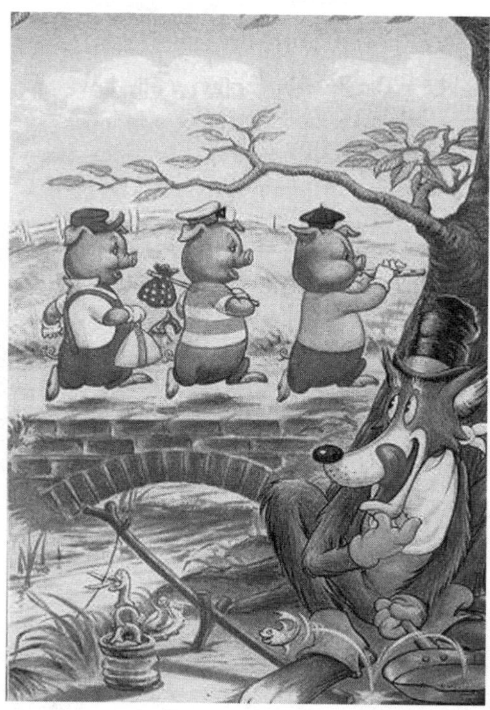

Source: Illustration by Vera Southgate, from the cover of *The Three Little Pigs (Well Loved Tales)*. Copyright © Ladybird Books Ltd., 1965. Reprinted by permission of Ladybird Archive.

THREE DEAF PIGS

The first pig built a house of straw.
The wolf came.
He yelled for the pig to come out.
The pig could not hear him.
The wolf blew down the house and ate the pig.

The second pig built a house of sticks.
The wolf came.
He yelled for the pig to come out.
The pig could not hear him.
He thought it was a tornado.
The wolf blew down the house and ate the pig.

The third pig built a brick house with flashing lights and all the necessary deaf devices.
The wolf rang the bell and the lights flashed.
He called the zoo, using the TTY relay service.
A zoo keeper came and put the wolf in a sign language class.
The wolf learned to communicate and became friends with the pig.

Author Unknown

Appendix 14–B
State Programs for the Hearing-Impaired

State	Program	Voice	TTY	Fax
Alabama	Department of Rehabilitation Services Vocational Rehabilitation Services Deaf/Hard of Hearing Services	800.441.7607	800.499.1816	
	Web site: http://www.rehab.state.al.us/Home/default.aspx?url=/Home/Main			
Alaska	Department of Labor and Workforce Development Division of Vocational Rehabilitation	907.465.2814 800.478.2815		907.465.2856
	Web site: http://labor.state.ak.us/dvr/home.htm			
Arizona	Department of Economic Security Rehabilitation Services Administration	602.542.3332	602.542.6049	602.542.3778
	Web site: https://www.azdes.gov/rsa/default.asp			
Arkansas	Rehabilitation Services	501.296.1600 800.330.0632	501.296.1600 800.330.0632	
	Web site: http://www.arsinfo.org/			
California	Department of Rehabilitation Assistive Technology	916.558.5775	916.558.5778	
	Web site: http://www.rehab.cahwnet.gov/			
Colorado	Department of Human Services Commission for the Deaf and Hard of Hearing	303.866.4824	303.866.4734	303.866.4831
	Web site: http://www.cdhs.state.co.us/DeafCommission/index.htm			
Connecticut	Bureau of Rehabilitation Services Vocational Rehabilitation Program	800.537.2549 860.424.4844	860.424.4839 800.537.2549	
	Web site: http://www.brs.state.ct.us/index.html			

Delaware	Department of Labor Division of Vocational Rehabilitation Office for the Deaf and Hard of Hearing		
	Voice: 302.761.8275	TTY: 302.761.8336	Fax: 302.761.6611
	Web site: http://www.delawareworks.com/dvr/services/dodhh.shtml		
District of Columbia	Rehabilitation Services Administration		
	Voice: 202.442.8629	TTY: 202.442.8629	Fax:
	Web site: http://www.rsa.dhs.dc.gov/rsa/site/default.asp?rsaNav=|		
Florida	Department of Education Division of Vocational Rehabiliation		
	Voice: 850.245.3399 800.451.4327	TTY: 850.245.3399 800.451.4327	Fax:
	Web site: http://www.rehabworks.org/		
Georgia	Department of Labor Rehabilitation Services		
	Voice: 404.232.3910 866.489.0001	TTY: 404.232.3911	Fax:
	Web site: http://www.vocrehabga.org/		
Hawaii	Department of Human Services Division of Vocational Rehabiliation		
	Voice: 808.692.7719	TTY:	Fax:
	Web site: not listed		
Idaho	Division of Rehabilitation Services		
	Voice: 208.334.3390	TTY:	Fax: 208.334.5305
	Web site: http://www.vr.idaho.gov/		
Illinois	Department of Human Services Rehabilitation Services		
	Voice: 800.843.6154	TTY: 800.447.6404	Fax:
	Web site: http://www.dhs.state.il.us/page.aspx?item=27893		
Indiana	Family and Social Services Administration Division of Disability and Rehabilitative Services		
	Voice: 800.962.8408	TTY: 800.962.8408	Fax:
	Web site: http://www.in.gov/fssa/ddrs/index.htm		

Iowa	Vocational Rehabilitation Services		
	Voice: 515.281.4211	TTY: 515.281.4211	Fax: 515.281.76459
	Web site: http://www.ivrs.iowa.gov/index.html		
Kansas	Department of Social and Rehabilitation Services Kansas Commission for the Deaf and Hard of Hearing		
	Voice: 785.368.8034 800.432.0698	TTY: 785.368.8046 800.432.0698	Fax: 785.368.7467
	Web site: http://www.srskansas.org/kcdhh/		
Kentucky	Vocational Rehabilitation Deaf and Hard of Hearing Services		
	Voice: 800.372.7172	TTY: 800.372.7172	Fax: 502.564.6742
	Web site: http://ovr.ky.gov/programs_services/deaf_services.htm		
Louisiana	Department of Social Services Rehabilitation Services		
	Voice: 225.219.2225 800.737.2958	TTY:	Fax: 225.219.4993 225.219.2942
	Web site: http://www.dss.state.la.us/index.htm		
Maine	Bureau of Rehabilitation Services Division of Deafness		
	Voice: 207.623.7958	TTY: 207.623.7998 888.755.0023	Fax: 207.623.7965
	Web site: http://www.maine.gov/rehab/dod/index.htm		
Maryland	Department of Education Division of Rehabilitative Services		
	Voice: 410.554.9442 888.554.0334	TTY: 410.554.9411	Fax:
	Web site: http://www.dors.state.md.us/dors		
Massachusetts	Health and Human Services Commission for the Deaf and Hard of Hearing		
	Voice: 617.740.1600 800.882.1155	TTY: 617.740.1700 800.530.7570	Fax: 617.740.1880
	Web site: http://www.mass.gov/mcdhh		

Michigan	Labor and Economic Growth Division on Deaf and Hard of Hearing		
	Voice: 800.605.7277	TTY: 888.605.6722	Fax: 517.335.7277
	Web site: http://www.michigan.gov/dleg/0,1607,7-154-28077_28545_28559-23760—,00.html		
Minnesota	Department of Employment and Economic Development Rehabilitation Services		
	Voice: 651.259.7366 800.328.9095	TTY: 651.296.3900 800.657.3973	Fax: 651.297.5159
	Web site: http://www.deed.state.mn.us/rehab/		
Mississippi	Department of Rehabilitation Services		
	Voice: 800.443.1000	TTY:	Fax:
	Web site: http://www.mdrs.state.ms.us/		
Missouri	Commission for the Deaf and Hard of Hearing		
	Voice: 573.526.5205	TTY: 573.526.5205	Fax: 573.526.5209
	Web site: http://www.mcdhh.mo.gov/		
Montana	Department of Public Health and Human Services Disability Services Division Deaf and Hard of Hearing Services		
	Voice: 406.444.5622	TTY: 406.444.2590	Fax: 406.444.1970
	Web site: http://www.dphhs.mt.gov/dsd/medicalcounseling/montandeafandhardofhearingservices.shtml		
Nebraska	Commission for the Deaf and Hard of Hearing		
	Voice: 402.595.3991 877.248.7836	TTY: 402.595.3991 877.248.7836	Fax: 402.595.2509
	Web site: http://www.ncdhh.ne.gov/		
Nevada	Department of Health and Human Services Office of Disability Services		
	Voice: 775.687.4452	TTY:	Fax: 775.687.7560
	Web site: http://dhhs.nv.gov/ODS_Programs.htm		

State	Agency	Voice	TTY	Fax	Web site
New Hampshire	Department of Education Vocational Rehabilitation	603.271.3743	603.271.3743	603.271.1953	http://www.ed.state.nh.us/education/index.htm
New Jersey	Department of Labor and Workforce Development Division for the Deaf and Hard of Hearing	609.984.7281 800.792.8339	800.792.8339	609.984.0390	http://www.state.nj.us/humanservices/ddhh/index.html
New Mexico	Division of Vocational Rehabilitation	505.954.8500 800.224.7005		505.954.8562	http://www.dvrgetsjobs.com/DVRInternet/Clients/ServToClients.aspx
New York	Education Department Vocational and Educational Services for Individual with Disabilities	518.474.5652	518.474.5652		http://www.vesid.nysed.gov/lsn/deaf.htm
North Carolina	Department of Health and Human Services Division of Vocational Rehabilitation	919.855.3500	919.855.3579	919.733.7968	http://dvr.dhhs.state.nc.us/index.htm
North Dakota	Department of Human Services Disabilities Services Division	701.328.8930 800.755.8529	701.328.8968	701.328.8969	http://www.nd.gov/dhs/
Ohio	Rehabilitation Services Commission	800.282.4536 614.438.1252	614.785.5048	614.438.1257	http://www.rsc.ohio.gov/VR_Services/BVR/bvr.asp

Oklahoma	Department of Rehabilitation Services		
	Voice: 405.951.3400 800.845.8476	TTY: 405.951.3529	Fax:
	Web site: http://www.okrehab.org/		
Oregon	Department of Human Services Office of Vocational Rehabilitation Services		
	Voice: 503.945.5880 877.277.0513	TTY: 866.801.0130	Fax: 503.947.5010
	Web site: http://www.oregon.gov/DHS/vr/		
Pennsylvania	Department of Labor and Industry Vocational Rehabilitation		
	Voice: 800.442.6352	TTY: 800.233.3008	Fax:
	Web site: http://www.nepacil.org/OVR.htm		
Rhode Island	Department of Human Services Offices of Rehabilitation Services		
	Voice: 401.421.7005	TTY:	Fax: 401.222.3574
	Web site: http://www.ors.state.ri.us/		
South Carolina	Vocational Rehabilitation Department		
	Voice: 803.896.6500 800.832.7526	TTY: 803.896.6553	Fax:
	Web site: http://www.scvrd.net/index.html		
South Dakota	Department of Human Services Division of Rehabilitation Services		
	Voice: 605.773.3195	TTY:	Fax: 605.773.5483
	Web site: http://dhs.sd.gov/		
Tennessee	Department of Human Services		
	Voice: 615.313.4914 800.628.7818	TTY: 615.313.6601 800.270.1349	Fax: 615.313.6617
	Web site: http://www.state.tn.us/humanserv/rehab/dhhs.htm		
Texas	Department of Assistive and Rehabilitative Services		
	Voice: 800.628.5115	TTY: 866.581.9328	Fax:
	Web site: http://www.dars.state.tx.us/		

Utah	Office of Rehabilitation		
	Voice: 801.538.7530 800.473.7530	TTY: 801.538.7530	Fax: 801.538.7522
	Web site: http://www.usor.utah.gov/		
Vermont	Agency of Human Services Department of Disabilities, Aging and Independent Living Deaf and Hard of Hearing Services		
	Voice: 866.4105787	TTY: 802.241.3557	Fax:
	Web site: http://www.dail.vermont.gov/dhhs-temp/dhhs-temp-default		
Virginia	Department of Rehabilitative Services		
	Voice: 804.662.7000 800.552.5019	TTY: 800.552.5019	Fax: 804.662.9531
	Web site: http://www.vadrs.org/vocrehab.htm		
Washington	Department of Social and Health Services Division of Vocational Rehabilitation		
	Voice: 360.725.3636 800.637.5627	TTY: 360.725.3636 800.637.5627	Fax: 360.438.8007
	Web site: http://www1.dshs.wa.gov/index.html		
West Virginia	Division of Rehabilitative Services Department of Education		
	Voice: 800.642.8207	TTY: 800.642.8207	Fax:
	Web site: http://www.wvdrs.org/		
Wisconsin	Department of Workforce Development Vocational Rehabilitation		
	Voice: 608.261.0050 800.442.3477	TTY: 888.877.5939	Fax: 608.266.1133
	Web site: http://www.dwd.state.wi.us/dvr/jobseek.htm		
Wyoming	Department of Workforce Services Vocational Rehabilitation		
	Voice: 307.777.8728	TTY:	Fax:
	Web site: http://www.wyomingworkforce.org/how/vr.aspx		

15

Accessibility for People with Hearing Impairments: Legislation and Implementation in Israel

Orna Eran
Zvia Admon

Introduction

The rights of people with disabilities, including people with hearing impairments, to equality, inclusion, and accessibility received recognition in Israeli law only in recent years. Legislative developments in the United States and Europe in the 1980s and 1990s preceded the antidiscrimination and accessibility measures in Israeli law, and provided the blueprint for them. The enactment of the Americans with Disabilities Act (1990), and European legislation such as the Disability Ombudsman Law (1994) in Sweden, the Disability Discrimination Act (1995) in the United Kingdom, and the Amsterdam Treaty of 1997 promoted equality and accessibility in the public sphere. These legislative developments, along with disability advocacy by Israeli civil rights lawyers and disability nongovernmental organizations (NGOs), led to a growing awareness within the Israeli public for the rights and needs of persons with disabilities. Several Israeli laws on accessibility were enacted during the first half of the 1990s, with the Equal Rights for People with Disability Law of 1998 finally recognizing their right to equality.

Although the Equal Rights for People with Disabilities Law included antidiscrimination measures in employment and some accessibility requirements, it was not until the enactment of the Accessibility Chapter (Equal Rights for People with Disability Law [amendment no. 2] 2005, S.H. p. 288) of the Law, in 2005, that the right to full accessibility in public premises and services for persons with disabilities was recognized. The draft Accessibility Regulations, drafted in accordance with the chapter, contain extensive accessibility measures, including requirements for hearing assistive technologies (HATs) in public buildings, premises, and services.

The current chapter surveys the history of the legislation and advocacy dealing with accessibility for persons with hearing impairment in Israel, and the contribution of government agencies, disability NGOs, and audiologists to the evolution of this legislation, including current accessibility regulations, and its provisions for HATs.

Part I. Legislation Prior to Drafting of the Accessibility Regulations

Until the 1990s, most of the legislation regarding people with disabilities focused on providing them with adequate care, including health care, education, and welfare pensions. This legislation was based on a paternalistic model that perceived people with disabilities as weak, needy, and unable to work for a living or care for themselves, whose needs were best served by professionals such as physicians, social workers, and special education teachers (Admon, 2007).

The welfare approach to people with hearing disability is reflected in the provisions for their social benefits. For instance, since 2002, adults with hearing impairment (age 18–65 with 70 dB or more in better ear) who lost their hearing prior to age 3, have been eligible for a monthly benefit and also for a refund once in four years covering a number of assistive devices (Eran, 2004b).

This paternalistic approach in the legislation was also reflected in the high unemployment rates among people with disabilities, in the negative stereotypes held by many in society toward them, and in an almost complete lack of accessibility to most public places and activities.

The Planning and Building Law and its regulations, were the only source for legislative accessibility provisions until the mid-1980s. The law was amended (1981) to include a chapter on accessibility in public buildings. The Planning and Building Regulations were amended, accordingly, to include requirements for accessibility in public buildings (K.T. 1970, No. 1851 and Planning and Building Regulations—Public Building, 1981, K.T. No. 1065).

These requirements were far from adequate. They were partial, relating only to public buildings while ignoring accessibility in public services, and required accessibility only for people with a mobility disability, who used a wheelchair. No provisions were made for people with hearing impairment, blindness, or cognitive disability. In addition, the requirements related only to "new" buildings constructed after 1972, and some public buildings, such as government offices, local municipal offices, and schools were required to make only one floor accessible. Moreover, the regulations did not apply to public premises not defined as "buildings," such as public bomb shelters, public parks, cemeteries, or archeologic or historical sites open to visitors.

Consequently, the majority of public buildings in Israel remained inaccessible. The inaccessibility of these public buildings left most public services, which are provided in these buildings, inaccessible to most people with disabilities, including people with hearing impairment (Admon, 2007). For example, banking services, emergency services, public education at all levels—from kindergarten to universities, including classrooms and schools for children with hearing impairment—were essentially inaccessible (Eran, 2004c).

Public dissatisfaction with the lack of accessibility and the inadequacy of the legal requirements increased in the late 1980s and early 1990s. The public Committee for Examination of Comprehensive Rights Legislation for People with Disabilities (Katz Committee, 1997), established by the government, published a report exposing the multiple inadequacies and lacunas in the law, which, according to the Committee, essentially legitimized segregation of people with disabilities and perpetuated discrimination against them. Consumer groups of people with disabilities began to demand accessibility to public places and services, and participation in the legislation process leading to accessibility provisions.

As a result of the increased dissatisfaction, several accessibility laws were enacted in the early 1990s. This legislation was not systematic or comprehensive, but reflected the growing awareness of the right to equality for persons with disabilities, including their right to accessibility. One of these new accessibility laws was the Deaf Assistance Law (1992), which required television channels to provide subtitles to some of their programs—initially one-quarter of non-live broadcasts—and simultaneous translation into Hebrew Sign Language for at least one weekly news bulletin.

The Equal Rights for People with Disability Law, which was enacted in 1998, established for the first time the right of people with disabilities to equality and full participation. The draft law was based on antidiscrimination laws in other countries, principally the Americans with Disabilities Act (1990), and included provisions for accessibility in public premises and services, based on the realization that equality and full participation can be attained only when the environment is designed with the needs of people with disabilities in mind (Draft Proposal, 1996).

At the time, only some of the draft law's chapters were adopted: the declarative clauses on the rights to equality, inclusion, and self-determination; the prohibition on discrimination in employment, including the right to accommodations in the workplace; accessibility in public transport; and the establishment of the Commission for Equal Rights of Persons with Disabilities. Although full accessibility to public premises and services was not expressly required by the law, at that stage, the right to inclusion required that "the implementation of rights and provision of services for people with disabilities will be made . . . through the services given and designed for the public at large and accommodations will be made, if relevant" [Equal Rights for People with Disability Law, 1998, clause 6(a)(2)]. This policy implies that the environment must be designed with the public at large in mind, including people with disabilities (Admon, 2007).

Inasmuch as little reference was made to accessibility at the time, in the Equal Rights for People with Disability Law, most public services have remained inaccessible. A survey conducted by the Szold Institute on behalf of the Commission for Equal Rights of Persons with Disabilities (Hiss-Yuness, Fridman, & Herkovitz, 2003) showed that most banks and medical clinics were not accessible for persons with hearing impairment (98.6% and 97.4%, respectively). These findings were consistent with the State Comptroller's report (2002), which described a very dismal socio-environmental situation regarding accessibility for persons with disabilities in all aspects of life. Limited accessibility to people with disability, including people with hearing impairment, was provided by the welfare authorities, especially the National Insurance Institute, as described below.

Part II. Accessibility Provisions Prior to 2005

The National Insurance Institute of Israel (NII), the equivalent of the Social Security Administration in the United States, is one of the pillars on which social policy in Israel is built. The activities of the NII in the development of social services are anchored in the National Insurance Law (1995). The NII was created to provide disadvantaged populations, who face temporary or long-term difficulties, with benefits and services in order to ensure their economic security. In addition to the benefit payments to eligible citizens, the NII also subsidizes the development of welfare services in the community through the Division for Service Development, which consists of five separate funds, one of which is the Fund for Development of Services for People with Disabilities.

The Fund for Development of Services for People with Disabilities provides funding to develop new services targeting persons with disabilities and to upgrade existing services in the fields of education, employment, and leisure time activities, in order to help these individuals utilize their potential to the fullest. The fund draws its budget from the annual allocation earmarked for the General Disability Insurance branch of the NII. It provides allocations for a wide range of disabilities—including people with visual, motor-function, and hearing disabilities, developmental and emotional disabilities including autism and learning disabilities—as well as people who are disabled due to illness (National Insurance Institute of Israel, 2007). Since the 1970s, the fund has provided assistance in purchasing equipment, renovating facilities, and constructing new buildings for a variety of governmental agencies, municipal bodies, and non-profit organizations.

The activities of the fund, whose main explicit goal is to foster integration of people with disabilities into the community, began prior to the enactment of the Equal Rights for People with Disability Law. To a certain extent, the areas of the fund's activities reflect the many changes that have occurred in Israeli society and the new egalitarian attitudes towards people with disabilities: an emphasis on promoting their rights; changing professional perceptions regarding their integration into the workplace, the family, the community, and society as a whole; and the development of unique services for those who are perceived as incapable of integration into the community.

In acknowledgment of the rights of persons with hearing loss to equal opportunities and accessibility, the fund has assisted in the development of over 100 facilities and services all over the country in order to help these individuals realize their potential to the fullest (Eran, 2007b; NII, 2007). The fund's policy is based on the notion that accessibility to one's surroundings is crucial for integration of persons with hearing impairment into society and for their equal opportunities. With this in mind, in 1998 the Fund began to design and finance accessibility programs for people with hearing impairment. These programs have included construction and renovation of governmental and municipal buildings and provision of educational services, such as schools for the deaf, classrooms for children with hearing impairment, and accessible higher education services in universities and colleges and in informal educational settings such as community centers and libraries. In addition, the fund supports vocational and rehabilitation projects such as the project for lending hearing aids and FM systems, and the Accessibility and Hearing Assistive Technologies Demonstration Center, as well as recreational and leisure activities such as social clubs for the deaf and accessibility in national parks, museums, and theaters (Eran, 2007b).

Part III. The Accessibility Chapter and Drafting of the Regulations

In 2005, the Knesset passed the Television Broadcasting (Subtitles and Sign Language) Law (S.H. 5765), which extends the accessibility of television broadcasts for people with hearing impairments, by requiring broadcasts to be accompanied either by subtitles or by sign language. In March of 2005, the Knesset passed an amendment to the Equal Rights for People with Disability Law, adding a Chapter to the Law on accessibility to public facilities, premises, and services. The amendment was made as a result of growing public awareness to the issue of accessibility and the involvement of the NII in funding accessibility projects. The chapter requires every public building and service to be fully accessible to people with disabilities, including people with hearing disabilities. In addition to the general requirements, some subchapters require specific accessibility measures in particular services, including health, education, insurance, and emergency services.

In accordance with the chapter, the Israeli Ministry of Justice has drafted Accessibility Regulations, relating to existing public buildings and services. (Accessibility regulations to new buildings are drafted by the Ministry of Interior.) The Accessibility Regulations, both to public buildings and to public services, require accessibility for people with hearing impairment. The Accessibility Regulations to Public Services include detailed requirements on the specific accessibility measures needed in various services, as described below.

The Accessibility Regulations to Public Services was drafted based on similar legal provisions in other countries and on input from disability experts, including audiologists—disability NGOs, other government ministries and agencies, and several public sectors including the Hotels Association and the Banks Association. The regulations were drafted with the aim of making the Israeli accessibility standards at least equal to the most advanced measures adopted in other countries. Toward that aim, the drafting drew on legal sources and standards such as the Americans with Disabilities Act (1990) and its regulations and the United Kingdom's Disability Discrimination Act (1995). In addition to the foreign legislation, the regulations drew on the experience and knowledge of experts on disabilities, including experts on accessibility for persons with hearing impairment. Among these experts was the first author of this paper, who planned and followed accessibility projects for persons with hearing loss that were supported by the NII.

In line with the requirements of the Accessibility Chapter in the Equal Rights for People with Disability Law and the principles of Israeli administrative law, the Ministry of Justice consulted with disability NGOs throughout the drafting process. These NGOs provided invaluable information about the needs of people with disabilities and about how these needs should be met in an egalitarian inclusive setting to promote integration into all facets of society and culture. Among these NGOs were several organizations for hard of hearing and Deaf people. In all, approximately 25 NGOs operate in Israel advocating for people with hearing impairment (Alon & Gidron, 2007). One NGO that participated in the consultation process, Bekol (the Hebrew word for "With Voice"), the Israeli organization for hard of hearing and deafened adults, promotes the interests of the estimated 600,000 individuals with hearing impairment in Israel. Bekol's representatives were very active in advocating for the rights of people with hearing impairment during the drafting process; however, the presence of Deaf organizations was less prominent.

The process of consulting with disability NGOs was challenging for both sides. The mandatory consultation with NGOs, especially in drafting regulations pertaining to human rights laws, has been previously criticized as unnecessarily complicated and unreliable. The NGOs must also invest precious time and resources into the process (Feldman, 2007a, 2007b). Yet, the major challenge for the Commission for Equal Rights of Persons with Disabilities was finding the balance between the demands of the disability NGOs, the interests of service providers and other government ministries, and the limitations set in the law on the scope of the regulations. Although the purpose of Commission for Equal Rights of Persons with Disabilities was promoting the rights of people with disabilities and to ascertain that their needs are met, drafting legislation means taking into account interests of other parties as well. As part of the mandatory consultation process, the Commission also consulted with various sectors of the industry and relevant government ministries. The draft regulations were challenged by providers of public services—such as hotels, cinema theaters, and banks—who pointed out the practical, financial, and attitudinal limitations to implementing the very broad regulations. For instance, the Association of Cinema Theaters, which represents not only cinema owners but also film distributors, initially objected to the provisions for HATs in cinemas and for subtitles in locally-produced films, on the grounds that these accommodations were an undue burden on them. Finding the balance between these limitations, the demands of the NGOs, professionals' recommendations, and the legal limitations on the scope of the regulations was the Commission's biggest challenge.

Part IV. Provisions for HATs in the Regulations and Current Accessibility Projects

The final draft of the regulations includes several provisions for HATs in public services for people with hearing disability. Assembly areas that use audio-amplification systems and house at least 50 fixed seats—such as theaters, movie houses, arenas and stadiums, auditoriums, meeting and lecture rooms, concert and performance halls, places of worship, and courtrooms—are required to install a permanent assistive listening system for people with hearing impairment.

There are three general types of assistive listening systems, which are appropriate for various applications and are named for their method of signal transmission: induction loop (IL), frequency modulation (FM), and infrared (IR). Assembly areas are advised to consult with a professional before purchasing any system.

Sales and service counters (including information points and checkout counters) are also required to install assistive technology to promote effective communication with people who have hearing loss. The regulations distinguish between closed counters or teller windows, with security glazing to separate personnel from the public, and open counters, where there is no such partition. At open counters, the regulations require installation of an IL system, whereas closed counters are required to provide a two-way voice communication system in addition to the IL. Closed counters are also required to allow the customer to clearly view the face of the attendant (Eran, 2007b; Eran, & Neustadt, 2007).

Regulations require clearly visible signs posted, including the international symbol of access for hearing loss (Figure 15–1), indicating the availability of assistive technology and the location in the facility where the appropriate receivers can be obtained.

Assistive technologies also must be provided in public transportation, guided tours, during police interrogations and—by request—in vocational training courses, in informal education settings, and in all other public services where audible communication with the public is used.

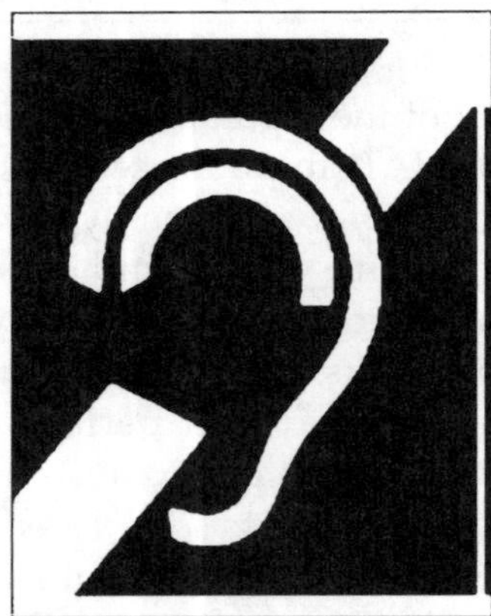

Figure 15–1. International symbol of access for hearing loss.

At the time of this writing, the final draft of the regulations has been submitted formally to the Knesset Welfare Committee, whose approval is needed for the regulations to be passed, but hearings are yet to be conducted by the Committee. Concurrent with the drafting process, many accessibility projects of the NII were expanded and new projects established. From 2005 through 2007, the Fund for Development of Services for People with Disabilities continued in its efforts to expand accessibility in public places and services all over the country (Eran, 2007b). Through these efforts, which the fund intends to continue until the full implementation of the Accessibility Regulations, the Fund aspires to raise public awareness to the need for accessibility to all services and to serve as a catalyst for additional funding sources.

The following are two of the many NII projects that facilitated accessibility to public services for hearing-impaired individuals, in recent years: the Masada archeological site and the Jerusalem Center for the Performing Arts (Eran, 2001, 2004a, 2007a).

Masada

Overlooking the Dead Sea, Masada is one of the most popular tourist destinations in Israel. Since 2005, this ancient site offers the visitor who has a hearing impairment full accessibility to all facilities and services on the premises (Eran, 2007a).

The box office is equipped with an IL system and a two-way amplification system (Figure 15–2). A large-area IL system is installed at the introductory film hall on the passageway to the cable car ride. The film has open captions in Hebrew and English. The upper and lower car ride lobbies are equipped with plasma monitors that provide the visitors with written information such as cable car arrival and departure times, special events, or an emergency evacuation warning if needed. Organized groups can borrow, with no additional fee, an FM tour guide system with 20 headsets or personal loop receivers. On the west side of Masada, at the "Masada" sound and light show, spectators sit in an open-air theater equipped with a large-

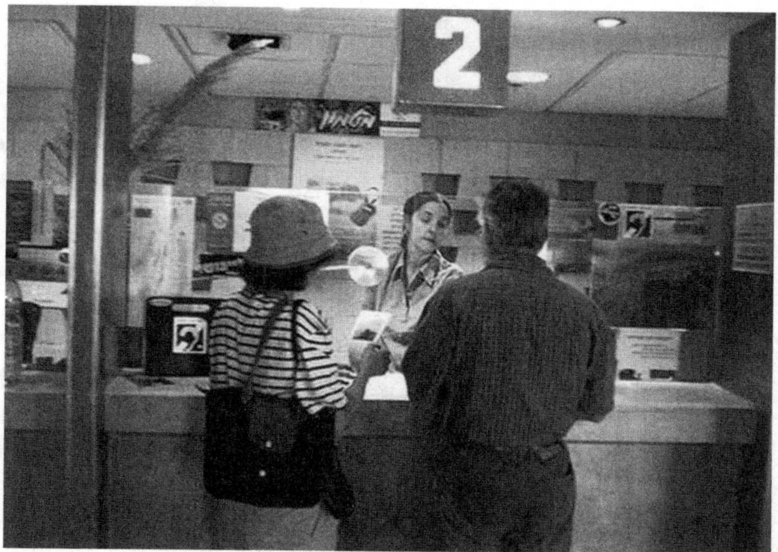

Figure 15–2. Box office equipped with an induction loop and a two-way amplification system.

area FM system with personal receivers (either headsets or IL). All accessible locations and services are indicated with the international symbol for accessibility for the deaf.

The Jerusalem Center for Performing Arts

The Jerusalem Center for Performing Arts is the largest and most active cultural center in Israel. The Jerusalem Center, which offers varied cultural activities, was the first of 39 Israeli theaters that were made accessible for patrons who have hearing impairments via the support of the NII Fund. The center encompasses three halls: the Sherover Theater with 950 seats, the Henry Crown Symphony Hall (home of the Jerusalem Symphony Orchestra) with 750 seats, and the Rebecca Crown Auditorium with 450 seats. Each was equipped with a large-area IR assistive listening system. Personal IR receivers, either stethophone (under the chin) or induction neckloop, are distributed free of charge on a first-come, first-serve basis at all performances. One of the box-office counters is equipped with an IL system (Eran, 2001).

The accessibility requirements established for the NII, which were later incorporated into the regulations, included the requirement that in each assembly area where audible communication system is integral to the use of the space, an assistive listening system must be installed (Eran, 2007b). Each assistive listening system must provide full coverage to the entire assembly area, so that a listener can use the borrowed receiver from any seat in a seating area. The number of receivers provided is at least 5% of the total number of seats. Coupling options include headphone and hearing-aid compatible receivers (neckloops). At least one neckloop is available for every three air conduction type receivers.

The process of raising awareness and assimilating acceptance of the available technology by the target population with hearing impairments was accompanied by a successful campaign by Bekol and the HATs' dealer under the slogan "Hearing from every row" (Figure 15–3). In collaboration with volunteers from Bekol, a proactive approach of informing and offering the personal receivers to elderly patrons was implemented. This proactive approach has proven to be very successful and was followed by increased demand

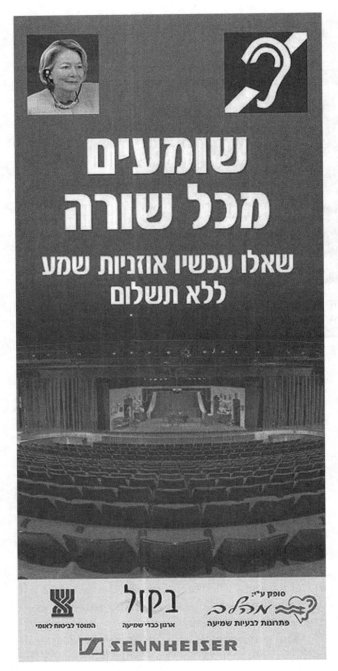

Figure 15–3. "Hearing from every row" campaign.

for assistive listening systems in other theaters, as well as a reported renewal of subscriptions by elderly patrons who previously may have complained about the "incoherence" of the young generation of actors.

Summary

Awareness among Israelis concerning the right of people with disabilities to accessibility, as a means to their full integration into society, has increased dramatically since the 1990s. Accessibility projects supported by the NII, and accessibility legislation, have created new opportunities for people with hearing impairment to fully use and enjoy the many varied services and activities offered to the general public, from which they were previously spurned. A first step toward accessibility in workplaces is taking place as of November 2007, after the government allocated a budget for accommodations in the workplace. The Accessibility Regulations are currently pending, and it will likely take years until they are fully implemented. Yet, along with the continuing support of the NII for accessibility projects throughout the country, the regulations have already created a shift in the public perception of people with disabilities and their rights in civil society. It remains to be seen how this shift will support the implementation of the Accessibility Regulations and increase the opportunities for participation in all social activities for people with hearing impairment.

References

Admon, Z. (2007). The right to accessibility in the international and Israeli legislation. In D. Feldman, Y. Danieli Lahav, & S. Haimovitz (Eds.), *Israeli society's accessibility for persons with disabilities on the threshold of the 21st century* (pp. 177–221). Israel: Government Advertising Agency.

Alon, Y., & Gidron, B. (2007). Characteristics and trends of the development of the third sector in the area of persons with disabilities in Israel: A macro perspective. In D. Feldman, Y. Danieli Lahav, & S. Haimovitz (Eds.), *Israeli society's accessibility for persons with disabilities on the threshold of the 21st century* (pp. 295–316). Israel: Government Advertising Agency.

Americans with Disabilities Act of 1990, 42 U.S.C. § 12101 et seq. (West 1993).

Berg, B. (2007). The role of the Commission for Equal Rights of Persons with Disabilities in implementation and enforcement of the Accessibility Chapter in the Equal Rights Law. In D. Feldman, Y. Danieli Lahav, & S. Haimovitz (Eds.), *Israeli society's accessibility for persons with disabilities on the threshold of the 21st century* (pp. 249–259). Israel: Government Advertising Agency.

Deaf Assistance Law of 1992, *S.H.* p. 116.

Disability Discrimination Act of 1995, ch. 50, Stationary Office 1995.

Disability Ombudsman Law (1994), Swedish Code of Statues—SFS no. 1994:749.

Draft Proposal for Equal Rights for People with Disability Law, 1996, *H.H.* p. 628.

Equal Rights for People with Disability Law of 1998, *S.H.* 1988, p. 252.

Equal Rights for People with Disability Law (amendment no. 2) 2005, *S.H.* p. 288.

Eran, O. (2001). *Assistive listening devices for patrons with hearing loss: A guide for the Jerusalem Center for Performing Arts.* Unpublished manuscript, National Insurance Institute of Israel, Jerusalem.

Eran, O. (2004a). *Accessibility guiding principle for visitors with hearing impairment at national parks.* Unpublished manuscript, National Insurance Institute of Israel, Jerusalem.

Eran, O. (2004b). *Aging and hearing loss: Accessible adult day care centers.* Unpublished manuscript, SHEKEL Community Services for People with Disabilities, The Israeli Center for Accessibility, Jerusalem.

Eran, O. (2004c). *Making classrooms accessible for hearing impaired children: Recommendations for making educational institutions accessible for hearing and visually impaired.* Jerusalem: State of Israel Commission for Equal Rights of People with Disabilities.

Eran, O. (2007a). *Assimilation of hearing assistive technologies at Masada National Park: Progress report.* Jerusalem: National Insurance Institute of Israel.

Eran, O. (2007b). Principles in environmental accessibility for persons with hearing impairment. In D. Feldman, Y. Danieli Lahav, & S. Haimovitz (Eds.), *Israeli society's accessibility for persons with disabilities on the threshold of the 21st century* (pp. 499–524). Israel: Government Advertising Agency.

Eran, O., & Neustadt, N. (2007). Principles in environmental accessibility for people who are dual sensory impaired. In D. Feldman, Y. Danieli Lahav, & S. Haimovitz (Eds.), *Israeli society's accessibility for persons with disabilities on the threshold of the 21st century* (pp. 547–556). Israel: Government Advertising Agency.

European Union. *Treaty of Amsterdam amending the Treaty of the European Union, the Treaties establishing the European Communities and certain related acts,* Official Journal (C340), 10 November 1997.

Feldman, D. (2007a). The contribution of the Equal Rights of Persons with Disability Law, 5758—1998 to the promotion of environmental justice for persons with disabilities in Israel. In D. Feldman, Y. Danieli Lahav, & S. Haimovitz (Eds.), *Israeli society's accessibility for persons with disabilities on the threshold of the 21st century* (pp. 31–79). Israel: Government Advertising Agency.

Feldman, D. (2007b). Environmental justice and persons with disabilities in Israel. *Disability Studies Quarterly, 27*(4). Available from: http://www.dsq-sds.org

Hiss-Yuness, A., Fridman, Y., & Herkovitz, A. (2003). *The accessibility of schools, primary health clinics, malls and banks in Israel: A survey.* Jerusalem: Henrietta Szold Institute for the Commission for Equal Rights of Persons with Disabilities, Ministry of Justice. Jerusalem.

Katz Committee. (1997). *Report of the committee for examination of comprehensive rights legislation for people with disabilities.* Jerusalem: Ministry of Justice, Ministry of Welfare.

National Insurance Institute of Israel. (2007). *Summary of trends and developments in social security—2006* (pp. 33–35). Jerusalem.

National Insurance Law [Consolidated Version], 5755—1995. *S.H.* p. 1522.

Planning and Building Law (amendment no. 15), 1981, *S.H.* no. 109.

Planning and Building Regulations of 1970, *K.T.* no. 1851.

Planning and Building Regulations (Public Buildings), 1981, *K.T.* no. 1065.

State Comptroller, Annual Report 52B for 2001 and the 2000 Fiscal Year (2002). *Integration of persons with disabilities in society and at work.* Jerusalem: State Comptroller's Office.

Television Broadcasts (Subtitles and Sign Language) Law, 5765—2005, *S.H.* p. 956.

16

Peer Support Groups: Promoting Treatment Effectiveness in Partnership with Consumers

Anne T. Pope
Carren J. Stika

Peer support organizations play an important role not only in personal audiologic rehabilitation (AR), but also in creating a wider, more realistic understanding of the consequences of hearing loss in the public at large. They provide information and support to people with hearing loss in a way that reinforces and builds on the information and support provided by audiologists. They counteract the myths, provide peer group role models who have made the adjustment to hearing loss, and teach self-advocacy to individuals with hearing loss. In addition, the membership of the groups comprises an effective consumer advocacy force to bring about policy change and awareness in the public arena.

Living with hearing loss is a journey with its own set of challenges—both intellectual and emotional. It is a journey for which we have no preparation. It is complicated by a lack of good information and exacerbated by misinformation acquired over a lifetime. Normal hearing is so much taken for granted that its essential role in our daily lives and the consequences of losing it are seldom considered and frequently misunderstood. Most important, hearing loss requires not only that we adjust to new and unfamiliar technology and shed well-ingrained biases, but also that we change a lifetime of communication habits. And because communication is, minimally, a two-party exchange, we need to use our new knowledge to educate others about the best way to enhance our ability to receive messages. Knowledge, role models, and the time to learn, practice, and incorporate new strategies into our thinking are necessary complements to the constantly improving technology. We need to become active listeners and constant educators. We have a lot to learn.

Howard P. (Rocky) Stone, the founder of the Hearing Loss Association of America under its former name Self-Help for Hard of Hearing People (SHHH), first described hearing loss as an invisible condition (Stone, 1993). Invisible condition and invisible disability are phrases that are used frequently today, but not in the sense meant by Stone. Most often, they refer to the fact that you can't see the damaged hearing mechanism or can't readily pick out a person with hearing loss in the way you can instantly recognize the disability of someone in a wheelchair or with a guide dog. However, Stone coined the phrase because there was little understanding of hearing loss by the general public or even by those who suffered from it.

This is still the case today. The widely held myths about hearing loss as well as the pervasive lack of information about its causes and effects still impact the willingness of many of us to seek treatment as soon as we need it and complicate the satisfactory adjustment for many of us who have done so.

How many positive messages about hearing loss do we hear in the course of our lives? None. Negativity prevails.

The Stigma of Hearing Loss

"Let's get one thing straight. I'm much too young for a hearing aid. I wouldn't even consider it if the people I live and work with would only speak louder and more clearly" wrote Melinda Beck in the *Wall Street Journal* (January, 2008). Although written tongue-in-cheek, those words reflect the generally held negative perception of hearing loss throughout our western culture.

In 1996, when former President Clinton turned 51 years old, the Associated Press circulated a picture of the president standing in a crowd with his hand cupped behind his ear, leaning forward, and obviously straining to hear. "President is fitted for hearing aids at physical exam" the headline of the article announces. Upon reading this piece of news, many people with hearing loss undoubtedly smiled to themselves and nodded in approval. We thought, "See, even the President of the United States can have a hearing loss! And he's only 51 years old." Somehow the image of the President straining to hear made having a hearing loss a bit more acceptable. Indeed, the Hearing Industries Association reported that following the announcement that President Clinton was getting a hearing aid, sales in hearing aids increased significantly, almost 25 percent from the year before (Rewick, 1997). However, negativity does not die easily. In the article about the President receiving hearing aids, we learn that over 28 million Americans suffer from a hearing loss, although less than half of those who could benefit from hearing aids actually use them. We are informed that technology has come a long way over the years, and many options are now available for those with hearing difficulty. It is clear that the article aims to erase the stigma attached to hearing loss—as it must, as it is the President of the United States with a hearing loss. But it is only partly successful. "Midlife is catching up with Clinton," notes the caption under the picture. The article explains that President Clinton has been "complaining for years about his hearing." Only now, however, after being encouraged by his doctors during his recent annual physical exam, is he fitted with hearing aids. But, don't worry, the public is informed, President Clinton will be prescribed "two nearly undetectable hearing aids, which will fit in his ear canals." No one will even be able to see them! Moreover, President Clinton "will use them only when he thinks he needs them." The article further assures the public, that apart from his "damaged ears," the President is "in excellent overall health and feeling pretty good." (For additional information on stigma and hearing loss, the reader is referred to Chapter 4 of this text.)

So, what is the message regarding hearing loss conveyed to the public in this article? Essentially, that hearing loss is something you put off dealing with for years (How long has the President been complaining?); that only after the suggestion of others do you actually do something about it; that hearing aids are best "hidden" from public view; and that hearing aids, like glasses, can be put on and taken off, and used only when you think they are needed. Unfortunately, even the news that the President of the United States wears hearing aids isn't enough to shake us free of the stigma associated with hearing loss.

This is not simply an American issue. In 2003, when the Ecology Minister said that French President Jacques Chirac was a hearing aid wearer, the news caused a flurry of attention in the press. The item brought a swift denial by Chirac's spokesman, and the *New York Times* reported that the Minister of Culture, presumably an intelligent and educated man, said that he did not want to know who was right, adding: "It's none of my business, and I would not allow myself to make such derogatory observations" (Sciolino, 2003).

Derogatory observations? What other disease or disability would evoke such a comment? This is an attitude that is intellectually indefensible, but all too embedded in our culture. Emotionally, if not intellectually, we believe that hearing loss is a condition of the elderly, that anyone suffering from it is over the hill and less than mentally sharp, and that it is something shameful and to be avoided. The result, of course, is that these negative perceptions create stress, worry, anxiety, even panic. Will I ever be promoted again? Will I be able to hold onto my job? Will my wife, husband, children, partner, friend still think I am worthwhile? What will my colleagues think? Will I slip silently into old age? Emotional assumptions learned over a lifetime affect our lives in ways we don't consider and are far more difficult to counteract than incorrect fact.

Small wonder, then, that there is a reluctance to admit and address hearing loss. The statistics paint a discouraging picture. On average, a person waits seven years after becoming aware of a hearing problem before taking steps to remedy it. Most people who seek treatment—75%—are doing so at the urging of someone else, typically family members (O'Mahoney, Stephens, & Cadge, 1996). And, most important, only 20% of those who might benefit from hearing aids actually use them (Kochkin, 2005).

Emotional bias is not the only obstacle to recognizing and accepting our hearing loss. The wonderful plasticity of the human brain, although it contributes to our recovery, also contributes to our initial difficulties. Most often, hearing loss is gradual—so gradual that it isn't immediately obvious. There is a little decline and the brain adapts; as hearing loss increases, we develop further adaptations. Unfortunately, any compensatory efforts are more likely than not negative and maladaptive ones. Without even being aware, we slip into the habit of smiling, nodding, and pretending to hear even though we haven't, or gradually withdrawing from activities we once enjoyed without really analyzing why. All too often, these dysfunctional strategies mask the communication difficulties in our own minds and contribute to the belief, or hope, that we aren't really having trouble hearing. The truth, however, is frequently more evident to our family members than it is to us.

Coming to Grips with Hearing Loss

When we finally acknowledge our own hearing loss for the first time, most of us don't understand that putting on hearing aids will not solve our problem. We will need to shed biases we aren't even aware that we have before we can be open and honest about our hearing loss. We will have to abandon old habits and develop new ones. We will have to acquire new and initially uncomfortable behaviors, as well as learn about and become comfortable with new technology. What we need to know is that, although we may feel lost at sea in the beginning, we can, in fact, make all of those changes.

Whether audiologists are able to communicate all of this information to us in addition to the necessary instruction and support about our newly acquired technology is questionable. The American Speech-Language-Hearing Association (ASHA) now identifies counseling as an essential component in the scope of practice for audiology (ASHA, 2004). However, many audiologists report not feeling comfortable or adequately prepared to address the psychosocial ramification of hearing loss with their clients, and they are not sure how to incorporate counseling into their clinical practice (Gagné, Jennings, & Southall, 2009; Martin, Barr, & Bernstien, 1992).

Although audiologists may be well aware that hearing loss places individuals at risk for mental health difficulties, they are less certain about how to assess these risks. What should they say? How do they ask about an individual's adjustment difficulties without seeming intrusive? And, most importantly, what should they do if issues come up? With so little time and so much to cover, audiologists wonder how they can possibly do it all. Consequently, most audiologists tend to shy away from discussing these "personal" issues with their clients and focus instead on what they feel most competent doing, that is, evaluating, selecting, and fitting hearing assistive technology (Clark & English, 2004; Stika, Ross, & Cuevas, 2002). Unfortunately, although audiologists may do an excellent job in serving the audiologic needs of the individual, the profound ways in which hearing loss may impact a person's social and emotional adjustment, employment status, and general well-being are seldom adequately addressed. In a study designed to investigate areas of quality of life impacted by adult-onset hearing loss (Stika, in preparation), one participant provided the following comment that describes the lack of attention given by her hearing healthcare providers to the emotional impact of her hearing loss:

> My hearing impairment was diagnosed by an MD, FACS and I was tested by and fitted for hearing aids by a degreed and certified audiologist. (With a geographical move, I saw doctors and audiologists in two states.) No one—absolutely no one!—addressed the emotional impact of adult-onset hearing loss, nor suggested ways to cope. The emotional aspect of what was happening totally blind-sided me! And, although I was told that even with bilateral hearing aids (expensive top-of-the-line aids!) my hearing ability would not be perfect, nothing truly prepared me for the difficulty I'd continue to face. Nor was I informed of ways to get help coping and/or learn speech reading. Only by speaking up and asking about it was I able to know where to begin to look for help. Doctors and audiologists need to address these issues as a matter of course and/or have information available to patients. *(49-year-old female, bilateral severe hearing loss)*

There may be multiple reasons audiologists fail to address these issues. Perhaps, audiologists are not comfortable addressing emotional issues; or, given the current medical model, there is insufficient time to teach communication strategies. In addition, perhaps those of us new to hearing loss may be unable to assimilate so much information at one time. Regardless of the origins of difficulty, we do find in our peer support groups that most new participants don't understand key things we need to know.

Many of us have had the experience of putting on glasses and seeing perfectly again. Few, if any, of us feel that we can hear perfectly when we first put on a hearing aid. The sound we hear is not what we would describe as "normal" sound. We may hear too much of what we don't want to hear and understand too little of what we do want to hear. Until the hearing aid is invented that replicates human ear, we need to take additional steps and use new strategies to understand what we are hearing.

What We Need to Know

Most of us know very little about hearing or think about its impact on our lives. We have little knowledge of the physics of sound, how it is processed and ultimately understood by the brain—or even of the important contributions hearing makes in our lives. We haven't thought about the crucial role of hearing in connecting us with others or the fact that our days are filled with communication. We haven't thought about the importance of hearing as a warning system. We don't know that distance and direction make a difference in our perception of sound. We aren't aware that whether the room has a carpet and curtains or a tile floor and bare windows affects the acoustics. We don't realize that the pitch or speed of the talker can affect our understanding. We don't know that the very act of listening with less than normal hearing can be tiring. Or, that whether we are feeling energetic or tired can have an impact on how well we hear. We don't know that our brains play a crucial role in how and what we "hear." Or, that our brains, even older brains, are still learning all the time, and that there are many strategies we can learn and use to maximize our understanding.

Yet, until we learn how hearing loss affects our communications and take whatever steps we can to counteract the disruptions, hearing loss can profoundly damage our lives, our relationships, and our aspirations. Those of us with hearing loss are susceptible to a long list of negative feelings—anxiety, sadness, anger, isolation, loss of control, and low self-esteem, among others—that can wreak havoc on the quality of our lives and relationships (Hallberg & Barrenäs, 1993; Hetu, Jones, & Getty, 1993; Stark & Hickson, 2004; Trychin, 2001, 2007; Wallhagen, Strawbridge, Shema, & Kaplan, 2004). These experiences are noted in the comments provided by individuals who were asked to describe ways in which their hearing impacts their quality of life (Stika, 2008). For example:

> While I still rate my quality of life as excellent, my hearing loss impacts me each and every day. I am constantly making adjustments. And while I am a very social person, I find that I must now spend more time alone, in quiet, to let my brain rest. The 24–7 tinnitus also impacts the quality of my life during the day and at times during sleep. *(52-year-old female, moderate-to-severe bilateral hearing loss, sudden-onset at age 50)*

> I've become much more withdrawn. I don't enjoy social gatherings like I used to. I'm much less patient than I used to be. And I get frustrated easily, especially when someone I'm close to says "never mind" when I've asked them to repeat something. I truly understand how frustrating it must be for someone to have to keep repeating something. But on the other hand, I wish people would understand how frustrating and uncomfortable it is for me to have to ask them to repeat. *(55-year-old male; profound, bilateral hearing loss; sudden onset at age 53 due to meningitis)*

Although studies have shown that hearing loss does not lead directly to psychiatric disorders, research does suggest that hearing loss can place the individual *at risk* for adjustment difficulties. Indeed, reported adjustment problems and associated functional disability by individuals who have acquired hearing loss later in life are considerable and common. Adverse effects on physical, emotional, behavioral, occupational, and social function have all been reported in the literature (cf. Hallberg, 1996; Hetu, Lalande, & Getty, 1987; Kochkin & Rogin, 2000; Mulrow et al., 1990; Stika, 1997a, 1997b; Thomas, 1984). Even when the actual hearing loss according to audiological measures is categorized as "mild," individuals frequently describe the associated disabling effects as being significant (Bess et al., 1989; Mulrow et al., 1990).

The Benefits of Peer Support Groups

Peer support groups are readily available and can play a vital complementary role to the expertise of the audiologist. These groups have proved invaluable for many of us. The advantage of a group of peers is that every member is in the same predicament. We know what it is like to start wearing a hearing aid or to adjust to a cochlear implant. We have all experienced the discomfort of not hearing during a meeting or the annoyance with a spouse who tries to carry on a conversation from another room. We are all familiar with the urge to bluff our way through a conversation, and have all experienced the sometimes disastrous results. We all know the strain and exhaustion of trying to hear at a cocktail party or in a noisy restaurant. At the same time, we know that being assertive about understanding has improved our lives and relationships. We know that making use of the appropriate technology can make our lives easier. And although we will be at different points in the continuum of adjustment, we can provide models and encouragement for those just beginning the journey or in need of additional information and support. (For a discussion of support groups from another perspective, the reader is referred to Chapter 13 of this text.)

In every good group, information, support, and inspiration are intertwined. There is no way to emphasize enough how much hearing loss impacts the everyday lives of people or the ways it complicates their functioning. For people who feel that somehow their hearing loss is shameful, learning to be comfortable discussing it takes time. Describing the problem and identifying the solution so that the listener is at ease takes skill. Even acquiring the language with which to discuss it is important. Peer role models and support are critical for this kind of learning. Equally important is professional input and knowledge. Most peer support groups do involve professionals to a great extent both as program presenters and as advisors. In addition, family members can play a significant role in peer support groups, because they share on a daily basis the consequences of hearing loss and must learn to cope with them.

Support groups can also ease adjustment to hearing loss issues in the workplace. Working-age adults with hearing impairment often feel at a loss knowing how to manage their communication difficulties in the workplace (Hetu & Getty, 1992; Stika, 1997b, in preparation). It is one thing to request accommodations from family and friends, but it can be more daunting to deal with a hearing loss in the competitive arena of work. It is true, there is the American with Disabilities Act (ADA), but many of us still feel apprehensive about disclosing our hearing loss to employers and coworkers, fearing possible dismissal, stigmatization, being viewed as less capable, and loss of potential career advancement (Hetu, Riverin, Getty, Lalande, & St-Cyr, 1990; Stika, 1997b). So, we often hide it, hoping that if we work even harder, we can compensate for not being able to hear as well as others. Sometimes these efforts are successful, but the price we pay for our lack of openness and assertiveness is a high level of stress that often leads to physical and emotional exhaustion. Some of us choose simply to retire early. Accommodations that could help are often not requested, not so much because we don't know what is available (although that too is frequently the case) but mostly because we don't want to draw attention to our hearing difficulty. We don't want to be perceived as less capable than our coworkers and, possibly more important, less capable than we know ourselves to be (Stika, 1997b; in preparation). Participants commented that:

> The biggest challenge for me is admitting my hearing loss to others at work. Why do I feel ashamed? Why do I see my hearing loss as a flaw when I can give every argument and the opposite? Why do I hesitate to ask for assistance when I have every reason telling me to and no good reason telling me not to? I wish I had the privilege in my youth, when my hearing loss first began, of meeting other young people with hearing loss and learning that it's okay and there's not something 'wrong' with me. *(25-year-old female; progressive, moderate-to-severe, bilateral hearing loss; diagnosed at age 10)*

> I am *always* unsure and doubting myself at work. I know I am capable and all but sometimes I grow weary of trying so hard. There is the constant stress: Did I get that right? Did she say "2" or "3"? Did he say "9" or "10"? etc., etc., etc! The greatest challenge is keeping up your spirits when you are constantly being forced to question your capabilities. *(23-year-old female; moderate-to-severe, bilateral hearing loss; diagnosed at age 19)*

Does having a hearing loss automatically mean that an individual is no longer a viable employee or capable of carrying out work responsibilities at a high level? "Of course not," you would say. (Don't forget that former presidents of both the United States and France have had hearing losses.) We know that the issue is not hearing loss. The challenge is to figure out how best to accommodate the individual with the hearing loss in the workplace. What assistive technologies would be helpful? What coping strategies are needed? And, importantly, how can the person with the hearing loss learn to educate supervisors, coworkers, and clients regarding his or her communication needs. Unfortunately, working-age adults with hearing loss rarely are provided this kind of information by their audiologists (Stika et al., 2002).

This is where peer support programs can be of benefit. Programs for people in the workplace might focus on assistive technology. What kinds of captioned telephones or Internet captioning services exist to help you hear on the telephone? What kind of equipment exists to help you hear in large and small meetings? Peer support groups must also focus on strategies for effectively communicating your needs and social skills. How do you go about explaining why you need the equipment, how it will help, and how it is used so that those who must use it are comfortable?

Support group meetings might educate you about your rights under the ADA. But you will also learn the strategies necessary for success. How do you tell your boss or colleague about your hearing loss in such a way that she or he is comfortable that you can continue to do your job? And how do you go about getting accommodations in a diplomatic and nonthreatening way?

Your relationship with your boss and your peers will be key to how well you can do your job. How do you stay connected to the informal information network—the water cooler talk? How do you ensure that you are getting the information you need to do your job? How do you function optimally at a lunch meeting in a restaurant? How do you ask for clarification when you haven't heard something or make sure that you have heard correctly even when you think you have? How can your secretary and your peers help you out, and what is the best way to enlist them? If you are looking for a new job, should you tell your interviewers about your hearing loss?

Another important area is safety and well-being. Programs might focus on technology. Many people don't know that there is equipment that provides information in an alternative way. Many of us don't know that there are flashing lights that can tell us when the baby is crying, or alert us when the telephone or doorbell is ringing. In our groups we hear too many stories of people who sit for hours near the doorbell in order to hear when the repairman arrives. We hear stories of sleepless nights for travelers unsure that they will wake up on time for an important meeting and know nothing about vibrating travel alarm clocks or flashing lights. We hear stories of people who are hesitant to use the telephone when talking with strangers and don't know that they can access captioning over the Internet. We talk about strategies to use at home to stay tuned into the family conversation or ways of watching TV without driving everyone else out of the room because of the volume. And in a much more tragic vein, we discuss safety alerts. We know people who have died because the carbon monoxide detector couldn't be heard. Support groups provide information and solutions for all these problems. (For additional information on hearing assistive technology systems, the reader is referred to Chapter 14 of this text.)

Other programs might focus on activities with family and friends. The background noise at a large gathering inevitably creates a problem. How do you enjoy a large family gathering whether it is for Thanksgiving, a wedding, a graduation, or a family reunion? How do you interact with the teen who talks too fast or the three-year-old whose voice is high and speech not quite precise, or Uncle John who has a mustache, or cousin Sadie who insists on talking to you as she is rummaging in the refrigerator? Knowing what you can do to make the most of your hearing will certainly increase your enjoyment. Understanding that there are ways of positioning yourself or ways of taking a "hearing breather" will let you be part of the group with less stress. When you go to a restaurant, are there strategies that will make it easier for you to understand the waiter and keep up with the conversation? When you travel, what can you do to make sure you hear the tour guide or the reservations clerk or know that the airline gate has been changed? Technology can be key here, of course. But, always, always, we discuss how you ask for accommodations and clarifications in a matter of fact and pleasant way.

Effectiveness of Peer Support Groups

Healthcare has witnessed a substantial growth in peer support groups since the early 1980s. These groups, also called self-help groups, offer a way for people with a mutual problem or health condition to take control of circumstances that affect their lives (Finn, 1999). The effectiveness of peer support groups is now widely documented in the literature (Kyrouz, Humpreys, & Loomis, 2002). Research has identified a number of benefits from participation in peer support groups, including enhanced self-esteem and general well-being; greater acceptance of a disability or health condition; increased optimism and control; and higher levels of self-efficacy (Kurtz, 1990; Roberts et al., 1999).

Certainly, those of us who have experienced the benefit of a hearing loss support group have offered a plethora of testimonials to its effectiveness. Talking about how troublesome the sound of a new hearing aid is with someone who uses one and receiving encouragement to stick with it carries a weight far greater than a message from someone with normal hearing. Seeing a person with hearing loss use an assistive device openly and without embarrassment makes a far greater impression than a demonstration in an office. Hearing a confident peer use a corrective strategy to get a conversation back on track shows both the strategy and the result in one easy lesson. And the group offers a variety of people from different walks of life offering the opportunity to learn strategies that seem analogous to our own.

Found in a variety of configurations, peer support groups can be large, encompassing all degrees of hearing loss (e.g., Hearing Loss Association of America, HLAA), or small and specialized (e.g., Association for Late Deafened Adults, ALDA). They can specialize in a single condition (e.g., American Tinnitus Association, ATA) or focus primarily on one aspect such as technology (e.g., Beyond Hearing). They can hold meetings in person or on the Internet (e.g., http://www.saywhatclub.com). They can be local or national or international in scope. But, no matter the size, format, or specifics of the group membership, the essential purpose of peer support groups remains the same—to empower its members through the exchange of knowledge, encouragement, and the sharing of experiences.

Although limited attention has been given to evaluating the advantages of participating in peer support groups for individuals with hearing loss, there is now some empirical data available indicating that participation in these groups, including online groups, result in emotional and informational benefits for its members (Cummings, Sproull, & Kiesler, 2002). Stika (in preparation) asked individuals to identify things that have helped them adjust to their adult-onset hearing loss. The variables most frequently noted were supportive family and friends and association with a peer support group:

> From the beginning, I began assertively to seek out new information and new assistive devices and methods—and, most importantly, I began to seek out other people who share my experience of hearing loss. I found online newsgroups, forums, and E-mail message lists such as Beyond Hearing. I discovered organizations that focused on hard of hearing and late deafened adults such as HLAA. Even more to my delight, I discovered a local HLAA group and began attending local monthly meetings and state conventions. In this wonderful group of people, I've found ideas and information that helped me adjust. I've also found understanding, support, and reassurance that I'm not alone. *(59-year-old male; severe bilateral hearing loss; diagnosed at age 35)*

> Feeling the despair and isolation of a hearing loss forced me to find support groups in my area. I was lucky enough to stumble across a few and they saved my life. I was able to see that there are other working-age adults coping with hearing loss; I'm not the only one. Now these people are my best friends. They are quality people I probably never would have met otherwise. So that's the very good thing! *(48-year-old female; severe bilateral hearing loss; diagnosed at age 35)*

Leading Peer Support Groups

HLAA (http://www.hearingloss.org) is the largest consumer group in the United States, with over 200 chapters and state organizations, as well as a national presence in the Washington D.C. area. Members have hearing losses ranging from mild to total, use hearing aids and/or have cochlear implants, and range widely in age. Some affiliates focus on a particular age cohort—young adults or retirees—or a particular segment—people with cochlear implants. But, most include people of a variety of ages and degrees of hearing loss.

HLAA sponsors state and regional conferences as well as a national convention. These events feature research seminars and technology exhibits as well as workshops focusing on adjustment strategies and use of technology. HLAA conducts an increasing number of walkathons around the country to disseminate information and awareness to the general public. The organization produces a wide variety of publications, including a bimonthly magazine, an Internet newsletter, and a Web site, with various specialized groups and forums. Professionals in the field are closely involved with the organization as members, advisors, and educators at the local, state, and national levels.

ALDA (http://www.alda.org) is primarily for people with profound hearing loss acquired as adults. Most members are unable to understand speech without visual aids such as speechreading, sign language, or computer-assisted real-time transcription (CART), and many are learning American Sign Language. ALDA has 14 chapters and groups and holds an annual conference with workshops and speakers.

Specialized groups exist for people whose main concern may not focus on hearing loss itself, but on another more bothersome condition related to it. There are groups for people with tinnitus (e.g., American Tinnitus Association; http://www.ata.org) and Ménière's disease (e.g., http://www.menieres.org; Vestibular Disorders Association; http://www.vestibular.org) as well as for those with acoustic neuromas (e.g., Acoustic Neuroma Association; http://ANAusa.org).

In person and online support groups offer different advantages. Although each provides information and support, face-to-face meetings can provide show and tell instruction whereas the Internet can only tell. On the other hand, some people are far more likely to discuss a problem if they can do it with the kind of anonymity that the Internet provides. And the interaction is available on a flexible timetable that accommodates any schedule. Some people participate in both forums.

Peer Mentoring Program

A new, credentialed program for peer counselors has now been developed at Gallaudet University to expand the effectiveness of peer support. In this program, people with hearing loss take a combined on-site and Internet training course and, upon completion, work under the direct or indirect supervision of an audiologist as paid staff or volunteers. As Ross and Bally (2005) have noted, peer counselors will serve as an extension of the audiologist's office. Most importantly, their presence in the office will address one of the intractable problems audiologists face. Those of us who come for treatment remember a shockingly low percentage of the information received (Margolis, 2004; Martin, Kreuger, & Bernstein, 1990). Even immediately after we leave the office, we recall only half of what we have been told. And of the information we do remember, only half is correct. Brochures and pamphlets just don't have the same impact as face-to-face communications and may, in fact, remain unread. So, peer mentors will supplement and reinforce information given by an audiologist, most of which is new and daunting to those of us who aren't technophiles.

With a sound knowledge base, the peer mentors will be able to explain the auditory challenges we face and help create realistic expectations in both the person with the hearing loss and the family as to what hearing aids can actually do. They also will be able to help those who do need technical adjustments articulate their problems to the audiologist. Peer mentors will be particularly valuable for people who either prefer not to be part of a hearing loss support group or who don't realize that they might benefit from additional information. They will provide an opportunity to discuss situational challenges, evaluate whether assistive devices might be helpful, and instruct in their usage. Equally important, peer mentors, as people who live with hearing loss themselves, can offer an empathetic ear to the problems and challenges presented (Ross & Bally, 2005). Although there is not yet any research documenting the effectiveness of individual peer mentors for people with hearing loss, based on what is known in other fields, the expectation is that they will be effective complements to audiologic treatment. Peer mentors and peer support groups can work well together. Peer mentors, working in conjunction with our audiologists, are invaluable for all of us seeking treatment for the first time, as well as offering on-going support for those of us who prefer not to be part of a group. On the other hand, peer support groups offer the advantage of sharing the experience of many different people. We are often unaware of what we don't know until we hear someone else ask the question.

Educating the Public

Hearing loss support groups do more than help with personal adjustment. They function as important advocacy and interest groups to educate legislators and opinion makers about the challenge of hearing loss and its impact. In addition to teaching self-advocacy, the HLAA and its members have an effective and successful history of advocating for accommodations. Beginning with founder Rocky Stone, who was the first to teach policy makers in Washington that those of us who live in the hearing world have challenges that are different from those in the Deaf community, the organization has taken the lead role in advocating for people with hearing loss. The organization is the contact point for initiatives with the hearing aid, television, movie, theater, cell phone, and traditional telephone industries. The national office also provides advice, guidance, and training to members for advocacy at the state and local levels.

But, that is not enough. We will never counteract the stigma of hearing loss until we all begin working together. Hearing health professionals, educators, students, corporations, foundations, support groups, and consumers with hearing loss, our families and friends need to take the message to the public through basic education in schools, articles in the media, enlightened advertising, public service announcements, walkathons, and health fairs. There needs to be widespread understanding that hearing loss is an important health and economic issue; that without treatment, it can have a devastating effect on the quality of life; and that with sufficient treatment, education, and support, people with hearing loss can live full and rewarding lives. Our friends, colleagues, the clerk at the grocery store, and the agent at the airport need to understand it so well that the simple things that can make our lives better—such as facing us when they talk—are automatic in the same way that everyone knows today that you don't feed a friend with a cardiac condition steak and French fries or give a cousin with diabetes ice cream and cake.

Unlike members of the Deaf community who have a culture and language of their own, the overwhelming majority of people with hearing loss have lived their lives in the hearing world, within mainstream society, and will continue to do so. What we need are the skills, abilities, and accommodations to meet the challenge. Peer support helps us acquire the necessary skills. Group advocacy helps educate those who communicate with us about the accommodations we need. Support groups are important parts of both efforts.

Our aim in this chapter was to demonstrate ways in which peer support groups reinforce and complement the audiologist in securing the best possible rehabilitation outcome. We have also explained the role of support groups in overcoming the stigma associated with hearing loss and encouraging people with hearing loss to seek professional help. By passing along the information in this chapter, and explaining how groups like these can help speed their adjustment to a satisfying and productive life, you will provide your patients with additional resources in their ongoing quest to overcome hearing loss. By associating your practice with one or more support groups, you can help spread the message that hearing loss is neither shameful nor embarrassing, but a widespread health problem that can be treated with success.

References

American Speech-Language-Hearing Association. (2004). *Scope of Practice in Audiology* (Scope of Practice). Available from http://www.asha.org/policy

Beck, M. (2008, January 29). Getting an earful: Testing a tiny, pricey hearing aid. *The Wall Street Journal*, D1.

Bess, F. H., Lichtenstein, M. D., Logan, S. A., Burger, M. C., & Nelson, E. (1989). Hearing impairment as a determinant of function in the elderly. *Journal of Geriatrics Society*, *37*, 123–128.

Clark, J. G., & English, K. M. (2004). *Counseling in audiologic practice: Helping patients and families adjust to hearing loss.* Boston: Pearson Education.

Cummings, J. N., Sproull, L., & Kiesler, S. B., (2002). Beyond hearing: Where real-world and online support meet. *Group Dynamics: Theory, Research, and Practice*, *6*(1), 78–88.

Finn, J. (1999). An exploration of helping process in an online self-help group focusing on issues of disability. *Health and Social Work*, *24*(3), 220–231.

Gagné, J. P., Jennings, M. B., & Southall, K. (2009). The International classification of functioning: Implications and applications to Audiologic rehabilitation. In J. J. Montano & J. B. Spitzer (Eds.), *Adult audiologic rehabilitation* (pp. 37–62). San Diego, CA: Plural.

Hallberg, L. R. (1996). Occupational hearing loss: Coping and family life. *Scandinavian Audiology*, *28*, 313–325.

Hallberg, L. R., & Barrenäs, M-L. (1993). Living with a male with noise-induced hearing loss: Experiences from the perspective of spouses. *British Journal of Audiology*, *27*, 253–261.

Hetu, R., & Getty, L. (1992). Overcoming difficulties experienced in the work place by employees with occupational hearing loss. *Volta Review*, *95*(4), 391–402.

Hetu, R., Jones, L., & Getty, L. (1993). The impact of acquired hearing impairment on intimate relationships: Implications for rehabilitation. *Audiology*, *32*, 363–381.

Hetu, R., Lelande, M., & Getty, L. (1987). Psychosocial disadvantages due to occupational hearing loss as experienced in the family. *Audiology*, *26*, 141–152.

Hetu, R., Riverin, L., Getty, L., Lalande, N., & St-Cyr, C. (1990). The reluctance to acknowledge hearing difficulties among hearing impaired workers. *British Journal of Audiology*, *24*, 265–276.

Kochkin, S. (2005). MarkeTrak VII: Hearing loss population tops 31 million people. *Hearing Review*, *12*(7), 16–29.

Kochkin, S., & Rogin, C. M. (2000). Quantifying the obvious: The impact of hearing instruments on quality of life. *Hearing Review*, *7*(1). 8–34.

Kurtz, L. F. (1990). The self-help movement: Review of the past decade of research. *Social Work with Groups*, *13*(3), 101–115.

Kyrouz, E. M., Humpreys, K., & Loomis, C. (2002). A review of research on the effectiveness of self-help mutual aid groups. In B. J. White & E. J. Madara (Eds.), *American self-help clearinghouse self-help group sourcebook* (7th ed., pp. 1–16). Washington, DC: Department of Veterans Affairs Mental Health Strategic Health Group.

Margolis, R. H. (2004, January 5). In one ear and out the other—what patients remember. *Hearing Journal* [On line]. Available from www.audiologyonline.com/articles.

Martin F. N, Barr, M. M, & Bernstein, M. (1992). Professional attitudes regarding counseling of hearing-impaired adults. *American Journal of Otology*, *13*, 279–287.

Martin, F. N., Kreuger S., & Bernstein, M. (1990). Diagnostic information transfer to hearing-impaired adults. *Texas Journal of Audiology and Speech Pathology*, *16*(2), 29–32.

Mulrow, C. D., Aguilar, C., Endicott, J. E., Velez, R., Tuley, M. R., Charlip, W. S., et al. (1990). Association between hearing impairment and the quality of life of elderly individuals. *Journal of American Geriatrics Society*, *38*, 45–50.

O Mahoney, C. F., Stephens, S. D. G., & Cadge, B. A. (1996). Who prompts patients to consult about hearing loss? *British Journal of Audiology*, *30*, 153–158.

Rewick, C. J. (1997, November 10). President's announcement rings up new sales. *Crain's Chicago Business*, *2*(45), 59.

Roberts, L. J., Salem, D., Rappaport, J., Toro, P. A., Luke, D. A., & Seidman, E. (1999). Giving and receiving help: Interpersonal transactions in mutual help meetings and psychosocial adjustment of members. *American Journal of Community Psychology*, *27*(6), 841–868.

Ross, M., & Bally, S. J. (2005). Peer mentoring: It's time has come. *Hearing Journal* [On line]. Available from http://www.audiologyonline.com/articles

Sciolino, E. (2003, November 21). Chirac has a hearing aid (At least that's the whisper). *New York Times* (Late Edition, East Coast), p. A8.

Stark, P., & Hickson, L. (2004). Outcomes of hearing aid fitting for older people with hearing impairment and their significant others. *International Journal of Audiology, 43*, 390–398.

Stika, C. J. (1997a, September/October). Living with hearing loss—focus group results; Part I: Family relationships and social interactions. *Hearing Loss*, pp. 22–27.

Stika, C. J. (1997b, November/December). Living with hearing loss—focus group results; Part II: Career development and vocational experiences. *Hearing Loss*, pp. 9–32.

Stika, C. J. (Manscript in preparation). *The impact of hearing loss on quality of life for working-age adults.*

Stika, C. J., Ross, M., & Cuevas, C. (2002, May/June). Hearing aid services and satisfaction: The consumer viewpoint. *Hearing Loss*, pp. 25–31.

Stone, H. P. (1993). *An invisible condition: The human side of hearing loss.* Bethesda, MD: Self Help for Hard of Hearing People.

Thomas, A. J. (1984). *Acquired hearing loss: Psychological and psychosocial implications*. London: Academic Press.

Trychin, S. (2001). *Living with hearing loss: What people who are hard of hearing and their significant others should know and do.* Presented at the Adult Aural Rehabilitation Conference. Portland, Maine.

Trychin, S. (2007, May/June). Living with hearing loss program: What we learned about people with hearing loss and their relationships. *Hearing Loss*, pp. 24–28.

Wallhagen, M., Strawbridge, W., Shema, S., & Kaplan, G. (2004). Impact of self-assessed hearing loss on a spouse: A longitudinal analysis of couples. *Journals of Gerontology: Series B: Psychological Sciences and Social Sciences, 59B*(3), S190–S196.

Part IV

Expanding the Scope of AR: Special Issues

17

Music and Cochlear Implants in Audiologic Rehabilitation

Geoff Plant

Introduction

The past 30 years have seen great advances in the communication opportunities available for adults with acquired profound hearing losses. Prior to the 1970's, the range of options available to adventitiously deaf adults was extremely limited. Hearing aids provided varying degrees of assistance, but many adults received little, if any assistance from these devices, and were forced to rely solely on lipreading for perception of spoken language. Unfortunately, lipreading abilities varied widely from person to person, and there was little evidence that training in visual speech perception resulted in significant improvement in the performance of individual subjects. As a result, many adults with acquired profound hearing loss found themselves cut off from all but the most basic conversational interchanges, and from other acoustic events in their environment.

It was against this background that single-channel cochlear implants (CIs) were introduced in the 1970s. Although the information provided by these devices was extremely limited, and restricted primarily to time and intensity cues, they did provide implantees with access to their acoustic environment, and many users reported great satisfaction with the outcome. Only a few exceptional users were capable of auditory-only speech perception, but the simple signal provided by single-channel implants did serve as a useful adjunct to lipreading, and this often resulted in greatly improved face-to-face speech understanding. Single-channel CI users also reported other benefits, such as feedback of their own speech and voice production, and access to environmental sounds.

The first multichannel CI's appeared in the early 1980s and resulted in greatly improved speech perception skills. Many adventitiously deafened adults with CIs were able to understand some speech via listening alone, and some were able to once again use the telephone. In the intervening 25 or so years, innovations in the design of CI hardware and software have led to substantial improvements in the speech perception performance of adults with CIs. Dorman and Wilson (2004) cite the example of an exceptional CI user, Scott N, who was able to recognize "100 percent of more than 1,400 words, either in sentences or alone, without any prior knowledge of the test items" (p. 436). Although the authors note that such performance levels are exceptional, they cite average scores for adult CI users of 80 to 100% for sentence materials and 45 to 55% for words in isolation (p. 439). These performance levels certainly allow adult CI users to communicate effectively via audition alone, or auditory-visually in everyday life.

This chapter reviews the current situation concerning music perception by cochlear implant users. It includes an overview of research findings, and a description of a program designed to enhance music enjoyment by adults with cochlear implants.

Music and Cochlear Implants

One quite surprising consequence of these improvements in speech perception has been a concomitant increase in demand for improved *perception of music*. It is quite tempting to see this surge in musical interest over the past 10 or so years as a direct consequence of improved processing and presentation of the speech signal—speech sounds better and better, so why not music? This is not a particularly surprising trend, but it seems that there is no easy solution to the challenges created by music for many CI users.

Dorman and Wilson (2004) note that Scott, the exceptional subject cited above, reported that "speech sounds natural and clear through the implant" (but) "no patient (in our experience) has described music in this fashion." (Dorman & Wilson, 2004, p. 443). They make the point that music requires much greater frequency precision than speech, and few CI users seem to have reliable and accurate access to some of music's important "components" such as melody, interval, and timbre.

Hilbert (1912) showed that an acoustic signal can be decomposed into a slowly varying envelope (amplitude modulation) and a high-frequency carrier of constant amplitude—the temporal fine structure of the signal. The work of Smith, Delgutte, and Oxenham (2002) has shown that *fine time structure* is critical for music perception, whereas speech is well transmitted by the more slowly changing *temporal envelope structure*. At this time, the information available to implant users is, by and large, restricted to envelope cues, and as a result, many CI users are frustrated in their desire to once again listen to and enjoy music.

Oxenham (2005) believes that "coding temporal fine structure is likely to remain difficult for cochlear implants, especially if fine structure relies heavily on place coding in the normal auditory system." In the long term, improvements in electrode configurations and processing strategies will almost certainly lead to improvements in access to fine structure cues, which should in turn lead to enhanced access to music. At the present time, however, it seems that at least 50% of adult CI users are dissatisfied with the sound of music, and there appears to be no technological "quick fix" to this problem.

Reactions to Music

A number of studies have looked at the reactions of adult CI users to music. Tyler, Gfeller, and Mehr (2000), for example, noted that 83% of 63 respondents in a previous study (Tyler & Kelsay, 1990) "reported a decline in musical enjoyment postimplantation (while) 51% characterized the sound of music postimplantation as unpleasant or difficult to follow" (Tyler et al. 2000, p. 83). Brockmeier (2004) reported on a questionnaire completed by more than 100 users of the MED-EL COMBI 40 or 40+ cochlear implant, and found that only 30% of their respondents felt that music sounded "natural." When the same users were asked if music sounded pleasant, however, around 48% responded positively. There are a number of other studies which have looked at the reactions of CI users to music, and the response seems to be uniform, regardless of the type of implant used. Overall, the results of all studies indicate that there is a 50/50 "split" in the responses of CI users to music: around half of CI users are satisfied with the sound of music, and the remainder are not. The following quote seems to sum up the situation for many of adult CI users. *"I'm very happy with my implant when it comes to speech . . . but the one disappointment is music which just doesn't sound right at all. It's often difficult to recognize even familiar stuff, let alone enjoy new stuff"* (Stevew, 2004).

"Cheesecake or Nutritional Necessity?"

There are some people who would not see this as any great problem. Pinker (1997), for example, suspects (his word) that *"Music is auditory cheesecake, an exquisite confection crafted to tickle the sensitive spots of at least six of our mental faculties"* (Pinker, 1997, p. 534), and seems to believe that *"music could vanish from our species, and the rest of our lifestyle would be virtually unchanged."* I have great difficulty with this point-of-view, however, as I have found that many adults regard the loss of access to music as one of the most traumatic consequences of their acquired profound hearing losses. Speech perception is, of course, of primary importance for most people. It plays a critical role in many aspects (social, vocational, informational, etc.) of our everyday lives, but music also appears to have many important functions. The great Chinese philosopher Confucius believed that, *"Music produces a kind of pleasure which human nature cannot do without,"* and this seems to more accurately describe the reaction of adults to the loss of easy access to musical experiences. Levitin (2006) is another, more recent advocate for the importance of music. He devotes a chapter in *This Is Your Brain on Music* to presenting arguments against Pinker's conclusions. This is recommended to readers who would like to pursue the topic in more detail.

If we accept that music is an important part of the life of most people, then something needs to be done to optimize the music listening experience of adults with CI's. CI technology is continually improving, but it appears that around 50% of users are denied acceptable access to music, and there is a need to provide assistance and support for this group. This chapter represents an attempt to provide clinicians/therapists with some ideas that can be used to help CI users have better access to, and derive enjoyment from, music.

Access to the Components of Music

Music is sometimes divided into its various "elements" such as *tempo and rhythm, pitch interval and melody, and timbre and instruments* (Zeng, 2004). A number of studies have found that while tempo and rhythm are relatively well perceived by CI users (Gfeller & Lansing, 1991; Gfeller, Woodworth, Robin, Witt, & Knutson, 1997), the latter two elements are not (Fearn, 2001; Galvin & Zeng, 1998; Gfeller, Turner, Mehr, Woodworth, Fearn, Knutson, Witt, & Stordahl, 2002; Gfeller, Witt, Woodworth, Mehr, & Knutson, 2002. Gfeller, Turner, et al., (2002), for example, presented 49 adult CI users with 12 "familiar melodies," such as "Happy Birthday," and "The Wedding March" ("Here comes the bride") played on a synthesized piano. The mean score for the CI users was 12.6% correct (range = 0–43.75%), which was significantly poorer (p <0.0001) than the performance of a control group of adults with normal hearing (mean = 55.1%; range = 13–68.9%).

Although previous research indicated that "experienced implant recipients preferred the tone quality of piano to that of seven other commonly heard instruments" (Gfeller, Turner, et al., 2002, p. 36), it should be noted that CI's were developed specifically for the human voice, and that a "fairer" test of the ability of CI users to detect melody would involve singing. The obvious limitation of such a study, however, is that listeners could use the lyrics to identify the song. One alternative is to substitute the nonsense syllable [da] for each syllable/note in a song or tune to determine whether this led to improvements in the ability of CI users to identify familiar tunes.

To evaluate this concept informally, 15 familiar songs, such as "Happy Birthday," "Twinkle, Twinkle Little Star," and "Yankee Doodle," were recorded using this technique, and were played to

12 adult CI users. They were told that they would hear a number of familiar songs, and asked to name as many as possible. They were also told that if they didn't know the name of the song, but knew the words, they should sing or say them. A third option was to hum or sing the tune. The responses were scored correct if they indicated the subject knew the identity of the song. Two of the songs used, "On Top of Old Smokey" and "Stars and Stripes Forever" are the basis of popular parodies, and several subjects named these works as "On Top of Spaghetti" and "Be kind to your web-footed friends, 'cause that duck may be somebody's mother," respectively. These responses were marked correct, as they indicated that the subject was able to correctly identify the tune.

The scores obtained by the 12 subjects are presented in Figure 17–1. The mean score for the subject group was 65% correct (range = 20–100%), which is considerably higher than the scores obtained in the Gfeller, Turner, et al. (2002) study. There are several possible factors that may have contributed to these scores, such as the access to temporal cues, but the use of a male voice with a relatively low pitch is probably the most important.

Zeng (2004) notes that "cochlear implant subjects . . . have a great deal of difficulty identifying timbres associated with different musical instruments," and this obviously creates difficulties in music listening. Gfeller, Witt, et al. (2002) presented a group of 51 cochlear implant users with a forced-choice task involving eight different musical instruments—trumpet, trombone, flute, clarinet, saxophone, violin, cello, and piano. The mean identification score obtained by the implant users was 47% correct. A control group of listeners with normal hearing scored around 90% correct for the same task.

Studies focusing on these individual musical components have yielded much useful information, which helps to explain the difficulties that many implant users have with music. In the end, however, music must be seen as a *multifaceted* experience that *combines* tempo and rhythm, pitch

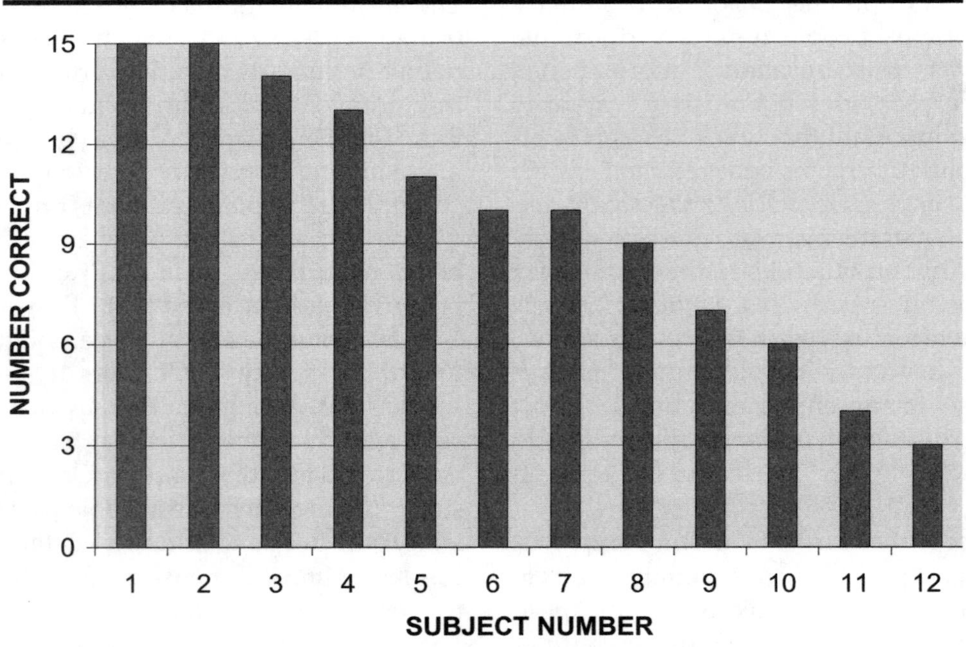

Figure 17–1. Scores obtained by 12 CI users for a test of song/tune recognition.

interval and melody, and timbre and instruments. It should also be noted that access to one of the parameters may help recognition of another. Gfeller, Turner, et al. (2002) for example, cite the case of an implant user who "stated that she often listened to the rhythmic pattern at the beginning of an item. As the item continued, she would then try to match that pattern with her memory of familiar melodies" (p. 49).

Kraemer, Macrae, Green, and Kelley (2005) provide some insights into the processes that may be involved in this type of "remembered listening." They played familiar and unfamiliar songs and tunes to a group of normal hearing listeners while monitoring brain activity using functional magnetic resonance imaging (fMRI). Short segments, ranging from 2 to 5 seconds in duration, were extracted from the musical pieces and replaced with a period of silence. They found that "familiar songs induced greater activation in auditory association areas than did silent gaps embedded in unknown songs" and that "simply muting short gaps of familiar music was sufficient to trigger auditory imagery that indicates the obligatory nature of this phenomenon. Corroborating this observation, all subjects reported subjectively hearing a continuation of the familiar songs, but not of the unfamiliar songs, during the gaps in the music" (Kraemer et al., 2005, p. 158).

CI users often report that they prefer to listen to familiar music, at least initially, and the CI signal may trigger a similar reaction to that described by Kraemer et al. That is, a CI user may be able to "evoke" similar auditory memories of a familiar song or tune. The "auditory imagery" could be triggered by aspects of the melody, a distinctive rhythm pattern, or the lyrics, and serve to "fill out" the user's auditory experience.

Music Tests

There are few test instruments to assess the music perception skills of individual clients. The Mu.S.I.C. Test (Fitzgerald & Fitzgerald, 2006) contains six modules, which assess specific musical skills (pitch, rhythm, melody, chord discrimination, instrument identification in isolation, and instrument identification in small groups). There are also two modules that require the CI user to give subjective ratings of short musical pieces. These look at the individual's rating of emotion or degree of dissonance in original musical pieces.

The Clinical Assessment of Music Perception (CAMP Test) developed by Nimmons, Kang, Drennan, Longnion, Ruffin, Worman, Yueh, and Rubinstein (2008) consists of three subtests, which measure a CI user's pitch discrimination, melody identification, and timbre identification. In the pitch test, the CI user hears two tones and has to indicate which one was higher. The melody test presents familiar melodies without temporal cues (isochronous) using digitally synthesized musical tones. "The tones had 500-millisecond duration and were presented at a tempo of 60 beats per minute" and "all melodies were truncated at 8 seconds to prevent song length as a potential cue" (Nimmons et al, 2008; p. 151). The timbre identification task requires the listener to discriminate between eight instruments (piano, violin, cello, acoustic guitar, trumpet, flute, clarinet, and saxophone) playing the same tune. The melody test and the timbre identification test are presented using a closed-set format. That is, the CI user is told the names of the melodies, and the instruments, and has to determine which one is heard after each presentation.

The Appreciation of Music in Cochlear Implantees (AMICI) Test (Spitzer, Mancuso, & Cheng, 2008) is another recent test. The AMICI test consists of four subtests, which use either a closed-set or an open-set format. The tasks presented in the subtests are:

1. discrimination of music and noise (closed set).
2. instrument identification (closed set consisting of trumpet, piano, drum, flute, drums/tympani, tuba, guitar, violin/strings, female singer, and male singer).
3. identification of musical styles (closed set of five styles—classical, Latin, country and western, jazz, rock and roll/popular).
4. identification of specific musical pieces (open set).

Neither the CAMP Test nor the AMICI Test is currently available for general distribution, but it is hoped that these potentially valuable resources will eventually be released for clinical use.

Music Training for Adults with Cochlear Implants: Starting Points

This section is designed to provide the reader with a description of some of the methods that I use in my music work with adult CI users at the Hearing Rehabilitation Foundation (HRF) and for MED-EL. The essential elements of this approach include the use of familiar melodies, simple musical arrangements, auditory-visual presentations, live performances, original music composed for CI users, Music Focus Groups, and musical exercises.

Use of Familiar Melodies

In working with adult CI users, the first step is usually to introduce music using a familiar song presented on either CD or DVD. One song that I have found particularly useful is Johnny Cash's "I Walk the Line," which seems to fulfill several important criteria for CI users. These include:

- It is familiar to a wide cross-section of adult listeners.
- Cash's bass/baritone voice is in the frequency region where CI users may be able to use envelope cues to access voice pitch (Oxenham, 2005).
- The singing style is close to that of speech (Cleveland, Sundberg, & Stone, 2001), the signal for which CI processing systems were developed.
- The instrumentation is very sparse—guitar, bass, and drums—and at a level that does not obscure the singer's voice.

The listener is provided with a copy of the lyrics to make sure that he or she does not have to devote extra attention to speech perception, which allows the listener to relax and focus on the overall musical experience. Copies of lyrics can usually be found on the Internet, but clinicians should check that the lyrics match those on the recording being used.

On some occasions, music may be introduced by the clinician singing a familiar song to a client. This is usually done without any accompaniment, although I do sometimes also use a simple hand drum to provide a simple rhythmic background. I usually sing well-known folk songs such as "Yankee Doodle," and "This Land Is Your Land," but always check to make sure that the client is familiar with the song before singing it.

Simple Musical Styles

There is often a hint of the pejorative when "simple" is used to describe music, but that is certainly not the intention here. "Simple" is used to describe music that has "easy-to-access" lyrics, a strong well-defined beat, and does not contain complex harmonies. The recording "mix" can also be critical, with preference given to recordings with a favorable "signal-to-noise-ratio." That is, the instrumental accompaniment is at a relatively low level, giving the voice extra prominence. Examples of music forms that fall into this category include folk, country, and other popular music forms such as rock, and blues. Individual performers used in introductory exercises include John Denver, Arlo Guthrie, and James Taylor, as these male singers are usually the easiest for CI users to hear initially. If a client has a preference for a particular female singer, however, it is worthwhile to use one or more of that artist's works as well. The preference for solo male singers at this point is that their voice pitch is in the range where envelope cues may afford some access to melodic information, thus enhancing the overall musical experience.

Auditory-Visual Presentation

This may seem to be a unusual category, as music is usually seen as an auditory art form, but there is a great deal added to the overall experience when CI users can both *hear* and *see* the performer(s). Vision can provide lipreading cues, which help in understanding the lyrics. It also allows the viewer to see the instruments being used, and, in some cases, featured in a particular performance. I have a large collection of DVD's of live music performances, and often use them in my work with adult CI users. Many of these are captioned, which means that the CI user can focus her or his whole attention on the screen, and not have to look at a separate printed sheet providing the lyrics. It is interesting to note that clients often complain about recordings, even when they are captioned, where the performer's lips are obscured by the microphone. The lipreading cues seem to provide a "framework" that helps the viewer to determine exactly what is occurring during the song, and serve to enhance the overall listening "experience."

Live Performance

One of the most effective ways to introduce music to CI users is via live performance. This could involve the clinician/therapist singing a familiar song, or playing an instrument for her or his client(s), or using outside musicians to provide the experience. Musicians who have performed for clients at the HRF'S Music Focus Groups (a more detailed description follows) include a keyboard player, a flautist, a saxophonist, and a tabla (Indian hand drums) player. All have been rated highly by the CI users who have enjoyed the opportunity to see music being played.

Original Music Composed for CI Users

On February 14, 2008, a special performance took place at the Royal Scottish Academy of Music and Drama (RSAMD) in Glasgow, Scotland. An ensemble of musicians from the RSAMD performed "Noise Carriers," an original work for adult CI users by the Scottish composer Oliver Searle. This work, commissioned by MED-EL, consisted of 13 short pieces inspired by several works of the 18th century Scottish poet and songwriter Robert Burns. In writing this piece, Searle attempted to use available research findings to create a work that would be accessible to CI users. These included:

- the use of an ensemble made up of instruments with low frequency timbres, including cellos, double bass, drums, horns, and saxophones.
- settings which involved extensive use of single instruments, or small groups of instruments.
- an avoidance of complex harmonies, even in movements that included several instruments.
- a male singer who sang in a "folk" rather than a "classically trained" style.

At the completion of the performance, a questionnaire was distributed to the audience members, who were asked to rate several aspects of the performance. The questionnaire was completed by 44 CI users with an average age of 55 years (range = 21–88 years), and their responses to the event were very positive. Figure 17–2 presents the CI users' overall rating of the performance. The 7-point scale used ranged from "Terrible" (1) to "Excellent (7). All but one of the CI users rated the work as being "Acceptable" or better, and the mean rating of 5.6 corresponds to a rating of "Good" to "Very Good." Written comments provided by the CI users included:

> *"Excellent event!! More please!!"*
>
> *"My first time and I think that it was very good, would like to go again in the future."*
>
> *"I thank you all for such joy you brought me . . . Excellent . . . I heard every instrument."*
>
> *"Less instruments make pleasurable music as they do not overpower each other."*

It should be mentioned that the audience was not "hand-picked," but rather reflected the overall caseload of the local CI center. This is well illustrated in Figure 17–3, which presents the CI users' responses to the question, "How often do you listen to music?" The 7-point scale used ranged from "Never" (1) to "a Great Deal" (7). The mean

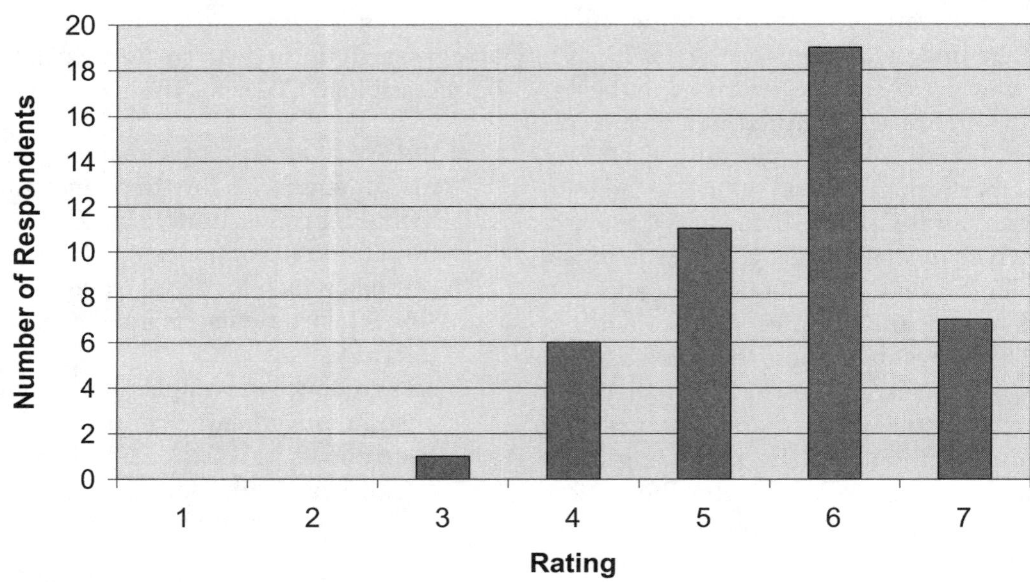

Figure 17–2. Distribution of responses for the overall rating of "Noise Carriers." The response categories used were: Terrible (1), Very bad (2), Bad (3), Acceptable (4), Good (5), Very good (6), and Excellent (7).

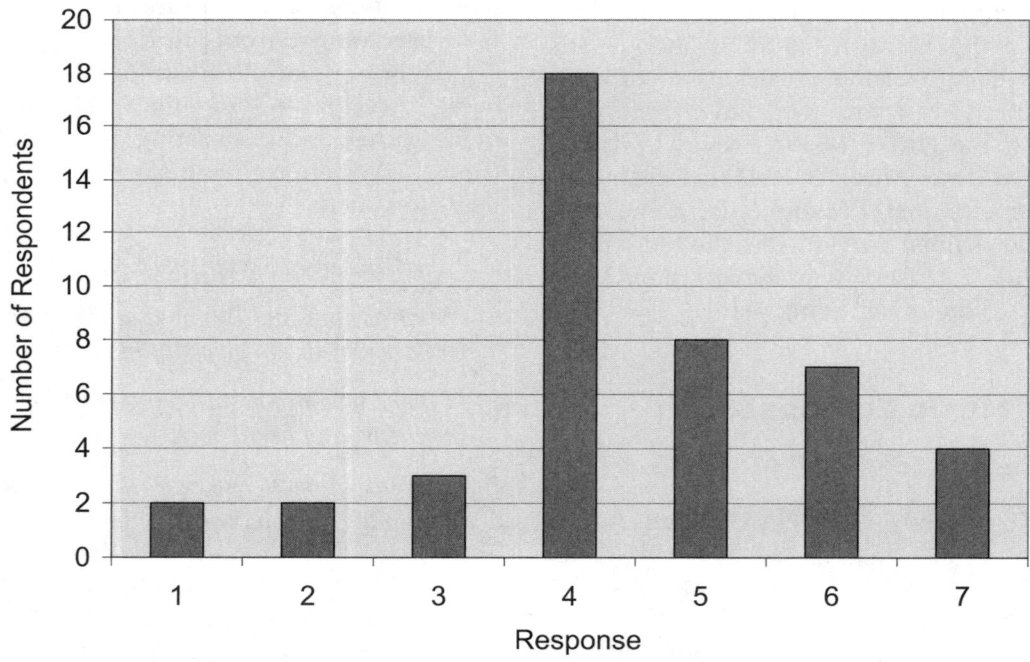

Figure 17–3. Pattern of responses to the question, "How often do you listen to music?" for the 44 cochlear implant users. The response categories used were: Never (1), Very rarely (2), Rarely (3), Sometimes (4), Often (5), Very often (6), and A great deal (7).

response was 4.5, which is in the range "Sometimes" to "Often."

Although such an event is probably not feasible for most CI facilities, small "concerts" that include local musicians who volunteer to perform could be a viable alternative. Another possible way to provide "live" music opportunities would be to play a selection of DVD's of concert performances.

Music Focus Groups

The success of approaches aimed at adults with hearing loss such as Hickson, Worrall, and Scarinci's (2007) ACE (Active Communication Education) has highlighted the value of "interactive group programs that focus on communication (not just hearing) and that take an active approach to problem solving" (Hickson, 2007, p. 10). Music Focus Groups are designed to provide opportunities for adults with cochlear implants to meet, share their musical experiences, and take part in musical activities.

The Music Focus Groups run at the HRF in Somerville, Massachusets are held on a Saturday afternoon, and are scheduled to last for three hours. The number of people in each group is restricted to five, and each participant is encouraged to bring along family members or friends. Few take up this offer, however, which may reflect the participants' initial reservations about music and their ability to access it.

Although no strict timetable is used, several different activities and exercises are covered in each group. At all times, the participants are encouraged to make comments, ask questions, etc., and I try to confine my role to that of facilitator rather than group "leader." Each group also has at least one live musical performance. My wife has played an electronic keyboard at every group that we have held, and we have also had a number of musical "guests" playing flute, table, and saxophone.

Musical Background

Each participant is asked to provide a brief description of her or his musical background. This includes her or his musical experiences, preferences, etc., prior to the onset of hearing loss, and pre- and postimplant. During this segment of the program, participants often ask questions of each other, and such sharing of experiences is very valuable, as it is often the first time that they have had the opportunity to discuss music with other adults with CIs. Many group members seem to be "pleased" or "relieved" to discover others with CI's are having similar difficulties with music—that it is not "just me"—and this sharing of experiences is a very valuable part of the overall program. (*Editors' note:* For further information on group dynamics, the reader is referred to Chapter 13 of this text).

Musical Exercises

In this segment of the program, several musical exercises are presented to the group. Although these do test the individual member's ability to perceive musical differences, care is taken to ensure that it is presented in an informal and relaxed manner. The exercises presented during each session are presented below.

Exercise 1: Three-Note Sequences

Three notes are played on the keyboard. The first two notes are always Middle C (261.6 Hz), while the third can be the same (Middle C), a higher or lower note. The participants are asked to indicate whether the third note is *lower*, *same*, or *higher* than the reference notes. The notes presented with their frequency in Hz are:

C2	D2	A3	C3
130.8 Hz	146.8 Hz	220 Hz	261.6 Hz
E3	**G3**	**B4**	**C4**
329.6 Hz	392 Hz	493.9 Hz	523.2 Hz

Exercise 2: Five-Note Sequences

The starting note for these sequences varies between C1, C2, C3, C4, and C5. The subsequent four notes can be the same (C C C C C), rising

(C D E F G), or falling (C B A G F). The participants are asked to judge whether the notes in each sequence are *constant*, *rising*, or *falling*.

Exercise 3: Tune Identification

The melodies of 10 familiar tunes ("Twinkle, Twinkle, Little Star," "Frere Jacques," etc.) are presented on the keyboard (right hand only with the starting note always in the octave of Middle C) and the participants are asked to write down the name of each tune.

These three exercises are presented via listening alone. That is, the participants are asked to not watch the keyboard player. At the completion of each exercise, each item is repeated, with the participants encouraged to watch each sequence being produced. The participants "score" each item, but no attempt is made to collect these, as this may lead to the tasks being regarded as formal "tests."

Rating of Familiar and Unfamiliar Music

In many ways, this is the "core" activity in each Music Focus Group, and usually occupies around half of the session.

Live Music. As mentioned previously, live music experiences at Music Focus Groups have included performances on keyboards, flute, saxophone, and tabla. Where required, the musicians have been asked to tailor their performance to attempt to meet the needs of CI users. For example, the flautist was asked to transpose her pieces to a lower octave. The participants are asked to rate how each piece sounded through their implants, using the 7-point scale shown in Figure 17–4.

In all cases, these "performances" have been very well rated by the participants, and it is felt that this results from them being able to both hear and see the musician(s) playing.

Recorded Music. The second segment consists of around 10 recordings, presented on either CD or DVD, of familiar or unfamiliar songs. The lyrics of each song are provided on a sheet of paper, or via captions on the television monitor. Following each recording, the participants are asked to indicate whether they are familiar with each song, and to rate it, using the 7-point scale shown below. The songs chosen represent a range of *popular* music genres including folk, country, rock, and blues, and include both male and female singers.

Although audio-only (CD) presentations of Johnny Cash's "Walk the Line" and Arlo Guthrie's "City of New Orleans" were rated very highly, there is an overall preference for DVD performances. The value of DVD presentations is perhaps best illustrated by the uniformly positive reaction of group members to a Chinese instrumental group—The Twelve Girls Band. This group plays a repertoire of Chinese and western music using traditional Chinese instruments such as the pipa (a plucked four-string lute), ehru (a two-stringed bowed fiddle), dizi (bamboo flute), and yangqin (hammered dulcimer. Possible reasons for the positive response to this music include the use of a well defined bass line and rhythm, the unique timbres of the instruments, the use of a pentatonic scale (five notes to the octave), and an absence of harmony. Although these may all contribute in varying degrees to the clients' reactions, I feel that the ability to both see and hear the instruments being played is paramount, and doubt that there would have been such a positive response had the

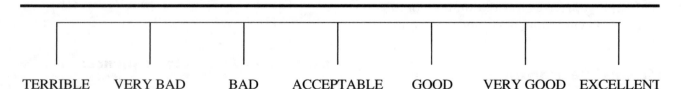

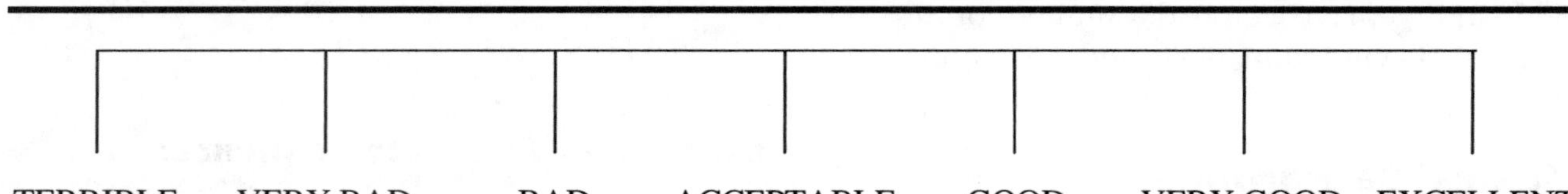

Figure 17–4. 7-point scale to rate how each musical piece sounds through their implants.

group been presented via CD. The ability to observe the musicians and pinpoint the instrument(s) being played seems to make the experience more acceptable for CI users and this is an area that warrants further investigation.

Response to Music Focus Groups. A few days after a Music Focus Group, a message is sent to the participants asking for feedback and reactions to the session. These could be collected at the end of the session, but I prefer to give the participants some time before seeking their opinions. The feedback received has been extremely positive, and many participants mention that the session provided them with their first positive music experience with their CI(s). The comments of several participants in Music Focus Groups are provided below:

> *"Thanks for the eye-opening (or ear-opening) experience."*
>
> *"The focus group removed my trepidation about listening to music, and allowed me to realize that there are other ways to appreciate music than trying to get it to sound the way I remember."*
>
> *"Makes me think that I need to hear the same thing over and over again. When CI was first switched on, it sounded like Smurfs or Donald Duck, but quickly changed to normal. Feel that the same process may occur if I listen to more music."*
>
> *"I very much enjoyed the Music Focus Group for a variety of reasons. For one, I believe that it is important to understand not only objective differences when it comes to music appreciation with a CI, but also subjective differences/similarities."*

These comments highlight the value of Music Focus Groups for adults with CI's. Clinicians wishing to learn more are referred to "Music Notes" (Plant, 2006), which provides detailed information to assist in planning and providing Music Focus Groups for adults with CIs.

Follow-Up Activities. Although the activities outlined here may serve as a good reintroduction to music, many clients require ongoing support. The HRF has provided follow-up groups for interested clients. These have offered the participants the opportunity to share their musical experiences and to be exposed to other musical forms. Clinics could also consider building up collections of CDs and DVDs, and providing opportunities for clients to either listen to these "in house," or allow them to be borrowed for home use.

Although sometimes difficult to arrange, live performances by volunteer musicians are another way to provide follow-up musical experiences. Local music schools or conservatories are potential sources of musicians who would be willing to volunteer their skills.

One area that warrants further investigation is music making by adults with CIs. One of the items in the questionnaire distributed to the audience attending the premiere of "Noise Carriers" asked, "Do you play a musical instrument?" and provided three possible responses—"Yes," "No," and "I used to, but not now." The number of responses for each of these three categories was 4, 30, and 8, respectively. This is similar to the responses obtained for a questionnaire that I distributed in the United States, so it seems that, perhaps not surprisingly, many people discontinue playing musical instrument after the onset of a significant hearing loss.

There are, however, some notable exceptions to this trend. One CI user with whom I have worked has learned the tabla and drums since receiving his implant. He is an active amateur musician, and plays in a band he helped form with a number of hearing friends. Another client, a former professional keyboard player, returned to performing about two years postimplant, and has become an advocate for increased music opportunities for children and adults with CIs. Both derive great pleasure from their music-making activities, which seem to have encouraged them to listen to a progressively wider repertoire of music and musical styles.

Encouraging CI clients to experiment with simple percussion instruments and other tuned instruments—piano, keyboards, guitar, etc.—may help them improve their overall music listening.

Conclusion

Music remains an area of difficulty for many adults with CI's, and much more needs to be done to support them in their quest for improved access to this important part of our "auditory culture." Ongoing improvements in CI technology will almost certainly lead to enhanced music listening for users, but many clients will still require ongoing support and encouragement. This chapter provides readers with an introduction to this topic, and offers some suggestions for clinicians wishing to help their clients improve their access to music. While many clinicians may not have access to live music, a variety of musical instruments, or even a strong musical background, they should still be able to implement a music program for CI users. Training through the use of CDs and DVDs allows CI users to practice music listening in much the same way as listening to books on tape can enhance speech perception skills.

Acknowledgments. The author would like to thank Kerryn Plant for her invaluable contribution to and support of the Music Focus Groups and other musical activities provided by the Hearing Rehabilitation Foundation. Thanks, also, to Zack Moir for his musical contributions and support. Finally, thanks are due to RR for his unique insights into music listening and performance with a cochlear implant.

References

Brockmeier, S. J. (2004, January 27). *Music and cochlear implants.* Paper presented at MED-EL UK Workshop, Zell am Zimmer, Austria.

Cleveland, T., Sundberg, J., & Stone, R. E. (2001). Long-term-average-spectrum characteristics of country singers during speaking and singing. *Journal of Voice, 15,* 54–60.

Dorman, M. F., & Wilson, B. S. (2004). The design and function of cochlear implants. *American Scientist, 92,* 436–445.

Fearn, R. A. (2001). *Music and pitch perception of cochlear implant recipients.* Ph.D. Thesis, University of New South Wales.

Fitzgerald, D., & Fitzgerald, H. (2006). *Mu.S.I.C. Perception Test.* Innsbruck, Austria: MED-EL.

Galvin, J., & Zeng, F-G. (1998). Music instrument perception in cochlear implant listeners. *Proceedings of the 16th International Congress of Acoustics and 135th Meeting of the Acoustical Society of America, 3,* 2219–2220.

Gfeller, K., & Lansing, C. R. (1991). Melodic, rhythmic, and timbral perception of adult cochlear implant users. *Journal of Speech and Hearing Research, 34,* 916–920.

Gfeller, K., Turner, C., Mehr, M., Woodworth, G., Fearn, R., Knutson, J. F., et al. (2002). Recognition of familiar melodies by adult cochlear implant recipients and normal-hearing adults. *Cochlear Implants International, 3,* 29–53.

Gfeller, K., Witt, S., Woodworth, G., Mehr, M. A., & Knutson, J. (2002). Effects of frequency, instrumental family, and cochlear implant type on timbre recognition and appraisal. *Annals of Otology, Rhinology, and Laryngology, 111,* 349–356.

Gfeller, K., Woodworth, G., Robin, D. A., Witt, S., & Knutson, J. F. (1997). Perception of rhythmic and sequential pitch patterns by normally hearing adults and adult cochlear implant users. *Ear and Hearing, 18,* 252–260.

Hickson, L. (2007). Pull out an "ACE" to help your patients become better communicators. *Hearing Journal, 60,* 10–16.

Hickson, L., Worrall, L., & Scarinci, N. (2007). *Active Communication Education (ACE): A program for older people with hearing impairment.* Brackley, UK: Speechmark.

Hilbert, D. (1912). *Grundzüge einer allgemeinen Theorie der linearen Integralgleichungen.* Leipzig: Teubner.

Kraemer, D. J. M., Macrae, C. N., Green, A. E., & Kelley, W. M. (2005). Musical imagery: Sound of silence activates auditory cortex. *Nature, 434,* 158.

Levitin, D. J. (2006). *This is your brain on music.* New York: Dutton.

Nimmons, G. L., Kang, R. S., Drennan, W. R., Longnion, J., Ruffin, C., Worman, T., et al. (2008). Clinical assessment of music perception in cochlear implant listeners. *Otology and Neurotology, 29,* 149–155.

Oxenham, A. J. (2005, May 25). *Representation of pitch in the auditory system: Implications for cochlear implant and hearing aid processing*. Paper presented at the International Sensory Aids Conference (ISAC-05); Portland, ME.

Pinker, S. (1997). *How the mind works*. New York: Norton.

Plant, G. (2006). *Music notes: Introducing music to adults with cochlear implants*. Innsbruck, Austria: MED-EL.

Smith, Z. M., Delgutte, B., & Oxenham, A. J. (2002). Chimaeric sounds reveal dichotomies in auditory perception. *Nature, 416*, 87–90.

Spitzer, J. B., Mancuso, D., & Cheng, M-Y. (2008). Development of a clinical test of musical perception: Appreciation of Music in Cochlear Implantees (AMICI). *Journal of the American Academy of Audiology, 19*(1), 56–81.

Stevew. (2004). RNID Forum June 19, 2004. Retrieved 11/15/2005 from http://www.mid.org.uk/ubb/Forum1/HTML/002747

Tyler, R. S., Gfeller, K., & Mehr, M. A. (2000). A preliminary investigation comparing one and eight channels at fast and slow rates on music appraisal in adults with cochlear implants. *Cochlear Implants International, 1*, 82–87.

Tyler, R. S., & Kelsay, D. (1990). Advantages and disadvantages perceived by some of the better cochlear-implant patients. *American Journal of Otology, 11*, 282–289.

Zeng, F-G. (2004). Trends in cochlear implants. *Trends in Amplification, 8*, 1–34.

18

Evidence-Based Practice in Adult Audiologic Rehabilitation

Louise Hickson

Introduction

The rise of Evidence-Based Medicine (EBM) in the 1990s had a profound effect on all areas of health care, including audiology. Sackett, Rosenberg, Gray, Haynes, and Richardson (1996) defined it as "the conscientious, explicit and judicious use of current best evidence in making decisions about the care of individual patients" (p. 71). Now referred to as Evidence-Based Practice (EBP), thus incorporating disciplines beyond medicine, it involves the integration of the best available research evidence with clinical expertise and the patient's preferences and goals. In this chapter, EBP is defined, the evidence to date about adult audiologic rehabilitation (AR) is presented, and areas of need for future research are outlined. The process of applying EBP has four key steps (Worrall & Bennett, 2001).

EBP Step 1: Asking the Clinical Question

The first step involves forming a clinical question. It must comprise a patient or problem; an assessment, treatment or prognostic factor; an outcome; and, possibly, a comparison treatment. The best way to illustrate this is by example. A 66-year-old man with an acquired moderate to severe sensorineural hearing loss who wears bilateral well-fitted hearing aids presents to the audiology clinic seeking further assistance because he is feeling extremely stressed by his inability to communicate as well as he would like. He is becoming increasingly socially isolated. He has had a trial with assistive devices but decided not to purchase one. There are a range of possible interventions available through the clinic which would improve his communication—individual auditory training, fitting of an FM system, individual communication strategy training, and group communication education. Options are discussed with him and his preference is for a group program. The clinical question is: "Is group communication education effective in improving communication for people with acquired hearing loss?"

EBP Step 2: Gathering the Evidence

The second step in the EBP process is to assemble and evaluate the best evidence. This is accomplished by searching relevant databases using keywords such as hearing loss, group and communication. To locate research about amplification in audiology Cox (2005) suggests PubMed (www.pubmed.gov), ComDisDome (www.comdisdome.com) and CINAHL (www.cinahl.com) as the most useful. Such databases are also relevant for AR. PubMed is a popular, publicly available database that is primarily based on the Medline database. ComDisDome stands for Communication Sciences and Disorders Information Service and this service requires a subscription. CINAHL is the Cumulative Index to Nursing and Allied Health Literature and also requires a subscription. Some databases beyond these three may also be useful for searching topics related to AR and in Sweetow and Palmer (2005)'s review of individual auditory training, they searched Medline, CINAHL, Psych Info, EMBASE, Applied Social Science Index and Abstracts, and the Rehabilitation Literature Index. It is possible to search a number of databases at once by using systems such as Web of Science. Discussing search approaches initially with a librarian is recommended and can save valuable time in the long run.

EBP Step 3: Evaluating the Evidence

The next step involves determining the relevance of the articles you find to your clinical question, and then if they are relevant, critically reviewing them. Rating the quality of a particular piece of research is central to EBP. Table 18–1 shows a commonly used hierarchy with level 1 considered the highest level of research evidence and 5 the lowest (Straus, Richardson, Glasziou, & Haynes, 2005). Systematic reviews feature prominently in this Table. They are comprehensive evaluations of the literature that try to limit bias by systematically identifying, appraising and summarizing research on a particular topic. Primary data sources only are evaluated and criteria for inclusion in such a review are predetermined. Such synthesis of research is important because single studies can and do provide conflicting evidence and a systematic review can help establish why this occurs. They are also extremely useful for clinicians as they provide a summary of the evidence on a particular clinical question. For example, the question proposed earlier was "Is group communication education effective in improving communication for people with acquired hearing loss?" Hawkins (2005) completed a very relevant systematic review on the topic of counseling-based group rehabilitation, the results of which are discussed later in this chapter.

Table 18–1. Levels of Evidence Relevant to Therapy Studies

Level	Nature of Evidence
1a	Systematic review of Randomized-Controlled Trials (RCTs)
1b	Individual Randomized-Controlled Trials
2a	Systematic reviews of cohort studies
2b	Individual cohort study including low quality RCTs
3a	Systematic reviews of case-control studies
3b	Individual case-control study
4	Case series
5	Expert opinion

Source: Straus et al., 2005.

Levels of Evidence

Systematic reviews aside, there are three types of studies mentioned in Table 18–1 and it is important to understand the difference between these.

Many textbooks discuss these types of studies and Cox (2005) provides an excellent review relevant to audiology. The first and most rigorous from a scientific perspective is the Randomized Controlled Trial (RCT). In an RCT, participants who meet stated inclusion criteria are randomly allocated to groups receiving different forms of treatment or to a no-treatment or placebo-treatment group. Abrams, Hnath-Chisolm, Guerreiro, and Ritterman (1992) provide an example of this in AR where participants were allocated to receive no intervention, hearing aid fitting alone, or hearing aid fitting and counseling sessions. Participants and the researchers who assess them should be blind to group membership, that is, not aware of which treatment a participant is receiving. This is necessary to reduce any potential bias. If both participants and researchers are unaware of the treatment, the study will be described as a "double-blind RCT." If the researcher knows the nature of the treatment but the participant does not, this is referred to as a "single-blind RCT." Occasionally, the term "triple-blind" is used and this refers to the fact that the participant, the researcher, and the person doing the final analysis of the data are all blind to the different types of treatment. Randomization of individuals to groups should mean that the different groups will be equal on all variables, except the type of treatment, although this equality needs to be checked statistically. RCTs vary in quality depending on how careful the researchers have been to follow the guidelines for such studies (see the Consort group at www.consort-statement.org).

A crossover study is another type of RCT and has some advantages because participants can act as their own controls and all participants receive the treatment in the end. In this type of study, participants are first randomly allocated to different groups as they are for an RCT and then one group begins a particular type of treatment and the other groups begin other treatments. At a certain point in time, those who have completed one form of treatment begin the other, so that all participants complete all treatments. Such studies are not common in AR, however, there are examples in hearing aid fitting trials (e.g., Wood & Lutman, 2004). There are some examples of studies that used a simplified crossover design, where one group of participants receive the intervention from the start, and the other "control" group receives no treatment or a placebo initially, followed by the intervention (Hickson, Worrall, & Scarinci, 2007; Sweetow & Sabes, 2006).

The second level of evidence is available from cohort studies. These are common in AR and involve the examination of the effects of a particular intervention in a single cohort or group of participants. Results for the experimental cohort are compared to a group who did not receive the intervention. The major difference between a cohort study and an RCT is that random allocation to groups does not occur, so there is the potential for bias and for results to be influenced by variables other than the type of intervention. Norman, George, Downie, and Milligan (1995) described such a study in which they compared hearing aid outcomes for participants who received informational group sessions to a group who did not receive such additional sessions. Only those willing to undertake the intervention were included in the experimental group and the outcomes of this program may well have been influenced by factors other than the intervention, for example, general health, intelligence, and readiness for change.

Case controlled studies provide the next level of evidence. In studies of this kind participants with particular outcomes are studied retrospectively to investigate factors that influence outcomes. In AR, one group (cases) could be people who achieve high levels of benefit from auditory training and another group (controls) could be people who do not achieve benefit. Thus, the outcome is measured after the intervention and then the groups are compared on different variables to identify those that are predictive of group membership. No studies of this kind were evident in the AR research literature; however, there are examples in the hearing aid literature (Hickson, Timm, Worrall, & Bishop, 1999; Swan & Gatehouse, 1990). The lowest levels of evidence are studies that describe one or more outcomes for a series of cases with no comparisons to other groups and, finally, expert opinion that is not based on critical appraisal of the research evidence. An example of a case series study in AR is the paper by Hickson, Worrall, and Scarinci (2006) which describes the outcomes obtained by participants who completed a group communication education program. Although such research does not provide evidence of the effectiveness of one kind of intervention over another, they are useful as they provide a baseline for comparison of outcomes across studies. More detailed descriptions of levels of evidence, along with a number of other very useful tools, such as tips for finding the best evidence and critical appraisal worksheets, are available from the Center for Evidence-Based Medicine (www.cebm.net).

It is also important to point out that, although the level of evidence hierarchy is commonly used, it is not always the only way to rate the value of a particular piece of evidence. Sackett et al. (1996) makes the point that "Evidence-based medicine is not restricted to randomised trials and meta-analyses. It involves tracking down the best external evidence with which to answer our clinical question.." In the case of the question proposed initially in this chapter, "Is group communication education effective in improving communication for people with acquired hearing loss?" an RCT will provide the most appropriate evidence to answer the question. If, however, the question was "What are the barriers and facilitators to participation in a group communication education program?" a qualitative research methodology would be most appropriate. Thomas et al. (2004) provide an example of a systematic review that addresses such a clinical question in relation to a different topic (i.e., barriers and facilitators to healthy eating in children) and combines qualitative and quantitative research.

EBP Step 4: Informing the Patient

After the clinical question has been developed, the evidence sought and appraised, the fourth and final step in the EBP process is to discuss the information gained from this approach with the patient. The aim is to provide the patient with sufficient information so that they can make an informed decision. This is not always as easy as it sounds and Irwin, Pannbacker, and Lass (2008) suggest methods for this such as decision aids, graphic representations of data, and quantitative translations of research evidence. In the case described at the start of this section, the issue was the effectiveness of group communication education for an adult with acquired hearing loss who is using hearing aids. It would be helpful and appropriate in this case for the clinician to summarize the systematic review on this topic by Hawkins (2005) and to also include the highest level of available evidence since that time, an RCT of a group program by Hickson et al. (2007). This study is described in more detail later in this chapter.

Limitations of EBP

Although EBP is a worthy aim, Kent (2006) in his paper discussing EBP in speech-language pathology and audiology reminds us that "EBP is very much a work in progress, not a polished perfection" (p. 268). Worrall and Bennett (2001) list some of the barriers to EBP for speech language pathologists and many are equally applicable to audiology. Possible barriers are: (1) access and ability to use data bases for searching the scientific literature, (2) the fact that not all relevant literature is in some databases, (3) a lack of evidence in some topic areas, (4) the level of evidence is not high in some areas, and (5) the evidence does not always match the reality of clinical services. This last point relates to the fact that participants included in research studies are often highly selected cases (e.g., inclusion criteria mean that they have no other impairments, English as a first language, are willing to participate in research, etc.) and the treatment regimes used in research may be unrealistic in clinical settings where resources are limited. Nevertheless, it is important to aspire to EBP in AR and the remainder of this chapter focuses on a review of the available evidence to date.

Research on Adult AR

The starting point for this review of the existing literature are two systematic reviews published in a special issue of the *Journal of the American Acad-*

emy of Audiology in 2005 (Hawkins, 2005; Sweetow & Palmer, 2005). The review by Hawkins (2005) was concerned with group AR programs for adults and the one by Sweetow and Palmer (2005) with individual auditory training for the same patient group.

Systematic Review of Group AR

Hawkins (2005) provides a systematic review of effectiveness of group adult AR programs that focus on counseling and communication strategies. Effectiveness was measured as benefits of AR over those obtained with hearing aids alone, benefits in adjustment to hearing loss, or reductions in perceived "handicap" (i.e., the psychosocial impact of hearing loss). Studies were included if they used an RCT or cohort design of some kind, an appropriate outcome measure that related to the dimensions of effectiveness and had been published in a peer-reviewed journal. A search of three major databases (ComDisDome, PubMed, and CINAHL) as well as articles referred to in textbooks and by experts in the field revealed 12 studies that met the inclusion criteria from 1988 to 2004.

Overall, the research was variable in nature with different research designs, different programs and different outcome measures and Hawkins comments on "the lack of well-designed experiments" (p. 488). There were eight RCTs and three cohort studies, and one case series. Half of the studies compared results for participants who received hearing aids only to those who had hearing aids followed by group AR. The intervention varied significantly in length from 4 weekly sessions to 8 to10 weekly sessions of 2 hours per week. The number of participants in individual studies was small, ranging from 10 per group to 53. A range of outcome measures was used, with the most common being self-report questionnaires about the psychosocial impact of hearing loss (e.g., Hearing Handicap Inventory for the Elderly; Ventry & Weinstein, 1982) or about the use of communication strategies (e.g., Communication Profile for the Hearing Impaired; Demorest & Erdman, 1987) and the majority of studies measured outcome immediately postprogram with no long term follow-up. Although research findings were positive in that significant reductions were found in handicap postprogram, Hawkins was validly critical of studies in this area because of the failure to use an appropriate combination of outcome measures that assessed all the hypothesized benefits of a particular group program, a lack of measurement of long-term benefit, and the small number of participants in many groups. He concluded that " . . . one does not see overwhelming evidence to support the benefits of group AR programs" (p. 490).

Hawkins (2005) singled out only two of the 12 studies as being of high quality, and both of these had US veterans as participants. Abrams, Chisolm, and McArdle (2002) used an RCT to compare 52 participants fitted with hearing aids only to 53 who had hearing aid fitting followed by 4 sessions (i.e., 8 hours) of an AR group. Those who attended the group program showed greater improvements in the mental component score of the Short-Form 36 quality of life scale (SF-36; Ware & Sherbourne, 1992) than those who received hearing aids only. Although the difference in treatment effects between the two groups was not statistically significant, the authors conducted a cost-benefit analysis and reported that hearing aid fitting plus AR was more cost-effective than hearing aid fitting alone.

Chisolm, Abrams, and McArdle (2004) used a similar RCT design to compare two groups of 53 participants; one group received hearing aid fitting only and the other hearing aid fitting followed by 4 2-hour group rehabilitation sessions. The participants who attended the group program had a significant short-term gain in communication strategy use and personal adjustment compared to those who had hearing aid fitting only; however, at the one-year follow-up there was no significant difference between participant groups.

Recent Research on Group AR

Since this systematic review, there have been two further experiments involving group AR programs that warrant inclusion as they both address many of Hawkins (2005) criticisms of the earlier research.

The first is a case series study (Level 4 Evidence) by Heydebrand, Mauze, Tye-Murray, Binzer, and Skinner (2005) and the second is an RCT by (Hickson et al., 2007). Heydebrand et al. evaluated a structured group therapy program for 33 adults with cochlear implants and significant others. The program consisted of a 2-day intensive workshop focusing on improving communication and coping skills. A range of outcomes was measured that were directly relevant to hypothesised program benefits in communication strategy use, personal adjustment, assertiveness, depression, and conversational fluency.

Communication strategy use and personal adjustment were assessed with the Communication Profile for the Hearing Impaired (Demorest & Erdman, 1987); assertiveness with the Rathus Assertiveness Scale (Rathus, 1973); and depression with the Depression, Anxiety and Stress Scale (Lovibond & Lovibond, 1995). Conversational fluency was assessed by analysing numbers of breakdowns in conversation in a 20-minute period. All measures were taken preprogram and then 3, 6, and 12 months later. Improvements were found immediately postprogram in levels of assertiveness, number of conversational breakdowns and some coping behaviors and these were maintained over time.

Subject variability was noted and Heydebrand et al. investigated this further by examining relationships between personality traits, as measured with the Temperament and Character Inventory (Cloninger, Svrakic, & Przybeck, 1993), and program success. Participants who were more energetic, outgoing, and optimistic became more assertive after the program and were less depressed. Participants who were more resourceful and goal directed became more effective and adaptive with communication behaviours. High levels of inter-subject variability in response to treatment is a characteristic of AR research and it is important to investigate variables that predict success, as Heydebrand et al. did, so that future treatments can be appropriately targeted. Although the study by Heydebrand and colleagues had many strengths, the authors acknowledge some limitations. A control group was not included, the subject numbers were quite small and there was no comparison to other forms of treatment (e.g., individual psychotherapy).

Hickson et al. (2007) included a control group in their evaluation of a group program for adults with hearing impairment, called Active Communication Education (ACE). The program was designed for adults with and without hearing aids, and significant others are encouraged to attend. It runs for 2 hours per week for 5 weeks, with its focus on facilitating the development of participants' problem solving skills to help in a range of communication situations. A double-blind RCT was used (Level 1b Evidence), with one group of participants undertaking a placebo social program ($n = 78$) initially prior to ACE and the other group ($n = 100$) undertaking ACE only (Figure 18–1). The placebo social program was included to control for the confounding effects of treatment contact. It involved the same amount of contact in a group setting as ACE and the same group facilitator ran both the ACE and the social programs. The researchers addressed many of the concerns expressed by Hawkins (2005) in that they included a range of outcome measures relevant to the hypothesised benefits of the program, outcomes were measured immediately postprogram and 6 months later, and the participant groups were appropriately large.

Outcome measures were all self-report and included two sets of measures: (1) those administered both pre and postprogram—the Hearing Handicap Questionnaire (Gatehouse & Noble, 2004), the Quantified Denver Scale of Communicative Function (Alpiner, Chevrette, Glascoe, Metz, & Olsen, 1974), the Self-Assessment of Communication (Schow & Nerbonne, 1982), the Ryff Psychological Well-Being Scale (Hoen, Thelander, & Worsley, 1997), the Short-Form 36 health-related quality of life measure (Ware & Sherbourne, 1992); and (2) those administered postprogram only—the Client-Oriented Scale of Improvement (Dillon, James, & Ginis, 1997), the International Outcome Inventory-Alternative Interventions (Noble, 2002), and a qualitative questionnaire. The relationships between participant response to the ACE program and a number of client-related factors were also investigated. These factors were the participants'

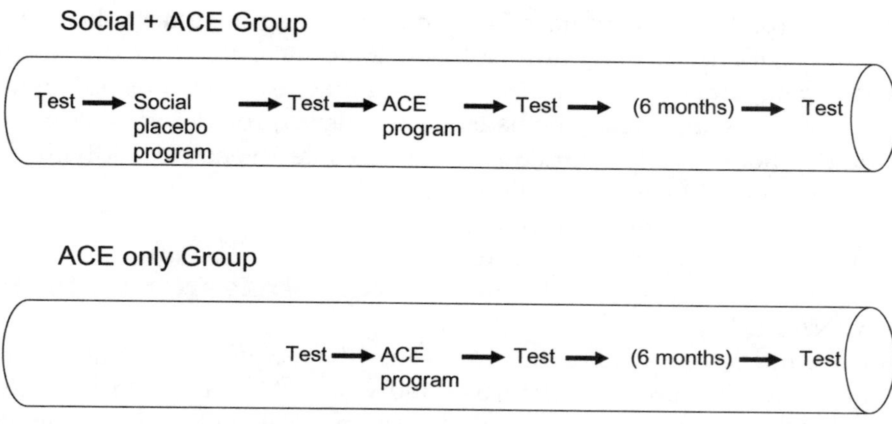

Figure 18–1. Research design used (Hickson et al., 2007) to evaluate the Active Communication Education (ACE) group program.

age, gender, hearing loss, hearing aid use, attitudes to hearing impairment (as measured using the Hearing Attitudes to Rehabilitation Questionnaire; Hallam & Brooks, 1996), and the involvement of significant others.

For those participants who completed the social program initially, significant improvements were found on the Quantified Denver Scale of Communicative Function and on the Mental Component Score of the Short-Form 36 only, when pre- and postprogram scores were compared. For those who completed the ACE program, there were significant pre-to-postimprovements on the Hearing Handicap Questionnaire, the Quantified Denver Scale of Communicative Function, the Self-Assessment of Communication, and the Ryff Psychological Well-Being Scale. These improvements following ACE were maintained at 6 months. Higher scores on the Hearing Attitudes to Rehabilitation Questionnaire prior to the ACE program were associated with greater positive change on a number of the pre-post program measures. Using the Client Oriented Scale of Improvement, 75% of participants reported some improvement on the primary goal they wished to achieve with the ACE. Positive outcomes were also recorded with the International Outcome Inventory-Alternative Interventions. Overall, these findings indicated that ACE was effective in reducing activity limitations and participation restrictions associated with hearing impairment and improving quality of life.

In summary, there is only a small body of high quality evidence to support group AR as an effective treatment for adults with hearing impairment. Although there have been nine RCTs, only one included a control group who received a program with the same amount of contact as the experimental program (Hickson et al., 2007). Likewise, the quality of many studies has been adversely affected by small participant numbers, the restricted range of outcome measures, and the fact that researchers conducting postprogram assessments are not blinded to preprogram results. Finally, another feature of these research evaluations that needs improvement is the description of the AR program itself. Programs differ in terms of content, structure and participants and it is not clear which approach is most effective for specific patients. Such evidence is critical for the clinician to be able to put EBP into practice in the clinic.

Systematic Review of Individual AR

In their systematic review, Sweetow and Palmer (2005) asked the question "Is there evidence of improvement in communication skills through individual auditory training in an adult hearing impaired populations?" (p. 986). The authors included studies of adults with hearing impairment who had received either analytic or synthetic auditory training or both combined, and who had been assessed using psychometrically sound outcome measures of some aspect of communication skills (e.g., speech perception, self-perceived communication ability). Studies of participants with cochlear implants were excluded. A specified term search of Medline, CINAHL, Psych Info, EMBASE, Applied Social Science Index, and Rehabilitation Literature Index identified six studies from 1970 to 1996 that met the inclusion criteria.

Of the six studies, three were RCTs with a comparison group that had received other kinds of training or no training, and three were case series. The number of participants in each study was small, ranging from 8 to 25, and all participants were hearing aid users. The type of training varied with two studies using analytic training, two using synthetic and two with a combination of analytic and synthetic. All studies included some kind of speech perception test as an outcome measure, but only two studies included a self-report questionnaire of hearing and communication (i.e., either Hearing Handicap Inventory for the Elderly or the Communication Profile for the Hearing Impaired). Thus, the research was variable in nature and pooling of findings across studies, which can form part of a systematic review, was not possible.

The two studies of analytic auditory training (Bode & Oyer, 1970; Walden, Erdman, Montgomery, Schwartz, & Prosek, 1981) found statistically significant improvements in speech perception with training; one of the synthetic training studies (Montgomery & Edge, 1988) found significant improvements on an auditory-visual speech test; and the two studies that employed a combination of training types (Kricos & Holmes, 1996; Rubinstein & Boothroyd, 1987) showed significant improvements in speech perception and self-perceived communication abilities, respectively. Sweetow and Palmer (2005) were critical of research to date for not providing information on the blinding of subjects or investigators, not including power calculations to determine appropriate sample sizes, not providing details of the treatment programs, not assessing long-term benefit and for using outcome measures that did not have published psychometric characteristics. They concluded that the review "provides very little evidence supporting the effectiveness of individual auditory training" (p. 501).

Recent Research on Individual AR

Since the review, additional research evidence for individual AR has come from Kramer, Allessie, Dondorp, Zekveld, and Kapteyn (2005), Sweetow and Sabes (2006), and Burk and Humes (2007). Each of these studies evaluates quite distinct forms of training in different ways, and as such make unique contributions to EBP in this area. Both Kramer et al. (2005) and Sweetow and Sabes (2006) have developed programs for home use by patients, a trend that has been driven by the fact that the uptake of AR in clinics has not been high, most probably because of concerns over cost-effectiveness. Kramer et al. (2005) evaluated a home education video program about communication strategies and lipreading for older adults with hearing impairment and their significant others. The program is in Dutch and consists of a total of five videotapes with an instruction booklet. Each video has a short film of an everyday situation (e.g., conversation at home, visit to a doctor, group meeting), some speechreading exercises and a demonstration of how speech sounds for a person with hearing impairment with and without hearing aids. The stated aim of the program is "to raise problem awareness for both the affected individual and the significant other, to enhance communication and to provide knowledge about the nature and consequences of hearing loss" (p. 256). The videos progressively increase in difficulty and participants do not receive the next video until they have returned the previous one. On average, participants took 11 weeks to complete the program.

Kramer et al.'s (2005) study was an RCT (Level 1b Evidence) in which participants were randomly allocated to one of two groups: a training group ($n = 24$) who received hearing aid fitting followed by the home education program and a control group ($n = 24$) who had hearing aid fitting only. A percentage of participants in both groups had previously worn hearing aids (50% of the training group and 63% of the control group). The authors used a range of outcome measures, and only those found to be associated with significant program change are discussed here. First, a self-report questionnaire, containing 8 items about the emotional response to hearing impairment and the use of communication strategies, was mailed to participants to complete prior to rehabilitation, immediately postrehabilitation and then 6 months after that. The results showed that the training group significantly improved their use of communication strategies postprogram and the control group did not. This improvement for the training group was maintained at the 6-month follow-up. Second, participants in the training group completed the International Outcome Inventory-Alternative Interventions (Noble, 2002) immediately postrehabilitation and at the 6-month follow-up, whereas those in the control group completed the International Outcome Inventory-Hearing Aids (Cox & Alexander, 2002). The training group showed significant improvement over time on two items (satisfaction and quality of life), whereas scores on these two items decreased over time for those in the control group. This suggests that the benefits of AR may accrue with time and highlight the importance of measuring longer term outcomes.

One of the difficulties with evaluating the evidence in this study by Kramer et al. (2005) is the confounding variable of previous hearing aid use. The effects of interventions differed for first time and experienced aid users and it was not possible in such a small study to make definitive conclusions about the effectiveness of the program for both groups. A number of participants who were experienced hearing aid users complained that the material in the home education program was not appropriate for them. This indicates that the program would best be targeted at new patients and an RCT including only these participants is recommended.

Another quite different home-based AR program, called Listening and Communication Enhancement or LACE (refer to Chapter 12 in this text for further information on LACE), has been developed and evaluated with experienced hearing aid users by Sweetow and Sabes (2006). LACE is an interactive and adaptive computer program for adults with hearing impairment with a focus on "better comprehension of degraded speech, enhancement of cognitive skills, and improvement of communication strategies" (p. 243). Participation involves trainings for 30 minutes per day for 5 days per week for 4 weeks (10 hours total). The program materials consist of three different types of degraded speech (time compressed speech, speech with a multitalker babble background, speech with a single competing speaker background), two different types of cognitive training exercises (auditory memory, processing speed), and hints for successful use of communication strategies. The listening exercises are adaptive, in that if the patient gives a correct response subsequent tasks increase in difficulty, and if they give an incorrect response, tasks become easier.

LACE has been evaluated using an RCT (Level 1b Evidence) in which 71 experienced adult hearing aid users were randomly allocated to one of two groups. One group ($n = 38$) received immediate LACE training and were assessed pre-intervention, immediately post-intervention and 4 weeks later. The other group ($n = 33$) received delayed LACE training. They were tested, then received no intervention for 4 weeks before being retested. After that, they began LACE and the testing protocol was the same as for the immediate LACE group. The period in which this group received no training served as the control condition. The researchers used a number of outcome measures: two tests of speech perception in noise (Quick Speech-in-Noise test, Killion, Niquette, Gudmundsen, Revit, & Banerjee, 2004; Hearing-in-Noise Test, Nilsson, Soli, & Sullivan, 1994), and two self-report measures (Hearing Handicap Inventory for the Elderly, Ventry & Weinstein, 1982; Communication Scale for Older Adults, Kaplan, Bally, Brandt, Busacco, & Pray, 1997). The difference between pre-post scores for the period of no intervention ($n = 33$ patients) was compared to the difference in pre-post scores for LACE ($n = 71$ patients). With the exception of one of the speech tests in noise (Hearing-in-Noise Test), all of the other outcome measures showed no change in the control condition and significant improvements with LACE. Although test results for all participants were not reported for the 4 week post-LACE assessment, the authors provide some preliminary results that indicate that the improvements obtained were maintained.

Overall, this study makes an important contribution to the evidence base for AR; however, there are some limitations that should be acknowledged. The authors themselves point out that the participants may not be representative of the population of adult hearing aid users. People attracted to participate in this research may be more positive and active than the general population and may have higher levels of computer use. In addition, the authors stress the need to measure outcomes long term, up to 12 months postintervention. There are two additional limitations that should be mentioned. First, the small sample size in the control condition compared to the treatment condition may explain why there were no effects during the waiting period and significant effects during the training period. Effect sizes for AR are typically small (e.g., .06 to .36 in Hickson et al., 2007 and .23 to .4 in Sweetow & Sabes, 2006) and larger participant groups are needed to show significant treatment effects. The evidence for LACE would be strengthened if a larger no-treatment group was compared to a similarly sized treatment group. Second, the fact that LACE is made up of a number of different types of training (degraded speech, cognitive skills, communication strategies) means that it is not possible to determine which aspect of the program is associated with the intervention effects. A study in which the different types of training are evaluated in isolation and in combination would provide potentially valuable evidence about the most effective treatment approach.

All of the AR research described thus far has been applied in nature, with evaluations of different forms of developed interventions with different populations. It is important to point out that evidence from more basic research may inform EBP in AR and the recent study by Burk and Humes (2007) is included as an example. In their study, both young normal-hearing (n = 16) and older hearing-impaired people (n = 7) were trained in a laboratory setting on 75 monosyllabic words over a 9- to 14-day period. All words used in training were spoken by the same female talker and participants' speech scores for this familiar talker were measured pre and post-training. In addition, performance on the trained words with the familiar talker was compared to performance for three other conditions: (1) the same words with three new unfamiliar talkers; (2) different words spoken by both familiar and unfamiliar talkers; and (3) the same words embedded in sentences. The aim of the research was to determine if word-based analytic auditory training using a single familiar speaker and a single set of trained words could improve word recognition for different speakers and on different sets of words. This issue of generalizability of training effects is highly relevant to AR.

The study findings were that both young and old participants performed significantly better on the trained words than the untrained words presented by the same talker. There were some small but significant improvements on the untrained words, but the improvements were not as great as for the trained words. On the positive side, improvements on the trained words were evident across different speakers and were maintained at a 6-month follow-up. Results indicate that the learning that is occurring is lexically rather than acoustically based. On the negative side, when the trained words were put in sentences (rather than tested in isolation), there was no difference in performance for trained and untrained words. The authors describe this research as "a preliminary step in the design of word-based training that ultimately could be produced as either a standardized or individually tailored training protocol" (p. 277), and their systematic evidence-based approach to developing such training is to be applauded.

Summary of AR Research

Systematic reviews of group and individual AR completed in 2005 highlighted the need for additional well-designed research to address the many questions likely to arise in a clinical setting (Hawkins, 2005; Sweetow & Palmer, 2005). Both groups of authors called for more larger scale RCTs that include blinding of participants and researchers, multiple outcome measures, and the assessment of long-term benefit. Since that time, some studies of this kind have appeared and they make an important contribution to the body of evidence. The RCT by Sweetow and Sabes (2006) using a computerized interactive individual AR program and the one by Hickson et al. (2007) using a group communication education program both identify positive benefits of AR for adults. Thus, although AR has been one of the cornerstones of audiology since the profession began, there is relatively limited high quality research evidence to support its use. Boothroyd (2007) concluded that "There is a pressing need for increased research effort—and for the training of clinical researchers to carry it out" (p. 69).

New Directions in Adult AR Research

Opportunities abound for future research on adult AR. Clearly, it is not possible at this point in time to conduct a systematic review of RCTs (Level 1a Evidence) as there are not sufficient studies of this kind. Therefore, a first step is for the systematic evaluation of different approaches to AR using RCTs. Studies need to be scientifically rigorous and adhere to the principles espoused in the Consort Statement (www.consort-statement.org). In addition, it is vital that researchers provide extensive detail about the content and nature of the rehabilitation program itself. AR is not a single entity and there are many possible types of interventions and combinations of interventions, which is clear from the studies reviewed in this chapter. If a treatment program uses more than one approach it would be useful to investigate which aspects of the program are most beneficial. For example, in the LACE program, what are the effects of the auditory exercises and/or the cognitive tasks and/or the communication strategy training? This information may well lead to better targeting of program content.

Another related question is what are the characteristics of participants who benefit from particular interventions? In this chapter, some treatments included only those with amplification (Chisolm et al., 2004; Heydebrand et al., 2005; Kramer et al., 2005; Sweetow & Sabes, 2006), whereas Hickson et al. (2006, 2007) included people with and without hearing aids. It is likely that different people will benefit from different types of interventions, depending on their communication difficulties and their goals for rehabilitation. Consideration could be given to conducting a "patient preference trial" which is a type of clinical trial where participants are first asked if they want to be randomized or not. If the answer is yes, they are randomized to the treatment options. If the answer is no, they are then asked for their treatment preference and they proceed with that treatment. It is possible then to compare the randomized and the preferred groups and to measure the preference effect, which is the difference in outcome for those who chose a particular intervention compared to those who were randomly allocated to it (McPherson, Britton, & Wennberg, 1997; Wingham, Dalal, Sweeney, & Evans, 2006). Such an approach recognizes the relationship between outcomes and a person's motivation, that is, people who are more motivated to try a particular intervention are more likely to achieve better results. This is certainly the case with hearing aid fitting (Brooks & Hallam, 1998; Hickson, Hamilton, & Orange, 1986; Hickson et al., 1999).

Effect sizes for AR interventions are typically in the low range, and an issue related to this that warrants further research is whether more appropriate outcome tools could be developed. Such measures may be more sensitive to the effects of the treatment being undertaken. The vast majority of the measures used in research to date were developed to evaluate the efficacy of hearing aid fitting (e.g., Hearing Handicap Inventory for the Elderly, Ventry & Weinstein, 1982; Communication Profile for the Hearing Impaired, Demorest & Erdman, 1987). They may therefore have more of a focus on hearing per se, rather than communication. The stated aim of AR is typically to improve a person's communication ability and not to improve their hearing, whereas the opposite is true of hearing aid fitting. Another useful approach for measuring outcomes that could be applied in aural rehabilitation is the inclusion of individualized measures such as the Client Oriented Scale of Improvement (Dillon et al., 1997). Although they include individual goals, the results can be aggregated to provide group data (Gagné, McDuff, & Getty, 1999).

Finally, a key component of EBP is the relaying of research information to patients so that they can make informed decisions. In audiology, little work has been done around developing appropriate processes and tools for this purpose. Sidani, Epstein, and Miranda (2006) describe a "patient-centred evidence-based" approach which consists of (1) identifying alternative treatment options on the basis of the best evidence available, (2) consulting with the patient to elicit their preference among the options, and (3) accounting for patients' preference in providing treatment (p. 118). The authors point out that patients' preferences are heavily influenced by the information that they are given. This information is in the form of written material (e.g., pamphlets, books), media (e.g., newspapers, Internet), verbal discussion with health professionals, family and friends, and/or personal experience. Decision aids can be developed to facilitate this provision of information and to encourage patients to express their treatment preferences (Charles, Gafni, Whelan, & O'Brien, 2005). Development and evaluation of decision aids is a priority for future AR research.

References

Abrams, H., Chisolm, T. H., & McArdle, R. (2002). A cost-utility analysis of adult group audiologic rehabilitation: Are the benefits worth the cost? *Journal of Rehabilitation Research and Development*, *39*(5), 549–557.

Abrams, H. B., Hnath-Chisolm, T., Guerreiro, S. M., & Ritterman, S. I. (1992). The effects of intervention strategy on self-perception of hearing handicap. *Ear and Hearing*, *13*(5), 371–377.

Alpiner, J. G., Chevrette, W., Glascoe, G., Metz, M., & Olsen, B. (1974). *The Denver Scale of Communicative Function*. Denver, Co: University of Denver.

Bode, D. L., & Oyer, H. J. (1970). Auditory training and speech discrimination. *Journal of Speech and Hearing Research*, *13*(4), 839–855.

Boothroyd, A. (2007). Adult aural rehabilitation: What is it and does it work? *Trends in Amplification*, *11*(2), 63–71.

Brooks, D. N., & Hallam, R. S. (1998). Attitudes to hearing difficulty and hearing aids and the outcome of audiological rehabilitation. *British Journal of Audiology*, *32*, 217–226.

Burk, M. H., & Humes, L. E. (2007). Effects of training on speech recognition performance in noise using lexically hard words. *Journal of Speech Language and Hearing Research*, *50*(1), 25–40.

Charles, C., Gafni, A., Whelan, T., & O'Brien, M. A. (2005). Treatment decision aids: Conceptual issues and future directions. *Health Expectations*, *8*(2), 114–125.

Chisolm, T. H., Abrams, H. B., & McArdle, R. (2004). Short- and long-term outcomes of adult audiological rehabilitation. *Ear and Hearing*, *25*(5), 464–477.

Cloninger, C. R., Svrakic, D. M., & Przybeck, T. R. (1993). A psychobiological model of temperament and character. *Archives of General Psychiatry*, *50*(12), 975–990.

Cox, R. M. (2005). Evidence-based practice in provision of amplification. *Journal of the American Academy of Audiology*, *16*(7), 419–438.

Cox, R. M., & Alexander, G. C. (2002). The International Outcome Inventory for Hearing Aids (IOI-HA): Psychometric properties of the English version. *International Journal of Audiology*, *41*(1), 30–35.

Demorest, M. E., & Erdman, S. (1987). Development of the communication profile for the hearing impaired. *Journal of Speech and Hearing Disorders*, *52*, 129–143.

Dillon, H., James, A., & Ginis, J. (1997). Client Oriented Scale of Improvement (COSI) and its relationship to several other measures of benefit and satisfaction provided by hearing aids. *Journal of the American Academy of Audiology*, *8*(1), 27–43.

Gagné, J.-P., McDuff, S., & Getty, L. (1999). Some limitations of evaluative investigations based solely on normed outcome measures. *Journal of American Academy of Audiology*, *10*, 46–62.

Gatehouse, S., & Noble, W. (2004). The Speech, Spatial and Qualities of Hearing Scale (SSQ). *International Journal of Audiology*, *43*(2), 85–99.

Hallam, R. S., & Brooks, D. N. (1996). Development of the Hearing Attitudes in Rehabilitation Questionnaire (HARQ). *British Journal of Audiology, 30*, 199–213.

Hawkins, D. B. (2005). Effectiveness of counseling-based adult group aural rehabilitation programs: A systematic review of the evidence. *Journal of the American Academy of Audiology, 16*(7), 485–493.

Heydebrand, G., Mauze, E., Tye-Murray, N., Binzer, S., & Skinner, M. (2005). The efficacy of a structured group therapy intervention in improving communication and coping skills for adult cochlear implant recipients. *International Journal of Audiology, 44*(5), 272–280.

Hickson, L., Hamilton, L., & Orange, S. P. (1986). Factors associated with hearing aid use. *Australian Journal of Audiology, 8*, 37–41.

Hickson, L., Timm, M., Worrall, L., & Bishop, K. (1999). Hearing aid fitting: Outcomes for older adults. *Australian Journal of Audiology, 21*(1), 9–21.

Hickson, L., Worrall, L., & Scarinci, N. (2006). Measuring outcomes of a communication program for older people with hearing impairment using the International Outcome Inventory. *International Journal of Audiology, 45*(4), 238–246.

Hickson, L., Worrall, L., & Scarinci, N. (2007). A randomized controlled trial evaluating the Active Communication Education program for older people with hearing impairment. *Ear and Hearing, 28*(2), 212–230.

Hoen, B., Thelander, M., & Worsley, J. (1997). Improvement in psychological well-being of people with aphasia and their families: Evaluation of a community-based programme. *Aphasiology, 11*(7), 681–691.

Irwin, D., Pannbacker, M. H., & Lass, N. J. (2008). *Clinical research methods in speech-language pathology and audiology*. San Diego, CA: Plural.

Kaplan, H., Bally, S., Brandt, F., Busacco, D., & Pray, J. (1997). Communication Scale for Older Adults (CSOA). *Journal of the American Academy of Audiology, 8*(3), 203–217.

Kent, R. D. (2006). Evidence-based practice in communication disorders: Progress not perfection. *Language, Speech and Hearing Services in Schools, 37*(4), 268–270.

Killion, M. C., Niquette, P. A., Gudmundsen, G. I., Revit, L. J., & Banerjee, S. (2004). Development of a quick speech-in-noise test for measuring signal-to-noise ratio loss in normal-hearing and hearing-impaired listeners. *Journal of the Acoustical Society of America, 116*(4 Pt. 1), 2395–2405.

Kramer, S. E., Allessie, G. H., Dondorp, A. W., Zekveld, A. A., & Kapteyn, T. S. (2005). A home education program for older adults with hearing impairment and their significant others: A randomized trial evaluating short- and long-term effects. *International Journal of Audiology, 44*(5), 255–264.

Kricos, P. B., & Holmes, A. E. (1996). Efficacy of audiologic rehabilitation for older adults. *Journal of the American Academy of Audiology, 7*(4), 219–229.

Lovibond, S. H., & Lovibond, P. F. (1995). *Manual for the Depression Anxiety Stress Scales*. Sydney, NSW: Psychology Foundation of Australia.

McPherson, K., Britton, A. R., & Wennberg, J. E. (1997). Are randomized controlled trials controlled? Patient preferences and unblind trials. *Journal of the Royal Society of Medicine, 90*(12), 652–656.

Montgomery, A. A., & Edge, R. A. (1988). Evaluation of two speech enhancement techniques to improve intelligibility for hearing-impaired adults. *Journal of Speech and Hearing Research, 31*(3), 386–393.

Nilsson, M., Soli, S. D., & Sullivan, J. A. (1994). Development of the Hearing-in-Noise Test for the measurement of speech reception thresholds in quiet and in noise. *Journal of the Acoustical Society of America, 95*(2), 1085–1099.

Noble, W. (2002). Extending the IOI to significant others and to non-hearing-aid-based interventions. *International Journal of Audiology, 41*(1), 27–29.

Norman, M., George, C. R., Downie, A., & Milligan, J. (1995). Evaluation of a communication course for new hearing aid users. *Scandinavian Audiology, 24*(1), 63–69.

Rathus, S. A. (1973). A 30-item schedule for assessing assertive behavior. *Behaviour Therapy, 4*, 398–406.

Rubinstein, A., & Boothroyd, A. (1987). Effect of two approaches to auditory training on speech recognition by hearing-impaired adults. *Journal of Speech and Hearing Research, 30*(2), 153–160.

Sackett, D. L., Rosenberg, W. M., Gray, J. A., Haynes, R. B., & Richardson, W. S. (1996). Evidence based medicine: What it is and what it isn't. *British Medical Journal, 312*(7023), 71–72.

Schow, R. L., & Nerbonne, M. A. (1982). Communication screening profile; use with elderly clients. *Ear and Hearing, 3*, 135–147.

Sidani, S., Epstein, D., & Miranda, J. (2006). Eliciting patient treatment preferences: A strategy to integrate evidence-based and patient-centered care. *Worldviews on Evidenced-Based Nursing, 3*(3), 116–123.

Straus, S. E., Richardson, W. S., Glasziou, P., & Haynes, R. B. (2005). *Evidence-based Medicine: How to practice and teach EBM* (3rd ed.). Edinburgh; New York: Elsevier/Churchill Livingstone.

Swan, I. R., & Gatehouse, S. (1990). Factors influencing consultation for management of hearing disability. *British Journal of Audiology, 24*(3), 155–160.

Sweetow, R., & Palmer, C. V. (2005). Efficacy of individual auditory training in adults: a systematic review of the evidence. *Journal of the American Academy of Audiology, 16*(7), 494–504.

Sweetow, R. W., & Sabes, J. H. (2006). The need for and development of an adaptive Listening and Communication Enhancement (LACE) Program. *Journal of the American Academy of Audiology, 17*(8), 538–558.

Thomas, J., Harden, A., Oakley, A., Oliver, S., Sutcliffe, K., Rees, R., et al. (2004). Integrating qualitative research with trials in systematic reviews. *British Medical Journal, 328*(7446), 1010–1012.

Ventry, I. M., & Weinstein, B. E. (1982). The Hearing Handicap Inventory for the Elderly: A new tool. *Ear and Hearing, 3*(3), 128–134.

Walden, B. E., Erdman, S. A., Montgomery, A. A., Schwartz, D. M., & Prosek, R. A. (1981). Some effects of training on speech recognition by hearing-impaired adults. *Journal of Speech and Hearing Research, 24*(2), 207–216.

Ware, J. E., & Sherbourne, C. D. (1992). The MOS 36-item short-form health survey (SF-36). I. Conceptual framework and item selection. *Medical Care, 30*(6), 473–483.

Wingham, J., Dalal, H. M., Sweeney, K. G., & Evans, P. H. (2006). Listening to patients: choice in cardiac rehabilitation. *European Journal of Cardiovascular Nursing, 5*(4), 289–294.

Wood, S. A., & Lutman, M. E. (2004). Relative benefits of linear analogue and advanced digital hearing aids. *International Journal of Audiology, 43*(3), 144–155.

Worrall, L. E., & Bennett, S. (2001). Evidence-based practice: Barriers and facilitators for speech-language pathologists. *Journal of Medical Speech-Language Pathology, 9*(2), xi–xvi.

19

Audiologic Rehabilitation for Older Adults

Patricia B. Kricos

The number of older Americans is increasing rapidly, with the fastest growing age group being individuals 85 years and older (U.S. Department of Health and Human Services, 2003). The predicted increase in the number of older adults with hearing loss, many of whom will have significant hearing impairments, will have a major impact on the profession of audiology and its service delivery models. Untreated hearing loss in elders may severely compromise their quality of life (Bagai, Thavendiranathan, & Detsky, 2006; National Council on Aging (NCOA), 1999) and audiologists can play an important role in ensuring quality of life for the senior population. To serve this population appropriately, it is critical that audiologists understand the special hearing health care needs of older adults. This chapter addresses the unique characteristics and needs of the older adult population and offers guidelines to provide effective treatment for elders who are challenged by hearing loss. These challenges include sensory aid prefitting concerns, such as lack of awareness of hearing problems and readiness for amplification; unique issues to be addressed during the hearing device fitting, such as increased likelihood of cognitive and/or psychoacoustic auditory processing components to the listening difficulties, as well as manual dexterity compromises, memory changes, and sensory difficulties beyond hearing loss (e.g., touch and vision). A comprehensive model of audiologic management is needed to assist older adults with their hearing problems.

Theories of Aging

Theories of aging related to progressive changes in physical and sensory characteristics abound. Attempts to answer the question "Why do we age?" have been made by biologists, physiologists, epidemiologists, and other bioscientists. According to one popular set of explanations referred to as "programmed theories," biological clocks are genetically programmed to follow a timetable that includes decline in maintenance, defense, and repair mechanisms (Weinert & Timiras, 2003). In contrast, "error theories" hold environmental assaults on the living organism responsible for cell damage, physical deterioration, and ultimately death. Although the causes of aging are not completely defined, the characteristics of aging have been documented and described in detail. Troen (2003) identifies five major characteristics of aging, including increased mortality after maturation, changes in biochemical composition in tissues, progressive decrease in physiologic capacity, reduced ability to respond adaptively to environmental stimuli, and increased susceptibility and vulnerability to disease.

Sources of Listening Difficulties for Older Adults

In order to provide effective audiologic treatment to help older adults manage their hearing losses, it is important to understand the sources of their communication challenges. Although the hearing loss itself obviously plays a huge role in the everyday communication dilemmas experienced by older adults with hearing impairments, a number of other sources can also negatively impact listening abilities. The contributions of peripheral and central hearing loss are discussed, as well as potential cognitive and visual speech perception compromises that may affect communication success.

The Aging Ear

There are a number of age-related changes in the auditory mechanism, including changes in the outer, middle, and inner ears (Chisolm, Willott, & Lister, 2003; Kricos, 1995). Of primary interest for considerations related to management of hearing difficulties for older adults are the age-related changes in the inner ear, first observed and described by Schuknecht (1955), who called these changes *presbycusis*. Although Schuknecht described four age-related patterns of presbycusis, the most common characteristic of presbycusis is a gradually sloping, high-frequency hearing loss that is bilateral and symmetric (Kricos, 1995) and results in decreased speech understanding, particularly in noisy environments. In the past few decades, researchers have tried to identify the origin of the speech recognition difficulties that older individuals experience in adverse conditions. Humes (1996) suggested that decreased hearing sensitivity accounts for much of the difficulty experienced by older adults, and in his more recent research (Humes, 2002, 2007), he has implicated both speech audibility and cognitive factors as major contributors to their speech recognition. Other researchers have identified central auditory system deterioration as a major contributor to the speech understanding problems of older adults (Craik, 2007; Jerger, Chmiel, Allen, & Wilson, 1994), whereas still others attribute much of the difficulty to cognitive dysfunction (van Rooij & Plomp, 1990). As Jerger (2006) points out, it is likely that a complex interaction of audibility deficits, central auditory processing compromises, and cognitive contributions is responsible for the speech perception difficulties of older individuals.

Potential Cognitive Effects on the Older Adult's Listening Difficulties

In recent years, researchers have delineated a number of ways that cognitive processing may contribute to the listening difficulties of older adults. Although many aspects of cognition are unperturbed by aging, others may decline with age. These include information processing speed, divided attention skills, ability to switch rapidly between multiple auditory inputs, sustained attention, selective attention, and working memory (Hooyman & Kiyak, 2005). Pichora-Fuller and Singh (2006) and Kricos (2006) have described how normal age-related changes in cognition, such as working memory, attention, and speed of processing, may contribute to everyday listening challenges of older adults. In challenging listening environments, for example, highly reverberant and noisy rooms, the reception of auditory information may be compromised because central cognitive resources are reallocated to support auditory processing. In turn, this may lessen the availability of cognitive resources for storage and retrieval functions of working memory (Larsby, Hällgren, Lyxell, & Arlinger, 2005; Tun, O'Kane, & Wingfield, 2002). In a situation in which the older adult is trying to understand a talker while also trying to ignore a nearby competing voice, there may be an increased load on attentional control, due to divided attention at the cognitive level (Tun et al., 2002). These may place a substantial demand on executive function, the working memory component responsible for scheduling, organizing, and allocating resources for attending to ongoing activities. Given the greater speech recognition problems, slower speed of processing, as well as other normal age-related cognitive abilities, it is not surprising that many older adults report feeling tired after communicating in noisy settings such as church halls or restaurants.

Auditory-Visual Speech Perception by Older Adults

For well over 50 years there has been research evidence regarding the usefulness of visual speech cues when individuals with normal hearing are trying to understand talkers in difficult listening situations (Kim & Grant, 2004; Sumby & Pollack, 1954). Thus, one could reasonably expect that older adults with hearing loss might benefit substantially from the visual cues of speech through lipreading. However, the findings of Tye-Murray and her coauthors (2005) regarding aging and audiovisual speech perception somewhat dampen expectations for how much assistance lipreading cues will provide to older adults with hearing impairments. These researchers conducted a set of coordinated investigations to study speechreading and aging, with their initial findings indicating that older adults did not benefit as much as younger adults from the addition of visual speech information. They then compared visual-only speech perception and found that older adults were poorer lipreaders than the younger research participants. Finally, they found slight but significant deficiencies in the older adults' abilities to integrate the auditory and visual cues of speech. As a result of their overall findings, Tye-Murray et al. recommend the inclusion of tests that assess both lipreading and audiovisual integration abilities during audiologic evaluations of older adults.

Factors Affecting the Audiologic Rehabilitation (AR) Needs and Outcomes of Older Adults

Many of the treatment protocols described in this book are relevant for older adults and should be applied to help this population reduce the effects of hearing loss on communication, lifestyle, and quality of life. However, there are several factors in particular that may affect the AR needs of older adults, and these should be considered when planning the treatment program for this population. Smith, Kricos, and Holmes (2001), as well as Smith and Kricos (2002) describe a number of ways that age may impact AR needs and outcomes, including vision problems, reduced manual dexterity, and the cognitive compromises described earlier in this chapter. Additionally, unlike most younger adults with hearing loss, older adults may have an auditory processing deficit in addition to their hearing losses, making speech recognition, particularly in noise, even more difficult (Kricos, 1995; Woods & Yund, 2007).

Manual Dexterity and Tactile Sense Compromises with Age

Many older adults have reduced manual dexterity and reduced tactile sensations, making the handling and placement of sensory aids and batteries particularly challenging. The term sensory aids may include hearing aids, assistive listening devices, and cochlear implants. Throughout this chapter, hearing aids are used as an example of the broader category of sensory aids. A patient with Parkinson's disease, for example, may have unsteady control of the arms, making it difficult to place the hearing aid in the ear. Similarly, a patient with arthritis may find if difficult to insert the hearing aid battery.

Vision Impairment in Older Adults

It is estimated that approximately 21% of older adults have both hearing and vision loss by the time they reach 70 years of age (Berry, Mascia, & Steinman, 2004; Brabyn, Schneck, Haegerstrom-Portnoy, & Lott, 2007). As the population ages, this number will increase dramatically. The impact of dual sensory loss is assumed to be greater than the sum of the impacts of visual impairment or hearing impairment alone because the individual cannot use compensatory strategies or redundancies in information that are available to individuals with single sensory impairment. Whereas many older adults with hearing loss can compensate, at least to some degree, for the loss of auditory information by using lipreading cues, facial expressions, written rehabilitation materials, captioning, and visual alerting systems, the individual with dual sensory loss cannot, at least to the same extent. When the older patient has a dual sensory loss involving poor audition and vision, care in selection of appropriate hearing aids must be taken. Brennan (2003) cited several studies in which functionality of individuals with vision impairment alone was compared to individuals who had both hearing and vision loss. He reported significant differences between these two populations in functional ability, such as managing medications, preparing meals, shopping, and using a telephone. The differences between the 2 groups magnified as the degree of the vision loss increased.

Central Auditory Processing Effects

If the older patient's pure tone thresholds and word recognition in quiet appear to be fairly good, but the patient complains of listening difficulties, word recognition in noise should be evaluated. Schneider, Daneman, and Murphy (2005) reported that older individuals with clinically non-significant hearing losses may need signal-to-noise ratios (SNRs) that are three to five dB higher than the SNR needed by young adults in order to asymptote in speech understanding. Because an auditory processing disorder (APD) typically results in difficulties understanding speech in noisy settings, speech-in-noise tests such as the Quick SIN (Etymotic Research, 2001) may be useful, both as pre- and postintervention measures. Strouse and Wilson (2000) suggest a number of advantages of using dichotic digit materials to determine auditory processing disorders in older adults, including the relative immunity of the digit stimuli to the effects of cochlear hearing impairment, high inter-test reliability, and the fact that digit stimuli generally are familiar to most listeners. Strecker and Dancer (2005) argue for APD screening to be included as part of the routine audiologic evaluation for older adults. They point out that patients will benefit from more appropriate recommendations and more realistic expectations for assistance from hearing aids, and thus be more satisfied with their hearing aids and with the professional services of audiologists.

Influence of Living Environments on Participation in Rehabilitation

When older adults are queried regarding their housing preferences and living arrangements, in all likelihood they will respond with a statement such as, "Right here in the house I've lived in for the past 45 years!" The "aging in place" concept has received considerable attention in communities throughout the United States, and with improvements in community transportation and home services for older citizens, the likelihood that they can remain in their own homes appears to be increasing. For those individuals who do not have the resources to live independently in their own residences, there are a number of options. One of the growing trends in senior housing is continuum-of-care facilities. This term refers to facilities and communities that offer the full continuum of care from independent living to assisted living, to skilled nursing care. According to government statistics, in the year 2000, less than 5% of the population 65 years plus lived in nursing homes (U.S. Department of Health and Human Services, 2006).

There is a myriad of ways that the living arrangements of older adults could affect participation in the AR program. If the individual lives alone, does not have family or community assistance to help with transportation, and either cannot drive or does not like to drive unless absolutely necessary, there may be difficulties in providing a treatment program that requires a number of visits. If the individual lives in an assisted living facility or nursing home, there may be complications in scheduling treatment sessions so they do not conflict with other facility activities. In a large continuum-of-care facility where the author at one time provided services, it was always a challenge to schedule hearing screenings and AR support programs around line dancing, water aerobics, book clubs, political action meetings, and other activities.

In terms of residential living with support, as well as institutional care, Gatehouse (2003) wisely pointed out that characteristics of the environment, particularly the acoustic environment, should be considered. A part of the treatment program should be to attempt to improve the signal-to-noise ratio in whatever ways are feasible, thus providing benefit not only to the resident with the hearing loss, but also to the caregivers, who often must repeat and rephrase their comments so that they are understood. Gatehouse recommends paying attention not only to room acoustics but also to the visual environment and the use of assistive technology in institutional settings.

Implications of Hearing Loss for Older Adults

Communication is essential for the older adult's well being, quality of life, independence, physical and mental health, and safety. The sensorineural hearing loss experienced by older adults may have dramatic effects on communication and psychosocial function. Weinstein (2000) described the potential consequences of hearing loss experienced by older adults. These include:

1. Altered psychosocial behavior
2. Strained family relations
3. Limited enjoyment of daily activities
4. Jeopardized physical well–being
5. Interference with the ability to live independently and safely
6. Interference with long-distance contacts on the telephone, potentially jeopardizing safety and security
7. Interference with medical diagnosis, treatment, and management.

Effects of Untreated Hearing Loss

The negative effects of untreated hearing loss on older individuals have been well documented. These include communication difficulties (Arlinger, 2003), compromised well-being and quality of life (Carabellese, Appollonio, & Rozzini, 1993; Mulrow, Tuley, & Aguilar, 1992; National Council, on Aging, 1999; Wallhagen, Strawbridge, Shema et al., 2004), cognitive function (Cacciatore, Napoli, & Abete, 1999), social interactions (Jang, Mortimer, Haley, Small, Chisolm, & Graves, 2003; Resnick, Fries, & Verbrugge, 1997), and deterioration of speech perception skills in unaided ears owing to auditory deprivation (Arlinger, 2003; Gelfand, 1995; Silman, Gelfand, & Silverman, 1984). Audiologic management such as dispensing of hearing aids and provision of counseling is critical to avoid the deleterious effects of untreated hearing loss.

Rowe and Kahn (1997), in their model of successful aging, described the three key determinants of successful aging as avoidance of disease and disability, high cognitive and physical function, and involvement in society. Clearly the ability to hear and communicate effectively would figure strongly in all three of these domains. Thus, AR for older adults with hearing loss is critically important to ensure the successful aging.

AR for Older Adults

A comprehensive model of audiologic management, one designed to help older adults deal more effectively with their hearing difficulties, is needed. AR is not just something to be tacked on after the fitting of hearing aids. In addition to consideration of decisional factors for selecting hearing aids and other assistive technology that are appropriate for older individuals, there should be prefitting education and counseling, as well as postfitting AR programming such as clear speech training, control of the listening environment, and auditory training.

Prefitting AR for Older Adults

Research conducted in the last decade has provided evidence to professionals in allied health disciplines that better outcomes with older patients are more likely to occur when a collaborative partnership is established with the patient, rather than having the patient assume a passive, compliant role (Haber, 2003). Many audiologists were educated in a traditional medical model, with the professional serving as the "expert," providing information to patients, rather than seeking the patient's input, and outlining a plan of intervention with little contribution of suggestions or perspectives from the patient or family. The current trend in health care is for professionals to provide education, not just care and rehabilitation, so that the health component of health care is emphasized. In the current model, the audiologist offers a collaborative relationship to patients, one designed to enhance self-management of their hearing losses. Unfortunately, the profession of audiology has had only modest success in attracting older adults to obtain hearing aids and to learn how to manage their hearing difficulties. According to MarkeTrak VII data, fewer than half of the 65+ age group who could benefit from hearing aids actually purchase them (Kochkin, 2005), and market research has shown that almost 20% of older adults who actually do purchase hearing aids discontinue their use and relegate them to the dresser drawer (Kochkin, 2000).

To at least some degree, one explanation for the high return rate for hearing aids may be that dispensing audiologists are not determining the older adult's degree of problem awareness and level of readiness for hearing aids before the fitting. Audiologists frequently point out that many older adults deny their hearing losses and blame their difficulties on mumbling speakers. Smith and Kricos (2003), however, conducted research showing that older adults with hearing loss actually do acknowledge their hearing losses, although they may downplay the *effects* that their hearing losses have. These results are consistent with the National Council on Aging (NCOA) (1999) research. Two-thirds of the older adults in the NCOA study who reported hearing loss but who did not use hearing aids stated that their hearing losses were not "bad enough to get a hearing aid." Similar to the results of Smith and Kricos (2003), the NCOA respondents acknowledged their hearing losses, but not their effects.

In the Smith and Kricos (2003) study, 91 older adults with no hearing aid experience answered a perceived hearing loss question ("Do you think you have a hearing loss?"), completed the Hearing Handicap Inventory for the Elderly-Screening Version (HHIE-S; Ventry & Weinstein, 1983), and were identified as likely having a hearing loss based on screening results at a 40 dB level for 1000 and 2000 Hz. Based on their findings, the authors speculated that there might be three broad levels of acknowledgment of hearing difficulties by the older adult population: complete acknowledgment, partial acknowledgement, and nonacknowledgment. Individuals were labeled complete acknowledgers if they stated that they perceived loss *and* if their HHIE-S score was high, indicating awareness of the social and/or emotional effects of hearing loss. Partial acknowledgers also indicated that they perceived a hearing loss but their HHIE-S results were low, indicating that they were not aware of or possibly not willing to admit that their hearing loss was affecting them socially or emotionally. Nonacknowledgers reported that they did not perceive a hearing problem and their low scores on the HHIE-S indicated that they were not experiencing any social or emotional effects of hearing loss. The authors described possible interventions for older individuals at each of the levels of problem awareness. For nonacknowledgers and partial acknowledgers, an intervention might be designed to help increase awareness of everyday communication difficulties. If nonacknowledging or partial acknowledging patients are fit with hearing aids before realizing the degree of difficulties caused by their hearing losses, the probability of the hearing aids being returned or relegated to the dresser drawer is likely to be significantly increased.

Consider the evidence provided by Kochkin (2002) via the MarkeTrak 6 data: close to 30% of individuals who discontinued use of hearing aids attributed their non-use to poor benefit. It is possible that lack of perceived benefit may have occurred for many of these new hearing aid users because they were fit *before* fully acknowledging the degree of difficulty their hearing loss was causing them. Kochkin's (1998) MarkeTrak IV results demonstrated that more than half of all new hearing aid users reported that family members had motivated them to obtain hearing aids. Thus, it is quite likely that many of the patients who schedule an appointment for a hearing evaluation actually acknowledge their hearing loss but do not accept the fact that their hearing losses are causing them significant problems in their every day lives. The risk entailed by fitting nonacknowledgers and partial acknowledgers with hearing aids before they are aware of the effects that their hearing losses are having on them, as well as on their families, friends, and coworkers, is that they do not appreciate how much the hearing aids are helping them. One way to identify older individuals who are not fully acknowledging their hearing difficulties is simply to ask them if they think they have a hearing loss. The nonacknowledger will state that they do not have a hearing loss and may make comments that most audiologists have heard time and again, such as "I can hear when (or what) I want to," or "Folks just don't speak clearly anymore." The partial acknowledger may say "I know I have a hearing loss, but it's not causing me any problems."

Babeu, Kricos, and Lesner (2004) provided a number of suggestions for effective audiologic management of patients with significant hearing loss who do not acknowledge their listening difficulties. These authors suggest that the audiologist can provide nonacknowledgers with information about the symptoms and effects of untreated hearing loss to increase their awareness of symptoms and effects of hearing loss besides communication breakdowns. The nonacknowledger may not realize, for example, that the reason he feels tense, or becomes tired more quickly, is because he is straining to understand what people are saying. Some sources of information for patients who do not fully acknowledge their problems are presented in Appendix 19-A. Dispensing audiologists could request that their community librarians obtain any of the bibliotherapy references listed in Appendix 19-A, and then refer patients to their community libraries.

When older adults fully acknowledge their hearing losses, the audiologist should ask for their perspectives on communication problems they may be experiencing. To determine their hearing assistive technology needs, it is important to assess what kinds of communication dilemmas they experience. There are a number of easily administered self-assessment measures, such as the Hearing Handicap for the Elderly (HHIE; Ventry & Weinstein, 1982) questionnaire. These take minutes to administer and help delineate the older adult's perception of communication difficulties. Well-validated self-assessment measures such as the HHIE are also helpful as a postfitting outcomes measure.

Hearing Assistive Technology Considerations for Older Adults

Earlier in this chapter, a number of factors were identified that should be considered when selecting and providing hearing assistive technology for older patients. Manual dexterity may be a problem for many older adults, especially given that arthritis is the most common chronic condition experienced by this population. Other sources of dexterity problems include Parkinson's disease, secondary effects of strokes, and other neurologic problems. Thus, it is essential to consider dexterity of the fingers, hand, and wrist, as well as the ability to raise the arms to the ears. An informal evaluation can be used, such as asking the patient to pick up a sample hearing aid, turn the controls, and lift the aid to the ear. Souza (2004) suggests that if physical dexterity is a problem, the audiologist may want to consider automatic directional hearing aids because a toggle switch or push button may be difficult to manipulate. Likewise, she suggests that hearing aids with automatic telecoils and hearing aids that automatically select the electroacoustic program for different listening situations might be considered for those with dexterity compromises. In addition to possible dexterity issues, older adults may also have reduced tactile sensation that may interfere with their abilities to manipulate hearing aid controls, insert hearing aid batteries, and position the hearing aids in their ears. The audiologist should use observing and/or interviewing the patient to determine if there may be issues with handling the hearing aids.

An important area to consider when fitting older adults with hearing assistive technology is whether there are sensory deficits besides hearing loss. Vision loss in particular must be addressed. Hearing aids with automatic features and raised volume controls may be helpful for the older patient with dual sensory loss. Magnification devices throughout clinical areas are also useful and may enable older patients to see hearing aid landmarks (e.g., microphone, volume wheel, telephone switch, battery door, etc.) more easily. These visual assistive devices may be handheld magnifiers that are on adjustable stands or closed-circuit television devices (CCTV). Written materials for older adults should have a larger (e.g., 14-point) font, dark print on a light background, an uncluttered design, and materials that are printed on non-glossy paper (Smith & Kricos, 2002). Detailed suggestions for helping older adults with dual sensory loss are offered by Kricos (2007) and Saunders and Echt (2007). The tactile sense may also be reduced in many older adults, which may affect the type of hearing aids that are chosen, and the ease with which hearing aids are inserted and removed.

As described earlier in this chapter, there has been increasing interest in the potential contributions of cognitive processing to the listening difficulties of older adults (Humes, 2007; Wingfield & Tun, 2007). Pichora-Fuller and Singh (2006) and Kricos (2006) reported that normal age-related changes in cognition impact older adults in everyday situations even when audibility has been restored via amplification. In acoustically hostile environments, auditory information may be denigrated due to central cognitive resources being reallocated to support auditory processing. As more research information becomes available regarding cognitive contributions to the unique listening challenges experienced by many older adults, the hearing aid industry has responded by offering hearing aid signal processing strategies for various subgroups of older adults with hearing loss, including those with cognitive and/or auditory processing disorders (Souza, 2004). One promising strategy appears to be use of a slower speech-processing algorithm (Cienkowski, 2003). There is some research evidence from audiology and related disciplines that older listeners with reduced cognitive abilities may obtain greater benefits from hearing aids when slow-acting compression is used (Gatehouse, Naylor, & Elberling, 2003). Several authors have studied the predictive value of cognitive tests, such as letter monitoring and reading span tests, relative to what the preferred hearing aid compression release time would be to improve an older individual's aided speech recognition in noise (Foo, Rudner, Rönnberg, & Lunner, 2007; Gatehouse, et al., 2003; Lunner, 2003). As research in this area continues, cognitive screening tests may be developed for use in audiology clinics to predict the best compression release setting for a given patient.

In addition to advising older patients about hearing aid options, information should be provided to them about other assistive devices for people with hearing loss, such as carbon monoxide detectors, amplified phones, flashing or vibrating fire alarms, and weather emergency alerts. When the older adult exhibits pronounced difficulties in speech recognition in noise, the audiologist needs to be proactive in recommending assistive devices beyond hearing aids. Although many older adults reject the use of FM devices (Boothoyd, 2004; Chisolm, McArdle, Abrams, & Noe, 2004), they should still be aware of the options available to help them understand speech in noisy settings.

Postfitting Interventions: Increasing the Likelihood of Successful Hearing Health Care

There are a number of postfitting interventions available to help ensure successful hearing aid use and maximum communication abilities for older adults. The importance of postfitting counseling and support for older adults and their significant others cannot be emphasized enough, given the complexities and challenges experienced by many older adults with hearing loss, as noted above. A collaborative problem-solving approach to helping older adults cope with their listening difficulties is likely to be far more successful than a one-way stream of information from the audiologist to the new hearing aid user (Abrahamson, 2000). In a collaborative model, audiologists and patients can identify the everyday listening challenges that are experienced, then work together to find solutions. There are a number of advantages for offering a collaborative problem-solving approach via group programs that are attended by patients and their frequent communication partners. New hearing aid users learn that other people have problems similar to theirs and receive support from them as well as from the group facilitator. Spouses and other family members achieve more realistic insights into the new hearing aid user's communication problems and they learn strategies for reducing communication breakdowns. Regardless of whether the postfitting support program is offered in a group, via individual counseling, or even through recommendations of reading materials or referral to Web sites such as HealthyHearing.com and the Better Hearing Institute, the important point is to *educate* the patient about how to manage their hearing losses. Despite phenomenal advance in hearing aid technology, the hearing aid alone is probably not going to be enough, especially with the older population. Ideally, the audiologist will provide communication tips and strategies, such as identifying the sources of everyday communication difficulties, controlling the communication environment to reduce listening difficulties, and positive and effective ways of repairing communication breakdowns.

Beyond postfitting collaborative problem solving, the older adult patient may benefit from other treatment options, including formal listening training, attention to the patient's self-efficacy for managing communication challenges and using hearing aids, and clear speech training for frequent communication partners. A formal listening training program was recently developed and the evidence so far appears promising for use with older adults. As Sweetow and Henderson Sabes (2007) point out, modern technology can provide audibility of sounds, but may not overcome changes in the patient's spectral, and temporal resolution, susceptibility to noise, or decline in cognitive skills that are associated with aging. The Listening and Communication Enhancement (LACE; Sweetow, 2005; Sweetow & Henderson-Sabes, 2004, 2007) program is described by its developers as a cost-effective home-based program to teach listening strategies, to build self-efficacy about communication, and to address some of the cognitive changes that may detrimentally affect the listening abilities of many older adults, as discussed earlier in this chapter. Using interactive and adaptive tasks, the LACE program provides exercises for listening to degraded speech such as rapid time-compressed speech, and speech in noise. To improve conversational fluency, the LACE includes adaptive training activities for cognitive tasks such as auditory memory and speed of processing, as well as interactive communication strategies. Results of initial investigations using the LACE suggest that it will be of significant benefit to older adults, regardless of whether they are hearing aid users or not (Sweetow & Henderson Sabes, 2007). For further discussion of auditory training options, see Chapter 12 in this text.

Woods and Yund (2007) conducted research that provided further evidence of the benefits of providing auditory training to older adults. Assessing older adults aged 50 to 80 years, they found that perceptual training in phoneme identification resulted in increased ability to detect phonemes that are difficult to hear, as well as reduced consonant confusions.

Self-efficacy is another consideration for the older adult who has just received hearing aids. Self-efficacy, as defined by Bandura (1986, 1989), is the domain-specific belief that one can complete a task successfully. Although an older adult may appear to be confident in many areas, such as social interaction, ability to golf, and self-independence, she may not necessarily feel confident in her ability to learn how to use hearing aids. Perhaps this is why audiologists frequently hear comments from new hearing aid users such as, "I *can't* figure out how to tell the right hearing aid from the left," or "I *can't* remember which program to use when I'm in church." These negative assertions regarding the ability to learn how to use hearing aids successfully can sabotage the best of hearing aid fittings. According to Bandura (1989), one of the best ways to avoid low self-efficacy is to avoid failure when learning a new task. In the case of the new hearing aid user, that means minimizing problems in handling the hearing aids and learning how to use and care for them. Hence, again we see the need for postfitting support in the form of education and counseling. Bandura (1986, 1989) also encourages vicarious learning, such as observing successful role models; thus, you may want to refer patients with low self-efficacy to venues where they could interact with highly self-assured and positive hearing aid users in the community, such as active members in local Hearing Loss Association of America chapters.

In recent years, there has been increasing research evidence regarding the significant benefits that production of clear, precise speech can provide for individuals with hearing loss and for their frequent communication partners. Talkers differ considerably in their rate of speech, precision of articulation, loudness, and use of pauses. Many talkers speak rapidly and drop the volume of their voices at the end of sentences. A sentence such as "My brother will be trying to catch a nap later on today" may sound like "My-brotherull be tryun tuhketcha bus lateron," with one word falling upon the next. This type of speech is encountered daily by individuals with hearing loss and often exacerbates their listening difficulties.

Clear speech is a method in which the speaker talks slightly slower and louder, uses frequent pauses, and enunciates speech sounds more clearly. It is not exaggerated speech, but rather a style of speaking that is adopted naturally by many talkers in difficult communication situations, such as conversing in noisy or reverberant environments, or when speaking to foreigners or to listeners who are hearing impaired. Several research studies have demonstrated that listeners with hearing impairment can more easily understand speech when the talker speaks in a deliberately clear manner (Helfer, 1998; Krause & Braida, 2004, 2005; Liu et al., 2004; Payton et al., 1994; Picheny, et al., 1986; Schum, 1996). Of particular relevance in this chapter are the findings by Helfer (1998) that the older the research participant, the greater the benefit from clear speech. Additionally, Helfer (1998) found no correlation between the degree of hearing loss in older adults and the amount of clear-speech benefit. This is not surprising, given the speech processing challenges experienced by older adults that were discussed earlier in this chapter. Many older adults need more time to process what a talker is saying, and hence the benefits from listening to a talker who speaks slowly and carefully and who articulates each sound.

In general, research results have indicated an increase of approximately 17 to 20% in speech intelligibility when speakers deliberately produce clear speech rather than use their more typical conversational speech (Krause & Braida, 2005). Researchers have determined that clear speech is characterized by specific acoustic changes, including a slower rate, frequent pauses, increased duration of phonemes, and fuller differentiation between phonemes. Many individuals with hearing loss report that a substantial number of people with whom they must communicate on a regular basis do not inherently know how to produce clear, visible speech. Research has shown that clear speech training may enable individuals who are hearing impaired to better understand their frequent communication partners (Caissie et al., 2005; Kricos et al., 2003; Schum, 1996, 2001). Caissie et al. (2005) compared a spouse who received approximately 45 minutes of instruction on how to produce clear speech to a spouse who did not receive instruction but who instead was simply asked to speak clearly. Sentence productions for each talker were recorded for conversational speech conditions at 1-week postintervention (intervention being provided for only one of the talkers) and for 1-month postintervention. The recordings were played back for identification by research participants, half of whom were hearing impaired and half of whom were normal hearing. Interestingly, research participants who were hearing impaired had im-proved results of 33% in the 1-week and 18% in the 1-month postintervention sentence perception testing when the talker was simply asked to use clear speech. Even more impressive, how-ever, were the 42% and 40% improvements, respectively, in the post intervention 1-week and 1-month sentence perception results for the individuals with hearing impairment who listened to the talker who had received clear speech training.

The production of clear speech can be accomplished using the following guidelines;

- All sounds are precisely and accurately articulated.
- Speech rate is slowed a bit.
- Slight pauses are used between phrases and thoughts.
- There is a modest increase in vocal volume.

In the example of typical conversational speech provided above, an utterance might be heard as "Mybrotherull be tryun tuhketcha bus lateron." The clear speech version of this sentence would be "My brother [pause] will be trying [pause] to catch a bus [pause] later on," with all sounds fully formed and pauses provided at syntactically appropriate intervals. Despite adjustments such as these, however, the talker must strive to maintain a lively voice. The likely results for older adults are more accurate and relaxed conversations with their frequent communication partners. The frequent communication partners also benefit. In all likelihood, they will have less need to repeat things, experience less frustration, and avoid misunderstandings. Oticon™ has a brochure available that helps communication partners learn how to produce clear speech for their family or friends who are hearing impaired (Oticon™, 2008). Additional guidelines for speaking clearly can be found in Clark and English (2004).

These interventions may provide significant help to older adults with hearing loss, as well as to their families and friends. The author acknowledges that the prefitting, fitting, and postfitting considerations for working with older adults require considerable time, something many audiologists in busy clinics do not have. To streamline the process, the reader may find the tool developed recently by Sandridge and Newman (2006) to be helpful. The nine-item instrument known as the Characteristics of Amplification Tool (COAT) is designed to help the dispensing audiologist consider important audiological and non-audiological prefitting issues, choose the best hearing aid fitting, and counsel the patient, in one hour or less. The COAT can be completed in 10 minutes or less, is easy to administer and interpret, and helps the audiologist obtain the important nonaudiologic information to determine the patient's technology needs. An attractive feature of the COAT for time-pressed audiologists is that the results provide a guide for realistic counseling during the hearing aid selection appointment.

Impact of Aging on Participation in Rehabilitative Services

In this chapter, a number of options have been described for AR with the older adult population. It is important to keep in mind, however, that, unlike the younger person with hearing loss, the older person may have greater challenges and obstacles to overcome when trying to participate in the rehabilitation process.

Cameron and Kurrle (2002) point out that comorbid chronic and acute health conditions may prevent or challenge the older adult's ability to participate in rehabilitation programs. These conditions, which might include arthritis, hypertension, stroke, vascular disease, ambulatory problems, to name only a few, may complicate and/or disrupt AR.

Besides health problems, older adults must confront and adjust to a number of life events that are not typically experienced by younger individuals, such as retirement, death of friends and spouses, increased dependence on others, reduction in finances, and change of residence. Having to cope with significant changes such as these may detract from the older person's abilities to complete an extended program of AR. Kricos, Erdman, Bratt, and Williams (2007) found that life events are related to continued hearing aid use. In their comparison of veterans who continued to use their hearing aids versus those who discontinued use of their hearing aids, the hearing aid users reported significantly fewer events that impacted their hearing aid use. In particular, participants who discontinued use of hearing aids were more likely to report major changes in life events such as retirement, increased dependence on others, and death of a spouse or partner. Major health-related events, however, did not appear to exert as great a negative impact on hearing aid use as lifestyle changes.

There are a number of other obstacles that may hamper the older adult's engagement in and completion of the intervention program. The older adult may no longer be able to drive, and thus there may be transportation issues if family, friends, and the community are not able to help. The older adult may tire more quickly and thus AR sessions may need to be shorter. Severe cognitive impairment is another risk factor for a poor response to rehabilitation programs (Cameron & Kurrle, 2002).

The audiologist must find creative ways to overcome the obstacles that may affect the older adult's participation in the AR program. Some strategies include providing well-designed, elder-friendly patient education materials, offering shorter sessions, counseling for realistic expectations, and quiet encouragement in order to build the person's self efficacy for AR. When appropriate and feasible, the family should be included so that there is continuity to the program of AR.

Conclusion

Although hearing aids can provide substantial benefit to older adults with hearing loss, there are a number of reasons why pre- and postfitting AR can provide benefits beyond those provided by amplification. Research evidence has substantiated that auditory training, collaborative problem-solving, education, and other AR strategies help people to manage their everyday communication dilemmas more effectively. In this chapter, the unique and daunting challenges faced by older adults with hearing loss, compared to younger adults AR with hearing loss, have been described. The likely results of a well-planned program of AR for older adults, from prefitting through post-fitting of hearing aids, will be older patients who are more satisfied and competent hearing aid users, and who are confident in their abilities to manage their hearing losses.

References

Abrahamson, J. (2000). Group audiologic rehabilitation. *Seminars in Hearing*, *21*, 227–235.

Arlinger, S. (2003). Negative consequences of untreated hearing loss: A review. *International Journal of Audiology*, *42*, 2S17–2S21.

Babeu, L., Kricos, P., & Lesner, S. (2004). Applications of the stages-of-change model in audiology. *Journal of the Academy of Rehabilitative Audiology*, *37*, 41–56.

Bagai, A., Thavendiranathan, P., & Detsky, A. (2006). Does this patient have a hearing impairment? *Journal of the American Medical Association*, *295*, 416–428.

Bandura, A. (1986). Self-efficacy. In A. Bandura (Ed.), *Social foundations of thought and action: A social cognitive theory* (pp. 390–453). Englewood Cliffs, NJ: Prentice-Hall.

Bandura, A. (1989). Regulation of cognitive processes through perceived self-efficacy. *Developmental Psychology*, *25*, 729–735.

Berry, P., Mascia, J., & Steinman, B. (2004). Double trouble. *Care Management Journal*, *5*, 35–40.

Boothroyd, A. (2004). Hearing aid accessories for adults: The remote FM microphone. *Ear and Hearing, 25*, 22–33.

Brabyn, J., Schneck, M., Haegerstrom-Portnoy, G., & Lott, L. (2007). Dual sensory loss: Overview of problems, visual assessment, and rehabilitation. *Trends in Amplification, 11*(4), 219–226.

Brennan, M. (2003). Impairment of both vision and hearing among older adults: Prevalence and impact on quality of life. *Generations, 27*, 52–56.

Cacciatore, F., Napoli. C., Abete, P., Marciano, E., Triassi, M., & Rengo, F. (1999). Quality of life determinants and hearing function in an elderly population: Osservatorio Geriatrico Campano study group. *Gerontology, 45*, 323–328.

Caissie, R., Campbell, M., Frenette, W., Scott, L., Howell, I., & Roy, A. (2005). Clear speech for adults with a hearing loss: Does intervention with communication partners make a difference? *Journal of the American Academy of Audiology, 16*, 129–139.

Cameron, I. D., & Kurrle, S. E. (2002). Rehabilitation and older people. *Medical Journal of Australia, 177*(7), 387–391.

Carabellese, C., Appollonio, I., Rozzini, R., Bianchetti, A., Frisoni, G. B., Frattola, L., et al. (1993). Sensory impairment and quality of life in a community elderly population. *Journal of the American Geriatrics Society, 41*, 401–407.

Chisolm, T. H., McArdle, R., Abrams, H., & Noe, C. M. (2004). Goals and outcomes of FM use by adults. *Hearing Journal, 57*(11), 28–35.

Chisolm, T. H., Willott, J. F., & Lister, J. J. (2003). The aging auditory system: anatomic and physiologic changes and implications for rehabilitation. *International Journal of Audiology, 42*, 2S3–2S10.

Cienkowski, K. (2003). Auditory aging: A look at hearing loss in older adults. *Hearing Loss: The Journal of Self-Help for Hard of Hearing People*, pp. 12–15.

Clark, J. G., & English, K. M. (2004). *Counseling in audiologic practice: Helping patients and their families adjust to hearing loss*. Boston: Pearson Education.

Craik, F. (2007). The role of cognition in age-related hearing loss. *Journal of the American Academy of Audiology, 18*, 539–547.

Etymotic Research. (2001). Quick SIN version 1.3 manual. Retrieved June 23, 2006, from www.etymotic.com/pdf/quicksin-manual.pdf

Foo, C., Rudner, M., Rönnberg, J., & Lunner, T. (2007). Recognition of speech in noise with new hearing instrument compression release settings requires explicit cognitive storage and processing capacity. *Journal of the American Academy Audiology, 18*, 618–631.

Gatehouse, S. (2003). Rehabilitation: Identification of needs, priorities, and expectations, and the evaluation of benefit. *International Journal of Audiology, 42*(Suppl. 2), 77–83.

Gatehouse, S., Naylor, G., Elberling, C. (2003). Benefits from hearing aids in relation to the interaction between the user and the environment. *International Journal of Audiology, 42*, 1S77–1S86.

Gelfand, S. A. (1995). Long-term recovery and no recovery from the auditory deprivation effect with binaural amplification: Six cases. *Journal of the American Academy of Audiology, 6*, 141–149.

Haber, D. (2003). *Health promotion and aging: Practical applications for health professionals* (3rd ed.). New York: Springer.

Helfer, K. (1998). Auditory and auditory-visual recognition of clear and conversational speech by older adults. *Journal of the American Academy of Audiology, 9*, 234–243.

Hooyman, N. R., & Kiyak, H. A. (2005). *Social gerontology: A multidisciplinary perspective*. Boston: Pearson Education.

Humes, L. (1996). Speech understanding in the elderly. *Journal of the Acoustical Society of America, 7*(3), 161–167.

Humes, L. (2002). Factors underlying the speech-recognition performance of elderly hearing-aid wearers. *Journal of the Acoustical Society of America, 112*(3), 1112–1133.

Humes, L. (2007). The contributions of audibility and cognitive factors to the benefit provided by amplified speech to older adults. *Journal of the American Academy of Audiology, 18*, 590–603.

Jang, Y., Mortimer, J. A., Haley, W. E., Small, B. J., Chisolm, T. E., & Graves, A. B. (2003). The role of vision and hearing in physical, social, and emotional functioning among older adults. *Research on Aging, 25*, 172–191.

Jerger, J. (2006). Behavioral studies of auditory aging. *Seminars in Hearing, 27*(4), 243–264.

Jerger, J., Chmiel, R., Allen, J., & Wilson, A. (1994). Effects of age and gender on dichotic sentence identification. *Ear and Hearing, 15*, 274–286.

Kim, J., & Grant, C. (2004). Investigating the audio-visual speech detection advantage. *Speech Communication, 44*, 19–30.

Kochkin, S. (1998). MarkeTrak IV: Correlates of hearing aid purchase intent. *Hearing Journal, 51*(1), 30–38.

Kochkin, S. (2000). MarkeTrak V: Why my hearing aids are in the drawer: The consumer's perspective. *Hearing Journal, 53*(2), 34–42.

Kochkin, S. (2002). MarkeTrak VI: Ten-year customer satisfaction trends in US hearing instrument market. *Hearing Review, 9*(10), 14 18–20, 22–25, 46.

Kochkin, S. (2005). MarkeTrak VII: Hearing loss population tops 31 million people. *Hearing Review, 12*(7), 16–29.

Krause, J. C., & Braida, L. D. (2004). Acoustic properties of naturally produced clear speech at normal speaking rates. *Journal of the Acoustical Society of America, 115*, 362–378.

Krause, J. C., & Braida, L. D. (2005). *The role of energy distribution in the benefit of clear speech at normal rates*. Paper presented at the Third International Adult Aural Rehabilitation Conference, Portland ME, May 9, 2005.

Kricos, P. (1995). Characteristics of the aged population. In P. Kricos & S. Lesner (Eds.), *Hearing care for the older adult: Audiologic rehabilitation* (pp. 1–21). Boston: Butterworth-Heinemann.

Kricos, P. (2006). Audiologic management of older adults with hearing loss and compromised cognitive/psychoacoustic auditory processing capabilities. *Trends in Amplification, 10*(1), 1–28.

Kricos, P. (2007). Hearing assistive technology considerations for older individuals with dual sensory loss. *Trends in Amplification, 11*(4), 273–280.

Kricos, P., Erdman, S., Bratt, G., & Williams, D. (2007). Psychosocial correlates of hearing aid adjustment. *Journal of the American Academy of Audiology, 18*(4), 304–322.

Kricos, P., Sapienza, C., Nandur, V., & Crandell, C. (2003). Acoustic correlates of clear speech: Training effects. *Proceedings of the Second International Adult Aural Rehabilitation Conference* (pp. 1–7). Portland, ME: The Hearing Foundation.

Larsby, B., Hällgren, M., Lyxell, B., & Arlinger, S. (2005). Cognitive performance and perceived effort in speech processing tasks: Effects of different noise backgrounds in normal-hearing and hearing-impaired subjects. *International Journal of Audiology, 44*, 131–143.

Liu, S., Del Rio, E., Bradlow, A. R., & Zeng, F. G. (2004). Clear speech perception in acoustic and electric hearing. *Journal of the Acoustical Society of America, 116*, 2374–2383.

Lunner, T. (2003). Cognitive function in relation to hearing aid use. *International Journal of Audiology, 42*, S49–S58.

Mulrow, C. D., Tuley, M. R., & Aguilar, C. (1992). Sustained benefits of hearing aids. *Journal of Speech and Hearing Research, 35*, 1402–1405.

National Council on Aging. (1999). *The consequences of untreated hearing loss in older persons*. Retrieved January 26, 2008, from http://www.ncoa.org/content.cfm?sectionID=105&detail=46

Oticon™. (2008). *Clear speech* [pamphlet]. Retrieved January 6, 2008 from http://otikids.oticonus.com/eprise/main/Oticon/US_en/SEC_AboutHearing/LearnAboutHearing/Products/SEC_OtiKids/Parents/Helping/DailyLifeHelp/CNT07_ClearSpeech

Payton, K. L., Uchanski, R. M., & Braida, L. D. (1994). Intelligibility of conversational and clear speech in noise and reverberation for listeners with normal and impaired hearing. *Journal of the Acoustical Society of America, 95*, 1581–1592.

Picheny, M. A., Durlach, N. L., & Braida, L. D. (1986). Speaking clearly for the hard of hearing II: Acoustic characteristics of clear and conversational speech. *Journal of the Speech and Hearing Research, 29*, 434–446.

Pichora-Fuller, K., & Singh, G. (2006). Effects of age on auditory and cognitive processing: Implications for hearing aid fitting and audiological rehabilitation. *Trends in Amplification, 10*(1), 28–59.

Resnick, H. E., Fries, B. E., & Verbrugge, L. M. (1997). Windows to their world: The effect of sensory impairments on social engagement and activity time in nursing home residents. *Journal of Gerontology: Social Sciences, 52B*, S135–S144.

Rowe J. W., & Kahn R. L. (1997). Successful aging. *Gerontologist, 37*, 433–440.

Sandridge, S. A., & Newman, C. W. (2006). *Improving the efficiency and accountability of the hearing aid selection process*. Retrieved June 21, 2006, from http://www.audiologyonline.com/articles/article_detail.asp?article_id=1541

Saunders, G. H., & Echt, K. V. (2007). An overview of dual sensory impairment in older adults: Perspectives for rehabilitation. *Trends in Amplification, 11*(4), 243–258.

Schneider, B. A., Daneman, M., & Murphy, D. R. (2005). Speech comprehension difficulties in older adults: Cognitive slowing or age-related changes in hearing? *Psychology and Aging, 20*, 261–271.

Schuknecht, H. G. (1955). Presbycusis. *Laryngoscope, 65*, 402–419.

Schum, D. (1996). Intelligibility of clear and conversational speech of young and elderly talkers. *Journal of the American Academy of Audiology, 7*, 212–218.

Schum, D. (2001). *Clinical applications of clear speech training*. Paper presented at the First International Adult Aural Rehabilitation Conference, Portland, ME, May 8, 2001.

Silman, S., Gelfand, S. A., & Silverman, C. A. (1984). Late-onset auditory deprivation: Effects of monaural versus binaural hearing aids. *Journal of the Acoustical Society of America, 76*(5), 1357–1362.

Smith, S., & Kricos, P. B. (2002). Rehab for the elderly patient. *Advance for Audiologists, 4*, 35–37.

Smith, S., & Kricos, P. (2003). Acknowledgement of hearing loss by older adults. *Journal of the Academy of Rehabilitative Audiology, 36*, 19–28.

Smith, S., Kricos, P., & Holmes, A. (2001). Vision loss and counseling in audiologic rehabilitation for elders. *Hearing Review, 8*(3), 28–33

Souza, P. (2004). New hearing aids for older listeners. *Hearing Journal, 57*(3), 10–17.

Strecker, N., & Dancer, J. (2005). Routine APD screenings needed. *Advance for Audiologists, 7*. Retrieved June 23, 2006 from http://audiology.advanceweb.com/common/Editorial/PrintFriendly.aspx?CC=50535

Strouse, A., & Wilson, R. (2000). The effect of filtering and inter-digit interval on the recognition of dichotic digits. *Journal of Rehabilitation Research and Development, 37*, 599–606.

Sumby, W. H., & Pollack, I. (1954). Visual contribution to speech intelligibility in noise. *Journal of the Acoustical Society of America, 26*, 212–215.

Sweetow, R. W. (2005). Training the adult brain to listen. *Hearing Journal, 58*(6), 10–16.

Sweetow, R. W., & Henderson-Sabes, J. (2004). The case for LACE (Listening and Communication Enhancement). *Hearing Journal, 57*(3), 32–40.

Sweetow, R. W., & Henderson Sabes, J. (2007). Listening and Communication Enhancement (LACE). *Seminars in Hearing, 28*, 133–141.

Troen, B. R. (2003). The biology of aging. *Mount Sinai Journal of Medicine, 70*, 3–23.

Tun, P., O'Kane, G., & Wingfield, A. (2002). Distraction by competing speech in young and older adult listeners. *Psychology and Aging, 17*, 453–467.

Tye-Murray, N., & Schum, L. (1994). Conversation training for frequent communication partners [monograph]. *Journal of the Academy of Rehabilitative Audiology, 27*, 209–222.

Tye-Murray, N., Sommers, M., & Spehar, B. (2005, July 12). Speechreading and aging: How growing old affects face-to-face speech perception. *ASHA Leader*, pp. 8–9, 28–29.

U.S. Department of Health and Human Services. (2003). *A profile of older Americans: 2003*. Retrieved July 7, 2005, from http://www.aoa.gov/prof/Statistics/profile/2003/4.asp

U.S. Department of Health and Human Services. (2006). *A statistical profile of older Americans age 65+*. Retrieved January 17, 2009, from http://www.aoa.gov/press/prodsmats/fact/fact.aspx

van Rooij, J., & Plomp, R. (1990). Auditive and cognitive factors in speech perception by elderly listeners. II: Multivariate analysis. *Journal of the Acoustical Society of America, 88*, 2611–2624.

Ventry, I., & Weinstein, B. (1982). The Hearing Handicap Inventory for the Elderly: A new tool. *Ear and Hearing, 3*, 128–133.

Ventry, I., & Weinstein, B. (1983). Identification of elderly with hearing problems. *Asha, 25*, 37–42.

Wallhagen, M. I., Strawbridge, W. J., Shema, S. J., & Kaplan, G. A. (2004). Impact of self-assessed hearing loss on a spouse: A longitudinal analysis of couples. *Journal of Gerontology Social Sciences, 59,* S190–S196.

Weinert, B. T., & Timiras, P. S. (2003) Invited review: Theories of aging. *Journal of Applied Physiology, 95,* 1700–1716.

Weinstein, B. (2000). *Geriatric audiology*. New York: Thieme.

Wingfield, A., & Tun, P. (2007). Cognitive supports and cognitive constraints on comprehension of spoken language. *Journal of the American Academy of Audiology, 18,* 548–558.

Woods, D. L., & Yund, E. W. (2007). Perceptual training of phoneme identification for hearing loss. *Seminars in Hearing, 28,* 110–119.

Appendix 19–A
Sources of Educational Materials for Nonacknowledgers and Partial Acknowledgers

Organizations and Support Groups

American Academy of Audiology
11730 Plaza America Drive Suite 300
Reston, VA 22102-3611
(800) 222-2336
http://www.audiology.org

American Speech-Language-Hearing Association
2200 Research Boulevard
Rockville, MD 20850-3289
(800) 638-8255
http://www.asha.org

Better Hearing Institute
1440 I Street, N.W.
Suite 700
Washington, D.C. 20005
Ph: (202) 449-1100 † Fax: (202) 216-9646 †
E-mail: mail@betterhearing.org
www.betterhearing.org

Healthy Hearing
www.Healthyhearing.com

Hearing Loss Association of America (formerly known as Self-Help for Hard of Hearing People, Inc.)
7901 Woodmont Ave, Suite 1200
Bethesda, MD 20914
(301) 657-2248-Voice
(301) 657-2249-TTY
http://www.hearingloss.org

Say What Club
http://www.saywhat.org

Reading Resources

Bauman, N. G. (2007). *Help! I'm losing my hearing: What do I do now? A Basic Guide to Hearing Loss.* Stewartstown, PA: GuidePost.

Burkey, J. M. (2006). *Baby boomers and hearing loss: A guide to prevention and care.* New Brunswick, NJ: Rutgers University Press.

Carmen, R. (2004). *The consumer handbook on hearing loss and hearing aids: A bridge to healing.* Sedona, AZ: Auricle Ink.

Dugan, M. (1997). *Keys to living with hearing loss.* Bethesda, MD: SHHH.

Dugan, M. B. (2003). *Living with hearing loss.* Washington, DC: Gallaudet University Press.

Harvey, M. A. (2004). *Odyssey of hearing loss: Tales of triumph.* San Diego, CA: Dawnsign Press.

Pope, A. (1997). *Hear: Solutions, skills and sources for people with hearing loss.* Bethesda, MD: SHHH.

Self-Help for Hard of Hearing People, Inc. (2002, March/April). Position statement on hearing aids for people with hearing loss. *Hearing Loss.*

Smith, R.D., Alpiner, J.G., & Mulvey, M. (2007). *The hearing aid decision: Answers to your many questions.* Denver, CO: Ramie.

Trychin, S. (2003). *Living with hearing loss workbook.* Can be ordered from Sam Trychin, 212 Cambridge Rd., Erie, PA 16511; (814) 897–1194.

Wayner, D. S. (1998). *Hear what you've been missing: How to cope with hearing loss.* New York: John Wiley.

20

Tinnitus Management

Craig W. Newman
Sharon A. Sandridge

Introduction

Tinnitus has become an increasing health concern (Henry, Dennis, & Schechter, 2005; Hoge et al., 2008), with as many as 42 million Americans experiencing some degree of chronic tinnitus. Approximately 10 million Americans have tinnitus severe enough to seek professional assistance from a hearing health care provider (Saunders, 2007). Yet, very few audiologists provide services to patients who suffer from tinnitus. Many audiologists feel ill-equipped to evaluate patients with tinnitus and to develop and execute a treatment plan for several reasons. First, there is no single unifying model describing the mechanisms underlying the symptom of tinnitus, making it difficult to develop specific treatment protocols. Second, available treatment options have minimal evidence-based data to support their efficacious use, with no single therapeutic modality sufficiently compelling to warrant its use above all others (Sandlin & Olsson, 2000). Third, there is a lack of specific training about tinnitus and its management even in today's Doctor of Audiology (Au.D.) programs. In general, students typically receive only a few lectures on the evaluation and audiologic treatment of tinnitus with limited clinical exposure to patients suffering from tinnitus (Henry, Zaugg, & Schechter, 2005a). Finally, there is considerable variability across patients in regard to their tinnitus and their ability to cope with it. Accordingly, the rehabilitative management of patients with tinnitus varies depending on the impact it has on the individual's health-related quality of life (HRQoL)—creating a less than straightforward treatment approach. Taking all of these issues into consideration, it is understandable that so many audiologists are reluctant to provide clinical management for this patient population in need of clinical services.

Tinnitus management, however, does fall within the scope of practice for audiologists (American Academy of Audiology, 2004; American Speech-Language-Hearing Association, 2004). Furthermore, it is the audiologist who is best positioned to function as the primary health care professional on a multidisciplinary tinnitus management team. As audiologists, we have the: (1) knowledge of auditory disorders and understanding of auditory system functioning; (2) expertise in selecting and fitting hearing aids (HAs) which remains a primary treatment method for providing tinnitus relief; (3) understanding of acoustic and psychoacoustic principles underlying tinnitus assessment (e.g., pitch and loudness matching) and intervention (e.g., sound therapy including tinnitus masking and habituation); (4) competency in using clinical instrumentation necessary to evaluate hearing and conduct the tinnitus psychoacoustic evaluation; (5) professional working relationship with physicians, psychologists, and other health care practitioners; and (6) counseling skills which serve as the cornerstone for all contemporary management programs (Henry, 2004; Henry, Zaugg, et al., 2005a).

Therefore, the purpose of this chapter is to provide an overview of the audiologic management of patients with tinnitus using a multistep, multidisciplinary model that can be implemented in a busy clinical practice. This chapter begins by providing the basics such as definitions, epidemiologic factors, perceptual attributes, perceived severity, classification schemes, and the mechanisms of tinnitus generation and perception; followed by the evaluation process and treatment options; and concludes with a discussion of the roles of other health care practitioners and alternative nonaudiologic treatment options for patients with tinnitus.

Underlying Principles of Tinnitus

Definitions

Tinnitus has been defined as a spontaneous and conscious expression of sound that originates in the head, is involuntary in nature, and occurs without an external acoustic source (McFadden, 1982). Some have described it as a "phantom" auditory perception resulting from tinnitus-related neuronal activity within the auditory pathways (Jastreboff, 1990, 1995). (It has been argued, however, that the use of the term "phantom" may not be helpful in a clinical context because it suggests that the perception is nonexistent [Noble & Tyler, 2007]).

Some authors have defined tinnitus in terms of its temporal course, indicating that tinnitus must exceed five minutes in duration (Coles, 1984; Davis, 1995; Hazell, 1995). Dauman and Tyler (1992) expanded this definition indicating that pathologic tinnitus should last at least five minutes and must occur more often than once a week. Using a broader perspective, Meikle, Creedon, and Griest (2004) suggested that tinnitus is an internal sound that is present most or all of the time.

Epidemiology

Obtaining a clear picture of the prevalence of tinnitus (i.e., number of individuals who experience tinnitus at a given time) is difficult because it has many forms and levels of severity causing different studies to yield widely different outcomes (Moller, 2007). Furthermore, methodological techniques to gather prevalence data have varied using diverse sampling methods (e.g., questionnaires sent by mail or asked during an interview) and study populations (e.g., clinical samples having otologic pathologies or lack of differentiation between "normal" ear noises from "pathologic" tinnitus). In addition, such factors as general health status, level of hearing loss, and noise exposure have not been well controlled (if at all) in most epidemiologic studies (Hoffman & Reed, 2004).

With an understanding of the aforementioned caveats, tinnitus has been estimated to affect approximately 10 to 15% of the adult population (Brown, 1990; Hoffman & Reed, 2004; Sindhusake et al., 2003). Generally speaking, the prevalence of tinnitus increases with age, occupational noise exposure, lower socioeconomic class, and hearing loss. The effects of gender on the prevalence of tinnitus are inconsistent across several studies (Davis & Rafaie, 2000). The latter factors, however, are not mutually exclusive and a complex relationship among the variables exist (Baguley, 2002; Davis & Rafaie, 2000; Hoffman & Reed, 2004).

Perceptual Attributes of Tinnitus

Tinnitus can be described in a multitude of ways including: intermittency; perceived location; quality descriptors; loudness magnitude ratings; loudness and/or pitch fluctuations; and number of sounds comprising the tinnitus, to name a few. An extensive database containing information about the perceptual attributes of tinnitus reported by 1,630 patients with *clinically significant tinnitus* has been created by Meikle and colleagues (Meikle et al., 2004). The reader is encouraged to visit their very resourceful Web site, www.tinnitusarchive.org.

Classification Schemes

Tinnitus is often categorized as being either *subjective* (i.e., heard only by the patient) or *objective* (i.e., produced by an internal source that can be heard by another person). It has been argued (Hazell, 1995; Dobie, 2004b), however, that the latter term is inappropriate in that some internally-generated acoustic sounds may not be heard by anyone except the patient. Accordingly, the term *somatosound*, ("body sound") has been proposed (Dobie, 2004b) as more suitable than the term *objective* for all sounds with internal acoustic sources whether or not they are audible to an external listener. The etiology of somatosounds may include such conditions as vascular pulsations, patulous eustachian tubes, palatal or intratympanic myoclonus, and jugular outflow syndrome (Perry & Gantz, 2000).

The site of generation has also been proposed as a classification scheme, similar to hearing loss categorization. In this manner, the terms *middle ear/conductive*, *sensorineural*, or *central tinnitus* (Tyler & Babin, 1986; Zenner & Pfister, 1999) are used to describe tinnitus.

On the other hand, Tyler and Baker (1983) proposed that tinnitus be described as a function of associated problems. Using the data obtained from 72 members of a tinnitus self-help group completing the Tinnitus Problem Questionnaire (TPQ), problems were assigned to one of four general categories: effects on hearing; effects on lifestyle; effects on general health; and emotional problems. Table 20–1 displays the 15 highest ranked tinnitus-related difficulties associated within each of the four general categories.

Our preference for classifying tinnitus, especially within the context of audiologic rehabilitation, is based on a *biopsychosocial* model. The World Health Organization's International Classification of Functioning, Disability, and Health (WHO-ICF, 2004) provides a conceptual framework for developing a tinnitus classification taxonomy (Henry et al., 2005; Newman & Sandridge, 2004; Tyler, 1993; Tyler, 2000). Table 20–2 summarizes the individual domains of the WHO-ICF schema describing how these categories pertain to tinnitus, and their application in the assessment

Table 20–1. Highest Ranked Difficulties (Percentage of Total Respondents) Associated with General Functional Consequence Categories for Individuals Attending a Tinnitus Self-Help Group (*n* = 72)

Effects on Lifestyle	Effects on Hearing	Emotional Problems	Effects on General Health
sleep (56.9)	understanding speech (37.5)	despair/frustration/ depression (36.1)	drug dependence (23.6)
persistence (48.6)	understanding TV (11.1)	annoyance/irritation/ inability to relax (34.7)	pain/headache (18.0)
worse on awakening (16.6)		concentration/confusion (33.3)	giddiness/balance/fuzzy head (13.8)
avoid noise (15.3)		insecurity/fear/worry (16.6)	
withdrawal/avoid friends (13.8)			
avoid quiet (11.1)			

Source: Adapted from Tyler and Baker (1983).

Table 20–2. Tinnitus Classification Taxonomy, Associated Functional Domains, and Representative Assessment Tools Based on the World Health Organization's International Classification of Functioning, Disability, and Health (WHO-ICF, 2004)

Category	Definition	Functional Domains	Assessment Tools
Impairment	Dysfunction of the auditory system resulting in the perception of tinnitus	Perception of pitch/loudness/ location/quality	Psychoacoustic measures/ direct estimation ratings/ visual analogue scales
Activity Limitation	Effect of impairment on reducing an individual's ability to function in a normal manner	Emotional effects (e.g., depression, annoyance)/hearing interference/intrusiveness or persistence of tinnitus/sleep disturbance/rest or relaxation interference/cognitive effects (e.g., reduced concentration)/ loss of control	Self-report tinnitus questionnaires/ psychological tests/ diaries
Participation Restriction	Psychosocial manifestations of impairment and activity limitation resulting in the need for extra effort and reduced independence	Participation in social events/difficulty performing work or home obligations/ interference with leisure activities/interference with relationships with family, friends, coworkers/reduced overall quality of life	Self-report tinnitus questionnaires/diaries

Source: Adapted from Newman and Sandridge (2004).

process. (*Note:* For further information about the WHO ICF, the reader is referred to Chapter 3 of this text.)

Mechanisms and Models

The precise origins of tinnitus and associated mechanisms involved in the generation of tinnitus are not well-understood. Based on current research findings, it seems most likely that multiple mechanisms (both peripheral and central) are involved in the generation of tinnitus, either simultaneously or interactively (Baguley, 2002; Bartels, Staal, & Albers, 2007; Georgiewa et al., 2006). In general, there is agreement that the mechanisms of tinnitus involve deprivation of input or abnormal input from the peripheral auditory system to the central auditory nervous system. Reduced neural activity from the cochlea (e.g., due to noise exposure or ototoxicity) may result in increased spontaneous neural activity in the central auditory nervous system (Salvi, Lockwood, & Burkhard, 2000) possibly due to a reduction in inhibitory influences (Kaltenbach et al., 2002; Kaltenbach, Zhang, & Zacharek, 2004). Because of neural plasticity, changes in neural input may result in structural and/or functional changes in the central pathways causing the perception of tinnitus (Kaltenbach, 2000; Lockwood, et al., 1998).

Currently, there is no single convergence of view regarding tinnitus mechanisms. In fact, several models, theories, and hypotheses of tinnitus have been proposed, based on anatomic sites, physiologic mechanisms, and psychologic influences. Table 20–3 provides a summary of current models and mechanisms of tinnitus involving the cochlea, auditory nerve, and central auditory nervous system. Note that the table includes both potential anatomic and physiologic sites of tinnitus generation as well as general psychological models of tinnitus development.

Table 20–3. Representative Models and Mechanisms Underlying the Generation of Tinnitus

Generator	Investigator	Mechanism
Peripheral contribution	Penner (1990)	Spontaneous otoacoustic emissions
	Jastreboff (1990)	Discordant inner and outer hair cells: Damaged outer hair cells with relatively intact inner hair cells result in increased neural spontaneous activity from the cochlea
	Patuzzi (2002)	Damaged outer hair cells cause excessive release of neurotransmitter (glutamate) from inner hair cells producing sustained cochlear activity
	Sahley & Nodar (2001)	Increase of endogenous dynorphins (associated with stress) potentiates excitatory function of glutamate resulting in increased spontaneous neural activity
	Chery-Croze, Truy, & Morgon (1994)	Loss of lateral efferent connectivity between inner and outer hair cells result in an imbalance between inhibitory and excitatory cochlear events causing an increase of spontaneous neural activity
	Moller (1984)	Cross-talk between nerve fibers results from ephaptic coupling (interneural synchrony)
Brainstem contribution	Kaltenbach (2000)	Hyperactive spontaneous activity in the dorsal cochlear nucleus
	Salvi, Wang, & Powers (1996)	Hyperactive spontaneous activity in the inferior colliculus and dorsal cochlear nucleus result in tonotopic reorganization (auditory plasticity) of these structures
Cortical contribution	Salvi, Lockwood, & Burkard (2000)	Cortical reorganization following changes in the auditory periphery result in a disproportionately large number of neurons becoming sensitive (tuned) to frequencies at the upper and lower borders representing peripheral hearing loss
	Arnold, Bartenstein, Oestreicher, Romer, & Schwaiger (1996)	Hyperactivity in the left transverse temporal gyrus
	Lockwood et al. (1998)	Abnormal activation of auditory cortex and amygdala
Somatic modulation	Levine (2004)	Modulation of tinnitus results from an interaction of auditory perception and somatosensory links between the dorsal cochlear nucleus and medullary somatosensory nucleus
Psychological factors	Sweetow (1986, 2000)	Cognition: Inappropriate ways of thinking about tinnitus result from maladaptive strategies and cognitive distortions
	Hallam, Rachman, & Hinchcliffe (1984)	Habituation: Intolerance to tinnitus results from individual's failure to habituate (adapt) to the tinnitus sensation
	Hallam et al. (1984); Hallam & McKenna (2006)	Attention: Disturbing tinnitus is a failure to shift attention away from tinnitus
	Hallam et al. (1984); Jastroboff & Hazell (1993); McKenna (2004)	Learning: Enhanced tinnitus perception is a learned response resulting from negative emotional reinforcement involving the limbic system and autonomic activation

Source: Adapted from Tyler (2006).

Components of the Clinical Pathway Model

Figure 20–1 illustrates a model that can guide the clinician in the management of patients with tinnitus. It is a multistep process allowing patients to be referred by several health care services and be discharged at various points within the clinical pathway. The presentation of a tinnitus management clinic (TMC) model will provide the framework for our discussion for the remainder of this chapter.

Step One: TMC Entry

Patients with tinnitus can be referred to the TMC from any health care specialty (i.e., primary care physician, gerontology). Yet, the initial entry point is when the patient has been seen by both otolaryngology and audiology. The importance of each service is described below.

Audiology

Results from the comprehensive audiologic evaluation (i.e., pure-tone and speech audiometry, immittance measurements, and otoacoustic emissions) provide information about the severity and type of hearing loss, audiometric configuration, and functional integrity of the auditory system and are critical to the medical diagnosis of any ear disease that may underlie the tinnitus symptoms. It is important to note, however, that many patients who have tinnitus also experience some degree of hyperacusis (i.e., hypersensitivity to sound). Thus, the clinician must be aware that the administration of specific tests in the audiologic battery, for example, acoustic reflex threshold determination and reflex decay testing, may need

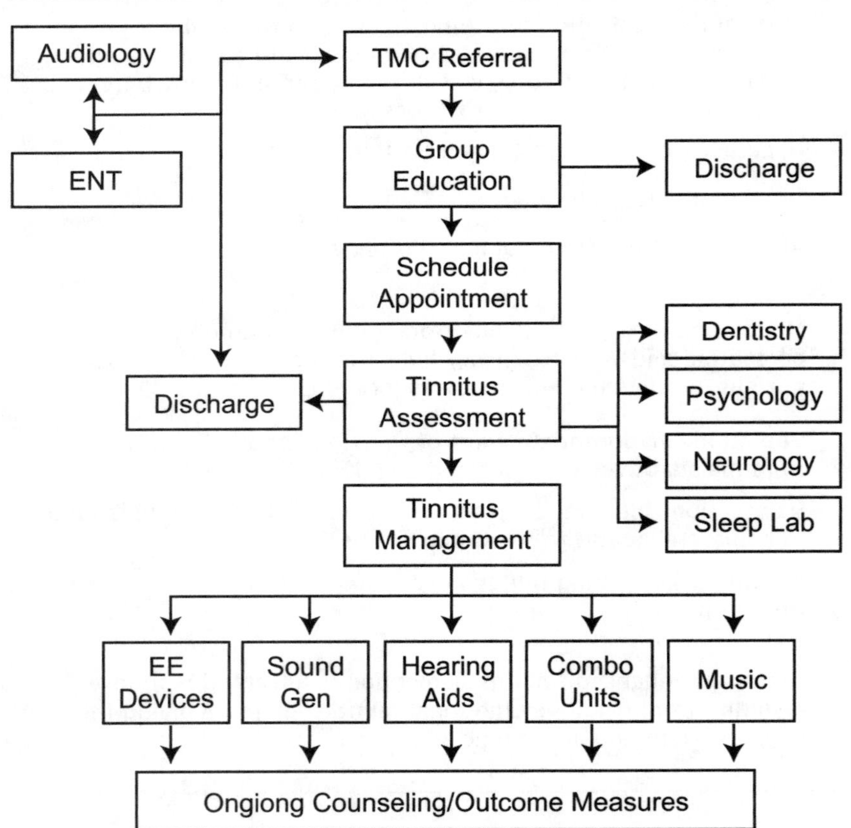

Figure 20–1. Tinnitus Management Clinic (TMC) clinical pathway. ENT = Ear, Nose, and Throat physician (otolaryngologist); EE = Environmental Enhancement; Gen = Generators; Combo = Combination. Adapted with permission from Newman et al., 2008 (p. 301).

to be abandoned to prevent patient discomfort due to loudness intolerance. (The reader is referred to Baguley and Andersson [2007] for a complete discussion of hyperacusis mechanisms, diagnosis and treatment.)

The results of the audiometric testing also serve an important role in the rehabilitation process by providing a basis for selection of the particular sound therapy in the treatment phase of the clinical pathway. For example, a patient with hearing loss and tinnitus may improve communication function and gain relief from tinnitus by using HAs or combination instruments (HA and sound generator housed in the same unit). In contrast, an individual with normal or near-normal hearing may benefit from sound generators alone without the need for amplification.

It would be prudent to incorporate a tool to screen for *clinically significant tinnitus* into every audiologic evaluation, not just when evaluating patients who are referred with tinnitus as their chief complaint. A quick and easy method to screen for clinically significant tinnitus is shown in Figure 20–2. Using this flow chart, the patient responds to each question guiding the clinician toward follow-up treatment recommendations. For example, if a patient indicates that his or her tinnitus is "not a problem" or a "small problem," the provision of some basic counseling within the context of the audiologic evaluation may be sufficient. This minimal level of counseling might include information about the causes of tinnitus and hearing loss, hearing loss prevention, some strategies to manage his or her reactions to tinnitus, and the need to maintain a sound-enriched environment. For many patients, this brief counseling is sufficient and negates the need to return for further intensive tinnitus treatment. In contrast, if a patient indicates that his or her tinnitus is chronic and causing him or her at least moderate problems, referral to the TMC may be indicated.

Another screening option is the Tinnitus Handicap Inventory-Screening Version (THI-S; Newman, Sandridge, & Bolek, 2008). This 10-item

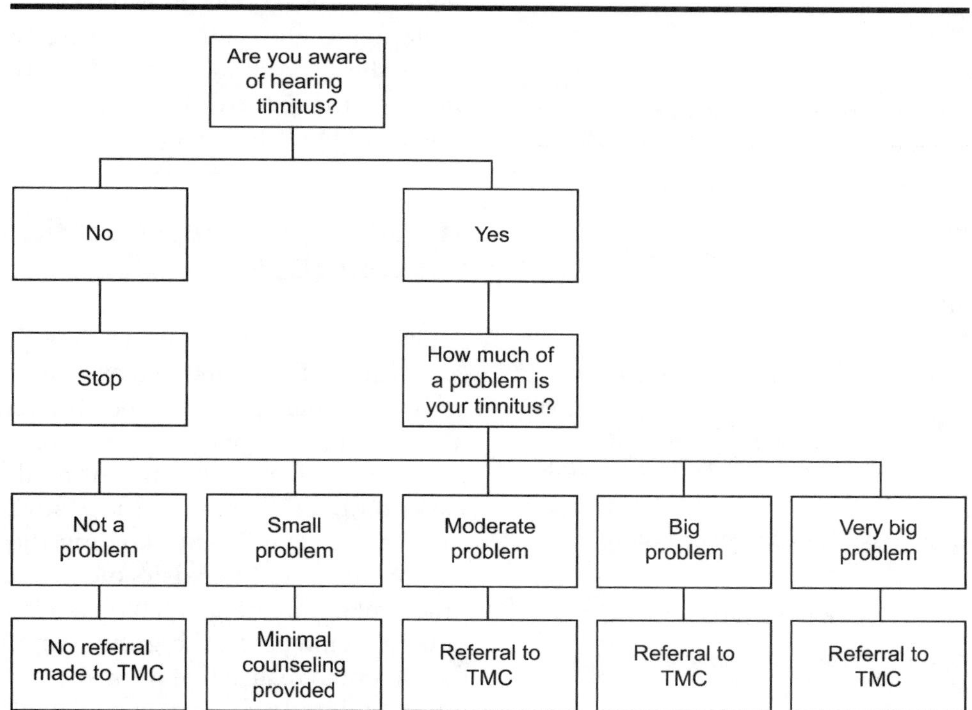

Figure 20–2. Flow chart used as screening model to determine need for enrollment in the Tinnitus Management Clinic (TMC).

questionnaire, shown in Table 20–4 is a shortened version of the 25-item THI (Newman, Jacobson, & Spitzer, 1996) using the same questions and same scoring process. Patients indicate a "yes," (worth 4 points), a "sometimes" (worth 2 points), or a "no" (worth 0 points) for each question asked, yielding a possible total score ranging from 0 to 40 points with higher scores representing greater perceived psychosocial problems as a consequence of tinnitus. The scores on the THI-S have been shown to be comparable ($r = .90$) to the full 25-item version of the THI and yielded adequate test-retest reliability ($r = .81$). Furthermore, a cutoff value of >6 points (out of a possible 40 points) was established as a fence for recommending follow-up. The THI-S is an attractive screening tool in a busy clinical practice because it is brief (i.e., it takes less than 2 minutes to complete) and is easy to administer, score, and interpret.

Otololaryngology

The primary goals of the examination conducted by the otolaryngologist are to: (1) rule out any health condition that requires further medical or surgical intervention; (2) alleviate the patient's fear that they might have a serious medical problem; and (3) provide medical clearance for audiologic management. The otologic physical examination is directed at identifying abnormalities of the cochleovestibular system and the head and neck (Wackym & Friedland, 2004). Table 20–5 summarizes the main components of the medical evaluation of tinnitus.

The medical or surgical management of the underlying pathology may help alleviate the symptom of tinnitus for some; however, for the majority of patients, the cause for the tinnitus cannot be identified, or if it is, it cannot be reversed (e.g., noise-induced hearing loss) or successfully treated. When this is the case, the physician needs to encourage the patient to seek non-medical treatments (e.g., sound therapy, cognitive behavioral therapy), reassuring their patients that help is available from other health care providers, rather than tell them to "learn to live with it." The later advice can lead to further distress and discourages the patient from seeking appropriate non-medical services that offer tinnitus relief. On the other hand, the physician's positive comments about the benefits of nonmedical treatments set the stage for successful management by the audiologist and psychologist.

Table 20–4. Ten Questions Comprising the Screening Version of the Tinnitus Handicap Inventory

Because of your tinnitus, is it difficult for you to concentrate?
Do you complain a great deal regarding your tinnitus?
Do you feel as though you cannot escape your tinnitus?
Does your tinnitus make you feel confused?
Because of your tinnitus, do you feel frustrated?
Do you feel that you can no longer cope with your tinnitus?
Does your tinnitus make it difficult for you to enjoy life?
Does your tinnitus make you upset?
Because of your tinnitus, do you have trouble falling asleep at night?
Because of your tinnitus, do you feel depressed?

Source: THI-S; Newman, Sandridge, and Bolek (2008).

Step Two: Group Education Session (GES)

Attending the Group Education Session (GES) is considered the first major component in the audiologic management process, as shown in Figure 20–1. The use of a group session offers a number of advantages. Briefly, from the clinician's viewpoint, conducting group sessions is very cost- and time-efficient allowing the same information to be delivered to more patients in less time—maximizing available resources. From the patient's viewpoint, the group experience allows the patient to realize that he or she is not alone, that others suffer from tinnitus as well. The group situation promotes a safe and supportive environment to share experiences with tinnitus and

Table 20–5. Components of the Medical Evaluation of Tinnitus

History
Characteristics of tinnitus: Duration, character, location, constant or intermittent
Otologic symptoms: Hearing loss, vertigo, otalgia, otorrhea
Head trauma
Use of medication/ototoxic agents
Central nervous system infections
Family history of otologic disease
Otologic surgery
Social history: Tobacco use, alchohol use, noise exposure (occupation/recreational)
Family history
Review of systems
Physical Examination
Otomicroscopy
Tuning fork examination
Tests of cranial nerve function
Oral cavity examination
Palpation of temporomandibular joint and inspection of dentition
Audiologic Studies
Pure-tone and speech audiometry
Immittance measurements (tympanometry, acoustic reflex testing, reflex decay)
Otoacoustic emissions
Auditory brainstem response
Additional Testing as Needed
Radiologic Evaluation
Carotid ultrasound
Gadolinium-enhanced magnetic resonance imaging
Contrast-enhanced computerized tomography
Magnetic resonance angiography
Magnetic resonance venography
Laboratory Evaluations
Blood work: Blood count; chemistry panel; blood glucose; lipid panel
Thyroid function testing
Screens for ototoxic drugs and pollutants: Solvents, heavy metals, carbon monoxide
Syphilis serology
Autoimmune workup: Rheumatioid factor, C reactive protein, serum antibody to inner ear antigens
For Pulsatile Tinnitus Need Also to Assess
Auscultation of ear canal, periauricular region, orbits, and neck to assess for bruits
Rate of tinnitus compared to patient's pulse
Effect of light digital pressure over internal jugular vein
Effects of turning heard (causes tinnitus of venous origin to subside)

Source: Adapted from Perry and Gantz (2000); Schleuning, Shi, and Martin (2006); Shiley, Folmer, and McMenomey (2005); Wackym and Friedland (2004).

how to cope—or not cope—with the handicapping nature of the tinnitus. The reader is referred to other sources such as Jacobs, Harvill, and Masson (1988) and Corey and Corey (1992) for more information on the different types and virtues of group therapy. (*Note:* For further information about group process, the reader is referred to Chapter 13 of this text.)

The ideal size for an educational group is 8 to 12 members with the session lasting approximately 1.5 to 2 hours in length (Childers & Couch, 1989). It is important to control the group size because a group that is too large or too small may inhibit individual participation and reduce opportunities for interaction. Spouses/significant others should be encouraged to attend the session so that they have a better understanding of the patient's problems and are better prepared to provide emotional support. The meeting room should be quiet and inviting, with chairs arranged in a circle where everyone feels a sense of equality with one another and the exchange of information is enhanced.

Although the primary goal of GES is to educate, there are specific aims for the session. The intent of GES is to:

- demystify tinnitus by providing fundamental information about hearing, hearing loss, and tinnitus;
- remove fears and concerns about tinnitus and clarify misconception (e.g., "Will I go deaf because of my tinnitus?);
- provide reassurance and hope for tinnitus relief balanced with realistic expectations for treatment outcome;
- offer self-help coping strategies and practical suggestions for immediate relief (i.e., sound therapy using environmental enhancement devices such as tabletop sound generators, fans, music, etc.);
- empower the patient to control his or her tinnitus rather than being controlled by the tinnitus; and
- establish trust and rapport between the patient and audiologist to promote adherence to and compliance with further treatment recommendations.

At the beginning of GES, participants are asked to provide a *brief* description of their tinnitus including quality descriptors, onset, duration, and etiology, if known. These introductions allow each participant to realize that he or she is not the only person to experience specific tinnitus difficulties and that the situation is not unique. This introductory portion of the session allows each member to feel more comfortable with the other participants. In addition, the audiologist leading GES must control the session so that individual members do not dominate the group by using it as a "sounding board" for personal problems. It is critical to the success of the group that all members understand this important ground rule.

The specific topics addressed during the education session should be selected carefully to include appropriate information for patients representing a wide range of tinnitus severity. The following topics serve as an outline for areas to be addressed during GES:

- definitions of tinnitus and related problems (e.g., hyperacusis);
- prevalence of tinnitus (e.g., age and gender distribution);
- hearing and hearing loss;
- mechanisms underlying the perception of tinnitus;
- common reactions to tinnitus;
- lifestyle factors affecting tinnitus (e.g., occupational/recreational noise exposure);
- benefits of sound therapy;
- application of different forms of sound therapy (e.g., environmental enrichment devices, hearing aids, sound generators, music);
- overview of "nonaudiologic" treatment options (e.g., diet, cognitive behavioral therapy, relaxation therapy) and the role of other health care professionals in the treatment process; and
- clarification of remaining steps in the clinical pathway for patients interested in pursuing additional treatment.

One way to convey the aforementioned information is through the use of a computerized, picture-based slide show presentation. The presentation, incorporating a series of animated picture sequences and sound clips (e.g., simulated tinnitus sounds), serves to: guide the flow of the counseling session; organize complex information in a logical sequence; keep group discussion focused; and provide visual and auditory interest to the patients. Figure 20–3 displays some examples of the pictures contained in the slide show presentation.

In addition to the formal presentation and the informal dialogue that may occur among the group members, take-home information should be provided. Resource materials reinforce and expand upon topics areas presented in GES. The take-home packet may include, but not limited to, the following:

- *Tinnitus: Questions and Answers* (Vernon & Tabachnick Sanders, 2001). This book is available from the American Tinnitus Association (ATA) and is an excellent resource for many aspects of tinnitus. Patients are counseled, however, not to read the book from cover to cover and only read those sections that pertain to their unique circumstances. Another option for a patient-oriented book is *The Consumer Handbook on Tinnitus* (Tyler, 2008).
- *Resource CDs.* There are a number of CDs available that promote relaxation including *Stress Management Program, Relaxation Programs for Sleep Disorders* developed by the Department of Psychiatry and Psychology at the Cleveland Clinic (available by calling: 216-445-7079);
- Fact sheet describing different forms of sound therapy including HAs, sound generators and music therapy;
- List of coping strategies to maintain sound-enriched environments including devices that can be used to promote sound therapy (e.g, fans, radios, television, talk-radio).
- Web site addresses for environmental enhancement devices such as tabletop

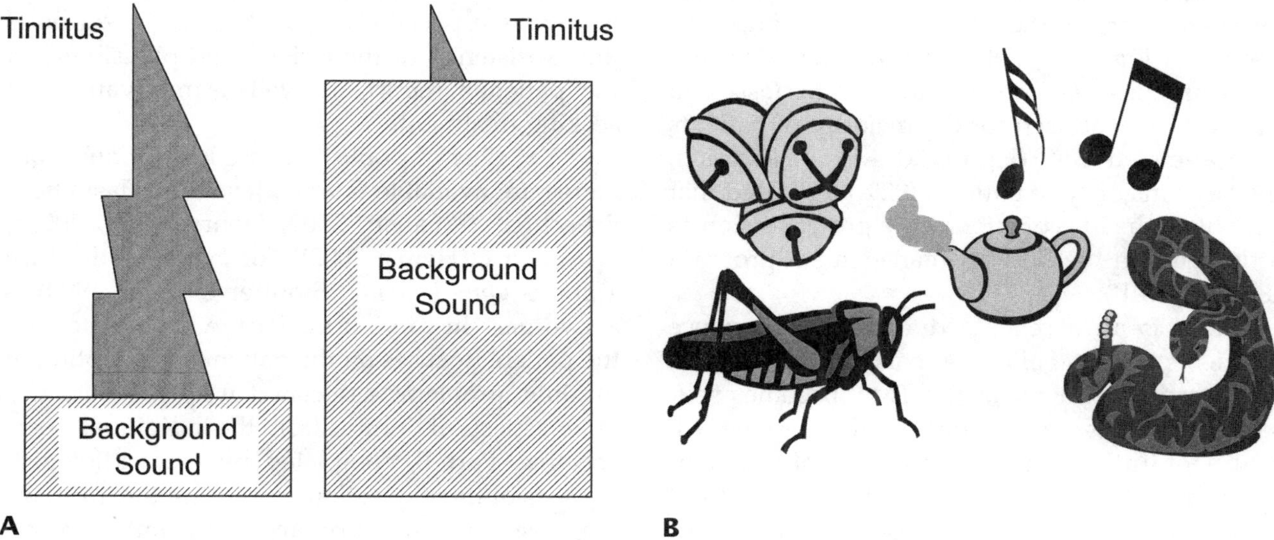

Figure 20–3. Examples of pictures used in the slide show presentation shown during the Group Education Session (GES). **A.** Illustration depicting the benefits of sound-enriched environment in providing tinnitus relief. **B.** Picture examples of tinnitus sound characteristics played with associated audio sound files (e.g., snake and teapot represents hissing sound; musical notes represent tonal quality).

generators, environmental/background sounds CDs, and delivery systems (e.g., pillows, headbands).
- Membership form and contact information for the American Tinnitus Association (www.ata.org; 800-634-8978 or 503-248-9985).

The concept of group counseling is not new to the process of audiologic rehabilitation (Kricos & Lesner, 1995). In fact, several investigators (Abrams, Hnath-Chisolm, Guerreiro, & Ritterman, 1992; Primeau, 1997; Taylor & Jurma, 1999) have demonstrated that patients who were enrolled in a counseling-based group education program while obtaining HAs experienced more significant reductions in activity limitation/participation restriction than those individuals who obtained HAs without the group counseling component. Related to tinnitus, Henry, Schechter, Loovis, et al. (2005) demonstrated that group intervention provided statistically significantly greater benefit in a sample of randomly-assigned veterans who received group counseling to those veterans who were assigned to the traditional support group or to the no-treatment group.

Newman, Sandridge, Meit, and Cherian (2008) also demonstrated the effectiveness of group education sessions. A statistically significant decrease in the psychosocial impact of the tinnitus (assessed by the THI) was seen for the majority of patients who attended GES (Figure 20–4A). In addition, the large majority of patients (92%) indicated that they liked the idea of attending a group session as a first step in the tinnitus management program (Figure 20–4B).

GES is an excellent educational experience for most patients. Following participation in GES, continued enrollment in the TMC becomes self-selective. That is, patients decide whether they will return for further individual assessment and management. Accordingly, GES is a process of natural separation for those patients just in need of informational counseling and those who require more intensive management. Continued participation in the clinical pathway requires the patient to be motivated, have realistic expectations for treatment outcomes, understand the nature of long-term treatment programs, and be willing to comply with treatment requirements.

Step Three: Individual Tinnitus Evaluation

The tinnitus evaluation protocol should include at least five areas of investigation: (1) an in-depth tinnitus case history; (2) assessment of tinnitus impairment; (3) evaluation of tinnitus activity limitation/participation restriction and cognitive reactions; (4) selection of the most appropriate form of sound therapy for a given patient; and (5) determination of the need for referral to other providers on the tinnitus management team (e.g., neurology, psychology, sleep clinic).

Case History

The intake case history provides information about the nature of the patient's complaints that cannot be measured objectively and support self-report measures. In addition, obtaining detailed historic information facilitates the development of the patient-audiologist relationship or rapport. For medicolegal cases, completion of the detailed history is especially critical because it supports the consistency, or the lack of, and plausibility of the patient's report, as well as motivation for seeking treatment.

A variety of published case history questionnaires are available (Henry, Jastreboff, Jastreboff, Schechter, & Fausti, 2002; Henry et al., 2005a; Schechter & Henry, 2002). For example, the *Iowa Tinnitus Questionnaire* (Stouffer & Tyler, 1990) is a two-part history form. Part A, completed by the patient, focuses on the patient's description of tinnitus, problems associated with tinnitus, and other aspects of tinnitus from the individual's perspective. Part B, completed by the audiologist, consists of three questions regarding the: primary diagnosis; patient's primary complaint; and air-conduction thresholds for each ear at 1000 Hz and 4000 Hz.

Many audiologists develop their own intake questionnaires. Table 20–6 summarizes the salient points that should be addressed during the history.

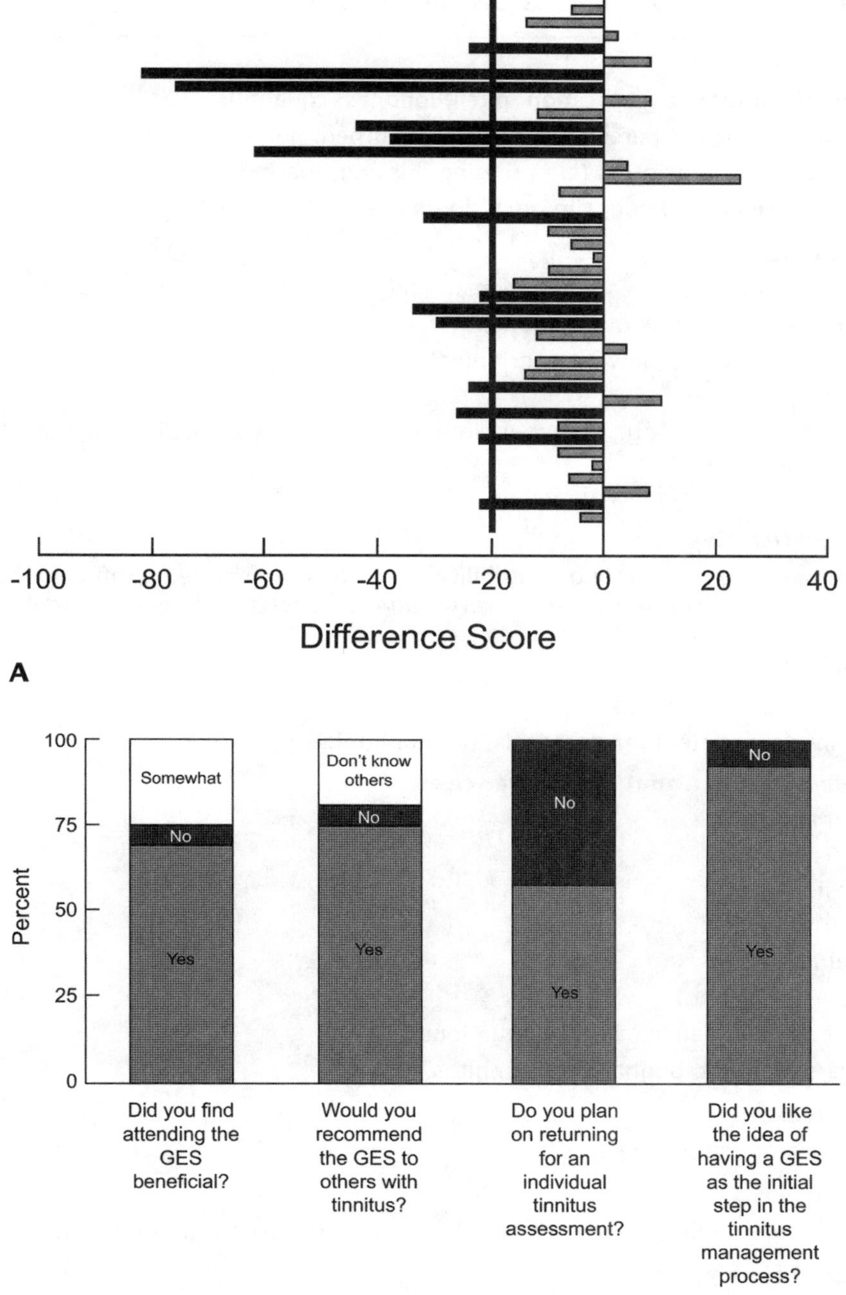

Figure 20–4. A. Individual difference scores (pre- and post-administration) for the Tinnitus Handicap Inventory (THI) for patients attending the Group Education Session (GES). Vertical line represents the 20-point cutoff score considered to a clinically significant change on the THI. **B**. Responses to selected items from a follow-up GES questionnaire mailed to participants (n = 52). Adapted with permission from Newman et al., 2008 (pp. 305–306).

Table 20–6. Elements of a Tinnitus Case History Questionnaire

Nature of tinnitus
Perceptual features (e.g., location, pitch, loudness, quality)
Duration (e.g., onset, percentage of time disturbed, percentage of time aware)
Tinnitus quality descriptors (e.g., ringing, hissing, roaring)
Recent experiences/changes in pitch, loudness, and/or quality
Tinnitus history
Noise exposure (e.g., vocational, recreational)
Drug use (e.g., ototoxic medications)
Dental problems (e.g., jaw pain, grinding)
Ear surgery/disease
Exacerbating factors (e.g., sound environment, diet, stress, medication, activity level, alcohol, smoking)
Reducing factors (same as above)
Hearing difficulties
Evaluation of *impairment* (e.g., audibility), *activity limitation* (e.g., difficulty hearing in background noise), *participation restriction* (e.g., relationships with family, friends, coworkers)
Hearing aid use
Ear protection/ear plug use
Sound intolerance (e.g., hyperacusis, phonophobia)
Psychosocial/functional consequences
Level of annoyance
Sleep disturbance
Depression
Concentration difficulty
Suicidal ideation
Stress
Interference/avoidance of social situations
Positive/negative thoughts about tinnitus
General health
Overall health status
Compensation
Currently pursuing compensation, disability, or other legal action related to tinnitus
Treatment history
Medical
Surgical
Rehabilitative
Benefits from previous treatment/s
Expectations from treatment
Past
Current

Source: Adapted from Newman and Sandridge (2004).

In general, history should include inquiry about: (1) descriptive attributes of the tinnitus; (2) specific behavioral, social, emotional, and interpersonal consequences of tinnitus; (3) factors that may increase or reduce tinnitus disturbance; (4) hearing, hearing loss, and sound tolerances issues; (5) previous tinnitus treatments; and (6) prioritization of concerns (e.g., hearing loss, tinnitus sound tolerance problems).

Evaluation of Tinnitus Impairment

Tinnitus impairment (i.e., perceptual characteristics of the tinnitus) may be quantified using two general approaches, namely scaling techniques or psychoacoustic measurement. Scaling techniques for tinnitus typically involve the application of a direct estimation method. The latter approach is designed to elicit from the patient a direct quantitative estimate of the magnitude of a tinnitus attribute such a pitch and/or loudness. Figure 20–5A illustrates examples of direct estimation rating scales. Using scaling technique, Stouffer and Tyler (1990) indicated that the average rating for subjective pitch estimates for their sample on a 10-point scale was 7.12 (*SD* = 2.3) with 65% of the subjects rating their pitch as 7 points or higher. The latter authors further noted that the average loudness rating was 6.3 on the 10-point scale (*SD* = 2.3) An alternative approach is the visual analogue scale (VAS) that often employs a line of fixed length, usually 100 mm, with anchors appropriate for the attribute being measured (Figure 20–5B).

Psychoacoustic measurement of tinnitus has a long history (Henry & Meikle, 2000) focusing on the development of specific techniques, test-retest reliability of the obtained data, and the extent to which different protocols might reflect differences among patient populations. In the clinical setting, psychoacoustic tinnitus measurements include pitch and loudness matching, minimum masking levels, residual inhibition, and loudness discomfort levels (Table 20–7).

Tyler (2000) proposed several reasons for conducting the aforementioned measures including: reassurance to the patient that the tinnitus is real; demonstration of the acoustic characteristics of the tinnitus to the patient's significant others; distinguishing different subcategories of tinnitus; determination of potential treatment benefit and

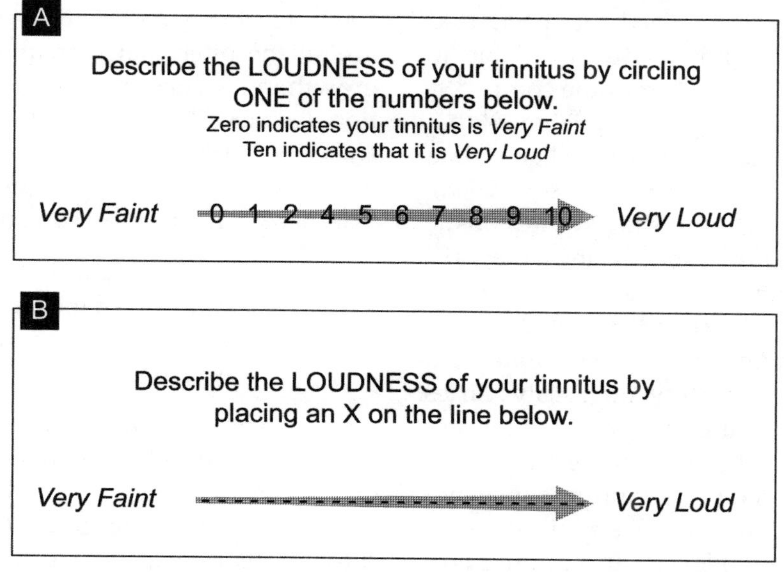

Figure 20–5. Examples of scaling techniques used to quantify tinnitus loudness including (**A**) direct estimation and (**B**) visual analogue scales.

Table 20–7. Psychoacoustic Measurements Conducted as Part of the Tinnitus Assessment

Measurement	Definition
Pitch match	Ability of the patient to equate the pitch of an externally generated pure-tone (or narrow band noise) to the most prominent pitch of his or her perceived tinnitus.
Loudness match	Ability of the patient to equate the loudness of an externally generated pure-tone (or narrow-band noise) to the overall loudness of his or her perceived tinnitus.
Minimum masking level	Minimum level of a broadband noise (BBN) required to completely mask the patient's tinnitus. If the tinnitus cannot be masked, the minimum level of a BBN that changes the perception of the tinnitus (e.g., louder or softer).
Residual inhibition	Period of time when the patient's tinnitus has been partially or completely suppressed after the externally produced masking stimuli has been turned off.
Loudness discomfort level	The threshold level of discomfort for pure tones, BBN, or cold running speech.

selection of specific treatment options; quantification of treatment outcome/effectiveness; and assistance in medico-legal issues.

Measurement protocols for assessing the psychoacoustic attributes of tinnitus are not currently standardized, although there have been several attempts to develop such procedures (Evered & Lawrenson, 1981; McFadden, 1982; Vernon & Meikle, 1988). A major drawback in the efforts to develop a test battery is the need for specialized instrumentation that is not readily available in most audiology clinics. There are some computer-assisted techniques currently being evaluated that hold promise for the acquisition of reliable data (Henry, Rheinsburg, Owens, & Ellingson, 2006). For further information about the psychoacoustic assessment of tinnitus impairment using a diagnostic clinical audiometer, the interested reader should consult Henry et al., (2005a) and Henry (2004).

The unit of measurement for each component for the psychoacoustic battery obviously varies depending upon the stimulus parameter. For example, pitch (psychoacoustic correlate of frequency) is measured in hertz (Hz) and loudness (psychoacoustic correlate of intensity) has typically been measured in dB sensation level (SL; amount in dB above the patient's threshold). It has been argued, however, that SL may not accurately reflect the patient's perception of tinnitus loudness (Tyler & Conrad-Armes, 1983, Tyler, Aran, & Dauman, 1992; Newman, Wharton, Shivapuja, & Jacobson, 1994). Tyler (2000) advocates that the use of sones, the conventional psychoacoustic unit for measuring loudness, would be a more appropriate measure than dB SL. The following example illustrates this point. Figure 20–6 displays the loudness growth function for a patient with normal hearing at 1000 Hz and a moderate sensorineural hearing loss at the pitch-match frequency. The predicted growth in loudness in sones is based on the equation described by Tyler and Conrad-Armes (1983): $L = k(P - P_0)^{0.6}$

Where: L = loudness in sones

k = constant that depends on the unit of measurement (with P measured in micropascals, $k = 0.01$)

P = equal-loudness match in dB sound pressure level (SPL).

Note that in Figure 20–6, SPL is converted into dB hearing level (HL) on the abscissa with loudness in sones on the ordinate. As can be seen, this patient's threshold at 1000 Hz was 20 dB HL.

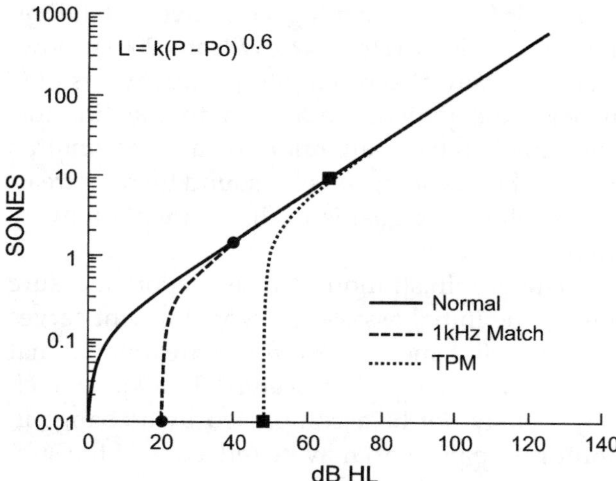

Figure 20–6. Loudness growth functions (sones) for an individual patient with normal hearing (20 dB HL) at 1000 Hz (●) and moderate hearing loss (48 dB HL) at the tinnitus pitch-matched (TPM) frequency (■). Adapted with permission from Newman, Wharton, Shivapuja, and Jacobson, 1994 (p. 56).

Tinnitus was determined to have an equal loudness match of 34 dB HL which was 14 dB SL and calculated to have a loudness judgment value of 0.88 sones. At the pitch-match frequency, however, this same patient had a threshold of 48 dB HL with an equal loudness match of 61 dB HL. The sensation levels for both frequencies were essentially equal, 14 and 13 dB SL, respectively. Yet, when the sone value was calculated for the pitch-matched frequency it was determined to be 5.68 sones—more than five times greater than the sone value at 1000 Hz. This case illustrates the appropriateness of estimating loudness with sones rather than simply reporting SL (Newman et al., 1994)

Self-Report Measures

The use of self-report measures to assess the impact of tinnitus on the patient's every day life is a critical component of the evaluation process. Newman and Sandridge (2004) outlined a number of reasons for inclusion of these measures in the evaluation process:

- There is a low correlation among psychoacoustic measures of tinnitus (e.g. loudness and pitch rating), with perceived severity and annoyance (Jakes, Hallam, Chambers, & Hinchcliffe, 1985; Meikle, Vernon, & Johnson, 1984) indicating that the sole utilization of psychoacoustic assessment is inadequate in assessing the patient's reactions to the perceived tinnitus sensation(s). For example, a loudness rating of 9 on a 10-point scale (indicating very loud) may be associated with a minimal annoyance rating or vice versa—a low loudness rating (3 on the 10-point scale) may be causing significant stress in the patient's life.
- Tinnitus is fundamentally a self-report phenomenon and is not readily apparent to others except through the complaints of the sufferer, similar to chronic pain. That is, others cannot see it, feel it, hear it, or touch it and therefore cannot appreciate the impact that tinnitus has on one's life.
- Self-report tinnitus questionnaires allow the patient to self-realize the extent that the tinnitus is impacting his or her day-to-day lives. The questionnaires also allow the audiologist to identify those patients who are especially bothered by their tinnitus and who may benefit from treatment.
- Specific problems areas may be identified by conducting an item-analysis of the self-report measures.
- Treatment efficacy can be quantified when questionnaires are administered in a pre and post-treatment paradigm, promoting evidence-based practice.

Prior to the selection of a particular instrument for inclusion in the tinnitus assessment, the clinician needs to have a good understanding of the psychometric characteristics of that instrument. When evaluating a "candidate" tool, the clinician should be aware of the following psychometric standards (Hyde, 2000): overall methodology of development, validation, and norming; reliability; validity; responsiveness; and feasibility of practical application.

Over the years, several questionnaires have been developed. Table 20–8 summarizes some of the readily available questionnaires that evaluate a broad spectrum of activity limitation, participation restriction, cognitive reaction to tinnitus, and coping. As shown, for each questionnaire there is a short description of its content domains, scoring/interpretation, psychometric properties and strengths/weakness as viewed by the current authors. The self-report measures summarized in Table 20–8 are all quantitative in nature or score-driven (i.e., responses can be summed and/or averaged resulting in a total score or subscale scores). (*Note:* For additional discussion of self-report measurement, the reader is referred to Chapter 5.)

In contrast, *qualitative* tinnitus questionnaires are not score-driven and provide the clinician with information that is more descriptive in nature. For example, the TPQ developed by Tyler and Baker (1983) employs an open-ended format. The patient is simply asked, *"Please make a list of the difficulties that you have as a result of your tinnitus. List them in order of importance, starting with the biggest difficulties. Write down as many of them as you can."* The primary advantage of the open-ended approach (e.g., TPQ) in contrast to structured measures (e.g., THI; Tinnitus Reaction Questionnaire [TRQ; Wilson, Henry, Bowen, & Haralambous 1991]), is that they allow the patient to list their own specific tinnitus problems instead of limiting the patient to a fixed set of responses that may or may not be of relevance. This is similar to the benefits offered by the hearing aid tool, Client-Oriented Scale of Improvement (COSI; Dillon, James, & Ginis, 1997) where the patient reports his or her own specific hearing difficulties, rather than select from among a closed-response list.

Maintaining diaries has been used as a technique for assessing the patterns of tinnitus complaints over time (e.g., changes in pitch, loudness, annoyance, sleep disturbance) and factors that may be associated with those changes (e.g., noise exposure, medication use, diet). Daily diaries have been helpful in designing cognitive behavioral therapy sessions (Henry & Wilson, 2001); however, they may also be counterproductive as they increase the patient's attention to the tinnitus. Continued shifts in attention toward the tinnitus may not be advantageous for sound therapy treatments where the goal is to direct attention away from the tinnitus.

The administration of a self-report measure during the initial assessment appointment serves as the baseline measure for future treatment. That is, a reduction in self-perceived HRQoL (which may or may not be accompanied by a change in tinnitus impairment) may be reflective of the subjective benefit derived from a particular audiologic treatment approach (e.g., hearing aids, sound generator). In contrast, no change or an increase in perceived problems may suggest that the treatment is not providing sufficient benefit, and additional or alternative options should be considered.

One of the most widely used self-report measures for tinnitus is the THI. It is popular because it is brief, easily scored/administered/interpreted and assesses the domains of function that can be remediated by the clinical pathway model. Newman, Sandridge, and Jacobson, (1998) determined that a change in the total score of at least 20 points suggested that treatment is clinically effective. Furthermore, the four severity categories (0 to 16 points—no handicap; 18 to 36 points—mild handicap; 38 to 56 points—moderate handicap; 58 to 100 points—severe handicap) provide a method for clinicians to quantify changes in perceived participation restriction. (A fifth category, a *catastrophic* category, has been proposed by McCombe et al. (2001) for scores >76 points.) That is, it is possible to monitor movement from one category to another over time with or without intervention. In addition, the THI, can be used with its companion scales, the Hearing Handicap Inventory for the Elderly (HHIE; Ventry & Weinstein, 1982), Hearing Handicap Inventory for Adults (HHIA; Newman, Weinstein, Jacobson, & Hug, 1990), and the Dizziness Handicap Inventory (DHI; Jacobson & Newman, 1990) to quantify HRQoL for a variety of patient populations, such as those with Ménière's disease (Kinney, Sandridge, & Newman, 1997).

Table 20–8. Examples of Self-Report Tinnitus Questionnaires

Questionnaire/Authors	Content	Scoring/Interpretation	Psychometrics	Strengths/Weaknesses
Tinnitus Questionnaire/ Tinnitus Effects Questionnaire (TQ/TEQ; Hallam, Jakes, & Hinchcliffe, 1988)	52 items: sleep disturbance; emotional distress; auditory perceptual difficulties; inappropriate or lack of coping skills ("absolutist" beliefs)	Level of agreement to each statement: true (2 points); partly true (1 point); not true (0 points) Score range: 0–104 points with higher scores reflecting greater tinnitus complaints	High internal consistency reliability (Cronbach's α = .91–.95) High test-retest reliability (r = .91–.94) Convergent validity with the THQ and TRQ	Stable measure over time making it a useful outcome measure No data available regarding what is considered a clinically or statistically change in score following intervention for a given patient
Tinnitus Handicap Questionnaire (THQ; Kuk, Tyler, Russell, & Jordan, 1990)	27 items: **factor 1:** physical, emotional, social consequences of tinnitus; **factor 2:** effects on hearing; **factor 3:** patient's view of tinnitus	Level of agreement to each statement between 0 (strongly disagrees) and 100 (strongly agrees) Mean scores calculated with higher scores reflecting greater handicap Individual scores can be compared against normative percentile data	High internal consistency reliability for total scale (Cronbach's α =.95 with factors ranging from .47–.95) High test-retest reliability for total (r = .89), factor 1 (r = .89), and factor 2 (r = .90); low for factor 3 (r = .50) Adequate construct validity (r >.50) with tinnitus loudness judgments, life satisfaction, hearing, depression, and general health	Percentile ranking for given patient is useful in determining individual severity Application of factor 3 as an independent measure is questionable Scoring on a 100-point scale may be difficult for some individuals
Tinnitus Severity Scale (TSS; Sweetow & Levy, 1990)	15 items: intrusiveness; distress; hearing loss; sleep disturbance; and medication	Multiple choice format for each item range in score 1 (no impact) to 4 (most impact) Each item weighted 1 to 3 points (total = 39 points) Total score calculated by multiplying item score × weight and summing products	Adequate test-retest reliability (r = .86)	Item analysis may be useful in determining treatment goals Limited psychometric data available

continues

Table 20–8. *continued*

Questionnaire/Authors	Content	Scoring/Interpretation	Psychometrics	Strengths/Weaknesses
Subjective Tinnitus Severity Scale (STSS; Halford & Anderson, 1991)	16 items: severity defined as intrusiveness, prominence, and distress	YES/NO response format 10/16 items earn 1 point for YES response; 6/16 items earn 1 point for NO response Scores range: 0–16 with high scores reflecting greater overall severity	High internal consistency reliability (Cronbach's $\alpha = .84$) Criterion validity determined by significant correlations with clinician rating of severity	Brief and simple to administer and score No severity classification schemes developed No test-retest reliability available required for measuring outcome
Tinnitus Reaction Questionnaire (TRQ; Wilson, Henry, & Bowen, Haralambous, 1991)	26 items: distress consequences including anger, confusion, annoyance, helplessness, activity avoidance, and panic	5-point scale (0 = not at all; 4 = almost all of the time) Score range: 0–104 with higher scores reflecting greater distress	High internal consistency reliability (Cronbach's $\alpha = .96$) High test-retest reliability ($r = .88$) Construct validity supported by moderate to high correlations with clinician ratings and self-report measures of anxiety and depression Four factors emerged using principal components analysis: general distress; interference; severity; avoidance	Global measure of distress Brief and simple to administer and score Test-retest data helpful in determining treatment outcome; however only short-term (3 day to 3 weeks) data available No data available regarding what is considered a clinically or statistically change in score following intervention for a given patient
Tinnitus Handicap/ Support Scale (TH/SS; Erlandsson, Hallberg, & Axelsson, 1992)	28 items: **factor 1:** perceived attitudes or reactions of others; **factor 2:** social support; **factor 3:** personal and social handicaps	5-point scale (1 = strongly disagree; 5 = strongly disagree)	Construct validity assessed with the TSQ showing significant relationships between tinnitus severity and perceived attitudes (factor 1) and between severity and personal and social handicaps (factor 3)	Only questionnaire assessing influence of significant other in management process Lacks test-retest reliability data Factor 2 is not sufficiently sensitive to quantify complexity of social support

Questionnaire/Authors	Content	Scoring/Interpretation	Psychometrics	Strengths/Weaknesses
Tinnitus Handicap Inventory (THI; Newman, Jacobson, & Spitzer, 1996; Newman, Sandridge, & Jacobson, 1998)	25 items: **functional subscale:** role limitations in mental, social/occupational, physical functioning; **emotional subscale:** anger, frustration; irritability; depression; **catastrophic subscale:** desperation; loss of control; inability to cope and escape; fear of grave disease	Response format: YES (4 points); SOMETIMES (2 points); NO (0 points) Total score range: 0–100 points with higher scores reflecting greater handicap Handicap severity categories: no handicap (0–16 points); mild (18–36 points); moderate (38–56 points); severe (58–100 points)	Excellent internal consistency reliability (Cronbach's α = .96) High test-retest reliability: total (r = .92) and subscales (r = .84–.94) 95% confidence interval = 20 points Convergent validity with THQ and TQ Construct validity with Beck Depression inventory, Modified Somatic Perception Questionnaire, symptom rating scales (e.g., sleep, annoyance), tinnitus pitch and loudness	Brief, easy to administer and score Useful as a companion to the Hearing Handicap Inventory for the Elderly/Adults and Dizziness Handicap Inventory Available in languages other than English (e.g., Danish, Spanish) Psychometrical robust; however, only short-term (3 week) retest data available Should be considered unifactorial (distinctness of subscales questioned)
Tinnitus Coping Style Questionnaire (TCSQ ; Budd & Pugh, 1996a, 1996b)	33 items: maladaptive coping subscale; effective coping subscale	7 point scale (1 = never; 7 = always) Higher scores on maladaptive subscale reflect poor coping skills Higher scores on effective coping subscale reflect better acceptance of tinnitus	Excellent internal consistency reliability for maladaptive subscale (Cronbach's α = .90) and coping subscale (Cronbach's α = .89) Coping subscale significantly associated with measures of tinnitus severity, depression and anxiety Effective coping subscale significantly associated with tinnitus adjustment measures	Helpful in identifying behaviors and through patterns affect by tinnitus and coping strategies used Test-retest data are not available limiting application for evaluating treatment outcome

continues

Table 20–8. *continued*

Questionnaire/Authors	Content	Scoring/Interpretation	Psychometrics	Strengths/Weaknesses
Tinnitus Cognitions Questionnaire (TCQ ; Wilson & Henry, 1998)	26 items: positive and negative thoughts	5-point scale: 0 = never; 4 = very frequently Negative items are scored 0 to 4 Positive items reversed scored 4 to 0 Total score range: 0–104 with higher scores reflecting greater tendency to engage in negative thoughts and low engagement in positive thoughts	Excellent internal consistency reliability (Cronbach's $\alpha = .91$) Excellent test-retest reliability ($r = .88$) Factor analysis supported positive and negative subscales Construct and convergent validity assessed: TCQ showed moderate correlations with TRQ, THQ and TQ TCQ-negative subscale showed high correlations with tinnitus (tinnitus related distress, handicap, complaint behavior) and non-tinnitus (general depression, automatic thoughts, locus of control) measures	Useful index of cognitive responses Psychometrically robust Useful as an outcome measure Measures the extent to which patients actually engage in the reported cognitions/thoughts
Tinnitus Functional Index (TFI; Meikle, Henry, et al., 2008; Meikle, Steward, et al., 2008)	25 items 8 domains/subscales: intrusive, feeling, thinking, hearing, relaxing, sleeping, managing, quality of life	11-point scale (0 to 10) All responses summed, divided by number of questions answered, multiplied by 10 Total score range: 0–100)	High test-retest reliability (short-term, $r = 82$; long-term, $r = 0.76$) Excellent internal consistency reliability (Cronbach's $\alpha = .98$) Good construct validity with THI ($r = .87$), visual analogue scale for severity ($r = .75$), THQ ($r = .83$) High responsiveness to treatment-related changes in the severity of tinnitus (.79 effect size for overall TFI score)	Developed in a large sample of patients (327 for Prototype 1; 347 for Protype 2) Excellent measurement and psychometric properties Valid for measuring treatment-related changes

Sound Therapy Device Selection

A number of sound therapy devices (to be discussed later in the chapter) are available to provide relief from the annoying and bothersome consequences of tinnitus. These include assistive sound enrichment devices, HAs, ear-level sound generators, combination instruments, and other personal listening devices. In general, the goal for using any device is to decrease the perception of the tinnitus thus reducing the signal (tinnitus)-to-background noise ratio. That is, the goal is to reduce the contrast between the environment and the patient's tinnitus percept. In this way, the brain interprets the tinnitus as less noticeable, and therefore, less annoying and troublesome. Henry, Zaugg, Myers, and Schechter (2008) propose that sounds can provide not only relief (soothing) from the tinnitus but can also act as a distracter either through passive *background* sound or active *interesting* sound.

A problem faced by many clinicians is the selection of the specific sound therapy device for a given patient. As an aid in this process, Henry, Zaugg, and Schechter (2005b) developed a Sound Treatment Work Sheet. The work sheet requires the patient to list 3 specific situations when the tinnitus is most bothersome and is followed by a checklist that recommends specific types of sound treatment such as tabletop sound generators, wearable CD player, ear-level sound generators. On the worksheet, the patient reports how helpful (i.e., 5-point checklist ranging from "not at all" to "extremely") he or she found the device, providing feedback about treatment effectiveness to the clinician. Furthermore, the audiologist can note if the sound therapy was used primarily for enriching the sound environment or was used as a distracter to the tinnitus.

The Sound Therapy Option Profile (STOP; Newman & Sandridge, 2006) is an 11-item tool (see Appendix 20–A) that guides the audiologist in the selection of the optimal sound therapy device for the patient's individual needs. More specifically, completion of STOP creates a profile of the patient including his or her motivation, willingness to seek treatment and pay for that treatment, preference for specific types of sound generators, expectation level (i.e., realistic or not), and the need for referral to psychology. Within a few short minutes, the profile directs the clinician to the selection of broadband noise versus music, ear level devices versus body worn/handheld devices, or custom versus noncustom products, for example. STOP is a useful tool during the tinnitus evaluation; however, it is important to note that the profile is best administered after the patient has been counseled about tinnitus treatments and different forms of sound therapy. The patient must be an informed consumer to answer the queries regarding specific devices or treatments.

Listening Experiences

It is a valuable experience for patient's to listen to the various available sound therapy options during the evaluation session. Clinic-stock devices can be used to determine if tinnitus relief can be achieved from environmental enrichment devices (e.g., tabletop sound machines, CD recordings of nature/environmental sounds, fans), HAs, sound generators, or other personal listening devices (e.g., Neuromonics sound processor, or MP3 players).

The availability of open-fit behind-the-ear (BTE) digital signal processing (DSP) HAs and open-fit BTE or noncustom in-the-ear (ITE) sound generators now allows for efficient demonstrations. Some patients may experience immediate relief during the demonstration because of complete or partial masking; however, this is not the sole purpose of the demonstration. The in-clinic trial also allows the patient an opportunity to listen to different types of sounds and indicate which form of sound therapy might be more acceptable over the long term.

If the patient has hearing loss in addition to the tinnitus, it is important to determine which is more problematic to the patient—the hearing loss or tinnitus. As the patient's response will influence the device selection, it is important to add a tool that will assess the psychosocial impact of the hearing loss. The HHIA/E can determine to what degree the hearing loss impacts the patient's communication and/or psychosocial function. For example, if the patient's hearing loss has little or no impact (e.g., <18 out of 100 points on the

HHIE/A), the use of sound generators alone may be an appropriate first choice. In contrast, if the HHIE/A exceeds 18 points, reflecting significant activity limitation/participation restriction, the use of HAs or combination units would be more appropriate options.

Need for Referral

As shown in the clinical pathway (see Figure 20–1), the audiologist serves as the gatekeeper for further referral to other health care professionals. Therefore, it is incumbent upon the clinician to determine the need and urgency for further referral and treatment following the tinnitus evaluation.

There are several available tools that can be used to help triage patients for psychological treatment, especially for depression and anxiety. For example, the Beck Depression Inventory-Fast Screen for Medical Patients (Beck, Steer, & Brown, 2000) is a 7-item scale reflecting the cognitive and affective symptoms of depression making it a quick and effective way of screening for depression. For each item the patient is asked to read a group of statements about a single dimension of depression (e.g., pessimism; sadness; loss of interest) and to select one statement that best describes how he or she felt over the past 2 weeks. An example of the responses to the pessimism item is shown in Table 20–9. Scores range from 0 to 21 points, with higher scores reflecting greater perceived depression.

Table 20–9. Responses to the "Pessimism" Item on the Beck Depression Inventory-Fast Screen*Score*

Value (points)	Response
0	I am not discouraged about my future.
1	I feel more discouraged about my future than I used to be.
2	I do not expect things to work out for me.
3	I feel that my future is hopeless and will only get worse.

Source: Beck, Steer, and Brown, 2000.

The Hospital Anxiety and Depression Scale (HADS; Zigmond & Snaith, 1983) has been evaluated as a screening tool for anxiety and depressive disorders in patients with tinnitus (Zoger, Svedlund, & Holgers, 2004). The HADS is comprised of 14 items (7 items on the anxiety subscale; 7 items on the depression subscale) with ratings on a 0- to 3-point scale. Zoger et al. (2004) recommended using a cut-off score for each subscale of ≤5 points for patients with tinnitus.

A relationship between tinnitus and psychologic/psychiatric disorders has long been recognized (Folmer, Griest, Meikle, & Martin, 1999; Harrop-Griffiths, Katon, & Dobie, 1987; Sullivan, Katon, & Dobie, 1988) with the extreme cases being reports of suicide. Jacobson and McCaslin (2001) indicated that it is not the tinnitus per se that results in suicide, but concomitant psychiatric disorders that amplify the effects of tinnitus. The latter authors indicate that it may not be necessary to question specifically the patient as to whether they have attempted or are considering suicide; however, they suggest that it is important to be attentive to suicidal ideations offered by the patient.

As shown in the clinical pathway (see Figure 20–1), the patient may also be referred to neurology, especially if the tinnitus is somatically modulated. Somatic modulation of tinnitus is the phenomenon where, most often loudness, can be transiently modulated (increased or decreased) with various muscular contractions of the neck and/or jaw (Levine, 2004). As described in a latter section of this chapter, patients with somatically-modulated tinnitus are currently being treated with novel physical therapy approaches. Referral to dentistry may also be warranted because tinnitus has been associated with temporomandibular disorders (TMD; Camparis, Formigoni, Teixeira, & de Siqueira, 2005; Gelb, Gelb, & Wagner, 1997; Steigerwald & Verne, 1996).

Patient Disposition

At the conclusion of the tinnitus evaluation, recommendations are made for specific sound therapy devices, referrals are made to other health specialties, if warranted, and follow-up audiology appointments are made, if needed. If no further treatment is indicated or chosen, the patient may be discharged from the TMC.

Step Four: Individual Audiologic Treatment

The focus of audiologic treatment is the provision of the selected sound therapy device. Yet, it is critical to be cognizant that the device is only one component in the management process. Similar to hearing assistive technology, the device is a tool in the process and not the complete solution. The remaining portions of this section focus on: (1) advantages and benefits of sound therapy; (2) applications of sound therapy approaches; and (3) sound therapy treatment efficacy.

Sound Therapy: Advantages and Benefits

Inclusion of sound therapy devices within the management plan is important because they:

- provide immediate relief for many patients reducing the emotional consequences such as frustration, anxiety, and even depression;
- provide a means of allowing patient control over the tinnitus rather than tinnitus control over the patient;
- promote habituation to the tinnitus by neutralizing the threatening quality of the tinnitus;
- act as an attention-getting sound that distracts the listener away from the tinnitus;
- are noninvasive and have no adverse side effects;
- allow some patients to experience residual inhibition (i.e., tinnitus suppression or temporary disappearance after exposure to external sound);
- contribute to the reorganization of the central auditory nervous system pathways and centers responsible for tinnitus generation and perception (Folmer, Martin, Shi, & Edlefsen, 2006b; Henry et al., 2005b, Shiley et al., 2005).

Sound Therapy: Device Options

As shown on the bottom of Figure 20–1, there are several different forms of sound therapy strategies. Regardless of the type of sound treatment, each device provides a "sound-enhanced" environment by maintaining a low level of background noise whether it is delivered via sound field or coupled to the ears.

Environmental Enrichment Devices. A variety of simple-to-use, inexpensive techniques and devices can be used to increase the level of background sound to decrease the tinnitus signal-to-noise ratio. The exposure to pleasant external sounds promotes relief, provides distraction, and decreases the patient's awareness to tinnitus. Many patients find it beneficial, for example, to play the TV or radio at home in the background. A number of other environmental enrichment devices are available and include: (1) tabletop sound machines that can generate different types of sounds (e.g., rain, wind, waterfall); (2) CDs that contain recordings of music and nature/environmental sounds; (3) tabletop water fountains; (4) fans; and (5) water purifiers (Folmer et al., 2006b). For patients with sleep disturbance, the sound generated by tabletop sound machines and CDs may be delivered effectively using the commercially available Sound Pillow (www.soundpillow.com), pillow speakers (small flat speakers) or headband speakers (headband with speakers sewn inside the band originally developed for athletes). Headphones/earbuds coupled to CD or MP3 players efficiently direct sounds to the ear canals; however, they may restrict mobility and may be impractical or too conspicuous to be worn in certain situations such as at work (Folmer et al., 2006b).

Hearing Aids. The use of HAs in the management of tinnitus is a common and acceptable practice (Kochkin & Tyler, 2008; Sheldrake & Jastreboff, 2004; Vernon & Meikel, 2000). It is estimated that up to 90% of patients experience a reduction in the loudness of the tinnitus from the use of HAs

(Johnson, 1998; Schechter, Henry, Zaugg & Fausti, 2002). An additional benefit is improved communication gained from amplifying the inaudible speech sounds. Although the exact mechanisms involved in the success of HAs for tinnitus treatment are unknown, there are a few proposed theories. The most common theory suggests that HAs provide sufficient amplification of ambient sound to mask or "cover up" the tinnitus. In this connection, it has been suggested that HAs increase stimulation in the auditory pathway which, in turn, decreases the difference between the tinnitus and the background neuronal activity. Furthermore, the amplification provided by HAs decreases the "strain to hear," thereby reducing overall stress and anxiety associated with the tinnitus (Sheldrake & Jastreboff, 2004).

Regardless of the exact mechanisms responsible for providing benefit from the use of HAs, it is important for patients to understand the relationship between hearing loss and tinnitus and to appreciate the differences between the two auditory symptoms. For patients with both hearing loss and tinnitus, Shiley et al. (2005) suggested that the following points be addressed:

- Tinnitus does not cause hearing loss; however, hearing loss may increase the chances for individuals to have tinnitus.
- Even when relief is provided for tinnitus, residual communication breakdown will remain due to hearing loss.
- HAs do not amplify the tinnitus. On the contrary, the use of HAs often provides relief.
- Improvement in communication function due to HA use will help the individual feel less frustrated, isolated, and withdrawn.

It is interesting to note that of the use of "high-end" HA technology incorporating sophisticated noise reduction algorithms may be counterproductive for patients with tinnitus. Some amplification of environmental noise is indeed helpful for these patients. On the other hand, DSP HAs provide flexibility in manipulating the signal. For example, "soft" sounds can be enhanced by lowering the compression kneepoint in the DSP HAs creating a masking effect which, in turn, will reduce the perception of tinnitus. Open-fit HAs may be especially beneficial as they permit normal entry of environmental sounds into the ear canal.

Sound Generators. Ear-level sound generators are a choice for patients who do not benefit or require amplification because they have normal or near-normal audiometric thresholds. BTE or ITE sound generators are the most portable and inconspicuous method for patients to receive a stable broadband signal to the ear. This contrasts with the use of tabletop sound machines, for example, where the effectiveness of the sound is lost when the patient leaves the room. During the fitting of sound generators, it is important for the clinician to describe the signal in positive terms (e.g., "gentle shower sound") and to avoid negative terms such as "noise" or "static."

Combination Tinnitus Instruments. Combination devices contain a HA circuit and a noise-producing circuit in the same instrument, allowing patients who have both a hearing loss and suffer from tinnitus to use one device. A critical feature in the combination device is the ability to control the volume of the sound generator portion independent of the volume control of the HA.

Sound Therapy: Device Applications

Sound therapy devices can be used in a variety of approaches. No matter which application is used by the clinician, it is important that the patient understand the rationale for its use.

Masking. Masking therapy has a long history and the readers are referred to the following works for historic reference (Hazell et al., 1985; Vernon, Griest, & Press, 1990; Vernon & Meikel, 2000; Vernon & Schleuning, 1978). The key features of tinnitus masking are summarized in Table 20–10.

For many patients, sound generators can provide total or partial masking resulting in immediate relief. The broadband sound is found to be more acceptable than their own tinnitus. Some patients use maskers on an "as-needed" basis when they

Table 20–10. Comparison of Salient Features Underlying Masking Therapy and Habituation/Retraining Therapy

Feature	Masking Therapy	Habituation/Retraining Therapy
Rationale	To mask or partially mask perception of tinnitus.	To promote habituation of tinnitus.
Counseling	Not to attend to tinnitus; provide control.	Do not fear tinnitus.
Types of ear-level devices used	Maskers or tinnitus instruments (masker + HA housed in same device). Used monaurally or binaurally. Trial-and-error procedure in clinic to determine most effective device.	Sound generator or combination unit (sound generator + HA housed in same device). Used binaurally. Device selection based on prescribed category (0, 1, 2, 3, or 4).
Spectral characteristics of sound	Noise varies depending on patient's perception of most effective.	Stable broadband noise.
Sound therapy regimen	Use of ear-level device with masking noise adjusted to patient's preference, typically at the lowest level to mask (or partially mask) tinnitus. Wear as desired.	Use of ear-level device with noise adjusted just below "mixing point" at the beginning of the day. Use during waking hours.
Follow-up visits	Typically at 6 months and 1 year to ensure proper use of maskers.	Typically at 3 and 6 weeks, and 3, 6, 12, and 18 months.
Long-term use	Use as long as necessary to provide masking relief.	Use until habituation is achieved, typically 1 to 2 years.

Source: Adapted from Henry, Schechter, Nagler, and Fausti (2002).

are most bothered by the tinnitus. Hazell (1987), however, suggested that long-term use of masking may produce beneficial effects even when the masker is removed.

There are a few caveats regarding sound generators as maskers that must be discussed with the patient. It is important when counseling patients that they be cautioned that sound generators set too loud might interfere with communication. They might even cause damage to hearing if used for extended periods of time at too intense a setting. In addition, sound generators can increase the tinnitus so it is suggested that patients should give themselves rest periods from using the devices (Tyler & Bentler, 1987).

Habituation/Retraining. In contrast to the immediate relief produced by total or partial masking, sound generators can be used to promote habituation of the tinnitus over the long term. Sound generators provide a continuous and monotonous sound stimulus, one identified as nonthreatening. The brain habituates to the nonthreatening sound as well as the tinnitus. Jastreboff (1990) and Jastreboff and Hazell (1993) have defined habituation as an adaptation process of the auditory system to reduce perceived signal intensity. By reducing the perceived signal intensity, the negative consequences of tinnitus, including emotional and automatic reactions, will decrease. Accordingly, the application of sound generators in this type of habituation treatment focuses on the disappearance of tinnitus awareness as the tinnitus becomes an essentially irrelevant signal. Hallam and McKenna (2006), however, proposed several "roadblocks" to the habituation process, including an elevated arousal state, avoidance of exposure to external noise and/or tinnitus; and negative beliefs about tinnitus.

Tinnitus Retraining Therapy (TRT), developed by Jastreboff and colleagues (Jastreboff, 2000; Jastreboff & Hazell, 2004; Jastreboff & Jastreboff, 2004) is based on the concept of habituation along with neuroplasticity and may involve 18 to

24 months of treatment (see Table 20–10). The treatment is composed of two major components: (1) the use of low level white noise generators; and (2) directive counseling (Jastreboff & Jastreboff, 2004). The white noise generators are used for approximately 6 to 8 hours per day set specifically at the "mixing point." The mixing point is the level where the noise is just below the patient's perception of his or her tinnitus and is considered important for facilitating habituation (Jastreboff & Hazell, 1993). Directive counseling includes ongoing explanations and education about the causes of tinnitus and identification of specific anxieties relating to tinnitus in order to challenge the patient's perception of "harm" or "threat."

Criticism of TRT has included failure to acknowledge that there may be a need for additional psychological intervention, such as cognitive-behavioral therapy/cognitive restructuring techniques. In addition, there remains a paucity of data from well-controlled studies (Kroener-Herwig et al., 2000; Wilson, Henry, Andersson, Hallam, & Lindberg, 1998) supporting its efficacy.

Combined Approach. Another treatment option that we have found to be beneficial involves a combination of masking and habituation approaches. That is, if a patient requires immediate relief from the tinnitus, complete masking is attempted during the initial phases of treatment. This relief provided by the masking promotes a reduction in stress and thereby helps to reduce the perception of the tinnitus, which in turn promotes a sense of hope. Yet, masking may not be effective for long-term treatment, therefore, after a short period, approximately one month, the patient is transitioned into a more long-term management approach using the habituation model (Hallam, Rachman, & Hinchcliffe, 1984). In this approach, patients are now counseled not to "cover up" the tinnitus (total masking) but to set the device to deliver the signal at a level slightly below the tinnitus (partial masking) to facilitate habituation. The salient differences between tinnitus masking and TRT are summarized in Table 20–10.

Music Therapy. Music has been used therapeutically in a number of different applications and has been shown to be successful in addressing the physical, emotional, cognitive, and social needs of individuals of all ages (Standley, 1995). In this connection, music therapy interventions have been designed to promote wellness, manage stress, alleviate pain, and promote physical rehabilitation. (The reader is referred to www.musictherapy.org Web site for further information regarding the benefits of music therapy.) Like other forms of sound enhancement, music may be very helpful to patients with tinnitus and can be delivered using a personal listening device (e.g., CD player or MP3 player). Any music that the patient finds to be distracting from the tinnitus and/or provide relaxation may be beneficial. Examples of music that have been selected with the tinnitus patient in mind can be found at, www.soundpillow.com .

Recently, Davis (2006) extended the known benefits of music into the arena for treatment of tinnitus and developed an acoustic desensitization protocol, currently known as the Neuromonics Tinnitus Treatment (NTT). Figure 20–7 shows the Neuromonics sound processor that delivers the signal to the patient though a set of earphones with extended frequency response.

The NTT combines the use of the music with ongoing education, monitoring, support and counseling. As shown in Figure 20–8, the NTT is composed of two stages of treatment plus a maintenance

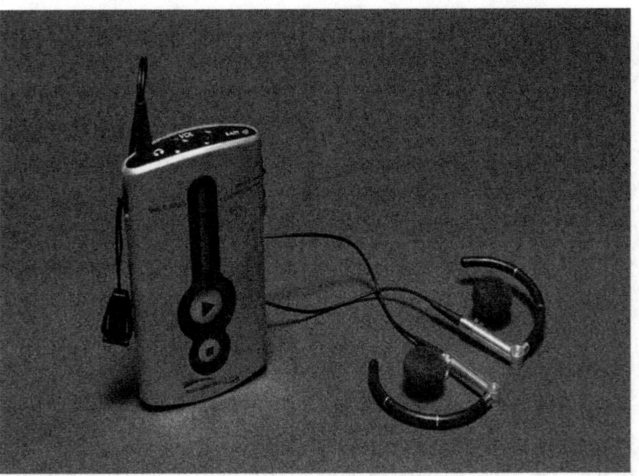

Figure 20–7. Neuromonics Tinnitus Treatment (NTT) sound processor.

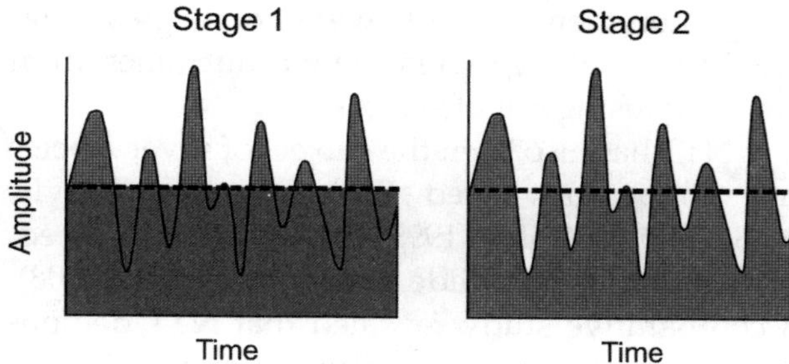

Figure 20–8. Schematic representation depicting the relationship between tinnitus perception (*dashed line*) and customized music stimuli (Stage 1 and Stage 2) produced by the Neuromonics Tinnitus Treatment (NTT) sound processor. The shaded area in Stage 1 represents the embedded "shower sound."

stage once treatment has been completed. Stage 1 (preconditioning stage) uses an embedded broadband noise (referred to as the "shower sound") in the spectrally modified music (i.e., compensating for the patient's hearing loss) and is delivered to the ears via the sound processor using extended frequency ear buds. The broadband noise is thought to increase interaction with the tinnitus (i.e., total masking, if possible) to help the patient attain relief and sense of control over the tinnitus at the beginning of treatment. Stage 1 is at least 2 months in duration. Volume of the acoustic stimulus is set to provide as much relief without being uncomfortable. In Stage 2 (active stage), the embedded broadband signal is removed from the music, otherwise the music is unchanged. Without the embedded masking signal, the volume of music is generally set so that the patient is aware of the tinnitus about one-half of the time. This provides more intermittent interaction with the tinnitus. The intention is that the intermittency helps retrain the brain to relegate the tinnitus signal to the background. The second stage of treatment is at least 4 months in duration, making the entire treatment last at least 6 months. The sound processor is used at least 2 to 4 hours per day (targeted at the times when the tinnitus is most disturbing) for both stages 1 and 2, followed by an "as needed" basis during the maintenance phase of treatment.

Sound Therapy: Efficacy of Options

Rigorous research designs evaluating sound therapy options should include the following characteristics: utilization of control group/s and blinding: appropriate statistical testing including "dropouts" that should be used in an "intention to treat" analysis rather than elimination from the data set; long-term follow-up of treatment effects; use of validated outcome measures; appropriate inclusion criteria and sample sizes based on a power analysis (Dobie, 2004b). In reality, however, research evaluating the efficacy of sound therapy devices is problematic. It is difficult to have a placebo group or conduct a blinded study. For example, subjects clearly know that they are using a sound generator when they hear the white noise or they clearly know when they are using HAs when their listening skills improved through amplification of the incoming sounds.

Despite the fact that there is a paucity of research showing clinical effectiveness of sound devices and therapy approaches, there is an extensive body of literature describing the underlying rational, clinical methodologies, and success rates for different sound therapy approaches. Although it would be more beneficial to have research to support our evidence-based practices, the different forms of sound therapy should not be abandoned on that basis alone. In fact, evidence-based practice's central message is one of flexibility and blending past clinical experiences with new research and knowledge as it becomes available to the practitioner (Law, 2002).

In general, HAs have been shown to be an effective treatment option, perhaps because they improved communication function which in turn reduced stress and consequently reduced the annoyance factor from the tinnitus (Surr, Kolb, Cord, & Garrus, 1999; Surr, Montgomery & Mueller, 1985). It has been observed that patients with greater degrees of hearing loss preferred the use of HAs over maskers (Mehlum, Grasel, & Fankhauser, 1984). Masking devices were shown to be superior to placebo devices (Erlandsson, Ringdahl, Hutchins, & Carlsson, 1987), provided greater improvement in sleep over HAs (Stephens & Corcoran, 1985), yet results were inconclusive when maskers were compared to nonacoustic treatments such as self-hypnosis (Attias, et al., 1993), acupuncture (Jansson, Warfvinge, Edensvard, & Wiberg, 1996), and cognitive behavior therapy (Jakes, Hallam, McKenna, & Hinchcliffe, 1992).

Recently, Henry and colleagues (Henry et al., 2006a, 2006b) conducted a controlled clinical study to evaluate the clinical efficacy of tinnitus masking and TRT in samples of veterans with clinically significant tinnitus using a repeated measures design. Several standardized outcome measures were used including the THI and Tinnitus Handicap Questionnaire (THQ; Kuk, Tyler, Russell, & Jordan, 1990). Qualifying patients were quasi-randomly (alternating placement) placed into the two groups: tinnitus masking group (TM) or TRT treatment (TRT). Outcome measures were administered at 0 (baseline), 3, 6, 12, and 18 months. Of the 123 patients enrolled in the study, 118 were included in the final analysis. Based on effect sizes, both the TM group and TRT group showed improvement, with TRT group showing greater improvement over the long term. Greater improvement for TRT when compared to TM occurred more strongly when the patients began treatment with a "very big" tinnitus problem. In contrast, when patients began treatment with a "moderate" tinnitus problem, benefits were not as great. Figure 20–9 displays representative outcomes from the study using data from the THI.

NTT has also been the subject of several peer- and nonpeer-reviewed clinical studies (Davis, 1998; Davis & Wilde, 1995; Davis, Wilde, & Steed, 1999, 2001; Davis, Wilde, Steed, & Hanley, 2008). A comparative study revealed that NTT demonstrated benefit over counseling alone or broadband noise presented at the "mixing point" plus counseling. These promising results led to a recent clinical study conducted by Davis, Paki, and Hanley (2007) wherein 35 subjects were randomly allocated to one of two treatment groups, corresponding to the two stages of the NTT. The TRQ was used as the primary outcome measure. Patients were followed at 2, 4, 6, and 12 months after the initiation of treatment. After 2 months of treatment, both groups displayed clinically and statistically significant improvement on the TRQ. After six months of treatment, 91% of the subjects exceeded the criteria considered as a significant improvement (i.e., reduction of at least 40% on the TRQ). Furthermore, the percentage of time that subjects reported being aware of their tinnitus progressively decreased as the mean usage of the device also decreased, suggesting a permanent

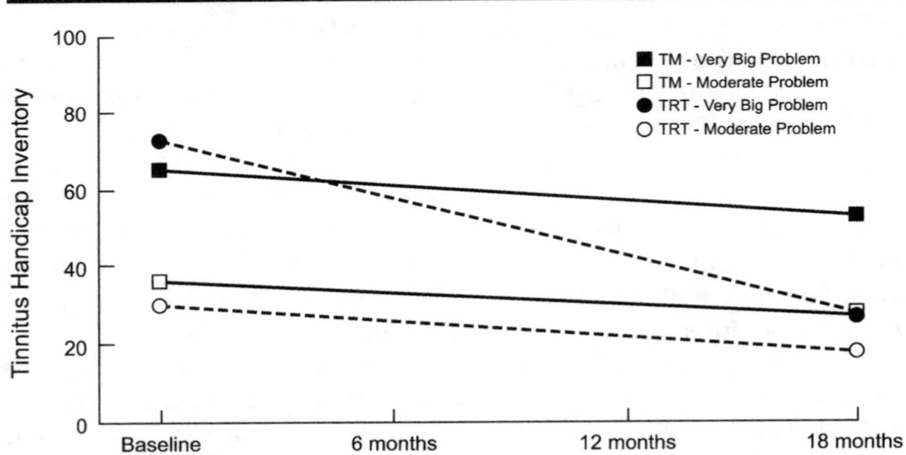

Figure 20–9. Representative outcome data (trajectories across 18 months) illustrating differences between tinnitus masking (TM) and tinnitus retraining therapy (TRT) using the Tinnitus Handicap Inventory (THI). Adapted with permission from Henry et al., 2006b (p. 120).

treatment effect. At present, there are no studies comparing the clinical effectiveness of NTT to other forms of sound therapy.

Ongoing Counseling

As previously noted, the use of sound therapy devices is only part of the management process. The most fundamental component of the treatment plan, regardless of device or approach (e.g., masking, TRT, NTT), is the provision of on-going counseling and encouragement. It is noteworthy that the interactions we have with our patients create expectations that ultimately influence the treatment. Tyler and colleagues (Tyler, Haskell, Preece, & Bergan, 2001; Tyler, Noble, Preece, Dunn, & Witt, 2004) developed a model that can be used to enhance patient expectations, improving treatment outcome. Expectations about the course of treatment for sound therapy must be realistic. The patient must understand that there is no singular "cure" for tinnitus and that the long-term goal is to provide relief from the distress nature of the tinnitus. Table 20–11 summarizes the attributes that influence patient expectations based on the nurturing patient expectations model.

Following device fitting, patients should be scheduled for follow-up appointments at regular intervals. Follow-up contacts may be face-to-face, via telephone or through email, depending upon the specific needs of the patient and treatment plan. As summarized in Table 20–12, several authors (Andersson & Kaldo, 2006a, 2006b; Folmer et al., 2006a, 2006b; Henry et al., 2005; Sizer & Coles, 2006; Tyler, Gehringer, Noble, Dunn, Witt, & Bardia, 2006) have offered areas of counseling that need to be addressed on a continuing basis during the audiologic management process (i.e., before, during and after the fitting of sound devices).

To quantify treatment effectiveness, measures of both tinnitus impairment and tinnitus activity limitation/participation should be administered on a regular basis as well. That is, information about the psychoacoustic attributes of tinnitus (obtained from impairment measurements) and HRQoL consequences of tinnitus (obtained from self-report measures) provide fundamentally different information and have somewhat different utility in assessing user benefit. Patients are discharged from the TMC once the tinnitus has become manageable; however, periodic contact with the patient provides support and evaluation of longitudinal benefit of the treatment program.

Table 20–11. Attributes Comprising the Nurturing Patient Expectations Model

Being perceived as a knowledgeable professional using jargon and examples that are understandable by the patient
Being sympathetic to the patient by listening and acknowledging problems
Demonstrating an understanding of the problem by providing relevant information about hearing, hearing loss, and tinnitus
Providing a clear treatment plan with realistic goals and expectations
Showing that you sincerely care about the patient
Providing feelings of mastery to the patient so that they gain a sense of control over the tinnitus
Providing hope which is not typically offered by other health care professionals to patients with tinnitus (e.g., too often a patient is told to learn to live with it)
Instilling confidence in your intervention efforts by believing in the treatment plan

Source: Adapted from Tyler, Haskell, Preece, and Bergan, 2001; Tyler, Noble, Preece, Dunn, and Witt, 2004.

Table 20–12. Example Topic Areas for Ongoing Counseling

- Lifestyle changes (e.g., stress management, adequate sleep, limiting alcohol, caffeine, and tobacco, avoid silence by maintaining safe levels of background noise, engagement in meaningful activities and hobbies, benefits of regular exercise)
- Informational counseling about hearing, hearing loss, hearing loss prevention
- Refocusing attention on the task (diverting attention away from tinnitus onto other tasks)
- Reassurance about the lack of a serious underlying cause (based on medical clearance for treatment program provided by otolaryngologist)
- Realistic expectations and perspectives about treatment outcome
- Promotion of relaxation including the use of relaxation exercise
- Benefits of sound therapy
- Ways to make tinnitus take on less importance
- Lack of quality control of information on the internet
- Improving sleep patterns (e.g., www.sleepfoundation.org)
- Actively listen to patient
- Provide patients with hope

Source: Adapted from Henry, Dennis, and Schecter, 2005; Sizer and Coles, 2006; Andersson and Kaldo, 2006a, 2006b; Folmer, Martin, Shi and Edlefsen, 2006a, 2006b; Tyler, Gehringer, Noble, Dunn, Witt, and Bardia, 2006.

Multidisciplinary Team Input

The TMC model includes a two-way communication between audiology and other health care practitioners including otolaryngology, psychology, neurology, and dentistry as shown in Figure 20–1. Typically, the audiologist serves as the gatekeeper for the latter three practitioners based on patient history and screening measures previously described. Referrals to other health care providers can occur at anytime; however, they occur most typically during the individual tinnitus evaluation as the audiologist assesses the patient. Following is an overview of the services offered by the psychologist, neurologist, and dentist on the team (medical assessment was addressed at the beginning of the chapter).

Psychology

The major focus of intervention by the psychologist may be to educate the patient about the "mind-body" connection. Most patients readily admit that stress in general, and negative emotions in particular, can increase the perceived severity of the tinnitus, ultimately affecting HRQoL. For some patients, the increased annoyance and distress they are experiencing may be triggered by major situational or emotional stress factors occurring in their everyday life. Patients seeking tinnitus treatments also typically report a fear of the long-term impact that tinnitus may have on their HRQoL. Specifically, the primary complaints that patients attribute to their tinnitus include: sleep disturbance; realization that there is "no quick cure" for tinnitus; difficulty adjusting to having a chronic condition; and the inability to relax secondary to attentional focus on internal tinnitus perception.

Important mediators and processes are involved in coping with stress of any chronic illness. The transactional model of stress (Lazarus & Folkman, 1984) points to three stress appraisals. That is, stress may be:

- perceived as a threat;
- experienced as a challenge; and
- expected to result in harm and/or loss.

Personality traits and/or social-cultural roles and expectations may influence a patient's construction of meaning and formulation of a model of their chronic condition (Pachter, 1994). Those patients with a strong internal locus of control (i.e., those who feel that they can impact the course of their treatment and ultimate prognosis) have advantages—often showing improved clinical and functional outcome.

Cognitive behavior therapy (CBT) is often helpful in overall treatment because it addresses problematic tinnitus-related cognitions, emotions, and behaviors. This approach provides patients with tools that help them to: (1) modify errors in logic; (2) recognize dysfunctional thoughts (i.e., beliefs, attitudes, and/or attributions); and (3) identify hypotheses that can be tested in relation to these thoughts. The psychologist helps the patient challenge (or test) the validity of his or her thoughts as a description of themselves, the world, or the future (Wilson et al., 1998). This approach focuses on helping patients identify cognitive distortions such as personalization (*Why did this happen to me?*), jumping to conclusions (*I woke up with tinnitus this morning so the rest of my day will be ruined*), or catastrophizing (*Because I have tinnitus, I must have a terrible disease*) and to alter those reactions and behaviors. The goal of treatment is not only to identify the cognitive distortions, but to change the way in which the patient interprets, feels and thinks; modify the patient's actions; and remove inappropriate belief, anxieties, and fears. (Sweetow, 2000). Fortunately, cognitive distortions respond well to behavior interventions such as scrutiny for "evidence" (which supports or does not support worrisome beliefs). Cognitive behavior therapy protocols for tinnitus treatment have also been developed using self-help books (Henry & Wilson, 2001, 2002) and Internet (Andersson, Stromgren, Strom, & Lyttkens, 2002) formats. A recently published Cochran Review (Martinez Devesa, Waddell, Perera, & Theodoulou, 2007) supports the application of CBT in the treatment of tinnitus patients and confirms that this approach has a positive effect on the patient's HRQoL.

In addition to CBT, other forms of behavioral therapy including imagery training (focusing thoughts on something pleasant thereby directing thoughts away from the tinnitus), attention control (learning to switch attention away from the tinnitus when it is bothersome), and relaxation training (progressive muscular relaxation using a guided protocol) are helpful in the treatment process (Tyler et al., 2004).

A meta-analysis of a variety of psychological treatments for tinnitus was conducted by Andersson and Lyttkens (1999). The outcome of 18 studies (because more than one treatment was tested in the same study, there were a total of 24 samples) including investigations of CBT (n = 11), relaxation training (n = 4), hypnosis (n = 2), biofeedback (n = 2), educational/information sessions (n = 2), and stress management/problem solving (n = 3) were included in the meta-analysis. In general, it was found that psychological treatments for tinnitus are more effective than previously reported in qualitative literature reviews. In particular, exploratory analyses revealed that CBT was more effective in reducing annoyance than any other form of treatment evaluated.

It is also important to consider the social support system for the patient in the overall management process. Social support by family members/significant others often requires education as to the nature of both hearing disturbance and tinnitus. The invisibility of tinnitus makes it difficult for social support networks to understand the degree of interference and distress that can be caused by the tinnitus. CDs (e.g., www.ata.org) and computer sound files (e.g., www.rnid.org.uk) that simulate tinnitus are helpful in conveying to significant others the annoyance of tinnitus.

Psychological treatment, although initially viewed with some apprehension and reluctance, has been very helpful for many patients. Noble and Tyler (2007) support an ongoing relationship between audiology and psychology as an optimal model for tinnitus treatment.

Neurology

Referral to neurology typically occurs when patients report somatic modulation of their tinnitus by contracting muscles of the head, neck, and/or jaw. Recall that somatic modulation of tinnitus is the phenomenon where some aspect of tinnitus, most typically perceived loudness, can be transiently modulated (increased or decreased) with contractions of the head, neck and/or jaw (Levine, Abel & Cheng, 2003; Sanchez, Guerr, Lorenzi, Brandao, & Bento, 2002;). Levine (1999a, 1999b, 2004) has indicated that musculature of the head and neck is involved in the pathogensis of tinnitus. Abnormal somatosensory feedback from muscle spindles or golgi tendon muscles in the head and neck muscles may release the dorsal cochlear nucleus from inhibition, resulting in tinnitus (Levine, 2004). Researchers have demonstrated that the dorsal cochlear nucleus receives somatosensory information in cats (Kanold & Young, 2001), demonstrating an anatomic link between the auditory and somatosensory sytems. Furthermore, studies have showed that reducing tension in jaw muscular (Wright & Bifano, 1997) or resolving vertebral subluxations are effective in reducing tinnitus (Alcantara & Plaugher, 2002; Whedon, 2006). Recent studies using positron emission tomography (PET) imaging have shown that movement of the jaw and lower face, activating only the somatosensory and motor cortex in normal individuals, actually activate regions of the auditory cortex in patients with severe tinnitus (Salvi, Lockwood, & Burkard, 2000).

At the initial visit with the patients, the neurologist conducts a physical examination. Based on the examination, specific physiotherapy protocols have been developed in conjunction with a physical therapist including treatment focusing on motion (e.g., repeated cervical and thoracic movements), manual manipulation (e.g., mobilizations to upper, mid and lower cervical spine, thoracic spine including extensions and rotations), exercise (e.g., strengthening of neck flexors/extensors), and patient education (e.g., body mechanics, ergonomics, spine care) components.

Dentistry

Tinnitus has been associated with temporal mandibular disorder (TMD; Lam, Lawrence, & Tenenbaum, 2001; Steigerwald & Verne, 1996). Access to a dentist with expertise in this area might be beneficial for a small select group of patients who might experience relief from tinnitus and TMD pain through dental treatments including bite realignment (Morgan, 1996). The goal of treatment is to improve abnormal jaw mechanics and tracking, as well as normalizing the internal and external soft tissue. Treatment is aimed at reducing tension in jaw muscular. For example, Wright and Bifano (1997) report that TMD therapy reduced tinnitus in individuals whose tinnitus worsened with teeth clenching.

Other/Alternative Treatment Options

Pharmacology Treatments

There are no drugs that have been specifically developed to "treat" tinnitus, *per se*; however, medications are often prescribed by physicians to treat insomnia, anxiety, depression, phobias, obsessive-compulsive behaviors, or other psychological problems (Shiley, Folmer, & McMenomey, 2005). The major classes of drugs that have been associated with the treatment of tinnitus include: antiarrhythmics (lidocaine); anticonvulsants (carbamazepine); benzodiazepines (diazepam; alprazolam); and antidepressants (nortriptyline; amitriptyline; floxetine; paroxetine). Results of randomized clinical trials with the aforementioned drugs have not been promising, with many of the medications having serious side effects (Dobie, 2004a). The most promising drugs affect the emotional status of patients through the reduction of anxiety, depression, and sleep disturbance (Brummett, 1989). It is noteworthy that the Food and Drug Administration (FDA) has not approved any specific drug specifically for the purpose of tinnitus treatment (Schleuning, Shi, & Martin, 2007).

Alternative Treatments

A variety of alternative tinnitus treatment options exist with a wide range of reported success rates. It is important for audiologists to at least be familiar with the various alternative and complementary treatments because patients often ask. Dobie (2004a) reported no beneficial effects from a range of physical treatments including acupuncture and devices purporting to deliver magnetic, electromagnetic, laser, or ultrasound stimulation through the skin over the mastoid area.

Electrical Stimulation

Electrical stimulation for tinnitus suppression includes a wide range of procedures. Electrical current is delivered from devices that are either external or internally implanted in the middle or inner ear. The reader is referred to Dauman (2000) and Rubinstein and Tyler (2004) for a summary of the history of electrical tinnitus suppression.

Currently, the most commonly used electrical stimulation is from cochlear implants. Mirz, Mortensen, Gjedde, and Pederson (2002) demonstrated the positive effect of the cochlear implant on the suppression of tinnitus through the use of PET. The PET scan revealed a reduction of tinnitus-related activity in the primary auditory cortex, associated cortex as well as areas associated with emotion (limbic system) and attention (dorsolateral prefrontal cortices). Quaranta, Wagsaff and Baguley (2004) conducted a literature search evaluating the effects of cochlear implants on tinnitus. They identified 32 papers meeting their search criteria. Although results were varied, the use of a cochlear implant was associated with a reduction in tinnitus intensity and awareness for approximately 86% of patients, and an exacerbation of the tinnitus occurred in only 9% of the patient population. Currently in the United States, cochlear implantation is limited to those individuals with severe to profound hearing loss; but for those individuals, the implant may have the secondary benefit of providing relief from tinnitus.

Nutritional Supplements

Currently, there are nutritional supplements on the market that have been touted to provide relief to the tinnitus sufferer. These include minerals such as magnesium or zinc, herbal preparations including ginko biloba, homeopathic remedies, and B vitamins (Seidman & Babu, 2003). Although there are many anecdotal reports associated with the aforementioned options, there is no conclusive evidence to support the use of supplements based on well-controlled trials.

Conclusion

Tinnitus is a distressing symptom that affects the HRQoL for many individuals. As audiologists, we have an obligation to help these patients overcome the psychosocial consequences of tinnitus impairment. Of course, not all patients require intensive audiologic management. Many patients will benefit considerably from minimal counseling about hearing, hearing loss, and tinnitus. For those patients requiring further treatment, the clinical pathway described in this chapter provides a "best practices" model to guide the audiologist through the management process. The sequencing of strategies provides differing levels of treatment to promote tinnitus relief for a wide variety of patients with tinnitus. In our TMC, we are fortunate to work hand-in-hand with a variety of other health care professionals including, otolaryngologists, psychologists, neurologists, and dentists. It may be necessary for some audiologists to develop working relationships with other health care practitioners in order to make appropriate referrals as needed.

One of the main contributions an audiologist can make in working with patients with tinnitus is to provide them with a sense of hope. This can be accomplished by offering education about tinnitus and the tools and management strategies designed to obtain relief. We believe that a multidisciplinary team approach represented by the provided clinical pathway provides the patient with the best clinical care.

References

Abrams, H., Hnath-Chisolm, T., Guerreiro, S., & Ritterman, S. (1992). The effects of intervention strategy on self-perception of hearing handicap. *Ear and Hearing, 13*, 371–377.

Alcantara, J., & Plaugher, G. (2002). Chiropractic care of a patient with temporomandibular disorder and atlas subluxation. *Journal of Manipulative and Physiological Therapeutics, 25*, 63–70.

American Academy of Audiology. (2004). *Audiology: Scope of Practice.* Retrieved June 12, 2008, from www.audiology.org/publications/documents/practice

American Speech-Language-Hearing Association. (2004). Scope of practice in audiology. *Asha Supplement, 24*, 27–35.

Andersson, G., & Kaldo, V. (2006a). Cognitive-behavioral therapy with applied relaxation. In R.

S. Tyler (Ed.), *Tinnitus treatment: Clinical protocols* (pp. 96–115). San Diego, CA: Thieme.

Andersson, G., & Kaldo, V. (2006b). Internet-based self-help treatment of tinnitus. In R. S. Tyler (Ed.), *Tinnitus treatment: Clinical protocols* (pp. 29–40). San Diego, CA: Thieme.

Andersson, G., & Lyttkens, L. (1999). A meta-analytic review of psychological treatments for tinnitus. *British Journal of Audiology, 33,* 201–210.

Andersson, G., Stromgren, T., Strom, L., & Lyttkens, L. (2002). Randomized controlled trial of Internet based cognitive behavior therapy for distress associated with tinnitus. *Psychosomatic Medicine, 64,* 810–816.

Arnold, W., Bartenstein, P., Oestreicher, E., Romer, W., & Schwaiger, M. (1996). Focal metabolic activation in the predominant left auditory cortex in patients suffering from tinnitus: A PET study with [18F]deoxyglucose. *Journal of Otorhinolaryngology, 58,* 195–199.

Attias, J., Shemsh, Z., Sohmer, H., Gold, S., Shoam, C., & Faraggi, D. (1993). Comparison between self-hypnosis, masking and attentiveness for alleviation of chronic tinnitus. *Audiology, 32,* 302–312.

Baguley, D. M. (2002). Mechanisms of tinnitus. *British Medical Bulletin, 63,* 195–212.

Baguley, D. M., & Andersson, G. (2007). *Hyperacusis: Mechanisms, diagnosis, and therapies.* San Diego, CA: Plural.

Bartels, H., Stall, M. J., & Albers, F. W. J. (2007). Tinnitus and neural plasticity of the brain. *Otology and Neurotology, 28,* 178–184.

Beck, A. T., Steer, R. A, & Brown, G. K. (2000). *BDI-fast screen for medical patients manual.* San Antonio, TX: Psychological Corporation.

Brown, S. C. (1990). *Older Americans and tinnitus: A demographic study and chartbook* (GRI Monograph Series A, No. 2). Washington, DC: Gallaudet Research Institute, Gallaudet University.

Brummett, R. (1989). Drugs for and against tinnitus. *Hearing Journal, 42,* 34–37.

Budd, R. J., & Pugh, R. (1996a). The relationship between coping style, tinnitus severity and emotional distress in a group of sufferers. *British Journal of Health Psychological, 1,* 219–229.

Budd, R. J., & Pugh, R. (1996b). Tinnitus coping style and its relationship to tinnitus severity and emotional distress. *Journal of Psychosomatic Research, 41,* 327–335.

Camparis, C. M., Formigoni, G., Teixeira, M. J., & de Siqueira, J. T. (2005). Clinical evaluation of tinnitus in patients with sleep bruxism: Prevalence and characteristics. *Journal of Oral Rehabilitation, 32,* 808–814.

Chery-Croze, S., Truy, E., & Morgon, A. (1994). Contralateral suppression of transiently evoked otoacoustic emissions and tinnitus. *British Journal of Audiology, 28,* 255–266.

Childers, J. H., & Couch, R. D. (1989). Myths about group counseling: Identifying and challenging misconceptions. *Journal for Specialists in Group Work, 14,* 105–111.

Coles, R. R. A. (1984). Epidemiology of tinnitus: Demographic and clinical features. *Journal of Laryngology and Otology,* (Suppl. 9), 195–202.

Corey, M. A., & Corey, G. (1992). *Groups: Process and practice* (4th ed.). Pacific Grove, CA: Brooks/Cole.

Dauman, R. (2000). Electrical stimulation for tinnitus suppression. In R. Tyler (Ed.), *Tinnitus handbook* (pp. 377–398). San Diego, CA: Singular Thomas Learning.

Dauman, R., & Tyler, R. S. (1992). Some considerations on the classification of tinnitus. In J. M. Aran & R. Dauman (Eds.), *Proceedings of the Fourth International Tinnitus Seminar* (pp. 225–229). Bordeaux, France.

Davis, A. C. (1995). *Hearing in adults.* London: Whurr.

Davis, A., & Rafai, E. A. (2000). Epidemiology of tinnitus. In R. Tyler (Ed.), *Tinnitus handbook* (pp. 1–23). San Diego, CA: Singular Thomas Learning.

Davis, P. B. (1998). *Music as therapy in the rehabilitation of tinnitus sufferers: Effects of spectral modification and counseling.* Ph. D. Thesis, Perth, Western Australia, School of Speech and Hearing Science, Curtin University of Technology.

Davis, P. (2006). Music and the acoustic desensitization protocol for tinnitus. In R. S. Tyler (Ed.), *Tinnitus treatment: Clinical protocols* (pp. 146–160). San Diego, CA: Thieme.

Davis, P. B., Paki, B., & Hanley, P. J. (2007). Neuromonics tinnitus treatment: Third clinical trial. *Ear and Hearing, 28,* 242–259.

Davis, P. B., & Wilde, R. A. (1995). Clinical trial of a new tinnitus masking technique. In G. E. Reich &

J. A. Vernon (Eds.), *Proceedings of the Fifth International Tinnitus Seminar,* (pp. 305–309). Portland, OR: American Tinnitus Association.

Davis, P. B., Wilde, R. A., & Steed, L. (1999). Changes in tinnitus distress over a four month no-treatment period: Effects of audiological variables and litigation status. In J. W. P. Hazell (Ed.), *Proceedings of the Sixth International Tinnitus Seminar* (pp. 384–390). London: Tinnitus and Hyperacusis Centre.

Davis, P. B., Wilde, R. A., & Steed, L. (2001). Relative effects of acoustic stimulation and counseling in the tinnitus rehabilitation process. *Australian and New Zealand Journal of Audiology, 23,* 84–85.

Davis, P. B., Wilde, R. A., Steed, L., & Hanley, P. J. (2008). Treatment of tinnitus with a customized acoustic neural stimulus: A controlled clinical study. *Ear, Nose, and Throat Journal, 87,* 330–339.

Dillon, H., James, A., & Ginis, J. (1997). Client-Orientated Scale of Improvement (COSI) and its relationship to several other measures of benefit and satisfaction provided by hearing aids. *Journal of the American Academy of Audiology, 8,* 27–43.

Dobie, R. A. (2004a). Clinical trials and drug therapy for tinnitus. In J. B. Snow (Ed.), *Tinnitus: Theory and management* (pp. 266–277). Hamilton, London: BC Decker.

Dobie, R. A. (2004b). Overview: Suffering from tinnitus. In J. B. Snow (Ed.), *Tinnitus: Theory and management* (pp. 1–7). Hamilton, London: BC Decker.

Erlandsson, S., Hallberg, L. R. M., & Axelsson, A. (1992). Psychological and audiological correlates of perceived tinnitus severity. *Audiology, 31,* 168–169.

Erlandsson, S., Ringdahl, A., Hutchins, T., & Carlsson, S. G. (1987). Treatment of tinnitus: A controlled comparison of masking and placebo. *British Journal of Audiology 21,* 37–44.

Evered, D., & Lawrenson, G. (1981). *Tinnitus. Ciba Foundation Symposium 85.* London: Pitman.

Folmer, R. L., Griest, S. E., Meikel, M. B., & Martin, W. H. (1999). Tinnitus severity, loudness, and depression. *Otolaryngology-Head and Neck Surgery, 121,* 48–51.

Folmer, R. L., Martin, W. H, Shi, Y., & Edlefsen, L. L. (2006a). Lifestyle changes for tinnitus self management. In R. S. Tyler (Ed.), *Tinnitus treatment: Clinical protocols* (pp. 51–64). San Diego, CA: Thieme.

Folmer, R. L., Martin, W. H, Shi, Y., & Edlefsen, L. L. (2006b). Tinnitus sound therapies. In R. S. Tyler (Ed.), *Tinnitus treatment: Clinical protocols* (pp. 176–186). San Diego, CA: Thieme.

Gelb, H., Gelb, M. L, & Wagner, M. L. (1997). The relationship of tinnitus to craniocervical mandibular disorders. *Journal of Craniomandibular Practice, 15,* 136–143.

Georgiewa, P., Klapp, B. F., Fischer, F., Reisshauer, A., Juckel, G., Frommer, J., et al. (2006). An integrative model of developing tinnitus based on recent neurobiological findings. *Medical Hypotheses, 66,* 592–600.

Halford, J. B. S., & Anderson, S. D. (1991). Tinnitus severity measured by a subjective scale, audiometry and clinical judgment. *Journal of Laryngology and Otolaryngology, 105,* 89–93.

Hallam, R. S., Jakes, S. C., & Hinchcliffe, R. (1988). Cognitive variables in tinnitus annoyance. *British Journal of Clinical Psychology, 27,* 213–222.

Hallam, R. S., & McKenna, L. (2006). In R. S. Tyler (Ed.), *Tinnitus treatment* (pp. 65–80). New York: Thieme.

Hallam, R. S., Rachman, S., & Hinchcliffe, R. (1984). Psychological aspects of tinnitus. In Rachman, S. (Ed.), *Contributions to medical psychology* (Vol. 3, pp. 31–53). Oxford: Pergamon Press.

Harrop-Griffiths, J., Katon, W., Dobie, R., Sakai, C., & Russo, J. (1987). Chronic tinnitus: Association with psychiatric diagnosis. *Journal of Psychosomatic Research, 31,* 613–621.

Hazell, J. W. P. (1987). Tinnitus masking therapy. In J. W. P. Hazell (Ed.), *Tinnitus* (pp. 96–117). London: Churchill Livingston.

Hazell, J. W. P. (1995). Models of tinnitus: Generation, perception, clinical implications. In J. A. Vernon & A. R. Moller (Eds.), *Mechanisms of tinnitus* (pp. 57–72). Needham Heights, MA: Allyn & Bacon.

Hazell, J. W. P., Wood, S. M., Cooper, H. R., Stephens, D. G., Corcoran, A. L., Coles, R. R. A., et al. (1985). A clinical study of tinnitus maskers. *British Journal of Audiology, 19,* 65–146.

Henry, J. A. (2004). Audiologic assessment. In J. B. Snow (Ed.), *Tinnitus: Theory and management* (pp. 220–236). Hamilton, London: BC Decker.

Henry, J. A., Dennis, K. C., & Schechter, M. A. (2005). General review of tinnitus: Prevalence, mechanisms, effects, and management. *Journal of Speech, Language, and Hearing Research, 48,* 1204–1235.

Henry, J. A., Jastreboff, M. M., Jastreboff, P. J., Schechter, M. A., & Fausti, S. A. (2002). The assessment of patients for treatment with tinnitus retraining therapy. *Journal of the American Academy of Audiology, 13*, 523–544.

Henry, J. A., & Meikle, M. B. (2000). Psychoacoustic measures of tinnitus. *Journal of American Academy or Audiology, 11*, 138–155.

Henry, J. A., Rheinsburg, B., Owens, K. K., & Ellingson, R. M. (2006). New instrumentation for automated tinnitus psychoacoustic assessment. *Acta Oto-Laryngologica, 126*, 34–38.

Henry, J. A., Schechter, M. A., Loovis, C. L., Zaugg, T. L., Kaelin, C., & Montero, M. (2005). Clinical management of tinnitus using a "progressive intervention" approach. *Journal of Rehabilitation Research and Development, 42*, 95–116.

Henry, J. A., Schechter, M. A., Nagler, S. M., & Fausti, S. A. (2002). Comparison of tinnitus masking and tinnitus retraining therapy. *Journal of the American Academy of Audiology, 13*, 559–581.

Henry, J. A., Schechter, M. A., Zaugg, T. L., Griest, S., Jastreboff, P. J., Vernon, J. A., et al. (2006a). Clinical trial to compare tinnitus masking and tinnitus retraining therapy. *Acta Oto-Laryngologica, 126*, 64–69.

Henry, J. A., Schechter, M. A., Zaugg, T. L., Griest, S., Jastreboff, P. J., Vernon, J. A., et al. (2006b). Outcomes of clinical trial: Tinnitus masking versus tinnitus retraining therapy. *Journal of the American Academy of Audiology, 17*, 104–132.

Henry, J. A., Zaugg, T. L., Myers, P. J., & Schechter, M. A. (2008). Using therapeutic sound with progressive audiologic tinnitus management. *Trends in Amplification, 12*, 185–206.

Henry, J. A., Zaugg, T. L., & Schechter, M. A. (2005a). Clinical guide for audiologic tinnitus management I: Assessment. *American Journal of Audiology, 14*, 21–48.

Henry, J. A., Zaugg, T. L., & Schechter, M. A. (2005b). Clinical guide for audiologic tinnitus management II: Treatment. *American Journal of Audiology, 14*, 49–70.

Henry, J. L, & Wilson, P. H. (1998). Tinnitus cognitions questionnaire: Development and psychometric properties of a measure of dysfunctional cognitions associated with tinnitus. *International Tinnitus Journal, 4*, 23–30.

Henry, J. L., & Wilson, P. H. (2001). *The psychological management of chronic tinnitus: A cognitive-behavioral approach*. Needham Heights, MA: Allyn & Bacon.

Henry, J. L., & Wilson, P. H. (2002). *Tinnitus: A self-management guide for the ringing in your ears*. Boston: Allyn & Bacon.

Hoffman, H. J., & Reed, G. W. (2004). Epidemiology of tinnitus. In J. B. Snow (Ed.), *Tinnitus: Theory and management* (pp. 16–42). Hamilton, London: BC Decker.

Hoge, C. W., McGurk, D., Thomas, J. L., Cox, A. L., Engel, C. C., & Castro, C. A. (2008). Mild traumatic brain injury in U.S. Soldiers returning from Iraq. *New England Journal of Medicine, 358*, 453–459.

Hyde, M. L. (2000) Reasonable psychometric standards for self-report outcome measures in audiological rehabilitation. *Ear and Hearing, 21*, (Suppl. 4), 24S–36S.

Jacobs, E. E., Harvill, R. I., & Masson, R. I. (1988). *Group counseling: Strategies and skills*. Pacific Grove, CA: Brooks/Cole.

Jacobson, G. P., & McCaslin, D. L. (2001). A search for evidence of a direct relationship between tinnitus and suicide. *Journal of the American Academy of Audiology, 12*, 493–496.

Jacobson, G. P., & Newman, C. W. (1990). The development of the Dizziness Handicap Inventory. *Archives of Otolaryngology-Head and Neck Surgery, 116*, 424–427.

Jakes, S. C., Hallam, R. S., Chambers, C., & Hinchcliffe, R. A. (1985). A factor analytical study of tinnitus complaint behavior. *Audiology, 25*, 195–206.

Jakes, S. C., Hallam, R. S., McKenna, L., & Hinchcliffe, R. (1992). Group cognitive therapy for medical patients: An application to tinnitus. *Cognitive Therapy Research, 16*, 83–94.

Jansson, G., Warfvinge, J., Edensvard, A., & Wiberg, A. (1996). The effects of acupuncture versus masker treatment in patients with tinnitus. In G. E., & J. A. Vernon (Eds.), *Proceedings of the Fifth International Tinnitus Seminar* (pp. 489–499). Portland, OR: American Tinnitus Association.

Jastreboff, P. J. (1990). Phantom auditory perception (tinnitus): Mechanisms of generation and perception. *Neuroscience Research, 8*, 221–254.

Jastreboff, P. J. (1995). Tinnitus as a phantom perception: Theories and clinical implications. In J. Vernon & A. R. Moller (Eds.), *Mechanisms of tinnitus* (pp. 73–94). Boston: Allyn & Bacon.

Jastreboff, P. J. (2000). Tinnitus habituation therapy (THT) and tinnitus retraining therapy (TRT). In R. Tyler (Ed.), *Tinnitus handbook* (pp. 257–376). San Diego, CA: Singular Thomson Learning.

Jastreboff, P. J., & Hazell, J. W. P. (1993). A neurophysiological approach to tinnitus: Clinical implications. *British Journal of Audiology, 27*, 7–17.

Jastreboff, P. J., & Hazell, J. W. P. (2004). *Tinnitus retraining therapy: Implementing the neurophysiological model*. New York: Cambridge University Press.

Jastreboff, P. J., & Jastreboff, M. M. (2004). Tinnitus retraining therapy. In J. B. Snow (Ed.), *Tinnitus: Theory and management* (pp. 310–313). Hamilton, London: BC Decker.

Johnson, R. M. (1998). The masking of tinnitus. In J. A. Vernon (Ed.), *Tinnitus treatments and relief* (pp. 164–186). Boston: Allyn & Bacon.

Kaltenbach, J. A. (2000). Neurophysiologic mechanisms of tinnitus. *Journal of the American Academy of Audiology, 11*, 125–137.

Kaltenbach, L. A., Rachel, J. D., Mathog, T. A., Zhang, J., Falzarano, P. R., & Lewandowski, M. (2002). Cisplatin-induced hyperactivity in the dorsal cochlear nucleus and it relations to outer hair cell loss: relevance to tinnitus. *Journal of Neurophysiology, 88*, 699–714.

Kaltenbach, J. A., Zhang, J., & Zacharek, M. A. (2004). Neural correlates of tinnitus. In J. B. Snow (Ed.), *Tinnitus: Theory and management* (pp. 141–161). Hamilton, London: BC Decker.

Kanold, P. O., & Young, E. D. (2001). Proprioceptive information from the pinna provides somatosensory input to cat dorsal cochlear nucleus. *Journal of Neuroscience, 21*, 7848–7858.

Kinney, S. E., Sandridge, S. A., & Newman, C. W. (1997). Long-term effects of Ménière's disease on hearing and quality of life. *American Journal of Otology, 18*, 67–73.

Kochkin, S., & Tyler, R. (2008). Tinnitus treatment and the effectiveness of hearing aids: Hearing care professional perceptions. *Hearing Review, 15*, 14, 16–18.

Kricos, P., & Lesner, S. (1995*). Hearing care for the older adult: Audiologic rehabilitation*. Newton, MA: Butterworth-Heinemann.

Kroener-Herwig, B., Biesinger, E., Gerhards, F., Goebel, G., Greimel, K. V., & Hiller, W. (2000). Retraining therapy for chronic tinnitus. *Scandinavian Audiology, 29*, 68–76.

Kuk, F. K., Tyler, R. S., Russell, D., & Jordan, H. (1990). The psychometric properties of a Tinnitus Handicap Questionnaire. *Ear and Hearing, 11*, 434–442.

Lam, D. K., Lawrence, H. P., & Tenenbaum, H. C. (2001). Aural symptoms in temporomandibular disorder patients attending a craniofacial pain unit. *Journal of Orofacial Pain, 15*, 146–157.

Law, M. (2002). *Evidence-based rehabilitation: A guide to practice*. Thorofare, NJ: Slack.

Lazarus, R. S., & Folkman, R. (1984). *Stress, appraisal and coping*. New York: Springer-Verlag.

Levine, R. A. (1999a). Somatic (craniocervical) tinnitus and the dorsal cochlear nucleus hypothesis. *American Journal of Otolaryngology, 20*, 351–362.

Levine, R. A. (1999b). Somatic modulation appears to be a fundamental attribute of tinnitus. In J. Hazell (Ed.), *Proceedings of the Sixth International Tinnitus Seminar* (pp. 193–197). London: The Tinnitus and Hyperacusis Centre.

Levine, R. A. (2004). Somatic tinnitus. In J. B. Snow (Ed.), *Tinnitus: Theory and management* (pp. 108–124). Hamilton, London: BC Decker.

Levine, R. A., Abel, M., & Cheng, H. (2003). CNS somatosensory-auditory interactions elicit or modulate tinnitus. *Experimental Brain Research, 153*, 643–648.

Lockwood, A. H., Salvi, R. J., Coad, M. L., Towsley, M. L., Wack, D. S., & Murphy, B. W. (1998). The functional neuroanatomy of tinnitus: Evidence for limbic system links and neural plasticity. *Neurology, 50*, 114–120.

Martinez Devesa, P., Waddell, A., Perera, R., & Theodoulou, M. (2007). Cognitive behavioural therapy for tinnitus. *Cochran Database of Systematic Reviews*, Issue 1 Art. No. CD005233. DOI: 10. 1002/ 14651858. CD005233. pub2.

McCombe, A., Baguley, D., Coles, R., McKenna, L., McKinney, C, & Windle-Taylor, P. (2001). Guidelines for the grading of tinnitus severity: The results of a working group commissioned by the British Association of Otolaryngologists Head and Neck Surgeons, 1999. *Clinical Otolaryngology and Allied Sciences, 26*, 388–392.

McFadden, D. (1982). *Tinnitus: Facts, theories and treatments*. Report of working group 89, Committee on

Hearing Bioacoustics and Biomechanics, Washington, DC: National Research Council National Academy Press.

McKenna L. (2004) Models of tinnitus suffering and treatment compared and contrasted. *Audiological Medicine, 2,* 41–53.

Mehlum, D., Grasel, G., & Fankhauser, C. (1984). Prospective crossover evaluation of four methods of clinical management of tinnitus. *Otolaryngology-Head and Neck Surgery, 92,* 448–453.

Meikle, M. B., Creedon, T. A., & Griest, S. E. (2004). *Tinnitus archive* (2nd ed.). Retrieved June 12, 2008, from www.tinnitusarchive.org

Meikle, M., Henry, J., Abrams, H., Frederick, E., Martin, W., McArdle, R., et al. (2008). *Development of the Tinnitus Functional Index (TFI): Part 1. Assembling and testing a preliminary prototype.* Poster presented at the Association for Research Otolaryngology [Abstract 395].

Meikle, M., Steward, B., Griest, S., Henry, J., Abrams, H., Martin, W., et al. (2008). *Development of the Tinnitus Functional Index (TFI): Part 2. Final dimensions, reliability and validity in a new clinical sample.* Poster presented at the Association for Research in Otolaryngology [Abstract 396].

Meikle, M., Vernon, J., & Johnson, M. (1984). The perceived severity of tinnitus. *Otolaryngology-Head and Neck Surgery, 92,* 689–696.

Mirz, F., Mortensen, M. V., Gjedde, A., & Pederson, C. B. (2002). Positron emission tomography of tinnitus suppression by cochlear implantation. In R. Patuzzi (Ed.), *Proceedings of the Seventh International Tinnitus Seminar* (pp. 176–181). Perth: University of Western Australia.

Moller, A. R. (1984). Pathophysiology of tinnitus. *Annals of Otology, 93,* 39–44.

Moller, A. R. (2007). Tinnitus: Presence and future. *Progress in Brain Research, 166,* 3–16.

Morgan, D. H. (1996). Tinnitus caused by a temporomandibular disorder. In G. E. Reich & J. A. Vernon (Eds.), *Proceedings of the Fifth International Tinnitus Seminar* (pp. 653–654). Portland, OR: American Tinnitus Association.

Newman, C., Jacobson, G., & Spitzer, B. (1996). Development of the Tinnitus Handicap Inventory. *Archives of Otolaryngology-Head and Neck Surgery, 122,* 143–147.

Newman, C. W., & Sandridge, S. A. (2004). Tinnitus questionnaires. In J. B. Snow (Ed.), *Tinnitus: Theory and management* (pp. 237–254). Hamilton, London: BC Decker.

Newman, C. W., & Sandridge, S. A. (2006, September 4). *Sound Therapy Option Profile (STOP): A tool for selecting devices used in tinnitus treatment.* Audiology Online, Article 1687. Available via the Articles Archive on http://www.audiologyonline.com. Direct access URL located at: http://www.audiologyonline.com/articles/article_detail.asp?article_id=1687

Newman, C. W., Sandridge, S. A., & Bolek, L. (2008). Development and psychometric adequacy of the screening version of the Tinnitus Handicap Inventory. *Otology and Neurotology, 29,* 276–281.

Newman, C. W., Sandridge, S., & Jacobson, G. (1998). Psychometric adequacy of the Tinnitus Handicap Inventory for evaluating treatment outcome. *Journal of the American Academy of Audiology, 9,* 153–160.

Newman, C. W., Sandridge, Meit, S., & Cherian, N. (2008). Strategies for managing patients with tinnitus: A clinical pathway model. *Seminars in Hearing, 29,* 300–309.

Newman, C. W., Weinstein B. E., Jacobson, G. P., & Hug, G. A. (1990). The Hearing Handicap Inventory for Adults: Psychometric adequacy and audiometric correlates. *Ear and Hearing, 11,* 430–433.

Newman, C. W., Wharton, J. A., Shivapuja, B. G., & Jacobson, G. P. (1994). Relationships among psychoacoustic judgments, speech understanding ability and self-perceived handicap in tinnitus subjects. *Audiology, 33,* 47–60.

Noble, W., & Tyler, R. S. (2007). Physiology and phenomenology of tinnitus: Implications for treatment. *International Journal of Audiology, 46,* 569–574.

Pachter, L. M. (1994). Cultural and clinical care: Folk illness beliefs and behaviors and their implications for health care delivery. *Journal of the American Medical Association, 271,* 690–694.

Patuzzi, R. (2002). Outer hair cells, EP regulation and tinnitus. In R. Patuzzi (Ed.), *Seventh International Tinnitus Seminar Proceedings* (pp. 16–24). Perth: Physiology Department, University of Western Australia.

Penner, M. J. (1990). An estimate of the prevalence of tinnitus caused by spontaneous otoacoustic emissions. *Archives of Otolaryngology-Head and Neck Surgery, 115,* 871–875.

Perry, B. P., & Gantz, B. J. (2000). Medical and surgical evaluation and management of tinnitus. In R. Tyler (Ed.), *Tinnitus handbook* (pp. 221–241). San Diego, CA: Singular Thomas Learning.

Primeau, R. (1997). Hearing aid benefit in adults and older adults. *Seminars in Hearing, 18,* 29–37.

Quaranta, N., Wagstaff, S., & Baguley, D. M. (2004). Tinnitus and cochlear implantation. *International Journal of Audiology, 43,* 245–251.

Rubinstein, J. T., & Tyler, R. S. (2004). Electrical suppression of tinnitus. In J. B. Snow (Ed.), *Tinnitus: Theory and management* (pp. 326–335). Hamilton, London: BC Decker.

Sahley, T. L., & Nodar, R. H. (2001). A biochemical model of peripheral tinnitus. *Hearing Research, 152,* 43–54.

Salvi, R. J., Lockwood, A. H., & Burkard, R. (2000). Neural plasticity and tinnitus. In R. Tyler (Ed.), *Tinnitus handbook* (pp. 123–148). San Diego, CA: Singular Thomas Learning.

Salvi, R. J., Wang, J., & Powers, N. L. (1996). Plasticity and reorganization in the auditory brainstem: Implications for tinnitus. In G. E. Reich & J. E. Vernon (Eds.), *Proceedings of the Fifth International Tinnitus Seminar* (pp. 457–466). Portland, OR: American Tinnitus Association.

Sanchez, T. G., Guerr, G. C., Lorenzi, M. C., Brandao, A. L., & Bento, R. F. (2002). The influence of voluntary muscle contractions upon the onset and modulation of tinnitus. *Audiology and Neurotology, 7,* 370–375.

Sandlin R. W., & Olsson R. T. (2000). Subjective tinnitus: Its mechanisms and treatment. In M. Valente, H. Hosford-Dunn, & R. J. Roeser (Eds.), *Audiology treatment* (pp. 691–714). New York: Thieme.

Saunders, J. C. (2007). The role of central nervous system plasticity in tinnitus. *Journal of Communication Disorders, 40,* 313–334.

Schecter, M. A., & Henry, J. A. (2002). Assessment and treatment of tinnitus patients using a "masking approach." *Journal of the American Academy of Audiology, 13,* 545–558.

Schechter, M. A., Henry, J. A., Zaugg, T., & Fausti, S. A. (2002). Selection of ear level devices for two different methods of tinnitus treatment. In R. Patuzzi (Ed.), *Seventh International Tinnitus Seminar Proceedings* (p. 13). Perth: Physiology Department, University of Western Australia.

Schleuning, A. L., Shi B. Y., & Martin, W. H., (2006). Tinnitus. In B. J. Bailey, J. T. Johnson, & S. D. Newlands (Eds.), *Head and neck surgery-otolaryngology* (4th ed., Vol. 2, pp. 2237–2245). Philadelphia: Lippincott Williams & Wilkins.

Seidman, M. D., & Babu, S. (2003). Alternative medications and other treatments for tinnitus: Facts from fiction. *Otolaryngologic Clinics of North America, 36,* 359–381.

Sheldrake, J. B., & Jastreboff, M. M. (2004). Role of hearing aids in management of tinnitus. In J. B. Snow (Ed.), *Tinnitus: Theory and management* (pp. 310–313). Hamilton, London: BC Decker.

Shiley, S. G., Folmer, R. L., & McMenomey, S. O. (2005). Tinnitus and hyperacusis. In C. W. Cummings, P. W. Flint, L. A. Harker, B. H. Haughey, M. A. Richardson, K. T., Robbins, Schuller, D. E., & J. R. Thomas (Eds.), *Otolaryngology head and neck surgery* (4th ed., pp. 2832–2846). Philadelphia: Elsevier Mobley.

Sindhusake, D., Mitchell, P., Newall, P., Golding, M., Rochtchina, E., & Rubin, G. (2003). Prevalence and characteristics of tinnitus in older adults: The Blue Mountain Hearing Study. *International Journal of Audiology, 42,* 289–294.

Sizer, D. I., & Coles, R. A. (2006). Tinnitus self-treatment. In R. S. Tyler (Ed.), *Tinnitus treatment: Clinical protocols* (pp. 23–28). New York: Thieme.

Standley, J. (1995). Music as a therapeutic intervention in medical/dental treatment: Research and clinical applications. In T. Wigram, B. Saperston, & R. West (Eds.) *The art and science of music therapy: A handbook* (pp. 484). Chur, Switzerland: Harwood Academic.

Steigerwald, D. P., & Verne, S. V. (1996). A retrospective evaluation of the impact of temporomandibular joint arthroscopy on the symptoms of headache, neck pain, shoulder pain, dizziness, and tinnitus. *Journal of Craniomandibular Practice, 14,* 46–54.

Stephens, S., & Corcoran, A. (1985). A controlled study of tinnitus masking. *British Journal of Audiology, 19,* 159–167.

Stouffer, J. L., & Tyler, R. S. (1990). Characterization of tinnitus by tinnitus patients. *Journal of Speech and Hearing Disorders, 55,* 439–453.

Sullivan, M. D., Katon, W., & Dobie, R. (1988). Disabling tinnitus: Association with affective disorder. *General Hospital Psychiatry, 10*, 285–291.

Surr, R. K., Kolb, J. A., Cord, M. A., & Garrus, N. P. (1999). Tinnitus Handicap Inventory (THI) as a hearing aid outcome measure. *Journal of the American Academy of Audiology, 10*, 489–495.

Surr, R. K., Montgomery, A. A., & Mueller, H. G. (1985). Effect of amplification on tinnitus among new hearing aid users. *Ear and Hearing, 6*, 71–75.

Sweetow, R. W. (1986). Cognitive aspects of tinnitus patient management. *Ear and Hearing, 7*, 390–396.

Sweetow, R. W. (2000). Cognitive-behavior modification. In R. Tyler (Ed.), *Tinnitus handbook* (pp. 297–311). San Diego, CA: Singular Thomas Learning.

Sweetow, R. W., & Levy, M. C., (1990). Tinnitus severity scaling for diagnostic/therapeutic usage. *Hearing Instrument, 41*, 20–46.

Taylor, K., & Jurma, W. (1999). Study suggests that group rehabilitation increases benefit of hearing aid fittings. *Hearing Journal, 52*, 48–54.

Tyler, R. S. (1993). Tinnitus disability and handicap questionnaires. *Seminars in Hearing, 14*, 377–384.

Tyler, R. S. (2000). The psychoacoustical measurement of tinnitus. In R. Tyler (Ed.), *Tinnitus handbook* (pp. 149–179). San Diego, CA: Singular Thomas Learning.

Tyler, R. S. (2006). Neurophysiological models, psychological models, & treatments for tinnitus. In R. S. Tyler (Ed.), *Tinnitus treatment: Clinical protocols* (pp. 1–22). San Diego, CA: Thieme.

Tyler, R. S. (2008). *The consumer handbook on tinnitus*. Sedona, AZ: Auricle Ink.

Tyler, R., S., Aran, J. M., & Dauman, R. (1992). Recent advances in tinnitus. *American Journal of Audiology, 1*, 36–44.

Tyler, R. S., & Babin, R. W. (1986). Tinnitus. In C. W. Cummings, J.-M. Fredrickson, L. Harker, C. J. Krause, & D. E. Schuller (Eds.), *Otolaryngology-head and neck surgery* (pp. 3201–3217). St. Louis, MO: Mosby.

Tyler, R. S., & Baker, L. J. (1983). Difficulties experienced by tinnitus sufferers. *Journal of Speech Hearing Disorder, 48*, 150–154.

Tyler, R. S., & Bentler, R. A. (1987). Tinnitus maskers and hearing aids for tinnitus. *Seminars in Hearing, 8*, 49–61.

Tyler, R. S., & Conrad-Armes, D. (1983). The determination of tinnitus loudness considering the effects of recruitment. *Journal of Speech and Hearing Research, 26*, 59–72.

Tyler, R. S., Gehringer, A. K., Noble, W., Dunn, C. C., Witt, S. A., & Bardia, A. (2006). Tinnitus activities treatment. In R. S. Tyler (Ed.), *Tinnitus treatment: Clinical protocols* (pp. 116–132). San Diego, CA: Thieme.

Tyler, R., Haskell, G., Preece, J., & Bergen, C. (2001). Nurturing patient expectations to enhance the treatment of tinnitus. *Seminars in Hearing, 22*, 15–21.

Tyler, R. S., Noble, W., Preece, Dunn, C. C., & Witt, S. A. (2004). Psychological treatments for tinnitus. In J. B. Snow (Ed.), *Tinnitus: Theory and management* (pp. 314–323). Hamilton, London: BC Decker.

Ventry, I., & Weinstein, B. (1982). The Hearing Handicap Inventory for the Elderly: A new tool. *Ear and Hearing, 3*, 128–134.

Vernon, J., Griest, S., & Press, L. (1990). Attributes of tinnitus and the acceptance of masking. *American Journal of Otolaryngology, 11*, 44–50.

Vernon, J. A., & Meikle, M. B. (1988). Measurement of tinnitus: An update. In M. Kitahara (Ed.), *Tinnitus: Pathophysiology and management* (pp. 36–52). Tokyo: Igaku-Shoin.

Vernon, J. A., & Meikle, M. B. (2000). Tinnitus masking. In R. Tyler (Ed.), *Tinnitus handbook* (pp. 313–356). San Diego, CA: Singular Thomas Learning.

Vernon, J., & Schleuning, A. (1978). Tinnitus: A new management. *Laryngoscope, 88*, 413–419.

Vernon, J. A., & Tabachnick Sanders, S. (2001). *Tinnitus questions and answers*. Boston: Allyn & Bacon.

Wackym P. A., & Friedland, D. R. (2004). Otologic evaluation. In J. B. Snow (Ed.), *Tinnitus: Theory and management* (pp. 205–219). Hamilton, London: BC Decker.

Whedon, J. (2006). Reduction of tinnitus by spinal manipulation in a patient with presumptive rotational vertebral artery occlusion syndrome: A case report. *Alternative Therapies in Health and Medicine, 12*, 14–17.

Wilson, P. H., & Henry, J. L. (1998). Tinnitus Cognitions Questionnaire: Development and psychometric properties of a measure of dysfunctional cognitions associated with tinnitus. *International Tinnitus Journal, 4*, 23–30.

Wilson, P. H., Henry, J. L., Andersson, G., Hallam, R. S., & Lindberg, P. (1998). A critical analysis of directive counseling as a component of tinnitus retraining therapy. *British Journal of Audiology, 32,* 272–286.

Wilson, P. H., Henry, J., Bowen, M., & Haralambous, G. (1991). Tinnitus Reaction Questionnaire: Psychometric properties of a measure of distress associated with tinnitus. *Journal of Speech Language and Hearing Research, 34,* 197–201.

World Health Organization. (2004). *International Statistical Classification of Diseases and Health Related Problems ICI-10* (10th ed.). Geneva, Switzerland: Author.

Wright, E. E., & Bifano, S. L. (1997). Tinnitus improvement through TMD therapy. *Journal of the American Dental Association, 128,* 1424–1432.

Zenner, H. P., & Pfister, M. (1999). Systematic classification of tinnitus. In J. Hazell (Ed.), *Proceedings of the Sixth International Tinnitus Seminar* (pp. 17–19). London: The Tinnitus and Hyperacusis Centre.

Zigmond A. S., & Snaith, R. P. (1983). The Hospital Anxiety and Depression Scale. *Acta Psychiatry Scandinavia, 76,* 361–370.

Zoger, S., Svedlund, J., & Holgers, K. (2004). The Hospital Anxiety and Depression Scale (HAD) as a screening instrument in tinnitus evaluation. *International Journal of Audiology, 43,* 458–464.

Appendix 20-A
Sound Therapy Option Profile (STOP)

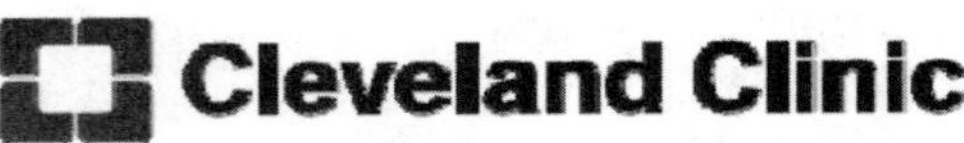

Name: ______________________ Date: ______________

CCF #: ______________________ Audiologist: ______________

Our goal is to help you find a method or combination of methods that will provide you with relief from your tinnitus. Treatments provided by our audiologists may include sound therapy using assistive devices, hearing aids, ear-level sound generators and/or an acoustic desensitization protocol using a form of music therapy. Other options may include behavioral modification therapy provided by our Tinnitus Management Clinic team members in the Department of Psychology. In order to reach our goal of providing you with tinnitus relief, it is important that we understand your perceived tinnitus and hearing problems, your personal preferences, and your expectations. By having a better understanding of your needs, we can use our expertise to recommend the form of sound therapy most appropriate for **you**. By working together **we** will find the best tinnitus treatment option for you.

Please complete the following questions. Be as honest as possible. Be as precise as possible. Thank you.

1. How much does your tinnitus affect your overall quality-of-life? Mark an X on the line.

   Not Very Much ______________________ *Very Much*

2. How important is it for you to hear better? Mark an X on the line.

   Not Very Important ______________________ *Very Important*

3. How motivated are you to use some form of sound therapy to help provide tinnitus relief? Mark an X on the line.

   Not Very Motivated ______________________ *Very Motivated*

4. Are you willing to use sound therapy:

   only at those times when your tinnitus is bothering you? ___ Yes ___ No

   at least 2–3 hours per day for at least six months? ___ Yes ___ No

   at least 6–8 hours per day possibly up to 12 to 18 months? ___ Yes ___ No

5. Do you expect the recommended sound therapy to be effective in providing you relief from tinnitus? Mark an X on the line.

   I expect sound therapy to:

   Not be helpful at all ______________________ *Provide a great deal of relief*

6. What is your most important consideration regarding sound therapy treatment? Rank the following factors with **1** as the most important and **4** as the least important. Place an **X** on the line if the item has no importance to you at all.

   ___ Improved hearing
   ___ Tinnitus relief
   ___ Improved hearing along with tinnitus relief
   ___ Cost of treatment

7. Answer this question ONLY after you have listened to the demonstration sounds.
   How acceptable did you find the each one of the following sounds?

   Nature sounds (e.g., waterfall, surf, wind, etc.)

   Not Very Acceptable ________________________________ *Very Acceptable*

   Gentle white noise

   Not Very Acceptable ________________________________ *Very Acceptable*

   Music

   Not Very Acceptable ________________________________ *Very Acceptable*

8. Would you be willing to pursue any of the following forms of treatment?

Wearable ear-level device for one or both ears	___ Yes	___ No
Wearable device that looks like an iPod or MP3 player	___ Yes	___ No
Assistive sound generating device (e.g., bedside masker, masking tapes/CDs, etc.)	___ Yes	___ No
Psychological forms of treatment (e.g., additional counseling, cognitive behavioral modification training, biofeedback)	___ Yes	___ No

9. How confident do you feel that you will be successful in using some form of sound therapy in the treatment of your tinnitus?

   Not Very Confident ________________________________ *Very Confident*

10. In the past, have you tried any of the following forms of tinnitus treatment:

Wearable (ear level) sound generators	___ Yes	___ No
Assistive (table top) sound generating device	___ Yes	___ No
Medical (medications, sleep therapy, surgery, other medical intervention)	___ Yes	___ No
Psychological	___ Yes	___ No

   Other form/s of treatment ______________________________

11. There is a wide range of available sound therapy options that may be used to help provide relief from your tinnitus. Devices are typically not covered by insurance. The selection of a particular form of sound therapy depends on a variety of factors including the type of device preferred (for example, assistive device versus customized wearable device), level and sophistication of device technology (for example, digital hearing aid versus compact disk vs. customized music therapy), length of time required for treatment (for example, six months versus 1 year), and personal finances. This information is helpful for us to select the most appropriate hearing device technology based on your budget. The costs for Categories B through Category D include the devices and related audiology appointments over the first year. Please check the cost category that represents the maximum amount you are willing to spend for your tinnitus treatment.

___ **Category A** Cost is between $XXX to $XXXX
Assistive sound generating devices

___ **Category B** Cost is between $XXXX to $XXXX
Noncustom wearable sound generators

___ **Category C** Cost is between $XXXX to $XXXX
Custom wearable sound generators

___ **Category D** Cost is between $XXXX to $XXXX
Custom hearing aids
Custom combination devices (sound generator and hearing aid)
Neuromonics Tinnitus Treatment (music therapy with processor)

Source: Adapted from Newman, C. W., & Sandridge, S. A. (2006, September 4). *Sound Therapy Option Profile (STOP): A tool for selecting devices used in tinnitus treatment*. Audiology Online, Article 1687. Available via the Articles Archive on http://www.audiologyonline.com . Direct access URL located at: http://www.audiologyonline.com/articles/article_detail.asp?article_id=1687 .

21

Central Auditory Influences in Audiologic Rehabilitation

Jack Katz

This chapter deals with the central nervous system (CNS) and audiologic rehabilitation (AR) for adults who (1) are hard of hearing, (2) have auditory processing deficits, or (3) experience both problems. First, is a brief introduction, a discussion of what central auditory processing (CAP; Katz, 1992) is, and its neural basis. This is followed by the importance of auditory processing in AR and screening for CAPD. Finally, four interesting rehabilitation cases are presented to illustrate the influence of central functions in different populations.

Introduction

An anecdote illustrates the importance of evaluating central auditory functions as part of an audiologic rehabilitation program. As a clinical supervisor at a university, my very first patient was an older woman who, when previously seen, was advised to get a hearing aid. She reported that for more than a year she received good results from her monaural hearing aid in her right ear. However, after a period of time, she noticed increasing difficulty understanding what was being said. Her amplification was operating normally, and yet her success with the hearing aid declined. Audiologic re-evaluation was consistent with previous results for both pure-tone and basic speech audiometry. Subsequently, the Staggered Spondaic Word (SSW) test, a measure of central auditory function, was administered. Results were essentially within normal limits in three of the four conditions, but a major reduction was noted in the right-competing condition. Thus, it seemed that the channel that the hearing aid information had to travel through was centrally impaired. We recommended that she see her physicians regarding the central signs and that a hearing aid be fit for the left ear. When she returned, she was very pleased with the left ear fitting. She reported that her medical doctor found no gross abnormalities and believed that the central changes were age-related. Although the problem may have resulted from normal aging, it adversely affected her performance when the hearing aid was delivering information to the defective central pathway. This case may be akin to binaural-interference (Silman, 1995; Walden & Walden, 2005). In this case, it appears that the auditory pathway that was impaired centrally interfered with the successful use of her hearing aid (and likely would have interfered with her use of binaural amplification).

This is by no means an isolated incident. Many of the poorest hearing aid and cochlear implant outcomes are likely to be for those persons who have weak central auditory skills (Rawool, 2007). If one does not screen for central auditory status prior to fitting with amplification or other forms of auditory rehabilitation, then surely when there is failure or frustration with these provisions, a strong consideration should be the status of the person's central auditory functions. For a review of other useful tests of central function, see Rawool (2006).

Central Auditory Processing

Central auditory processing (CAP) refers to the effectiveness and efficiency in using what is heard. Lasky and Katz (1983) define CAP as "what we do with what we hear" (p. 4). For example, some people can hear a very faint message and understand it completely, whereas others seem to hear speech loudly enough, but often fail to have a good sense of what was said. Because the functions of the central auditory nervous system (CANS) are enormously complex, it is easiest to appreciate its function by dividing auditory processing into categories. In the Buffalo Model, there are four auditory processing categories (Katz, 1992, 2007a): decoding (DEC), tolerance-fading memory (TFM), integration (INT), and organization (ORG).

The most prominent auditory processing skill is DEC. Decoding refers to the ability to understand speech quickly and accurately. DEC deficits are prevalent in both children and adults, and are related to many basic academic and communicative activities. Importantly, DEC problems are not difficult to identify or to remediate. Adults with longstanding auditory processing disorders (APD) associated with DEC difficulties often have histories of articulation problems early in life, difficulties in school with phonics, spelling, and/or oral reading.

Those who have hearing losses or auditory processing deficits frequently are unable to comprehend quickly and accurately what they hear. In this sense, they have auditory DEC problems. When determining if a hard-of-hearing person has CAPD, it is important to take into account the distortion associated with the hearing loss. Some central auditory tests are known to be relatively insensitive to peripheral auditory deficits (e.g., Dichotic Digits (Musiek, 1983), Synthetic Sentence Identification (Baran & Musiek, 1999, Jerger et al. 1968), or Staggered Spondaic Word test (Arnst, 1983)). Thus, the presence of a hearing loss need not contraindicate using tests to identify central auditory components.

Tolerance-Fading Memory (TFM), another important CAP category, is composed of two major subdivisions. The first is speech in noise, that is, the ability to extract speech from a background of noise; and the second is short-term auditory memory. These two characteristics are often seen together and are associated with other issues, such as distractibility and attention.

Integration (INT) is the most complex of the four categories. The common feature of INT is enabling different parts of the CNS to work together (e.g., auditory-visual integration; combining linguistic and affective components, see Medwetsky, in press). Integration problems are associated with very poor academic performance (especially, reading and spelling). Quite often those with the INT problems are also labeled dyslexic (Katz & Lawrence-Dederich, 1986).

Organization (ORG) is the final category in the Buffalo Model. It relates to sequencing and organizational performance. Those exhibiting difficulties with ORG are likely to mix up digit, letter, or even word sequences, especially when they are tired, inattentive or overloaded. These individuals tend to be disorganized, may have a sloppy appearance or frequently lose things (Lucker, 1981). Those who are referred for CAP evaluations generally demonstrate two or more CAPD categories.

The Neural Basis for Auditory Processing

The writings of Alexander Luria, the famous Russian neuropsychologist, have had a profound influence on my thinking about the neural basis of auditory processing. One of the most basic auditory functions of the brain is phonemic decoding. Luria (1966) studied soldiers with brain lesions that were caused by gunshot wounds during World War II. Importantly, he found that just one region of the brain was responsible for discriminating, remembering, and analyzing-synthesizing speech sounds (Luria, 1966, pp. 106–108). This area of the brain, commonly referred to as the auditory cortex, sits in the middle-posterior portion of the temporal lobe. Little wonder, when this area of the brain is damaged, in the left hemisphere (for right-handers and many left-handers), that we can expect receptive (Wernicke's) aphasia.

The anterior temporal lobe contributes significantly to auditory processing, for example, resulting in poor perception of speech under noise conditions (Efron, Crandall, Koss, Divenyl, & Yund, 1983). Efron et al. (1983) hypothesized that this region of the brain communicates with the auditory cortex and controls the lower brainstem gating functions by efferent pathways. One can also view speech in noise as a multitasking paradigm. That is, when we hear both foreground speech and background noise, we try to do one thing with the speech (attend to it) and quite another with the noise (ignore it). This function, in part, may be associated with the prefrontal cortex. Fuster (1980) pointed out that animals with lesions to this region cannot press one button for one stimulus and a different button for a second stimulus. That is, they cannot treat different auditory information differentially.

Short-term auditory memory is associated with the frontal lobes (Luria, 1966, pp. 276–279) as well as with the anterior temporal region (Fuster, 1997). The latter is due to the location of the head of the hippocampus within this region. The hippocampus is acknowledged to be the major memory center of the brain (Isaacson & Pribram, 1986). Short-term auditory memory is yet another critical auditory function and, like those mentioned above, may be trained as part of an auditory training program (Gillet, 1993). Other auditory functions that should be mentioned are sequencing, in the fronto-temporal parietal region (Efron, et al., 1983; Katz & Pack, 1975; Luria, 1970) and dichotic listening that is associated with the corpus callosum (Katz, Avellanosa, & Aguilar-Markulis, 1980; Musiek & Wilson, 1979).

Central Auditory Processing as an Element in AR

When I was a student; auditory training was called "ear training." We know now (and perhaps we knew even then) that the ear is not trainable. We cannot teach the ear anything—the most that we can hope do is teach the brain, or perhaps the brainstem, how to deal with the ear's problems. Those who are having difficulty as a result of hearing loss or APD often have similar challenges: for example, understanding in noise, speech is too quick to catch, and faint speech is tiring or stressful to follow. When a person with hearing impairment is in the best acoustic environment, with appropriately selected amplification and assistive technologies, successful communication could be expected (depending on the extent of loss, etc.). However, when communication is not up to expectations, then APD should be suspected as a potential reason for the limited success.

If we ignore CAPD for those who are hard of hearing, we ignore a potentially major contributor to their auditory limitations, as well as a powerful path for improving their performance. Hearing loss and CAPD each are important contributors to one's ability to communicate auditorily, but combined they are a formidable interference that limits the individual's potential for success. Fortunately, much can be done to maximize the person's hearing potential as described throughout this book as well as for CAPD that is discussed elsewhere (Chermak & Musiek, 2002; Geffner & Ross-Swain, 2007; Masters, Stecker, & Katz, 1998). Ignoring central factors in those with hearing loss can be just as serious as ignoring hearing issues with those who have CAPD.

Screening for Central Auditory Dysfunction as Part of the Intake Procedure for a Rehabilitation Program

Beck and Bellis (2007) indicate that auditory processing deficits may affect 75% of elderly adults and subsequently reduce the effectiveness of hearing aids. Therefore, it is likely that a high percentage of those who are seen for hearing aid evaluations have auditory processing deficits of some kind. Because so much depends not only on the person's hearing but also on how well they are able to process auditory information, it seems appropriate for audiologists to screen for CAPD.

Brody (1955) studied brain changes with aging and found the greatest change was in the auditory cortex. This corresponds to the region associated with auditory DEC. Jerger et al. (1993) and others (Walden & Walden, 2005) noted binaural interference in elderly cases. This might well be associated with deterioration of the corpus callosum (and possibly other regions) which could contribute to binaural interference. Patients with lesions of the corpus callosum have shown abnormalities on central auditory tests suggesting age-related deterioration (Katz et al., 1980). This is supported by the work of Jerger et al. (1995) based on dichotic listening and event-related potential measures.

Because of the vulnerability to change of the central auditory regions with aging, since most of the people seeking hearing aids are older adults, and because central problems can have a major influence on hearing aid success, it seems justified to recommend APD screening when considering amplification or other rehabilitative options. Dichotic speech tests are likely to provide the most practical information in the shortest amount of time.

Reduced Redundancy and Its Impact on AR

Those with normal hearing, language and cognitive functions can generally understand the spoken word in most situations with ease because of the considerable overlapping sources of information (e.g., phonemic, linguistic). However, when there is impairment of the auditory system anywhere along the path from the outer ear up to and including the brain, there is likely to be distortion and reduced internal redundancy. Distortion diminishes the amount of useful auditory information being processed by the CANS. This causes the person to spend more time and brain power to clarify meaning, if possible. Thus, despite the best hearing aids and assistive devices available today; we may still have major challenges in aural communications. Significant reductions in redundancy can make auditory training improvement more difficult to achieve. Despite the auditory obstacles that may impede progress; improvement can be made but perhaps to a more limited degree and/or requiring more time to achieve. If we ignore the plasticity of the CANS to improve understanding of the incoming signals, we likely are limiting the potential range of success with or without amplification (Hayes, Warrier, & Nicol, 2003; Musiek, Shinn, & Hare, 2002).

Case Studies

Over the years, I have learned so much from individual cases. Once sensitized to a problem, it is easier to recognize the characteristics or issues in other individuals. The following are some of these exemplar adult cases.

Case 1: Hearing Loss due to Alports Disease and a Central Connection

A 56-year-old man came for a central auditory evaluation from another city. For over a year he felt that he was not hearing as well as he had in the past and diagnosed himself as having CAPD. "RL" first noticed a hearing deficit when he was in college and subsequently wore hearing aids successfully since that time. As a young man, he was also diagnosed as having Alports disease, which is a kidney disorder associated with bilateral sensorineural hearing loss (Katz, 2000).

For more than a year before our evaluation, he noticed that he was not hearing well in noise and that people were speaking too quickly for him to follow. The problem got worse over the year but his hearing test results and word recognition scores remained unchanged. His audiologist attempted to optimize the hearing aids, but was unable to increase the patient's satisfaction. She referred him to our clinic for central testing.

Our tests showed that RL's results for pure-tone thresholds and word recognition had remained unchanged from the scores obtained over the previous 6 years. He had normal tympanograms and acoustic reflexes and a symmetrical, moderate, flat sensorineural loss in each ear. Recorded word recognition was 88%, bilaterally; however, central testing corroborated his complaints. Word recognition scores with ipsilateral noise were severely depressed, even when subtracting the word recognition in quiet scores. On the Phonemic Synthesis (PS) (a decoding) test, RL's scores were 10 standard deviations (S.D.) poorer than the mean. The SSW test has an effective correction factor for hearing loss in which the raw percent error is reduced by subtracting the word recognition percent error (Arnst, 1982; Katz, 1968). In this case, the significant percentage of error was offset by the correction factor and did not indicate clear evidence of central abnormality. The SSW was consistent with cochlear effects, but did not rule out central non-auditory reception abnormality (e.g., frontal lobe disorder).

These tests were strongly suggestive of a central auditory disorder. However, if one was unsure if the problem included a central component or was just a peripheral deficit, we could still assist RL with decoding and speech-in-noise training, plus strategies and assistive devices. Whether there was a central component or not, the therapy and accommodations would be the same in this case. Specific therapy approaches were recommended. Unfortunately, RL did not have access to therapy services close to his home.

Three years later, RL returned for reevaluation and therapy because he was having even more difficulty in noise and in following conversations. By this time, an MRI scan found "nonspecific subcortical white matter lesion within the frontal lobes." On retest, the basic (peripheral) findings remained the same; however, on the speech-in-noise test, the right ear was 5 S.D. poorer than the mean.

When RL returned the following year for testing and further therapy, his scores on the SSW test were clearly below normal limits (despite the correction for word recognition) and indicative of a central auditory problem involving non-auditory reception regions (likely in the anterior portion of the brain). In addition, speech-in-noise decreased further to 6 S.D. below normal in right ear and down to

4 S.D. below normal in the left ear. Although these scores are extreme compared to the typical CAPD cases, the type of problem (i.e., speech-in-noise) is consistent with the Tolerance Fading Memory category, which is associated with various anterior brain functions. It should be noted that despite the apparent worsening neurologic condition, each time RL came for therapy, his decoding performance subjectively improved and this was reflected on the PS test results. By the end of this second training program, his PS scores were within normal limits. The therapy included Phonemic Training Program (PTP) in which individual phonemes were taught and associated with specific letters (Katz, 2007a, 2007b); PS training (Katz & Harmon, 1981) dealing with sound blending, and speech-in-noise (Katz, 2007a; Medwetsky, in press), with speech presented at a constant level and the competing noise increasing from a mild to greater levels of challenge.

We learned from this experience:

1. It is important to be sensitive to the observations of the patient. In this case, RL's subjective observations were years ahead of medical and, perhaps, the audiological tests' ability to diagnose clearly aspects of his central auditory problem.
2. People who have hearing loss can have CAPD, whether long-standing or acquired.
3. Even if a clear distinction cannot be made between hearing loss alone or a coexisting CAPD, audiologists can still treat the auditory symptoms and consider assistive devices.

Case 2: Hearing Aid (HA) in One Ear and Cochlear Implant (CI) in the Other: Is This a Case for CAP Therapy?

A 78-year-old man who wore a hearing aid in his right ear and a cochlear implant in the left reported that until 13 years before he had had normal hearing. He suffered a sudden hearing loss in his left ear and, 10 years later, lost the hearing in his right ear over a period of months. Two years ago, he received a CI in his left ear and was quite pleased with his ability to hear and understand speech once again. At first, his complaint was just his inability to understand over the phone, but later he indicated that he also had difficulty in noise and in understanding rapid speech, especially on television.

"OV" is currently enrolled in our rehabilitation program. He was given six tests to assess his auditory abilities. Four of the six tests were from the Central Test Battery—CD.[1] These four recorded tests were presented via loudspeaker and two were given live voice. The recorded tests were: Speech in Quiet. Speech-in-Noise, Phoneme Recognition Test, Phonemic Synthesis, and live voice tests: CID Everyday Sentences and Speech in Quiet over the telephone. OV's scores with his CI were about equal to the means for 6 post-lingually deafened adults who were tested on the same procedures with their cochlear implants only. Table 21–1 shows OV's pre- and posttest scores.

[1]Precision Acoustics, 505 NE 87th Avenue, Suite 150, Vancouver, WA 98664; (360) 892–9367.

Table 21–1. Test Results for OV's Performance with Cochlear Implant in His Left Ear

Test Procedures and Measure	Pretest CI Left	Posttest CI Left
WRS—Quiet (W-22) % correct	36	44
WRS—Noise (W-22) % correct	20	32
CID Everyday Sentences % correct	84	96
Phoneme Recognition Test (PRT) % correct	38	68
Phonemic Synthesis (PS) Quantitative % correct	8	20
Phonemic Synthesis (PS) Qualitative % correct	0	16
Phonemic Error Analysis # errors	61	33
Telephone: WRS—Quiet (W-22) % correct	36	36

Pretest was prior to 15 sessions of therapy as described in text. All tests except CID sentences and telephone word recognition were presented via a single loudspeaker in front of patient.

The Phonemic Training Program (Katz, 1998), which is used to improve phonemic decoding, was the main procedure; however, after four sessions, we began teaching telephone strategies (PTP will be carried out over the phone in the next round of therapy). The Phonemic Synthesis (PS) task (a sound blending procedure) was so difficult for OV (and others with CIs) that 10 sessions of training were required for him to develop sufficient skill to begin the PS therapy. Another APD therapy that was delayed was speech in noise as this was far too difficult because OV's decoding skills were so weak. In addition, work on localization of sound is anticipated in the near future. Preliminary results suggest good improvement with both the CI-only and the HA-only but not as much on the binaural tests. In some ways, this appears to be associated with limited binaural interaction which would not be surprising for a man of 78 years. Nevertheless, the binaural scores are superior to those for each of the individual ears.

From this case it appears that:

- Although we have no evidence that OV had any CAPD characteristics earlier in life, speech through his hearing devices were not processed optimally. In this sense, it is a CAP limitation (although his CNS may be functioning normally for a person his age, it may not be functioning optimally for his current hearing situation).
- When hearing devices are used in both ears (whether two hearing aids or other devices) the binaural effect should be assessed (to understand the person's problems and potentials).
- Older/elderly individuals can benefit from therapy; which reminds us that plasticity remains a potential benefit even into the older years. Thus, we can conclude that neither age nor hearing status necessarily precludes CAPD therapy.

Case 3: Considering AR for Mentally Challenged Adults

Many wonder if it is legitimate to be doing AP evaluations and therapy with those who are mentally challenged. Surely, there are cognitive and other factors that must be considered in these cases. However, based on the author's years of experience evaluating individuals who are mentally challenged (Hadaway, 1968; Katz, 1969) and his more recent experiences providing therapy for them, it is clear that, in general, it can be done and to great advantage. In several cases, we have found essentially normal central test results in those with moderate or even severe intellectual deficits (Katz, 1969). We believe that IQ alone is not a sufficient reason for denying a person an AP evaluation or to assume that severe global results are a foregone conclusion (Katz & Tillery, 2006). In fact, the mentally challenged population, in addition to their other deficits, is a high risk group for CAPD. Because the brain is replete with auditory areas and pathways; any person with cerebral malfunction has a good chance of having some aspects of their AP performance compromised. With generalized brain problems, such as in mental retardation; involvement of important auditory areas is likely.

Until 10 years ago, this author suspected but did not have the opportunity to determine if AP training techniques would be successful with the mentally challenged. A speech-language pathologist (SLP) offered to have one of her mentally challenged patients, with a 31 IQ, treated for decoding issues as he appeared profoundly abnormal in decoding. This 24-year-old man ("AB") had not improved in speech therapy for 2 to 3 years. He knew perhaps a few dozen words, but they were unintelligible. He spoke in single-word sentences and the words were generally single brief sounds. For example, a brief /b/ meant to convey something about a "boy" or "book," but required accompanying gestures to be understood.

The only audiologic data that were available were AB's pure-tone threshold results, which showed essentially normal hearing. His extremely poor receptive language and severely limited speech articulation suggested an auditory decoding disorder in addition to his cognitive impairment. Because he did not understand oral instructions, this therapist and AB's SLP modeled (demonstrated) the procedures he was to follow. He had approximately one hour of therapy a week over a four-year period. AB slowly learned the procedures for the PTP (just as he slowly learned other therapy procedures initially). When we wanted to move from PTP to PS, it required several intervening steps (as in the case of OV, but breaking down skills into smaller steps is rarely necessary in learning-disabled children or adults with CAPD). We soon realized that improvement was restricted because of AB's very limited vocabulary. Thus, we decided that the most efficient way to increase his vocabulary would be to teach him to read and to put to practical use what he learned in associating sounds with letters of the alphabet in the PTP therapy. A little book was created with 285 simple, mostly predictable, phonically predictable words including some he already knew. It took 1½ years for him to finish the first book (not all the words were learned, but the words that AB did learn generally were understood in other reading and speaking contexts). He gradually built up a larger vocabulary and learned to pronounce correctly almost all of the words he was taught (although he continued to have intradental production of /s/ and /z/

which we did not address). The subsequent books required less time for him to master. AB mastered one of the books in just two weeks. We worked on increasing AB's memory span from 1 digit to 3 and eventually he learned to maintain them in proper sequence as well.

From this fascinating case we learned that:

- Even persons with severe mental retardation can improve their auditory processing deficits with training. Since working with AB, we have provided therapy to mentally challenged high school students who were able to demonstrate excellent test-retest improvement on standardized APD tests following therapy (Katz & Tillery, 2006).
- When performance is so severe that central tests cannot be administered, experienced clinicians are able to use working hypotheses regarding the types of APD so as not to deny the individual the opportunity to benefit from therapy.
- In this case, the therapeutic benefits helped to validate the working hypotheses. Those who are mentally challenged are high risk for CAPD and are able to make impressive improvements with therapy.

Case 4: No Hearing Loss but Major Auditory Challenges

This 35-year-old man, from out of state, requested an evaluation because he said that he had an adult onset of APD. "MK" had a lucrative job that required him to communicate quickly under very noisy conditions. In time, it became so difficult to understand what was said that he took a leave of absence to find out if anything could be done to correct his problem.

MK reported no history of academic or listening problems in the past, but did have 9 years of speech therapy in school. He also reported that over the past 10 years he had numerous bouts of otitis media (OM) in the right ear only and had seven pressure equalization (P.E.) tubes in that ear to remediate the problem. Over this period he had seen five Ear, Nose, and Throat physicians, and a Neurologist, and had three CT scans. MK also had many hearing evaluations and, in recent years, was administered two different complete APD test batteries prior to being seen by the author and his colleagues.

Both test batteries showed widespread CAP problems when testing each ear. The data indicated a severe deficit in auditory processing and likely involved at least Decoding and Tolerance-Fading Memory (TFM) categories. Prior to further evaluation by this author, the working hypothesis was that this was *not* a pure case of adult onset in view of the extensive history of speech therapy (which could have had a beneficial effect on CAPD during his school years) and the obvious signs of APD in each ear; however, the recent and numerous bouts of otitis media in one ear (especially the right ear in a right-handed individual) could have had an important disruptive influence (see Katz & Lawrence-Dederich, 1986; Katz & Illmer, 1972, pp. 554–556). Over the years, we have seen patients with slight unilateral conductive hearing loss acquired in adulthood who were greatly frustrated by these "minimal" losses, especially in noise. Furthermore, repeated bouts of OM during therapy have had a deleterious effect on auditory processing improvement. In addition to the long-standing difficulties, OM in the right ear may have disrupted binaural integration; perhaps, similar to those with binaural-interference problems (Walden & Walden, 2005).

MK came from his hometown for our evaluation plus therapy for one week. The first day was spent in testing by audiologists and speech-language pathologists. These results supported and extended the information that was obtained previously. The next 3½ days were spent in various forms of auditory training, and the last half day was set aside for retest of auditory skills. The training included the Phonemic Training Program, Phonemic Synthesis for Decoding issues, speech-in-noise desensitization (Katz, 2007a), and short-term auditory memory training were provided for the TFM issues. In addition, localization training was carried out when it was determined that this, too, was one of MK's auditory weaknesses.

The retest demonstrated impressive gains in each of the areas for which therapy was provided. However, it was clear that just one week of therapy would not be sufficient to serve MK's needs. Following therapy, MK was able to return to work and continued to do so for a number of years. Although handouts with follow-up procedures were provided to him, only a brief period of follow-up therapy was reported. Unfortunately, when MK returned home he continued to have many bouts of OM in the right ear and on five occasions P.E. tubes were again inserted. Perhaps for a number of reasons, he eventually had to give up his job.

This case suggests:

- Central functions may be compromised by transient OM, even in just one ear.
- The various associated symptoms e.g., speech decoding, speech-in-noise and localization of sound issues were treatable central conditions in this case.
- However, as we have frequently seen in therapy, when children or adults have continuing/transient middle ear disorder, this can disrupt therapeutic CAP benefits.

Summary

Central Auditory Processing is a common disorder not only in children, but in adults as well. It is most common in the elderly (Bellis, 2006). The impact of CAPD is increased with a hearing loss and vice versa. Almost any problem that can affect the CNS increases the chances that auditory areas or pathways will be involved. The good news is that generally CAPD is not very difficult to improve with therapy, and can be supplemented by hearing assistive technologies, as well as various accommodations and strategies. Therefore, it is important for audiologists to be aware of CAPD in their work and to realize the benefits their patients can receive by dealing with these issues.

References

Arnst, D. (1982). SSW test results with peripheral hearing loss. In D. Arnst & J. Katz (Eds.), *The SSW test: Development and clinical use* (pp. 287–293). San Diego, CA: College-Hill Press.

Baran, J., & Musiek, F. (1999). Beharioral assessment of the central nervous system. In F. Musiek & W.

Rintelmann (Eds.), *Contemporary perspectives in hearing assessment*. Boston: Allyn & Bacon.

Beck, D., & Bellis, T. (2007). (Central) auditory processing disorders: Overview and amplification issues. *Hearing Journal, 60*, 44–47.

Bellis, T. (2006). Differential diagnosis of (central) auditory processing disorder in older adults. In G. Chermak & F. Musiek (Eds.), *Handbook of (central) auditory processing disorder. Vol. 1, Auditory neuroscience and diagnosis*. San Diego, CA: Plural.

Brody, H. (1955). Organization of the cerebral cortex: Study of aging in the cerebral cortex. *Journal of Comparative Neurology, 102*, 511–556.

Chermak, G., & Musiek, F. (2002). Auditory training: Principles and approaches for remediating and managing auditory processing disorders. *Seminars in Hearing, 23*, 297–308.

Efron, R., Crandall, P., Koss, B., Divenyl, P., & Yund, E. (1983). Central auditory processing. III. The "cocktail party" effect and anterior temporal lobectomy. *Brain and Language, 19*, 254–263.

Fuster, J. (1997). *The pre-frontal cortex: Anatomy, physiology and neuropsychology of the frontal lobe* (3rd ed.). Philadelphia: Lippincott-Raven.

Fuster, J. (1980). *The prefrontal cortex*. New York: Raven Press.

Geffner, D., & Ross-Swain, D. (2007). *Auditory processing disorders: Assessment, management and treatment*. San Diego, CA: Plural.

Gillet, P. (1993). *Auditory process* (Revised ed., pp. 35–49). Novato, CA: Academic Therapy.

Hadaway, S. (1968). *An investigation of the relationship between measured intelligence and performance on the Staggered Spondaic Word test*. Masters thesis, Oklahoma State University.

Hayes E., Warrier C., Nicol T., Zecker S., & Kraus N. (2003). Neural plasticity following auditory training in children with learning problems. *Clinical Neurophysiology, 114*, 673–684.

Isaacson, R., & Pribram, K. (1986). *The hippocampus*. (Vol. 4). New York: Plenum Press.

Jerger, J., Alford, B., Lew, H., Rivera, V., & Chmiel, R. (1995). Dichotic listening, event-related potentials, and interhemispheric transfer in the elderly. *Ear and Hearing, 16*, 482–498.

Jerger, J., Silman, S., Lew, H, & Chmiel, R. (1993). Case studies in binaural interference: Converging evidence from behavioral and electrophysiologic measures. *American Journal of Audiology, 4*, 122–131.

Jerger, J., Speaks, C., & Trammell, J. (1968). A new approach to speech audiometry. *Journal of Speech and Hearing Disorders, 33*, 318–328.

Katz, J. (1968). The SSW test: An interim report. *Journal of Speech and Hearing Disorders, 33*, 132–146.

Katz, J. (1969). Differential diagnosis of auditory impairments. In R. Fulton & L. Lloyd (Eds.), *Assessment of the retarded and other difficult-to-test persons*. Baltimore: Williams & Wilkins.

Katz, J. (1992). Classification of auditory processing disorders. In J. Katz, N. Stecker, & D. Henderson (Eds.), *Central auditory processing: A transdisciplinary view* (pp. 81–92). Chicago: Mosby Yearbook.

Katz, J. (1998). Central auditory processing and cochlear implant therapy. In M.G. Masters, N. Stecker, & J. Katz (Eds.), *Central auditory processing disorders: Mostly management* (pp. 215–232). Boston: Allyn & Bacon.

Katz, J. (2000). The man with a hearing loss who said that he has CAPD. *SSW Reports, 22*, 14–18.

Katz, J. (2007a). APD evaluation to therapy: The Buffalo Model. www.AudiologyOnline.com

Katz, J. (2007b). Phonemic training and phonemic synthesis programs. In D. Geffner, & D. Ross-Swain (Eds.), *Auditory processing disorders: Assessment, management and treatment*. San Diego, CA: Plural.

Katz, J., Avellanosa, A., & Aguilar-Markulis, N. (1980). *Evaluation of corpus callosum tumors using the SSW, CES and PICA*. Presented at American Speech-Language Hearing Association convention, November 23; Detroit, MI.

Katz, J., & Harmon, C. (1981). Phonemic Synthesis: Diagnostic and training program. In R. Keith (Ed.). *Central Auditory and Language Disorders in Children*. San Diego, CA: College-Hill Press.

Katz, J., & Illmer, R. (1972). Auditory perceptual problems in children with learning disabilities. In J. Katz (Ed.), *Handbook of clinical audiology* (pp. 554–556). Baltimore: Williams & Wilkins.

Katz, J., & Lawrence-Dederich, S. (1986). Central nervous system, cerebral dominance and dyslexia. In P. Skov, S. Momme, & P. Kjeldsen (Eds.), *Dyslexia: Proceedings. Second Annual Conference on Dyslexia: Psychologic and Neurologic*. Aalborg, Denmark: Paedgogisk Psykologisk Radgiving.

Katz, J., & Pack, G. (1975). New developments in differential diagnosis using the SSW test. In M. Sullivan (Ed.), *Central auditory processing disorders*. Omaha, NE: University of Nebraska Press.

Katz, J., & Tillery, K. L. (2006). "Can central auditory processing tests resist supramodal influences?" *American Journal of Audiology, 14*, 124–127.

Lasky, E., & Katz, J. (1983). Perspectives on central auditory processing. In E. Lasky & J. Katz (Eds.), *Central auditory processing disorders: Problems of speech, language and learning*. Baltimore: University Park Press.

Lucker, J. (1981). Interpreting SSW test results of learning disabled children. *SSW Reports, 3*, 6–8.

Luria, A. R. (1966). *Higher cortical functions in man*. New York: Basic Books.

Luria, A. R. (1970). *Traumatic aphasias its syndromes: Psychology and treatment*. The Hague, The Netherlands: Mouton.

Masters, M. G., Stecker, N., & Katz, J. (1998). *Central auditory processing disorders: Mostly management*. Boston: Allyn & Bacon.

Medwetsky, L. (in press). Mechanisms underlying auditory processing. In J. Katz, R. Burkard, L. Hood, L. Medwetsky. (Eds.), *Handbook of clinical audiology* (6th ed.). Baltimore: Lippincott Williams & Wilkins.

Musiek, F. (1983). Assessment of central auditory dysfunction: The dichotic digit test revisited. *Ear and Hearing, 4*, 79–83.

Musiek, F., Shinn, J., & Hare, C. (2002). Plasticity, auditory training and auditory processing disorders. *Seminars in Hearing, 23*, 263–275.

Musiek, F., & Wilson, D. (1979). SSW and dichotic digit results pre and post commissurotomy: A case report. *Journal of Speech and Hearing Disorders, 44*, 528–533.

Rawool, V. (2006). The effects of hearing loss on temporal processing, part 2: Looking beyond simple audition. *Hearing Review, 13*, 30–34.

Rawool, V. (2007). The aging auditory system, part 3: Slower processing, cognition and speech recognition. *Hearing Review, 14*, 38–48.

Silman, S. (1995). Binaural interference in multiple sclerosis: Case study. *Journal of American Academy of Audiology, 6*, 193–196.

Walden, T. C., & Walden, B. E. (2005). Unilateral versus bilateral amplification for adults with impaired hearing. *Journal of American Academy of Audiology, 16*, 574–584.

22

Audiologic Rehabilitation with the Elderly Revisited: Research Needs

Barbara E. Weinstein

Introduction

Research is at the heart of any scientific or clinical endeavor. The importance of evidence-based science has been highlighted throughout this book and is an important need in the audiologic rehabilitation (AR). The purpose of this chapter is to expose the reader to areas of current thinking regarding the data-based management of older adults with hearing loss. As topics are identified throughout, a series of research questions will be proposed in order to stimulate the reader to consider possible avenues for scientific exploration.

Prevalence Estimates

Hearing loss is a growing public health problem for which effective interventions are available. The hearing-impaired population has been increasing steadily over the past several decades (Kochkin, 2005). In 1989, 24 million people reported hearing difficulty, in 2004, 31 million persons. It is projected that by 2020, 38 million people will experience hearing difficulty (Kochkin, 2005). Hearing loss affects Americans of all ages. Approximately three in 10 people over age 60 have hearing loss; one in six Baby Boomers (ages 41–59) or 14.6% have a hearing problem; one in 14 Generation Xers (ages 29–40), or 7.4%, already have a hearing loss; at least 1.4 million children (18 or younger) have hearing problems and 3 in 1,000 infants are born with severe to profound hearing loss. It is clear from epidemiologic studies that hearing loss is setting in at a younger age, increasing the number of years individuals will live with hearing loss. Additionally, adults continue to wait close to 10 years between first noticing hearing loss and seeking audiologic assistance. Detecting hearing loss at an earlier age, when the hearing impairment tends to be less severe, and encouraging adults to act earlier is an important priority for audiologists given the beneficial effects of our interventions and what we now know about brain plasticity and stabilization of word recognition scores with hearing aid use. Promoting hearing health literacy would most likely increase the ranks of first time users, close the gap between self ratings of hearing difficulty and measured hearing loss, and shorten time span between the existence of hearing loss and seeking assistance.

The number of older adults with severe to profound hearing loss is increasing, given changes in life expectancy among middle-aged and older persons. In fact, a 1994 report revealed that deafness is more prevalent among the elderly than in younger populations. Approximately 0.1% of the population under 45 years of age is deaf, compared to 2.5% of the population aged 65 and older (NCHS, 1994). For the latter group, cochlear implants are now a real possibility. Orabi et al. (2006) reported that the majority of elderly recipients of cochlear implants in their study reported improvements in quality of life with hearing ability improved beyond their expectations. Age should therefore not deter elderly patients from considering cochlear implants. Given the above prevalence figures and the changing demographics of hearing loss, data are needed to justify and design interventions that will meet the needs of emerging populations.

Research Question #1: What are preferences of older adults with profound hearing loss for hearing aids relative to cochlear implants?

Research Question #2: What are the health related quality of life benefits of cochlear implants for older adults with severe to profound hearing loss?

Research Question #3: What strategies can be used by audiologists to promote hearing loss awareness and earlier identification of adults and older adults with hearing loss?

Research Question #4: What are the benefits to the individual and society to identifying adults with hearing loss at a younger age and when the hearing loss is less severe?

Hearing Aid Use Patterns

Despite the high prevalence of hearing loss, the technologic explosion in hearing aids, the negative social and emotional effects of hearing instruments, and the fact that hearing impaired older adults who do not use hearing aids are more likely to report sadness and depression, hearing aid adoption rates over the years have not changed (Bagai, Thavendiranathan, & Detsky, 2006). Specifically, over the past 50 years, adoption rates have varied from 20 to 25% among those with a self-reported hearing loss. Interestingly, in 1955, five million Americans needed hearing aids, yet only 1.2 million wore them. In 2004, 24 million Americans with hearing impairment needed hearing aids, yet only 6.2 million actually owned them (Kochkin, 2005). The above numbers translate into a use rate of approximately 25% among those needing hearing aids who actually use them. Kochkin (2007) reported that the primary obstacles to hearing aid use include denial, stigma, uniqueness of hearing loss, financial constraints, and reports that the hearing loss is not bad enough. The above findings are quite telling, and underline the mandate for audiologists to develop creative strategies to change the status quo and encourage people to experience amplification earlier, so that they can continue to work productively, continue to enjoy leisure activities and contribute to society despite a hearing impairment.

Research Question #5: What protocols can be used effectively to change the *status quo* whereby the disparity between the prevalence of hearing loss and hearing aid utilization rates is reduced?

Research Question #6: How can audiologists be convinced that evidence based practice can be used to steer individuals toward concern for their hearing health care (Van Vliet, 2005)?

Research Question #7: Can data logging be used as an adjunct to the counseling process to demonstrate efficacy of hearing aids and, in turn, to promote hearing aid use?

Research Question #8: Can positive listening experiences with commercially available personal amplifiers and media amplifiers translate into increased hearing aid adoption rates?

Audiologic Rehabilitation Revisited

The fact that hearing aid adoption rates have remained stable over time is noteworthy and suggests that perhaps our approach to identifying, evaluating, and educating people about hearing loss and interventions for the hearing impaired should be re-evaluated. One possible jumping off point would be to revise the taxonomy we use in audiology, our conceptualization of the audiologic encounter and the role of the audiologist in the health care delivery system. Wellness programs targeting hearing related issues and consideration of the scope of the patient's audiologic needs from the outset are important first steps. To implement this goal, more audiologists should embrace the conclusions of the 2007 Clinical Research Summit that each patient is entitled to a holistic, client-centered therapeutic protocol which begins at the diagnostic evaluation and has as its focus their expressed needs (Sweetow, Corti, Edwards, Moodie, & Sabes, 2007).

Conceptualizing rehabilitation as an approach to preventing premature disability and thinking of AR as a process which begins at the time of identification may be ways to prevent the deleterious effects of hearing impairment on activity and participation. AR should not be considered an add-on, but rather a cost effective way of promoting success with technology and reducing the burden of hearing impairment (Sweetow, et al., 2007).

Alpiner (2008) recently suggested that today AR is the foundation of hearing health care. In his view, it should consist of the routine audiologic assessment, the hearing aid evaluation, consideration of amplification systems and hearing assistive technology, counseling and training to maximize hearing rehabilitation (Alpiner, 2008). Boothroyd (2006) asserts that AR should be aimed at promoting quality of life by reducing or circumventing communication difficulties. The most efficacious way of achieving positive results with AR is if it is delivered as follows: (1) diagnostic evaluation, (2) hearing aid selection and fitting, (3) instruction in the care and use of hearing aids, (4) AR and auditory training, and (5) comprehensive counseling based on patient self-assessment and diagnostic tests (Sweetow et al., 2007). Although hearing aids are at the heart of AR, we must keep in mind that we are recommending a "device" and a "process" to the hearing impaired which, when combined, will promote quality of life. Broadening our conceptualization of AR as part of the diagnostic process and not distinct from the hearing aid delivery system would help us move away from the medical model closer to including the human element, thereby promoting technology which actually can make a difference in the lives of persons with hearing impairment.

Research Question #9: What are the obstacles preventing hearing care professionals from embracing AR and the hearing aid fitting as part of the same process?

Research Question #10: What testing protocol during the diagnostic evaluation will enable audiologists to quantify the full range of communication challenges confronting patients so that the findings will dovetail with the design of a client-centered intervention program?

Research Questions #11: What counseling strategies included in the diagnostic process are most effective in moving individuals toward readiness to purchase rehabilitative services?

From Diagnosis to Rehabilitation

The first step in the rehabilitation process, namely, the diagnostic evaluation, should be seen as an opportunity to learn about the individual with hearing impairment in audiologic and nonaudiologic terms. We should select diagnostic tests that will help to unravel how and why signal processing is compromised and to understand the individual's perception of their situation and their stake in remediating that which can be remediated. The pure-tone audiogram and routine speech tests are insufficient if we are truly to realize our responsibility of identifying persons requiring our services. The diagnostic process should go beyond the routine, with every attempt made to gather information from the outset which will identify candidates able to benefit from some form of audiologic intervention. Information on speech processing abilities and cognitive function, performance on selected electrophysiologic tests, information about nonaudiologic variables (e.g. personality, motivational issues, stages of readiness), and self-report data on expectations, activity limitations and participation restrictions can inform decisions made at the time of the diagnostic assessment. The ability to predict hearing and health-related quality of life correlates of hearing impairment from electrophysiologic measures is potentially fruitful from a management perspective. Alternate ways of measuring the effects of aging on outer and inner hair cell function, including use of otoacoustic emissions and measurement of dead regions in the cochlea may hold considerable promise.

Several principles should govern our approach once we uncover hearing impairment and its sequelae during the audiologic evaluation: (1) the client should be involved from the outset in outlining their particular signal processing and communication challenges so that audiologists can try to measure the physiologic or psychoacoustic underpinnings of the problems; (2) findings from the diagnostic evaluation in concert with patient preferences should guide the design of the treatment plan; (3) audiologic and nonaudiologic variables should inform our recommendations; (4) the approach to treatment should be multifaceted, including provision of hearing instruments in the context of AR; (5) family members or caregivers should be involved in the process from the outset; and 6) the patient should know up front the value of our service, including evidence of plasticity, neural, and cognitive changes resulting from interventions, and should be armed with the appropriate expectations which in part are based on tests conducted at the diagnostic intake (AAA, 2006). Electrophysiologic tests may hold promise as an objective means to measure neural changes predictive of need for AR. In short, our diagnostic tests should inform our rehabilitative decisions and both audiologic, nonaudiologic and physiologic changes perhaps should be used to demonstrate the utility of our services. Of course, evidence must continue to emerge regarding the value of the available tools.

Research Question #12: What is the contribution of cognitive processing to hearing aid candidacy and rehabilitative outcomes?

Research Question #13: What measures of cognitive processing should serve as input and output measures in the hearing aid fitting/AR process?

Research Question #14: What aspects of cognitive processing are mediating variables in the success of the hearing aid fitting/AR process?

Research Question #15: Can auditory evoked potentials and MRI data assist in predicting candidacy and hearing aid outcomes as well as measure physiologic responses to AR treatments?

Research Question #16: What is the predictive value of otoacoustic emission measures in terms of candidacy and success of hearing aid fitting/AR?

Research Question #17: What is the relation between motivational level, expectations, and readiness for change assessed at the intake to hearing aid candidacy and success with amplification?

Research Question #18: Is the presence or absence of a dead region, as defined in terms of characteristic frequencies of the adjacent inner hair cells and neurons, predictive of disease-specific and generic measures of health-related quality of life?

Research Question #19: Do data from physiologic measures including otoacoustic emissions and auditory evoked potentials account for some of the variability in disease specific and generic measures of health-related quality of life?

Research Question #20: What is the relationship between behavioral, cognitive and electrophysiologic measures of the auditory pathway and responses to self-report scales used to quantify activity limitations, communication participation levels, and quality of life?

The Effects of Hearing Impairment: Role of Self-Report Measures in AR

There is considerable variability in terms of how hearing impairment affects the individual. These effects cannot be predicted from behavioral tests of auditory function. Information on the impact of hearing impairment however, is critical for both determining candidacy for services and for documenting the efficacy of interventions. It is now well accepted that hearing loss restricts one or more dimensions of quality of life, including communication function, mental status, and emotional and social function. The extent to which hearing impairment may affect such domains of function as psychosocial behavior, enjoyment of daily activities, independence, safety, productivity at work, and so forth, must be understood so that interventions can be designed to address directly "activities of daily living." Disease-specific self-report scales are gaining acceptance as a way of better understanding and meeting the needs of people with hearing impairment. Audiology is at a stage in its development where a detailed understanding of the individual's needs from a communication, psychosocial, and processing standpoint is critical to ensure a better match between the intervention and the individual. Open canal fittings, dual microphone technology, and digital noise reduction circuitry have broadened the pool of individuals for whom hearing aids are now an option and understanding the specific communication needs will help us fine-tune and target our interventions. The latter imperative is also clear because of the high cost of hearing aids and because of the sophistication of users.

As we look to the future, aging baby boomers will expect certain outcomes and audiologists will have to be accountable given the changing demographic characteristics and the economics of the health care system. Persons with hearing impairment should leave the audiologist's office with adequate information, a set of expectations and feedback regarding device- and patient-related variables. How the treatment is reducing activity limitations, decreasing participation restrictions and improving quality of life speaks to patient related expectations. Residual deficits in function and activity associated with hearing aid use also fall into the latter category (Boothroyd, 2006). Device-related expectations relate directly to care, maintenance, operation and use of the hearing aid. Setting patient expectations falls within the purview of the audiologist. Early on in the process is the time when expectations about realistic performance and satisfaction are enhanced.

Research Question #21: How do patient preference measures correlate with device-related patient satisfaction measures (Abrams, 2008)?

Research Question #22: What is the rank order of features of digital hearing aids which patients consider to be closely associated with hearing aid satisfaction and hearing aid benefit as measured using health-related quality of life metrics?

Research Question #23: What is the correlation between patient expectations of device- and patient-related benefit from and satisfaction with hearing aids?

Research Question #24: What is the relationship between hearing aid expectations prefitting and patient outcomes with hearing aids with advanced technologies, including feedback reduction technology, noise suppression, and directional microphone technology?

Research Question #25: What role does provision of strategies for encoding of information into long-term memory storage play in audiologic rehabilitation outcomes?

Research Question #26: Which prefitting audiologic and nonaudiologic measures are predictive of candidacy for and outcomes from AR and hearing aid fitting?

A Client-Centered Approach: What the Consumer Needs to Know

Self-report data regarding activity limitations, participation restrictions, and patient expectations provide information about the consequences of hearing impairment and are critical to measuring hearing and health-related quality of life outcomes (Johnson, Danhauer, Koch, Celani, Lopez & Williams, 2008). Interest in quality of life outcome metrics is gaining momentum from the perspective of health care costs. In short, it is incumbent on audiologists to demonstrate and inform the patient of the cost utility of our interventions as a way of increasing the number of individuals with hearing impairment who actually use hearing aids (Abrams, 2008). A systematic review of studies on the relation between hearing aids and health-related quality of life in adults with hearing loss was recently completed by a Task Force convened by the American Academy of Audiology (Hnath-Chisolm, Johnson, Danhauer, Portz, Abrams, Lesner, McCarthy, & Newman, 2007). The charge to the task force was to review and summarize the evidence regarding the nonacoustic benefits of hearing aids in light of the rise in prevalence of adult onset hearing loss, the increase in sophistication of hearing aids and the low proportion of adults using hearing aids. The conclusions of the task force, that hearing aids in fact are beneficial in several health and social domains, should be communicated to potential hearing aid users. This will help ensure that the patient knows what to expect and that the audiologist is conscious of what he/she should deliver. It should be emphasized that their positive impact on quality of life, and their impact on brain plasticity, is maximized when hearing aids are delivered close to the onset of hearing loss and in the context of a holistic AR process. This ensures and assumes that the consumer and hearing health care professional work collaboratively to maximize and optimize auditory function so that communication deficits, activity limitations, and participation restrictions are kept to a minimum. Outcomes must be achieved which ensure that the consumer's expectations meet or exceed performance levels with the hearing aids. Hence, quantification of patient expectations is at the heart of the counseling part of the AR process.

A systematic review of the effectiveness of short-term adult group AR conducted by Hawkins (2005) revealed beneficial outcomes, as well. Hearing aid users who participated in group rehabilitation sessions which focused on counseling and communication strategies did experience reductions in perceived hearing handicap, improvements in quality of life and improved communication. These short-term benefits were documented using questionnaires of proven reliability and validity which quantify aspects of personal adjustment, enhanced interpersonal communication and reductions in the social and emotional consequences of hearing loss. Abrams, Chisolm, and McArdle (2002) conducted a cost-utility analysis of adult group audiologic rehabilitation which revealed that the combination of hearing aid use and group aural rehabilitation was shown to be the most cost effective treatment approach. Statistically significant improvements were observed on mental component summary (MCS) scale measures of quality of life. Niparko (2007) convincingly argues that hearing care professionals have a responsibility to document the health-related quality of life benefits of hearing aids relative to their cost.

At the heart of each of the above studies were responses to some form of functional communication assessment (FCA) completed by the hearing aid user (Sweetow, 2007). According to responses to the FCA, the variable which emerges as central to successful outcome with audiologic interventions is self-efficacy. By quantifying residual auditory function we gain insight into information not gleaned from the audiogram. The concept of self-efficacy is integral to the decision to purchase hearing aids and is closely tied to the success of intervention with hearing aids. Self-efficacy, a belief system that influences motivation to learn and outcomes is of particular relevance to those with hearing loss as adjustment to hearing aids often requires some behavior and attitudinal changes. The self-efficacy framework suggests that treatment outcomes are directly dependent on one's beliefs about what they are capable of learning or activities they are capable of performing (Smith & West, 2006). For example, if a person with a hearing impairment believes that he or she can overcome the negative effects of this chronic condition by learning new skills and gaining mastery over a technology, this belief is important to goal setting and success. The health care provider must understand the motivation to seek professional assistance to overcome the activity limitations and participation restrictions associated with hearing loss. This enables the professional to work effectively on strategy setting and documenting that in fact the hearing aid is having the desired effect (Zimmerman & Kitsantas, 2007).

According to the self-efficacy model, the hearing health care professional actually has an obligation to share with the hearing aid user, tangible evidence of the value of hearing aids in promoting communication in the listening situations in which you experience the difficulty and in quantifying obstacles that remain despite hearing aid use. This can best be achieved by documenting how hearing aids actually improve or optimize audibility and speech understanding and how hearing aids actually impact the principal life domains beyond communication. Increasingly, insurance companies want to know how communication success through use of hearing technologies actually promotes involvement in leisure activities, socialization, emotional well-being, and cognitive ability. In order to strengthen self-efficacy, the hearing aid fitting, counseling, and orientation sessions must focus on performance accomplishment, encouragement, vicarious learning, and reinforcement. For example, the new hearing aid user must experience success in small group listening situations, and experience pleasure from the success in these situations. He or she must then be encouraged to undertake a new action, for example, use the device in large group situations after seeing other new users succeed in similar situations (vicarious learning).

Research Question #27: Is there a reliable and valid measure of self-efficacy that can be used to predict hearing aid candidacy and success?

Quality Indicators

Many audiologists argue that self-report measures are too time consuming yet patients frequently complain that they leave the fitting appointment without any objective evidence of the way in which the hearing aid(s) is(are) meeting the benchmarks important to them. If reliable and valid self-report measures are considered too time consuming, audiologists should be encouraged to use some form of checklist of quality indicators of benefit. A checklist that quantifies patient related benefits might include the following items: (1) audibility of sound; (2) improvements in speech understanding; (3) ability to tolerate loud sound; and (4) user comfort. Device-related variables might include: (1) ease of use, (2) frequency of feedback problems, (3) battery life, (4) removal and insertion difficulties, (5) ease of manipulation of controls, (6) effectiveness of the directionality of the hearing aid, and (7) ease of use of the telecoil. There are many ways in which you can evaluate any of the above domains. As suggested by the self-efficacy model, providing the patient with feedback helps to reassure that the hearing aids are meeting their needs and expectations and helps them to feel empowered by their new found abilities. When the hearing aid user is convinced that he or she has the ability to manipulate and troubleshoot the hearing aid, and to hear and communicate effectively with the hearing aid, they will most likely rate their experiences to be positive.

Table 22–1 displays a simple checklist which summarizes the device-related features the audiologist should review with patients prior to completion of the hearing aid fitting to help ensure mastery over as many of these functions as possible.

Table 22–1. Checklist on Knowledge of Device Related Aspects of Hearing Instruments

Did the dispenser:

1. Explain when to wear the hearing aids?
   ☐ yes ☐ no
2. Explain how to insert and use the batteries?
   ☐ yes ☐ no
3. Discuss where to purchase the batteries?
   ☐ yes ☐ no
4. Explain how to place hearing aid in the ear?
   ☐ yes ☐ no
5. Explain the controls and features?
   ☐ yes ☐ no
6. Explain how to use the volume adjustments if there is a volume control?
   ☐ yes ☐ no
7. Test how well you can hear/understand with the hearing aid(s)
   ☐ yes ☐ no
8. Make tuning adjustments based on your input?
   ☐ yes ☐ no
9. Explain cleaning and storage of hearing aid(s)?
   ☐ yes ☐ no
10. Explain precautions (e.g., not getting unit wet, wax blockage)?
    ☐ yes ☐ no
11. Explain how to use the telephone with the hearing aids?
    ☐ yes ☐ no
12. Have you practice using a telephone?
    ☐ yes ☐ no
13. Provide a copy of the hearing aid information brochure?
    ☐ yes ☐ no
14. Review the hearing aid information brochure?
    ☐ yes ☐ no
15. Explain your legal rights if you don't like the hearing aid(s)?
    ☐ yes ☐ no
16. Explain repair, loss, and damage warranties?
    ☐ yes ☐ no
17. Offer to sell you loss/damage insurance?
    ☐ yes ☐ no
18. Listen to your concerns regarding ease/difficulty of use?
    ☐ yes ☐ no
19. Answer your questions?
    ☐ yes ☐ no
20. Ask you to schedule a follow-up visit after the initial fitting?
    ☐ yes ☐ no

Responses to reliable and valid self-report questionnaires can be used to help the audiologist insure that hearing aids are meeting consumer needs and expectations as they relate to function, activity, participation and quality of life. Residual hearing difficulties and deficits often remain when first using hearing aids and questionnaires can help to identify the problems so that they can be addressed through counseling and communication strategies.

Candidacy for Hearing Aids

The desire to purchase hearing aids is directly linked to a number of nonaudiologic factors with which clinicians should be familiar. These include:

1. scores obtained on selected self-report scales
2. readiness for change
3. motivational level
4. self-efficacy

Bess (1995) reported that the extent of self-perceived hearing handicap on the 10-item screening version of the HHIE-S is predictive of hearing aid candidacy, in that it reliably distinguishes between people who ultimately purchase hearing aids and those who do not. Irrespective of the severity of hearing loss for pure-tone signals (e.g., mild or moderate sensorineural hearing loss), persons in their study who actually purchased hearing aids were more handicapped as evident by higher scores on the HHIE-S, than those who did not. Thus, the investigators concluded that when people perceive that a given hearing loss for pure-tone signals is interfering with participation in and enjoyment of various activities, they are motivated to purchase hearing aids to reduce some of their communication difficulties.

Similarly, a study reported by Kochkin (1996), who sampled many hearing aid owners and nonowners, revealed that an individual's total score on the HHIE-S statistically predicted ownership of hearing aids. For example, 5.7% of survey respondents who scored a "0" on their self-report measure owned a hearing aid whereas 49 percent of those with a score of "28" owned hearing aids. In general, this study revealed that the average score of nonhearing aid owners on the HHIE-S was 13.7 out of a total score of 40, compared to 20.8% for hearing aid owners. Clinically the sooner people come in for a hearing test, the more receptive they are to purchasing devices which may help overcome situation-specific difficulties such as understanding people on television or speech in large listening areas.

The transtheoretical stages of change model suggests that people are most likely to change their behavior if they are doing so for personal reasons without the prodding of outsiders. According to this model, which has been effectively employed in smoking cessation programs, there are approximately five to six stages that people tend to go through before behavior change is possible (Prochaska & DiClemente, 1983). These stages are depicted in Table 22–2. Individuals move from being uninterested, unaware or unwilling to make a change (precontemplation), to considering a change (contemplation), to deciding and preparing to make a change (preparation), to taking action (action), and finally maintaining the new behavior (maintenance). In my view, it is our responsibility through wellness programs (which include information about hearing loss, hearing assistive technologies, tips for communicating with the hearing impaired) and through public service announcements about hearing loss, to move collectively persons with hearing loss into the preparation phase, at which point they will be ready to undergo a hearing test for the purposes of considering possible interventions. When it is clear, based on the patient's own decisional balance sheet, that the benefits of seeking intervention are equal to or exceed the cost, people with hearing loss will be prepared to take action. We might assume that they perform their own cost benefit analysis and it is our responsibility to make them aware of the benefits to facilitate their analysis.

The assumptions that one must keep in mind when applying the model include the fact that change in behavior, especially in older adults, occurs gradually. Patients move through a series of stages and can be assisted in this process by a

Table 22–2. Stages of Change

Stage	Mental Set	Recommended Intervention
Precontemplation	Unwilling, uninterested in changing the status quo	Educational materials
Contemplation	Willing to consider a change	Provide positive listening experiences with HATs in selected listening situations (e.g., television, theatre); meet with new and satisfied hearing aid users
Preparation	Deciding and preparing to make a change	Counseling session regarding the value of hearing aids and the fitting process
Action	Taking action	Hearing aid fitting, orientation, counseling, follow-up; Listening and communication enhancement plan (LACE)
Maintenance	Maintenance or acclimatization to the new behavior	Short-term, medium-term, and long-term follow-up; send periodic E-mail communication with tips on hearing aids and hearing loss

Source: Prochaska and DiClemente (1983).

skilled clinician. People in different stages require different types of intervention and, by matching the stage to the intervention, we can help our patients progress toward acceptance. As suggested above, the decisional balance made by the patient mediates the decision to move from one stage to the next. Patients actually weigh the perceived advantages and disadvantages or the pros and cons of moving forward with an intervention (wearing hearing aids, purchasing hearing assistive technologies) prior to proceeding. In our role as counselors, during the various sessions with which we are working with our patients, clinicians should make sure to provide information that can be used to help weigh the issues. In my view, counseling about use of hearing assistive technologies when people are in the contemplation and preparation stage of readiness may be a strategy for helping the hearing impaired modify their behavior and become more accepting of audiologic interventions.

Research Question #28: What is the relation between stages of readiness and outcomes with hearing aids?

Research Question #29: What are the barriers to use of hearing assistive technologies for individuals who are not yet at the stage of readiness for audiologic intervention?

Maximizing Benefit from Questionnaires

Given the conclusions of the systematic review conducted by Hnath-Chisolm and colleagues (2007) confirming that: "Hearing aid use (a comparatively noninvasive, low-risk option with considerable potential benefits, which is the only viable treatment for sensorineural hearing loss) improves adults' health-related quality of life by reducing psychological, social and emotional effects of sensorineural hearing loss (p. 169)," audiologists are encouraged to obtain objective verification of outcomes with hearing aids. The feedback helps promote self-efficacy and motivation to use amplification technologies in a variety of situations.

Research Question #30: What are the short-term and long-term benefits of digital hearing aids with open mold technology in terms of reductions in activity limitations and participation restrictions?

Case Studies

The cases below exemplify the value of using patient responses to verify the adequacy of the fit for the short- or long-term, and possibly highlight the need for further intervention to reduce residual deficits. Furthermore, they highlight the value of hearing assistive technologies and the role the questionnaires can play in identifying older adults who require audiologic interventions.

Case 1

Mr. Schmidt, a 62-year-old businessman, presented with a bilateral moderate sensorineural hearing loss. His initial score on the HHIE-S was 30% with most of his difficulties manifesting in the social situational domains of function. He had purchased "TV Ears," an infrared system for the television so he would no longer disturb family members by raising the volume of the television. His difficulty understanding on his cellular phone and on the telephone at work led him to return to the audiologist for a consultation about hearing aids. During his first encounter with the audiologist, a pair of high-end digital hearing aids was recommended. He returned for a follow up and noted that he continued to have residual difficulties in a variety of listening situations. His score of 22% on the HHIE-S suggested that perhaps three to six weeks of counseling-oriented AR might be of long-term value.

Despite his busy schedule, he agreed and enrolled in group AR with new and experienced hearing aid users. He found the exchange with other group members to be quite fruitful and he found that being more assertive when speaking with co-workers and friends made a qualitative difference in his interpersonal exchanges. He also found that the encouragement and tips he received from others in the group served him well and afforded him a certain comfort level. The HHIE-S was readministered and a score of 10% achieved approximately three months following the initial purchase and the group sessions, confirming his impressions that the hearing aids were in fact making a difference. He became a strong advocate for hearing aids and, rather than continue to hide the fact that he had a hearing loss, he was proud to show others his state-of-the-art behind-the-ear hearing aids. He knew that when people could see that he wore hearing aids, they automatically modified their manner of speaking to facilitate communication.

Case 2

The reality that hearing aids can be very helpful in a variety of situations, and can alleviate feelings of isolation became apparent to Ms. Gordon, an 80-year-old woman who lived alone but was leading a very active life serving as a volunteer docent, a volunteer in a nursery school, and a volunteer visiting homebound older adults. At the time of her first hearing test, which revealed a mild-to moderate high-frequency sensorineural hearing loss typically associated with the aging process, she expressed her communication needs and the benefit she hoped to derive from hearing aids. Her expectations were a bit unrealistic, so prior to fitting her with hearing aids she was asked to return for one counseling session to ensure that her expectations were aligned with what she realistically could expect from the many situations in which she found herself experiencing difficulty. Well aware that a satisfied hearing aid wearer is one whose expectations match actual hearing aid performance, the audiologist chose to proceed with the hearing aid fitting once Ms. Gordon understood and accepted some of the situational limitations associated with hearing aids. Even though Ms. Gordon was not comfortable with technology and was living on a fixed income, it was possible to fit her with digital hearing aids. As part of the fitting, the audiologist conducted real-ear measurements to demonstrate the improvements in audibility immediately derived from the hearing aids. The visual feedback was quite reassuring, as was her improved ability to understand speech when the audiologist tested her before completing the fitting. Her initial score on the HHIE-S was 50%, suggesting that, in fact, she perceived her hearing loss to be handicapping socially, emotionally, and interpersonally.

More particularly, she reported feeling handicapped, upset, and embarrassed by and nervous from her inability to hear in a variety of situations, most notably when carrying out her many volunteer activities and when socializing with friends and relatives. When she returned to the audiologist for the three-week follow-up appointment, she indicated that the aids were helpful in the situations that mattered; however, she was annoyed by the sound of her voice and the occasional difficulty she continued to experience in noisy situations. The audiologist made an adjustment to the open mold, counseled her about expectations and conversational strategies, and readministered the HHIE-S. Her score of 24% verified that the hearing aids, in fact, were helpful in ameliorating some of the emotional consequences of hearing loss and of were of assistance on an interpersonal level as well. The audiologist reviewed device-related aspects of the hearing aids and encouraged her to return on an as-needed basis.

Responses to the HHIE-S confirmed the client's subjective reports. This case highlights the value of feedback from the client and the importance of objectively quantifying performance with given hearing aids. The importance of initial counseling about realistic expectations proved fruitful for this encounter and, given her fear of technology, the additional review of hearing aid use and operation provided her with a sense of confidence and self-efficacy as she embraced the challenges posed by the hearing aids and the successes she was experiencing.

Case 3

There are occasions when individuals who were previously functioning well with their hearing aids can experience a decline in performance. For example, Mr. Oz, an 80-year-old accountant who continues to work part-time, had worn analog behind-the-ear hearing aids for 10 years and up until recently was quite satisfied with them. They were alleviating his difficulties understanding speech, attributable to his bilateral moderate sensorineural hearing loss, first noted on his 65th birthday. Pure-tone findings at his most recent examination confirmed that his hearing loss had remained stable at the moderate level. Electrophysiologic and central auditory tests were informative. His problems understanding speech had declined dramatically, especially in noisy situations, and he was experiencing increasing difficulty on the telephone. A complete audiologic work-up revealed the possibility of an auditory processing problem. Noteworthy is the pattern of findings on the HHIE-S which confirmed Mr. Oz's subjective complaints in that he no longer was benefiting from the hearing aids. The initial HHIE-S score was 50% (prior to hearing aids), improving to 24% after the initial hearing aid fitting. His self-assessment score was between 24 and 30% over time, suggesting considerable reduction (improvement) in psychosocial handicap attributable to hearing aid use.

Four years later, at Mr. Oz's most recent visit, the HHIE-S score returned to 52%, confirming limited hearing aid benefit. The hearing health care provider recommended high-end digital behind-the-ear aids with a remote wireless FM receiver as an accessory. The advantages of remote wireless technology include elimination of the negative effects of talker distance, room noise, and room reverberation, and improved signal-to-noise.

Mr. Oz, at the urging of his wife, agreed to give the BTE with a remote wireless receiver a try and was immediately impressed with the clarity of the signal, especially with background noise. Mr. and Mrs. Oz were counseled on how to use the hearing aids, and upon their return visit were happy to report that speech understanding in the most difficult situations had improved dramatically. The HHIE-S score of 28% verified that Mr. Oz was deriving substantial benefit from the wireless technology.

A Final Word

Hearing aid fitting/audiologic rehabilitation are services that the audiologist is uniquely educated to provide. Given the changing demographics and the detrimental effects of hearing impairment, we have an obligation to reduce the gap between hearing loss prevalence and utilization of hearing health care interventions. We must expand the evidence base and make use of the tools in our armamentarium that may reduce the obstacles to hearing aid use. The earlier individuals learn about the detrimental effects of hearing impairment and come to understand the physiologic and psychosocial value of hearing aids, the sooner they will be ready to contemplate our services. Revisiting the purpose of the diagnostic protocol and conceptualizing AR as synonymous with the hearing aid fitting may help to close the gap between prevalence and hearing aid use. There is a growing need for research in the area of AR. One hopes this chapter has provided some focus for future research endeavors.

References

Abrams, H. (2008). What's the value of better hearing? Here are some ways to calculate it. *Hearing Journal, 61*, 10–15.

Abrams, H., Chisolm, T., & McArdle, R. (2002). A cost-utility analysis of adult group audiologic rehabilitation: Are the benefits worth the cost? *Journal of Rehabilitative Research and Development, 39*(5), 549–558.

Alpiner, J. (2008, May 6). Forecasting the future of aural rehabilitation. *ASHA Leader*, pp. 5–6.

American Academy of Audiology. (2006). Audiologic management of adult hearing impairment. *Audiology Today, 18*, 32–36.

Bagai, A., Thavendiranathan, P., & Detsky, A. (2006). Does this patient have hearing impairment? *Journal of the American Medical Association, 295*, 416–428.

Bess, F. (1995). Applications of the Hearing Handicap Inventory for the Elderly-Screening version (HHIE-S). *Hearing Journal, 48*, 51–57.

Boothroyd, A. (2004). Hearing aid accessories for adults: The remote FM microphone. *Ear and Hearing, 25*, 22–33.

Boothroyd, A. (2006). *Adult aural rehabilitation: What is it and does it work*? Paper presented at: State of the Science Conference on optimizing the benefit of hearing aids and cochlear implants for adults: The role of aural rehabilitation end evidence for its success; Sept. 18–20; Gallaudet University, Washington, DC.

Hawkins, D. (2005). Effectiveness of counseling-based adult group aural rehabilitation programs: A systematic review of the evidence. *Journal of the American Academy of Audiology, 16*, 485–493.

Hnath-Chisolm, T., Johnson, C., Danhauer, J., Portz, L., Abrams, H., Lesner, S., et al. (2007). A systematic review of health-related quality of life and hearing aids: Final report of the American Academy of Audiology Task Force on the Health Related Quality of Life benefits of Amplification in adults. *Journal of the American Academy of Audiology, 18*, 151–183.

Johnson, C. E., Danhauer, J. L., Koch, L. L., Celani, K. E., Lopez, I. P., & Williams, V. A. (2008). Hearing aid balance screening and referrals for Medicare patients: A national survey of primary care physicians. *Ear and Hearing, 19*, 171–187.

Kochkin, S. (1996). MarkeTrak IV: 10-year trends in the hearing aid market-has anything changed? *Hearing Journal, 49*, 23–33.

Kochkin, S. (2005). MarkeTrakVII: Hearing loss population tops 31 million people. *Hearing Review, 12*, 16–29.

Kochkin, S. (2007). MarkeTrak VII: Obstacles to adult non-user adoption of hearing aids. *Hearing Journal, 60*(4), 26–50.

National Center for Health Statistics. (1994). Data from the National Health Interview Survey, Series 10, #188.

Niparko, J. (2007). The cost of providing or not providing hearing care. *Hearing Loss Magazine, 28*, 21.

Orabi, A. A., Mawman, D., Al-Zoubi, F. Saeed, S. R., & Ramsden, R. T. (2006). Cochlear implant outcomes and quality of life in the elderly: Manchester experience over 13 years. *Clinical Otolaryngology, 31*, 116–122.

Prochaska, J. O., & DiClemente, C. C. (1983). Stages and processes of self-change of smoking: Toward an integrative model of change. *Journal of Consulting and Clinical Psychology, 51*(3), 390–395.

Smith, S., & West, R. (2006). The application of self-efficacy principles to audiologic rehabilitation: A tutorial. *American Journal of Audiology, 15*, 46–56.

Sweetow, R. (2007). Instead of hearing aid evaluation, let's assess functional communication ability. *Hearing Journal, 60*, 26–31.

Sweetow, R., Corti, D., Edwards, B., Moodie, S., & Sabes, J. (2007). Warning: Do NOT add on aural rehabilitation or auditory training to your fitting procedures. *Hearing Review, 14*(6), 48–51.

Van Vliet, D. (2005). The current status of hearing care: Can we change the status quo? *Journal of the American Academy of Audiology*, 16, 410–418.

Zimmerman, B., & Kitsantas, A. (2007). Reliability and validity of self-efficacy for learning from (SELF) scores of college students. *Journal of Psychology, 215*, 157–163.

Index

A

D

E

F

G

H

J

K

L

M

S

T

U

V

W